Ante Bilić
13.05. 1987.

Cellular Pathology Technique

Cellular Pathology Technique

Fourth Edition

C. F. A. Culling, MRCPath, FIMLS
Late Professor, Department of Pathology,
University of British Columbia, Vancouver, Canada

R. T. Allison, MSc, FIMLS, CMLM
Senior Chief MLSO, Department of Oral Pathology,
Dental School, University of Wales College of Medicine,
Heath Park, Cardiff, UK

W. T. Barr, FIMLS, CMLM
Senior Chief MLSO, Histopathology Department,
University Hospital of Wales, Heath Park, Cardiff, UK

Butterworths
London Boston Durban Singapore Sydney Toronto Wellington

First published, 1957
Second edition 1963
Reprinted 1966
Reprinted 1968
Third edition 1974
Reprinted 1975
Reprinted 1981
Reprinted 1983
Fourth edition 1985

© **Butterworth & Co. (Publishers) Ltd, 1985**

British Library Cataloguing in Publication Data

Culling, C. F. A.
    Cellular pathology techniques.—4th ed.
    1. Histology, Pathological—Technique
    I. Title II. Allison, R. T. III. Barr, W. T.
    IV. Culling, C. F. A. Handbook of histopathological
    and histochemical techniques
    616.07'583 RB43

ISBN 0–407–72903–8

Library of Congress Cataloging in Publication Data

Culling, C. F. A. (Charles Frederick Albert)
    Cellular pathology technique.

    Rev. ed. of: Handbook of histopathological and
histochemical techniques. 3rd ed. 1974.
    Includes bibliographies and index.
    1. Diagnosis, Cytologic—Technique. 2. Histochemistry
—Technique. 3. Pathology, Cellular—Techniques.
I. Allison, R. T. II. Barr, W. T. III. Culling,
C. F. A. (Charles Frederick Albert). Handbook of
histopathological and histochemical techniques.
IV. Title.
RB43.C94 1984   616.07'582   84-23164

ISBN 0-407-72903-8

Typeset by Mid-County Press, London SW15
Printed and bound by Butler & Tanner Ltd, Frome, Somerset

Preface

When the *Handbook of Histopathological and Histochemical Techniques* was first published in 1957, it represented a milestone in the development of histopathological technique. The unfortunate death of Charles Culling delayed the appearance of a Fourth Edition which the passage of time and consequent expansion in the body of knowledge necessitated. Presented with the challenge of thoroughly revising the entire text, the current authors sought to maintain the twin objectives of producing a comprehensive bench book and a text for candidates for the Special Examination in Cellular Pathology of the Institute of Medical Laboratory Sciences. These objectives we hope we have achieved in *Cellular Pathology Technique*.

Some areas of histopathology have seen much more dramatic advances than others. Thus the chapter on Lipids, for example, is little changed from the Third Edition; others, such as that on the Theory of Staining, have been greatly expanded and entirely new chapters are devoted to immunolocalization, the endocrine system and quantification. The organization of the book has also been reshaped. Some chapters retain the unmistakable stamp of Charles Culling, many are rewritten and reflect the new authors' bias. We have attempted to rationalize established areas in which, out of many alternatives, particular procedures have found favour. Where advances are still being made we have endeavoured to provide a wider variety of options. However, the scope and academic content of this field is now such that they cannot be comprehensively covered in a single text.

Whilst we do not claim our references to be error free, they have been checked meticulously, and, hopefully, the inaccuracies in the previous editions of this and the other textbooks, have been corrected. We have also tried to bring a consistency to the presentation of methods and trust the reader finds them clearly distinguished from the text.

We wish to record our appreciation to the authorities of the University of Wales College of Medicine and the University Hospital of Wales for allowing us the time and providing many of the facilities implicit in the authorship of this book.

R.T.A.
W.T.B.

Acknowledgements

During the preparation of this book, we have been fortunate to receive help and advice wherever we have sought it. In particular, Dr G. Cole, Dr A. R. Gibbs, Mr P. Gregory, Dr B. Jasani and Mr D. Williams provided helpful criticisms in reviewing chapters whilst Mrs K. Allsopp, Mr P. Cartwright, Mrs R. Davies, Miss H. Dewson and Miss M. Skinner evaluated many techniques and provided a variety of practical support.

Brian Amer, Department of Pathology, Southmead Hospital, Bristol wrote the chapter on Electron Microscopy.

Peter Langham helped with much of the photography and the Audio-Visual Aids Departments at the Medical School and Dental School of the University of Wales College of Medicine provided support whenever requested.

The library staff of both the Medical and Dental Libraries have proved as tenacious as we could possibly have hoped in pursuing the often tenuous leads we provided in our efforts to verify and expand every reference.

All of those named above deserve our gratitude, but none more so than Mrs O. Hancock and Mrs W. Williams who turned voluminous and often indecipherable handwritten notes into a recognizable typescript. We also appreciate the encouragement given to us to embark on this project by Professor E. D. Williams and Dr D. M. Walker of the University of Wales College of Medicine.

Finally, we should like to thank all the staff of both our departments for their patience and forebearance whilst we were immersed in our task.

Contents

Part I

Introduction

Cells and tissues

The basic unit of tissue structure is the cell and its products. It is essential to have an understanding of the cell and its functions to practise histopathological techniques successfully. Whilst there was a time when it was sufficient to recognize cell components, individual cells and cell organization into tissues, modern developments in technique require the practitioner to be acquainted not only with subcellular organelles but also to understand fully their biochemical roles in the particular specialized function in each cell type. It is becoming as common to recognize cell types on the basis of their biochemical or immunological properties as by their morphological appearance.

Historically, cells and tissues have been visualized in preparations owing more to technical expediency than to biological accuracy. This has not necessarily been a bad thing and a wealth of experience has been accumulated in the study of tissues under these conditions. Accuracy of diagnosis was not considered a major problem until technical advances showed that more detailed classification of diseases into subdivisions was possible and had clinical significance. This has led to a critical reappraisal of techniques adopted by universal approval as well as those of less popular appeal. The result has been that the well-equipped practitioner must have a wide-ranging knowledge and understanding of preparatory techniques.

Current concepts of the cell reflect a body of knowledge built on a variety of techniques from fixed, embedded sections to critical-point dried tissues, from light microscopy to scanning electron microscopy, from enzyme histochemistry to biochemical analysis of ultracentrifuged cell fractions, from immunocytochemistry to X-ray microanalysis and many others.

The cell (*Figures 1.1* and *1.2*) is to living tissue what the molecule is to chemistry; the unit of which larger masses are built, and which loses its individual identity if further divided. The most casual observation shows that the cell has two basic components:

(1) a nucleus, surrounded by
(2) a variable amount of cytoplasm.

Each is enclosed by a membrane. Even in the most bizarre diseased cell the nucleus and cytoplasm are easily identified, a reflection of profound structural and functional differences.

The static conditions under which cells are normally studied should not obscure the fact that they are dynamic organisms, often fluctuating between gel and sol states.

3

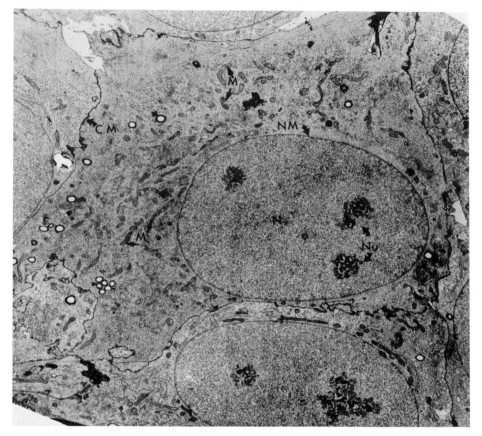

Figure 1.1 Normal cultured liver cell, as visualized in the electron microscope. N = nucleus; Nu = nucleolus; NM = nuclear membrane; CM = cell membrane; M = mitochondria. Original magnification × 2500. (Courtesy of Dr T. D. Allen)

The nucleus

Essentially, the nucleus is composed of nucleoprotein and nucleic acids as a colloidal solution. Deoxyribonucleic acid (DNA) comprises some 20% of the dry weight of the nucleus and acts as the basic genetic memory of the cell. This information is stored as a sequence of bases strung between two strands to form a double helix. It is the ability of this double helix to unwind and incorporate new bases onto exposed bases as complementary pairs, forming two new helices, that enables the cell to provide sufficient genetic material for two daughter cells. Individual nucleotides shed two of their three phosphate groups as bases are linked to form new DNA by the action of DNA polymerase. Prior to cell division, helices are folded, packed and condensed into recognizable structures—the chromosomes—of which there are 46 in normal human cells. Each chromosome carries hereditary characteristics which are thought to be dependent on the code of nitrogenous bases.

A further 20% of the dry weight of the nucleus is made up of ribonucleic acid (RNA), concentrated into one or more recognizable regions of the nucleus, the nucleolus or

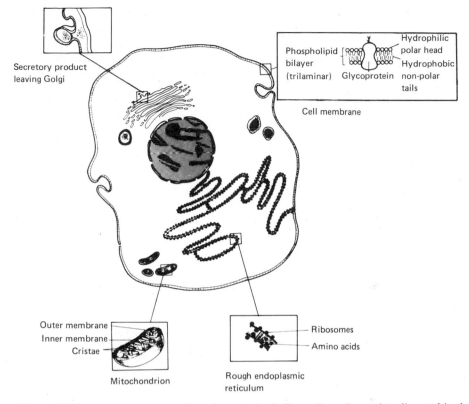

Secretory product leaving Golgi

Phospholipid bilayer (trilaminar) Glycoprotein

Hydrophilic polar head
Hydrophobic non-polar tails

Cell membrane

Outer membrane
Inner membrane
Cristae

Mitochondrion

Ribosomes
Amino acids

Rough endoplasmic reticulum

Figure 1.2 Diagrammatic representation of a typical cell, illustrating salient points discussed in the text

nucleoli. RNA is concerned with initiating cell metabolism in accordance with the information contained within the DNA double helix. These functions are fulfilled by messenger RNA leaving the nucleus with templates for protein production derived from DNA. Ribosomal RNA, present on the endoplasmic reticulum of cytoplasm, controls this production and influences cell metabolism because the proteins produced are enzymes. More dramatically, large amounts of RNA may be identified in the cytoplasm of immunologically active cells in which they are especially concerned with the production of globulins and hence antibody formation.

Messenger RNA has to cross the membrane limiting or surrounding the nucleus to carry out its cytoplasmic function. This is a relatively impermeable envelope, composed of a double membrane, punctuated by nuclear pores through which the RNA is thought to pass. The outer membrane is continuous with the endoplasmic reticulum, a complicated system of cytoplasmic membranes which may be seen to be smooth, or rough when bearing ribosomes—RNA-rich sites of protein synthesis.

The cytoplasm

The cell itself is bounded by a semipermeable membrane which, on the basis of three-dimensional reconstruction, has been called a 'fluid mosaic model' composed primarily of lipids and proteins. These phospholipids orientate themselves to form a double layer with the hydrophilic polar region of the molecule closest to the respective membrane surfaces, and the hydrophobic, non-polar regions in apposition between the two. Within this matrix, cell organelles are active. The most prolific is usually the membrane (glycoproteins), may either float or remain static, protruding through either side of the phospholipid bilayer.

The matrix of the cytoplasm is composed largely of water with variable amounts of soluble protein also present. It may also contain a variety of salts and carbohydrates. Within this matrix, cell organelles are active. The most prolific is usually the membrane system, composed of rough endoplasmic reticulum, smooth endoplasmic reticulum and the Golgi complex. Rough endoplasmic reticulum has already been described as ribosome-rich sites of protein synthesis. Ribosomes may also exist freely in the cytoplasm where their function is believed to be concerned with synthesizing the small amount of protein required by the cell for its own internal use. Areas of smooth endoplasmic reticulum permit the transport of ions through the cell and are also implicated in hormone synthesis.

The Golgi complex has been appropriately described as the 'packaging' area of the cell. Its structure is that of a series of flattened sacs with bulbous ends lying parallel to each other. Invariably having a curved configuration, the convex surface has been termed, in deference to function, the 'forming face' and the concave surface, the 'maturing face'. Protein synthesized by the ribosomes, is transported via the endoplasmic reticulum to the maturing face of the Golgi. Here it may be either packaged into sacs, or further processed by combination with locally produced carbohydrates (glycolysation). Once packed, the sacs of protein—or of mucopoly-saccharide, which may also be produced in the Golgi—are released into the cell cytoplasm and make their way to the cell membrane. At an appropriate time, the sacs, or vacuoles, expel their contents into the environment, following fusion of the vacuole membrane with the cell membrane. However, some protein is required by the cell itself for its own metabolism. This is prepared by a complex consisting of the Golgi, Endoplasmic Reticulum and Lysosomes (*see below*). The complex is referred to as GERL, an acronym of the component parts (*Figure 1.3*).

Amongst the vacuoles containing the products of cell metabolism are found two further organelles of specific function. Mitochondria are self-contained membrane structures responsible for respiration and thus providing the cell with its necessary energy. The structure of a mitochondrion is that of a double membrane, the inner of which is convoluted to form multiple cristae. Over 70 different enzymes and co-enzymes are present to complete the complicated process of oxidative phosphoryla-tion, culminating in the production of the energy reservoir, adenosine triphosphate (ATP). Their characteristic internal structure makes them the most easily recognizable cell organelle when viewed in the electron microscope. Each cell may contain up to several hundred mitochondria. Lysosomes although of similar size, and even shape, as mitochondria have contrasting functions. Of varying electron density, they display a finely granular internal structure surrounded by a single membrane in electron micrographs. They are produced in the rough endoplasmic reticulum and packaged by the Golgi complex in a similar manner to other secretory products. Lysosomes contain a number of enzymes, all of which are acid hydrolases capable of breaking down cell products. Acid phosphatase is one of the enzymes most commonly used as a marker of lysosomes in light microscopy. Obviously, the release of these enzymes within the cell cytoplasm would lead to severe damage of the cell itself. The role of the lysosome in intracellular digestion of foreign or effete material is facilitated either by the phagocytic action of the cell, or by packaging of unwanted cellular by-products. Phagocytosis is achieved by the cell extending cytoplasm around detected foreign material, which thus becomes membrane bound—a vacuole termed a phagosome. The phagosome then fuses with the lysosome and hydrolytic enzymes digest the foreign material. Undigested material is expelled from the cell by reverse phagocytosis—exocytosis. Alternatively, undigested material may be stored, membrane bound, within the cell when it is termed a residual body.

Other cytoplasmic inclusions include inert, non-protoplasmic substances which may be products of the cell's own activity or may be taken up from the surrounding medium.

The more important inclusions are:

(1) fat, which occurs as globules within the cytoplasm, often forcing the nucleus and other intracellular materials to one side;
(2) yolk, which is similar to fat but usually more yellow in colour. It may be differentiated by dissolving out the fat, the yolk having a protein base which is subsequently demonstrable;
(3) glycogen, which occurs in a watery solution of colloidal nature. After fixation it is seen as fine granules or an amorphous mass, dependent upon fixation;
(4) mucin, which is first demonstrable in mucin producing cells as minute granules known as mucigen. These become droplets of mucin which coalesce, producing the typical distension of the goblet cell;
(5) secretory granules, cell products or remnants of ingested material often seen in scavenger cells such as histiocytes.

Cell division

Introduction

A typical cell division consists first of an equal division of the nuclear material (DNA) known as *karyokinesis*, followed by division of the cell body known as *cytokinesis* in which each of the two daughter cells receives one of the daughter nuclei. Occasionally, *karyokinesis* will be seen without *cytokinesis* giving rise to a multinucleated cell.

With each complete turn of the cell through its life cycle, all the structural elements and functional capacities of the nucleus and cytoplasm must undergo a doubling. All of these events, such as mitochondrion and ribosome reproduction, must be so inter-related and coordinated that cell growth and function are assured.

This area of cell reproduction is still not completely understood, although many of the control mechanisms involved have been demonstrated. Developmental biologists divide the cell reproduction cycle into four periods, G_1, S, G_2 and D (or M), with the latter D (division) or M (mitosis) period being the only one that can be easily studied by histological or light microscope techniques, although the S, DNA synthesis or chromosome replication cycle can be seen by autoradiography using radio-isotope-labelled thymidine (*Figure 1.4*).

It has been shown that an initiator protein is produced that brings about the interaction between DNA and DNA polymerase necessary for DNA synthesis. A measurable G_1 phase may be absent during active cell proliferation, or prolonged when there is no apparent necessity or demand for cell growth, it is therefore an expendable time period. The S period is marked by DNA, RNA and protein synthesis. The G_2 period contains the events that link the end of chromosome replication with chromosome segregation. The mechanics of this segregation seem to involve a series of

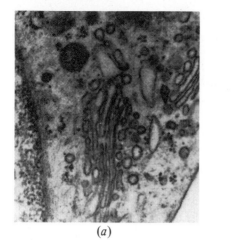

(a)

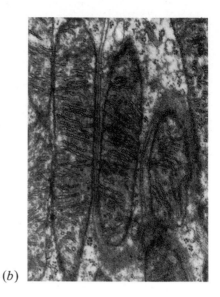

(b)

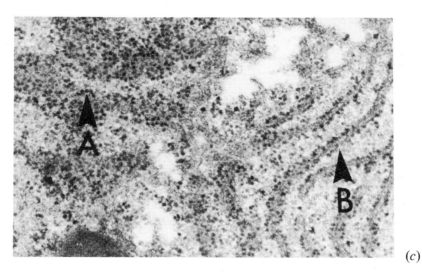

(c)

Figure 1.3 Electron micrographs showing (a) Golgi apparatus, (b) mitochondria, and (c) free ribosomes (A) and rough endoplasmic reticulum (B)

events, synthesis and assembly of the mitotic apparatus, alignment of the chromosomes on the apparatus, splitting of the centrioles, and so on. The G_2 period in animals is relatively short and of constant duration.

It will be evident that the subsections of this cycle, as described, are defined by what the chromosomes are, or are not, doing rather than by any necessary state of the whole cell.

Mitosis

This section is concerned with mitosis as it has been seen and known for a number of years by examination with the light microscope.

With the exception of certain specialized cells (e.g. nerve cells), cells multiply by division. The normal mechanism of division is a complicated one known as *mitosis*, but certain cells may possibly undergo simple division (*amitotic* division) like bacteria.

The process of mitosis is divided into four stages (*Figure 1.5*):

(1) prophase,
(2) metaphase,
(3) anaphase,
(4) telophase.

Prophase

The chromosomes become visible by concentration of the chromatin; they at first form a long continuous skein which later divides into separate chromosomes. At the same time the two centrioles move to opposite poles of the cell (if there is only one it first divides), and the nuclear membrane begins to disappear. Between the centrioles fine fibres appear, and it is on these fibres (the achromatic spindle) that the chromosomes arrange themselves, and appear to move after division (*Figure 1.5b*). The achromatic spindle, while not visible by normal staining methods, may be visualized with the polarizing microscope between crossed Nicol prisms or polaroids.

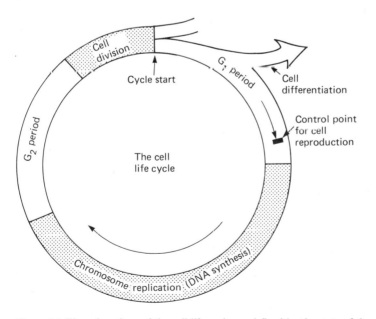

Figure 1.4 The subsections of the cell life cycle are defined by the state of the nucleus. Regulation of cell reproduction is achieved by interruption and arrest of cycle progress in G_1 (reproduced by courtesy of the Editor of *Cancer Research* and Dr D. D. M. Prescott)

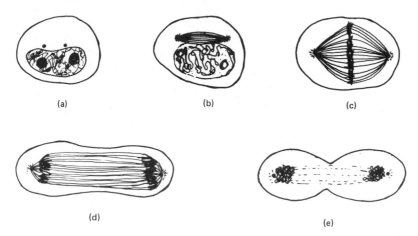

(a)   (b)   (c)

(d)   (e)

Figure 1.5 The stages of normal mitotic cell division. (a) Normal resting cell, with two centrioles illustrated above the nucleus. (b) Prophase: the spindle has formed between the centrioles and the chromatin condensed into a continuous thread. (c) Metaphase: the chromosomes have arranged themselves centrally across the spindle. (d) Anaphase: the chromosomes have divided equally and moved to opposite poles of the cell. (e) Telophase: the chromosomes coalesce and the cytoplasmic membrane begins to constrict, leading to the formation of two identical daughter cells

Metaphase

The centrioles are at opposite poles; the chromosomes are shorter and thicker and are arranged in the central region of the spindle. Each chromosome now splits into two (*Figure 1.5c*).

Anaphase

At this stage the chromosomes move along the spindle to opposite poles (*Figure 1.5d*).

Telophase

In this final stage, the sets of chromosomes having reached opposite poles, nuclear membranes are formed around each of the daughter nuclei, the chromosomes gradually expanding and dissolving. The cytoplasmic membrane itself divides, having become constricted during telophase and finally is only connected by a fine thread which ruptures as the cells move apart (*Figure 1.5e*).

Meiosis

Meiosis is a form of cell division which occurs only in sex cells during maturation. By a complicated system of coiling and splitting of the chromosomes, daughter cells, containing only 23 chromosomes are formed. The hereditary characteristics, carried on chromosomes by the genes, are rearranged during meiosis resulting in a random distribution amongst germ cells.

Organization of cells into tissues

During embryonic development, undifferentiated parental cells assume the position and characteristics necessary to perform specified functions during independent life. This process proceeds along a well-defined pathway in chronological order. It is knowledge of this orderly development that permits the exact age of immature tissues to be determined histologically. The process whereby cells develop from an aimless but multipotential state into one of specific function is termed differentiation.

All cells eventually work not as isolated units, but in groups, determined by function. Groups of cells so arranged are termed organs, and just as cells develop individual characteristics facilitating their identification, so do organs. Organs may be static, with little or no migration of the constituent cells, as for example the brain and kidney, or they may be more flexible and be composed of a constantly fluctuating population as, for example, in the case of blood or the spleen.

Cells may be held together by connections with one another, or they may require the presence of a second component, connective tissue, the function of which is to hold the various cells and organs together and to facilitate the movement of migratory cells and the transport of non-cellular substances. It consists of both cellular and non-cellular components. The maintenance of the connective tissue depends on the presence of specific cell types responsible for producing the connective tissue ground substance. The parental cell is the undifferentiated mesenchymal cell, few of which survive into adult life, although there always remains a pool of cells able to redifferentiate into certain cell types. The most important single cell type in connective tissue is the fibroblast, the secretory products of which are thought to provide the essential skeleton of most ground substances.

It can be seen, therefore, that histopathological technique is concerned with cells, their subcellular organization and their arrangement into organs and tissues. Although most conveniently grouped on morphological grounds there is increasing benefit in recognizing cell and tissue types by their behavioural characteristics.

Colloidal conception of tissue

In order to correlate the mobility of cells in certain conditions with the apparent immobility of tissues, it is necessary to have some knowledge of colloidal theory.

The cytoplasm of most cells allows free movement of granules within it, showing that it has a low viscosity, yet it maintains its shape by an outer area which is more of a gel. Both these areas are capable of reversal and the cell may, in certain circumstances, become almost liquid or, if injured or dead, may revert wholly to a stiff gel. Damage to the cytoplasmic membrane will normally result in gel formation under the damaged area until repair has taken place.

This reversion from sol to gel and vice versa is possible because of the colloidal nature of protoplasm.

Colloids

When a powdered solid is put into a fluid, it may remain suspended in that fluid and be easily removable by filtration through paper; or it may disperse as single molecules which cannot be removed by such simple means, in which case the solid will have gone into true solution. The physical properties of solutions differ greatly, some diffusing readily through collodion membranes, while others do not. These differences are due to the degree of dispersion of the material within the solvent or in other words, to the size of the dispersed particles. If there is a state of true molecular dispersion, the particles are smaller than one-millionth of a millimetre (10^{-6} mm), and the solution is a molecular solution. If the particles are so large that they can be seen microscopically, and can be removed by filtration through paper or porcelain, they are larger than one ten-thousandth of a millimetre (10^{-4} mm; 1 µm), and the solution is a coarse suspension. Between these limits there are the colloids, in which the dispersed material, while not in a state of true molecular dispersion, has been sufficiently reduced in size not to be classed, nor to act, as a coarse suspension.

Suspensoids and emulsoids

Colloids may be subdivided into two main types:

(1) suspensoids, and
(2) emulsoids.

The suspensoids with relatively large particles differ from coarse suspensions only in degree of suspension and size of particles, and do not combine to any degree with the solvent; they may be called anhydrocolloids.

In emulsoids, molecules of solvent (usually water) are firmly attached to the surface of the particles, rendering them miscible with water, or hydrophilic; they are therefore known as hydrocolloids. The two substances comprising a colloidal solution are known as phases, the solvent being the continuous phase, and the particles the dispersed phase.

Certain emulsoids, such as gelatin and protoplasm, are capable of reversal of their phases. In one phase they are liquid and are known as hydrosols, where semisolid globules are dispersed throughout a fluid; in the other phase they are semisolid and are known as hydrogels, where minute droplets of fluid are dispersed throughout the semisolid material.

It must be remembered that protoplasm is capable of rapid reversal from sol to gel, unlike gelatin in which a slow reversal takes place on heating and cooling.

Osmosis

If red blood cells are placed in water they will swell and burst; conversely, if they are placed in a strong salt solution, they will shrink; both of these reactions are due to osmotic pressure, a knowledge of which is essential to the understanding of the function and, especially, the preservation of cells and tissues.

Molecules of protein in colloidal solution are very much larger than those of simple salts or water, and it is possible to select membranes which will permit the passage of the small molecules but be impermeable to the larger ones. Such membranes are known as *semipermeable*, and may be natural animal tissue (e.g. pig's bladder), or artificial (e.g. collodion). If two solutions are separated by such a semipermeable membrane, small molecules will circulate freely between the two solutions, but large molecules, such as protein molecules, will be restricted to their own sides of the membrane; moreover, these large molecules will hinder the molecules of water attempting to pass through the membrane, the degree of hindrance being proportional to the concentration of protein in the solution. When the concentration of protein in the two solutions is different, water will pass more readily from the weaker to the stronger solution, and will continue

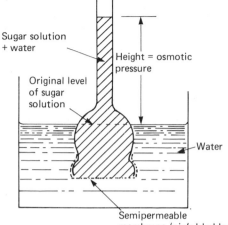

Sugar solution + water

Height = osmotic pressure

Original level of sugar solution

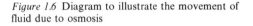

Water

Semipermeable membrane (pig's bladder)

Figure 1.6 Diagram to illustrate the movement of fluid due to osmosis

to do so until the two solutions are of the same strength; if the volumes of the two solutions are fixed the transfer of water molecules will increase the pressure in the stronger solution. This process is known as *osmosis*, and the pressure created is called *osmotic pressure*. The movement of fluid may be demonstrated by covering the open end of a thistle funnel with a semipermeable membrane, inverting this in a beaker of water and pouring sugar or protein solution into the funnel (*Figure 1.6*). The level of fluid in the stem of the funnel will rise, showing that water has passed through the membrane into the funnel; after several hours this level will become constant, and the height of this surface above the surface of the water in the beaker will be an indication of the osmotic pressure of the solution in the funnel. The effect of osmotic pressure in an enclosed space may be demonstrated by filling a pig's bladder with sugar solution and immersing this in water. The bladder will be distended and will ultimately burst.

The walls of all living cells are semipermeable membranes, and the cells contain colloidal solutions of protein. If such a cell is placed in a medium, the osmotic pressure of which is lower than that of the cell, water will pass into the cell and it will swell until it ruptures. This may be demonstrated with red blood cells. In the body these are surrounded by plasma which has osmotic pressure equal to that of the cells (about 7 atmospheres, 700 kPa), and they will retain their normal shape if placed in 0.85% sodium chloride solution, which has the same osmotic pressure as plasma (an *isotonic solution*). If placed in a weaker salt solution (a *hypotonic solution*) the red cells will be swollen by water passing through their cell walls, and will be ruptured (*lysed*), whereas if placed in a stronger salt solution (a *hypertonic solution*) water will leave the cells and they will become shrunken (*crenated*).

2

Outline of methodology

Preparation

Dissociation

The examination of thin pieces of tissue, gently separated in normal saline or other biologically inert medium is occasionally called for. The process is called 'teasing' and is performed in a watchglass using needles to gently pull the tissue apart. The specimen is transferred to a microscope slide while still wet, a coverslip is applied and the preparation is examined under the microscope with a reduced cone of illumination. More advantageously, a phase-contrast microscope may be employed, revealing a more detailed view of the structure of the unstained cells, often while the cells are still alive. Mitotic cells, especially in malignant tissue, may be clearly identified. This method may be of particular value in the study of vitally stained cells (*see below*) and especially in the examination of nerve endings in muscle. Modern phase-contrast microscopes provide exceptionally clear views of both stained and unstained cells, and in an inverted configuration are invaluable in the study of tissue cultures.

Although these methods enable details of individual cells to be seen clearly, they inevitably suffer from the disadvantage that anatomical relationships are destroyed.

Smears

To produce smears, the material to be examined is either pressed against a slide (impression smear), spread with a platinum loop, or crushed and spread with another slide. The preparation can then be fixed, stained to demonstrate specific structures and, after dehydration and clearing, mounted in a medium of high refractive index. This technique permits a much more detailed examination than a wet preparation. Although it may suffer from similar limitations, it is invaluable in the examination of exfoliated cells, or cells from lesions where it is not practical to remove a piece of tissue surgically. It is a method that has been re-evaluated and found to be a helpful adjunct to the study of lymphoid tissue and brain lesions amongst others.

Microtomy

Thick sections

In cases of emergency, very thin slices of fixed or unfixed tissue can be cut freehand with a sharp knife or razor. By restricting staining to the surface of the tissue an urgently required diagnosis may sometimes be made. Control of staining is effected by brushing a polychrome stain on the surface of the tissue and washing it off quickly. Although the method has been used with a great deal of accuracy, only if the operator has a wealth of experience can it be relied upon. In those cases where macroscopic examination of tissue is sufficient, whole organs such as breast, may be cut on a bacon slicer following embedding in gelatin, or freezing.

Paraffin-wax sections

To permit the microscopic examination of cells in their anatomical relationship with one another, thin (i.e. one cell thickness) slices or sections of tissue are required. To facilitate this, the tissue must be solidified and supported. Despite considerable experimentation paraffin wax, introduced for this purpose over 100 years ago, remains the support medium of choice. As a first stage the tissue must be preserved, and hardened, by treatment with a fixative, usually in aqueous solution. As this is not miscible with paraffin wax, the aqueous fixative must be removed and subsequently replaced by a wax solvent. Infiltration of the tissue by molten paraffin wax helps to ensure that this tissue is supported both internally and externally. There is probably no better way of preserving tissue for histological examination than in the final state—cast in a block of paraffin wax.

In an attempt to overcome some of the disadvantages of dehydrating and clearing tissues, certain water-soluble waxes have been substituted for paraffin wax. Sections obtained by such methods are more difficult to handle and rarely produce results comparable with paraffin-wax embedding. It has, however, been used with success by some workers with special requirements following freeze-drying.

Celloidin although apparently harder than paraffin wax, has a rubbery consistency which gives greater support to mixed tissues (e.g. skin with subcutaneous fat) and to very hard tissue such as bone. As processing of the tissues is performed at room temperature, it may be employed, with benefit, for tissues where the effects of heat may be deleterious, such as the central nervous system. It is technically more difficult to cut and stain celloidin sections, but persons with the time and patience will find the results superior to those achieved following paraffin-wax embedding.

Celloidin is usually obtained as LVN (low viscosity nitrocellulose) and is soluble in equal parts of alcohol and ether. Therefore, with celloidin embedding, clearing is avoided, the tissue being fixed and dehydrated before being infiltrated and finally embedded in celloidin. The blocks must be cut and stored in dilute alcohol, unless they are specially treated.

Resin embedding is a new, and in many ways, major development since the third edition of this book. The principal advantage of this method is the facility with which much thinner sections of tissue may be obtained, although there has been a concomitant improvement in the preservation of cellular relationships. Essentially, the method is a spin-off from sectioning methods for electron microscopy, although the full potential was not realized until developments in microtome and knife design were complete. There are many resins suitable for embedding, but it is the water-miscible ones that are proving most popular. The extra support provided by the resin permits thinner sections, and avoiding the rigours of clearing and infiltrating with hot wax results in improved morphology. Although never likely to replace paraffin-wax embedding, as some sages predicted, the method does have a definite place in the study of certain tissues, such as kidney and lymph node. The study of thin resin sections of these tissues has led to a greater understanding of certain pathological states, with definite clinical benefits.

Frozen sections are complementary to other methods of tissue preparation. They have a role either by providing a rapid diagnosis, or by permitting the study of tissue elements lost during more conventional processing. By freezing the tissue, the need for some external support during sectioning is obviated. Sections of frozen tissue may be cut on a specially adapted microtome, or, more commonly, on a microtome housed in a deep-freeze type cabinet—the cryostat. Apart from the facility to provide a rapid diagnosis, cryostats have found an increasing role in permitting the demonstration of labile substances, such as enzymes and the sites of immunological activity. Frozen sections are also the traditional methods for the demonstration of fats lost during conventional paraffin-wax processing, and elements of the central nervous system (*see Figure 2.1*).

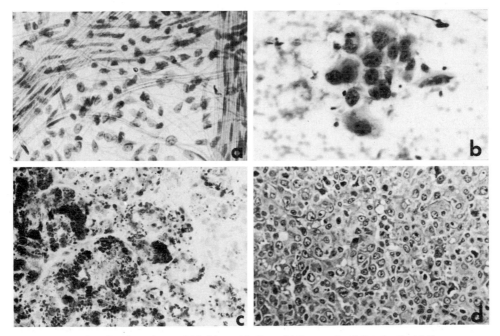

Figure 2.1 (a) Dissociated specimen of bladder epithelium. (b) Smear of exfoliated cells. (c) Frozen section stained to demonstrate fat. (d) Thin (2 µm) section to show increased cellular detail

Demonstration

Traditional histopathology depends upon pattern recognition of morphological features, almost all of which are only recognizable following colouring (staining) of tissue components. The study of stained tissue sections is the study of gross artefact, bearing little resemblance to living tissue. It is, nevertheless, a study which has created a considerable body of knowledge, easily communicated and reproducible. Even though a high degree of accuracy in diagnosis is achieved by these means, it remains a subjective art. To the general methods which impart tinctorial properties to tissue may be added methods which will demonstrate selectively certain tissue components and those that will, with appropriate controls, identify cell and tissue constituents on the basis of their chemical or immunological reactivity. An appreciation of these differences helps to differentiate between histological, histochemical and immunohistochemical techniques. These are all demonstration methods, the limitations of which have to be understood in terms of *selectivity* and *sensitivity*.

Selectivity refers to the extent to which a stain or reaction demonstrates the desired component to the exclusion of others. In histochemical and immunohistochemical techniques, the term *specificity* is preferred.

Sensitivity refers to the smallest amount or concentration of the substance that can be demonstrated by the chosen technique. The smaller the amount, the greater the sensitivity.

Obviously, the greater the selectivity and sensitivity of the procedure, the more helpful it is in reaching an unequivocal diagnosis. There is a definite relationship between the treatment tissue receives prior to the demonstration method and the success, clarity or brilliance of the result. Although it is probably inevitable that tissue received in the routine diagnostic laboratory will be fixed in formal–saline, it is as well to remember the benefits that may be gained by relating fixation to subsequent demonstration methods on those occasions when optimal fixation is possible. Indeed, specialized treatment of tissue is increasingly a prerequisite for the newer techniques providing specific identification and localization.

Staining

The general principles of the chemistry of staining will be found in Chapter 6. In this section it is intended to introduce the reader to why tissues are stained and the methods by which this may be achieved.

Early microscopists suffered a tremendous handicap because they worked before the use of dyes had been introduced to biology. It was the development of the textile dye industry in the second half of the last century that led to the application of commercial dyes to tissue sections. Today's microscopist would be at a complete loss without the very large range of biological stains and reagents available. Although a degree of change in cell and tissue contrast may be achieved by specialized techniques such as phase-contrast, polarizing and darkground microscopy, it is those methods that impart contrast on the basis of selective colouring which have proved most beneficial.

Biological stains are basically no different from commercial dyes, but often they have been adapted for use in biology. Special care and greater control may be used in their manufacture, and claims made that they are purer. There have been occasions, however, when difficulty has been experienced from using too pure a form since one of the apparent impurities has, in fact, acted as a mordant and therefore been an unacknowledged but necessary component. Impurities may be an unavoidable consequence of commercially acceptable manufacturing processes, or may be deliberately introduced as diluents of the dye powder. Examples of the latter include dextrin, sodium sulphate and borax. Laboratory workers often quote the reliability and brilliance of so-called 'Grubler's dyes' before the First World War. Good though these dyes undoubtedly were, it is a popular myth that they owed their success as much to the impurities present as to the actual dye. In fact Grubler was a most conscientious supplier who rigorously and conscientiously tested the dyes he received from his suppliers, and released for sale only those that met his own high standards. It was the unreliability of dyes once Grubler's became unavailable that led to the formation of the

Biological Stains Commission (BSC) in the USA. The BSC offers to test dyes for purity, total dye content and performance for manufacturers and suppliers. Those that prove satisfactory are approved and certified. Most reputable suppliers in the UK test their dyes 'in-house'. Nevertheless, unsatisfactory dyes do slip through and the Institute of Medical Laboratory Sciences has now introduced an independent Dye Approval Scheme on similar lines to the BSC.

Staining may be loosely defined as treating tissue or cells with a reagent or series of reagents so that it acquires a colour; usually, no particles of dye are seen and the stained element is transparent.

Staining techniques may be subdivided in the following ways.

Vital staining

Some living cells will take up certain dyes (*vital stains*) which colour selectively elements in the cells, for example, mitochondria take up Janus green. Such staining may be achieved in the body (*in vivo*) or in a microscopical preparation (*in vitro*). Where the technique is applied *in vivo* it is referred to as *intravital* and where *in vitro*, that is, living cells outside the body, *supravital.*

Particles of coloured matter may be engulfed by phagocytic cells from colloidal suspensions. This process is known as phagocytosis and the particle may be seen within the cytoplasm of the cell although no specific structure is demonstrated. An example would be reticuloendothelial cells phagocytosing Trypan blue or Indian ink. The method is included here purely for convenience as it is not truly staining as defined.

Histological stains

These impart a colour to tissue elements by methods that may often be quite selective but by a mechanism that is not always understood. Histological staining is by far the most common demonstration method employed in histopathology.

Fat stains

In these, the colouring agent is usually more soluble in the element to be demonstrated than in the vehicle (or solvent) in which it is applied, *elective solubility.*

Impregnation

Impregnation is not truly staining, but is, in fact, the deposition of salts of heavy metals over certain selected cell and tissue elements and processes. It cannot be classified as staining for the following reasons:

(1) The structures so demonstrated are usually rendered opaque. The only colours possible are shades of brown or black.
(2) The colouring matter is particulate.
(3) The metal salts are deposited *on* or *around* but not *in* the element demonstrated.

In spite of these differences, the wide use and frequent advantages of impregnation, either alone or in combination with staining techniques, are sufficient reason for its inclusion. Impregnation is indispensable for the satisfactory demonstration of many tissue elements.

Histochemistry

Histochemistry differs from staining in that it concerns reactions that are predicted with a knowledge of the chemical reaction that will occur. The specificity of histochemical methods is usually high. The reaction may take place between a colourless reagent and a specific tissue component, as in the Feulgen reaction (page 183) when a magenta dye is produced by the presence of induced aldehydes. A simpler example would be the combination of a tissue element with an applied reagent to give a coloured end-product as in the Perls reaction for iron (*see* page 279). A more sophisticated application is to introduce a 'missing link' to a chemical chain reaction and subsequent coloration of the end-product, as with the introduction of a specific substrate to demonstrate indirectly, by its activity, a viable enzyme.

Immunocytochemistry

Immunocytochemistry depends upon the specific affinity of an antibody for an antigen present in cells or tissue, or vice versa. Antigens are visualized by combining the antibody with a coloured substance, usually a fluorescent dye, or with an enzyme that may itself be subsequently demonstrated. Earlier methods, using the fluorescent dye technique, required the use of fresh frozen sections, but newer developments permit the localization of many antigens or antibodies in routine paraffin-wax sections. These methods are very much in vogue and hold great hope for reducing the degree of subjectivity previously inherent in histopathological diagnosis. The technique may be applied to electron microscopy by combining the antibody with an electron-dense reagent such as ferritin, or by rendering electron-dense the popular choice of the light microscopist—DAB (*see* Chapter 34)—by treatment with osmic acid.

Examination (*Figure 2.2*)

Light microscopy

As haematoxylin and eosin-stained sections are a universal cornerstone to diagnostic histopathology, so is bright-field microscopy. It is the premier method by which tissue is examined, other forms of microscopy having only a secondary role. The specialized methods enumerated below are useful and often indispensable adjuncts, but the bright-field examination of haematoxylin and eosin-stained sections is universal.

Fluorescence

Fluorescence is the property of certain substances, including a range of dyes, to convert light rays from the invisible (ultraviolet) spectrum into the visible spectrum. Fluorescent material, either natural, induced or stained, examined by this method will appear bright on a dark background. A special light source and filters are required, and protection must be given to prevent injury to the observer's eyes. The method is of limited value in the examination of the natural fluorescence of tissue components and there are probably few fluorescent staining methods of great value, except perhaps amyloid staining by thioflavine T (*see* page 469). Fluorescence microscopy is invaluable to the study of antibody/antigen reactions in tissue sections and is also increasingly applied to automatic methods of scanning for atypical cells and sorting of cell

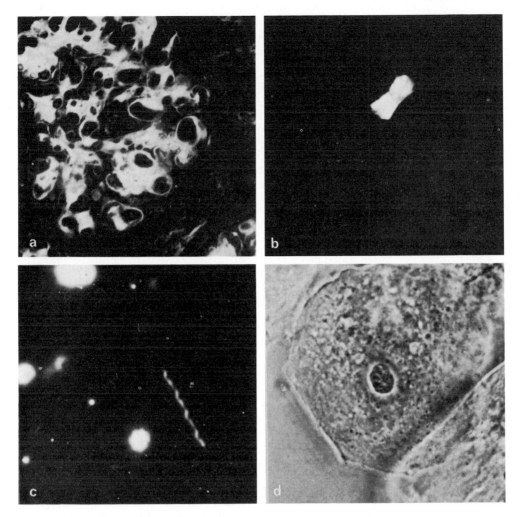

Figure 2.2 Examples of different methods of microscopic examination. (a) Fluorescence. Specimen illuminated by ultraviolet light revealing location of fluorochrome thioflavine T. (b) Positive birefringence of crystals photographed between crossed polars. (c) Micro-organisms visualized by the use of darkground microscopy. (d) Phase-contrast microscopy bringing extra detail to whole, unstained cells

suspensions. Both these latter methods make use of the differential staining of nucleic acids by the fluorochrome acridine orange.

Polarized light microscopy

This is particularly valuable for the detection and, often, the identification of certain foreign bodies, crystals and some lipids. Other structures, such as striated muscle, myelin and bone have characteristic appearances when viewed in this manner. Here it may be briefly stated, in simplistic terms, that light vibrating in a single plane is permitted to illuminate the specimen. Certain substances have the ability to alter the plane of vibration. If such altered planes of light are passed through a 'filter' or 'grille' which will allow the passage of that light only, the substance will appear light against a dark background. Such substances are described as being anisotropic, doubly refractile or birefringent.

Darkground microscopy

Darkground microscopy is of limited value to the cellular pathologist. By illuminating an object from a very oblique angle, only those light rays hitting the object and thereby deflected, will be collected by the objective lens of the microscope. Objects are therefore seen as a bright image, by the light they scatter, against a dark background. The method is used in the identification of spirochaetes and parasites in body fluids and in fluorescence microscopy.

Phase-contrast microscopy

This exaggerates slight differences in refractive index. Cell constituents, such as mitochondria, may be seen in detail and since living cells may be studied, this form of microscopy has proved invaluable in tissue culture work. Although specialized objectives are required for phase contrast, these are suitable also for bright-field microscopy with only minor readjustment to the microscope.

Electron microscopy

The transmission electron microscope (TEM) has an electron gun as an energy source in contrast to the light rays of the conventional light microscope. Optical lenses are replaced with electromagnetic lenses. As electrons pass less readily through tissue sections than do light rays, the specimen has to be correspondingly thinner. Electrons passing through the specimen may be retarded in exactly the same way as light rays; heavy metals, for example, being electron dense and producing a dark image when compared with, say, carbon. The actual image is formed by electrons hitting and exciting a fluorescent screen. Fortunately, electrons have exactly the same effect as light on photographic materials, so that photography in the electron microscope is essentially identical with that in the light microscope. The advantage of the electron microscope is found in the improved resolution and thus the magnification that is possible. The disadvantage, other than technical difficulties, lies in the small size of specimen it is possible to examine.

The scanning electron microscope (SEM) works on a very similar principle to the transmission instrument. Instead of sending electrons through very thin sections of tissue, electrons are reflected off the surfaces of more substantial structures, collected by an electron-sensitive detector and an image is formed on a cathode ray tube according to a processed electronic message. Specimen preparation is much simpler than that necessary for TEM; complete drying of the specimen is necessary, by such methods as simple desiccation, freeze-drying or freeze substitution, and the surface is coated with a thin layer of a heavy metal, usually gold. A major advantage of the SEM is the depth of field produced, yielding a three-dimensional image.

Analytical electron microscopy utilizes the property of all elements to emit characteristic X-rays as a result of bombardment by electrons. Analysis of these X-rays on the basis of energy dispersal, allows elements to be analysed as to their relative proportions in a specimen, or a spectral analysis can reveal the total content of a given element, if appropriate controls are included. These methods may be applied to both the transmission and scanning electron microscopes.

Quantitative methods

In recent years many attempts have been made to reduce the subjective nature of histopathological diagnosis. Most of these have centred on quantifying specific features of the disease process and, by statistical analysis, relating these to the clinical and histopathological diagnosis and progress of the disease. Not all of the methods involve the use of sophisticated instruments as will be found by reference to Chapter 28.

3
Fixation

Introduction

Tissue rots. For morphological examination this has to be prevented. More specifically, bacterial contamination leads to putrefaction of tissue, enzymes released from within the tissue cause autolysis, labile substances are destroyed and soluble substances are lost into the surrounding medium. The first aim of fixation is to prevent or, at least, arrest these changes. In choosing the most appropriate method of fixation it is also worth considering all the subsequent stages of preparing tissue for study with the microscope.

As a first step, it must be ensured, as far as possible, that those elements that are to be demonstrated remain at maximum concentration and precise localization. If tissue sections are to be prepared, an attempt must be made to stabilize labile elements so that they remain unaffected by subsequent treatment by organic solvents and, in the case of paraffin-wax embedding, heat; the tissue must be of sufficient rigidity to permit thin slices or sections to be cut, and optical contrast must be induced for worthwhile morphological examination. There are, however, occasions when fixation itself may destroy the element to be demonstrated. In such cases it may be necessary to perform the demonstration method prior to fixation, with stabilization of the tissue achieved subsequently. Such is the case with many enzymes and certain antigen/antibody reactions. The increasing use of these techniques has resulted in an increase in the number of specimens received in the laboratory unfixed. This situation demands that attention is given to these specimens as soon as possible. If the specimen is large enough, it should be divided immediately and receive the treatment appropriate to the manner of investigation. As much damage may be caused to a specimen by leaving it to dry as by immersing it in an inappropriate fixative. In certain quarters the use of a relatively inert transport medium has been introduced to overcome these problems.

The foundation of all good microscopic preparations is that the tissue should be appropriately and adequately treated as soon as possible after removal. Faults cannot be remedied at any later stage and the finished preparation can only be as good as the primary treatment.

If fixation is to be employed, it is essential that it is done as soon as possible after death or removal from the body, and for this reason screw-capped specimen jars containing appropriate fixatives should be kept permanently wherever tissues for histological examination are taken regularly, for example, in the operating theatre, post-mortem room or animal house. Good liaison between the clinician and the laboratory will help ensure that the fixative most appropriate to the required investigation is used. The amount of fluid used should, where practical, be 15 to 20 times the bulk of the tissue to be fixed.

Theoretical considerations of fixation

The commonest causes of poor cellular detail in histological preparations are as follows.

Autolysis

Literally autolysis means self-inflicted death or destruction. It is caused by the action of intracellular enzymes thought to be released by ruptured lysosomes. The enzymes responsible are cathepsins, some of which are proteinases which break down long-chain proteins to peptides, and others, carboxypeptidases and aminopeptidases which further break down peptides to individual amino acids. These changes are reduced by low temperature and eliminated by high temperature. Unfortunately, other tissue changes may accompany raising the temperature. Certain tissues, such as the central nervous system and the kidney, are more quickly affected than others, such as most connective tissues. The practical outcome is that nuclei may become intensely condensed or even break up, cytoplasm may become swollen and eventually the entire tissue architecture is lost. In the case of epithelium, the cells may be split off from the basement membrane, occasionally giving an appearance bizarre enough to suggest malignancy (*Figure 3.1*).

Putrefaction

Those tissues, such as the intestinal tract, which normally have a high bacterial content, will rapidly break down after removal or death, due to the action of the organisms.

Rate of fixation

Fixing solutions are chosen according to their different properties, included amongst which are the rate at which they penetrate, and fix, tissues. However, the greatest factor influencing the rate of fixation is the thickness of the tissue. It follows that whole organs should be sliced to expose the cut surfaces to the fixing solution as soon as possible. There have been several experiments aimed at determining the rate of penetration of fixatives, but it should be borne in mind that there are several factors that prevent this work from achieving absolute precision. For example, most, but not all, fixatives achieve the desired result by reacting with proteins, which may present in varying quantities in different tissues. The act of fixation may in itself hinder the further penetration of the fixative, as is certainly the case with osmium tetroxide. Fixatives may also find easier routes into tissue via loose connective tissue or along blood or lymphatic vessels. The rate of reaction between fixative and tissue will vary according to combination and penetration does not always equate with fixation. The reaction may also be reversible. It should also be noted that with mixtures of fixatives (e.g. Zenker's solution) each component will penetrate at its own individual rate.

Much of the experimental work has been performed on either relatively homogeneous tissues, such as liver and kidney, or on model systems such as protein gels. However, it has been established that fixatives penetrate tissue according to a

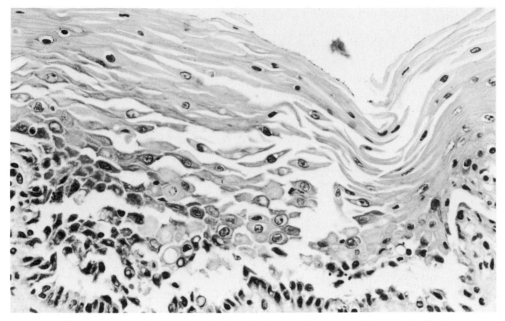

Figure 3.1 Fixation artefact of epithelium. Specimen inadvertently submersed in *normal* saline for 24 hours, with subsequent fixation in formal–saline. Note the bizarre appearance of the epithelial cells. Original magnification ×100

fairly standard form of diffusion. The depth of penetration (d) has a direct linear relationship with the square root of the time of exposure to fixative ($\sqrt{t}$). For each tissue there is a constant (k) representing the coefficiency of diffusion. Thus the general formula

$$d = k\sqrt{t}$$

may be applied.

Changes in tissue volume

Glutaraldehyde is one of the few fixatives that cause tissue shrinkage. Other fixatives cause tissue to swell, differing only in degree. A first, practical effect of this is that organs that may easily slip into wide-necked jars will not leave them so readily. It is not uncommon that a glass jar has to be smashed to retrieve an intact uterus immersed in formal*–saline, for example. Although ideally tissue volumes should remain unchanged during fixation, the swelling does go some way towards counteracting the shrinkage induced by dehydration and hot-wax infiltration during paraffin processing. A final shrinkage of some 33% may still ensue. Another noticeable effect may be that nuclei in paraffin-wax sections appear smaller than those in frozen sections prepared from the same tissue.

The mechanism causing these volume changes is not fully understood but is thought to be associated with changes in membrane permeability, inhibition of respiration and changes in sodium transport activity.

These volume changes have obvious implications for quantitative microscopy.

* *See* footnote on p. 30

Effects of osmolarity

Although it would appear that unless fixatives are isotonic, cells will become distorted, this is not necessarily the case. For example, acetic acid, which may be considered to be hypertonic in relation to body fluids, does, in fact, cause tissues to swell. Picric acid, which may be considered hypotonic and should therefore cause tissue to swell, in fact, shrinks tissue as it fixes. As a general statement it may be said that protein precipitants (*see below*) shrink tissue regardless of their osmotic pressure, and for non-protein precipitants the reverse is true.

In practice, the osmotic pressure need only approximate that of the tissue for routine work. There is little to be gained by exactly equating osmotic pressure and employing a complex physiological solution when 0.9% sodium chloride or 1% calcium chloride work equally well.

For more critical work it is often necessary to add a buffer and pay particular attention to osmolarity. This is particularly so in the more exacting area of ultrastructural preservation and in the precise localization of enzymes. Large-molecular-weight substances such as dextran and polyvinylpyrrolidone may be added with advantage, as may be sucrose.

Reagents employed as fixatives

Although there are important exceptions, most commonly, fixation is aimed at stabilizing the most ubiquitous tissue component, protein. This is achieved by insolubilizing the protein, the principal mechanism of which is cross-linking between end-groups. Horobin (1982) considers that the action of protein fixatives in breaking up secondary and tertiary protein structures to form insoluble derivatives is at least as important as cross-linking.

Formaldehyde (H.CHO)

Formaldehyde is a gas, commercially available as a 40% solution in water. This saturated solution is commonly termed formalin. A great deal of confusion has been caused by the careless use of these terms; a solution labelled '10% formalin' might contain 10% formal* (4% formaldehyde) or 10% formaldehyde (25% formalin). It is generally accepted that 40% formaldehyde is formalin and all references to it in this work will give actual percentages of this reagent. Thus, 10% formalin consists of:

Formalin (40% formaldehyde)	10 ml
Water	90 ml

Formalin consists mainly of the polymerized form of formaldehyde, whereas 10% formalin consists principally of the monohydrate methylene glycol $(CH_2(OH)_2)$

---

* There is continuing confusion over the terminology of fixative solutions containing formalin. Sometimes solutions containing formalin and isotonic sodium chloride, for example, are erroneously referred to as 'formol–saline'. We consider the views of Baker (1950) to be correct. He states: 'The word formaldehyde is often shortened to formol. This is not desirable, because the -ol termination suggests an alcohol or phenol. It is as illogical to write formol as it would be to write alcohal. The standard contracted terminology for aldehydes is -al (e.g. chloral, furforal), and formal is the logical contraction of the word.'

together with monomeric formaldehyde. Impurities in commercial formalin include methanol, added as a stabilizer but which may adversely affect enzyme reactions, and formic acid, which increases on storage. During long storage, particularly in the cold, concentrated formalin may become turbid due to the formation of a white precipitate of paraformaldehyde. This may be removed by filtration without noticeably affecting the efficiency of the formalin. Pure formaldehyde may be generated by heating paraformaldehyde powder, a property used in vapour fixation (*see below*).

The reaction of formaldehyde with protein end-groups to cross-link molecules giving rise to an insoluble end-product is well known (Hopwood, 1968a). Protein groups involved include amino, imino and amido, peptide, hydroxyl, carboxyl and sulphhydryl. Methylene bridges are also commonly formed between similar groups such as NH_2 and NH, but are thought to be reversible by washing in water (Pearse, 1980). This latter property may permit the demonstration of tissue components otherwise masked.

The reaction of formaldehyde with lipids has been investigated and it has been shown to react rapidly with phosphatidyl ethanolamine causing degradation; acid hydrolysis may have an effect in the very long term. Cholesterol, cerebrosides, sulphatides and sphingomyelin remain unaffected. Phospholipids, while not 'fixed' by formaldehyde, may remain localized by the addition of calcium (Baker, 1944; Lillie, 1965) which reduces their solubility in lipid solvents.

As the presence of formic acid as an impurity in formalin solution leads to a drop in pH, steps should be taken to neutralize this effect. For most purposes it should be made neutral or slightly alkaline before using as a fixative. This may be achieved by the use of either pH 7.2 phosphate buffer or by incorporating magnesium carbonate in the diluent. Magnesium carbonate should not be added to neat acid formalin (i.e. 40% formaldehyde) as a build up of carbon dioxide may result with the consequent danger of explosion within a closed container. Calcium acetate has also been advocated (Baker, 1944), although Drury and Wallington (1980) warn of the possible artefactual appearance of areas of calcification in soft tissue fixed this way.

The use of neutral formalin fixatives results in a marked increase in the frequency with which ferric iron can be demonstrated and an almost complete absence of the formation of formalin pigment.

Glutaraldehyde $((CH_2)_3CHO.CHO)$

Glutaraldehyde was introduced as a fixative by Sabatini, Bensch and Barrett (1963) following an investigation into nine aldehydes: it has been used principally for electron microscopy, usually in combination with osmium tetroxide. Although early supplies were often heavily contaminated with impurities, it is now commercially obtainable, at various concentrations, in relatively pure form.

It is obtainable commercially as a 25% solution in which form it contains various impurities; Hopwood (1967) noted that the glutaraldehyde could be fractionated from these impurities on Sephadex G-10. Chambers, Bowling and Grimley (1968) used activated coconut charcoal (10 g/100 ml 25% glutaraldehyde) for this purpose, they found that, after exposure to the charcoal for several days at 4 °C, the amber colour of the solution slowly diminished. It should be stored in the refrigerator without removal or change of the charcoal.

Studies by Bowes (1963) showed that, of several aldehyde fixatives tested, it was the most efficient cross-linking agent for collagen. Its cross-linking efficiency is said to give a better preservation of structure and a more rapid fixing action than formaldehyde, but poorer penetration. Hopwood (1968b) stated that at pH levels greater than 8.0 it undergoes rapid polymerization.

Glutaraldehyde, which is a bifunctional aldehyde, reacts chiefly with amino groups, its molecular size being particularly suited to bridge the gap between them on the polypeptide chain of collagen (Bowes and Cator, 1967). It also reacts with the amino acids tyrosine, tryptophan and phenylalanine (Hopwood, 1968b), but to a lesser degree than formaldehyde. Chambers, Bowling and Grimley (1968) recommended the use of 4% glutaraldehyde, in phosphate buffer at pH 7.4, as a routine fixative in histopathology. Non-specific PAS staining is encountered after glutaraldehyde fixation due to unbound (free) aldehyde groups which result from some 10–15% of the molecules being involved in unipointal fixation (only one end of the molecule bound or fixed). This false PAS positivity can be eliminated by blocking with acetic–aniline (see page 245).

Not only does glutaraldehyde give rise to marked shrinkage with paraffin-wax processed tissue, but it also results in a brittleness of the tissue that hinders successful microtomy.

Other aldehydes

Several other aldehydes used in the tanning industry have been evaluated as to their efficacy as histochemical fixatives, including acrolein, glyoxal, malonaldehyde and diacetyl. Acrolein has been shown to produce more cross-links than formaldehyde and to penetrate tissue well. Unfortunately it is an unpleasant compound to use and tends to be unstable at alkaline pH. Malonaldehyde is an interesting fixative in that it is reported to produce specific fluorescence by cross-linking peptide chains via amino-acid residues and reacts with DNA bases to form a fluorescent compound (Pearse, 1980).

Mercuric chloride ($HgCl_2$)

Mercuric chloride is a protein precipitant which rapidly penetrates and hardens. In general, like other metallic ions, it combines with the acid groups of proteins and the phosphoric acid group of nucleoproteins, it also reacts specifically with thiol (SH) groups (Pearse, 1980). While most protein reactions can be utilized after Hg fixation, it is not recommended where nucleoproteins or sulph-hydryl groups are to be investigated. Unfortunately, the rate of penetration is decreased after the first few millimetres and pieces of tissue exceeding 5 mm in thickness will usually tend to be hard and overfixed at the periphery, and soft and underfixed in the centre. Because of this, and the great shrinkage caused, mercuric chloride is seldom used alone; it is a constituent of many good routine fixatives when combined with reagents which combat these defects, such as acetic acid, formalin, potassium dichromate, and so on.

Fixatives containing mercuric chloride should be listed among the *intolerant fixatives*, in that exposure of tissues to their action in excess of recommended times, will produce excessive hardness and make the cutting of thin sections difficult.

Although mercuric chloride neither attacks nor preserves lipids, its presence in tissue inhibits adequate freezing and makes frozen sections difficult to prepare.

Because it is radio-opaque the presence of mercuric chloride in calcified tissue precludes the use of X-rays to determine the end-point of decalcification.

Staining, particularly of the cytoplasm, tends to be more brilliant following mercuric chloride fixation.

Tissues fixed in any mercury-containing fixative will require treatment to remove the brownish mercury precipitate which will be found throughout. This is done by oxidation with iodine to mercuric iodide, which can be removed by treatment with sodium thiosulphate. This converts it to mercuric tetrathionate which is readily water-soluble.

As a routine the incorporation of 0.25% iodine in the 80% alcohol used in dehydrating tissues is recommended, and the following routine advised for individual sections before staining:

(1) Place section in 0.5% iodine in 80% alcohol for 3 minutes.
(2) Rinse in water.
(3) Place in 3% aqueous sodium thiosulphate for 3 minutes.
(4) Wash in running water for 1–2 minutes.

Mercuric chloride corrodes metal and fixatives incorporating it must not be stored in containers with metal caps. There are suggestions that the use of mercuric chloride may enhance the demonstration of certain peptides by immunocytochemistry (Bosman *et al.*, 1977).

Precautions must be taken with the disposal of mercury-containing fixatives to avoid environmental pollution.

Potassium dichromate $(K_2Cr_2O_7)$

Potassium dichromate has a binding effect on protein similar to that of formalin, giving fixation of the cytoplasm without precipitation. It is thought that this is because chromium ions form complexes with water which combine with the reactive sites on adjacent protein chains. Their main affinity is for carboxyl and hydroxyl groups of protein which makes fixatives containing chromium ions unsuitable for histochemistry with the exception of the chromaffin reaction (page 285). It preserves phosphatides and is used for the fixation of mitochrondria. It has a pH of 3.75 and, although it is said that when acidified both chromatin and cytoplasm are precipitated as meshworks, chromosomes are well fixed, and mitochondria destroyed. *Champy's fluid*, which contains potassium dichromate, chromic acid, and osmium tetroxide with a pH of 2.5, preserves mitochondria. This may, however, be due to the direct fixing action of osmium tetroxide on lipids.

Following fixation in potassium dichromate (or chromic acid), tissue must be well washed in running water before dehydration. The transfer of chromate-containing tissue direct to alcohol results in the formation of an insoluble lower oxide which can be removed by treating with 1% HCl in 70% alcohol for 30 min.

Chromic acid

Chromic acid is prepared by dissolving anhydrous chromium trioxide (CrO_3) in distilled water.

It precipitates all proteins, and preserves carbohydrates. It is a powerful oxidizing reagent, and should it be contained in a compound fixative such as Orth's fluid, or Zenker's fluid, then reducing agents such as formalin should only be added immediately before use.

Chromic acid hydrolyses DNA with the conversion of its pentose sugar to an aldehyde; it also converts carbohydrates to aldehydes. DNA and carbohydrates will therefore give positive staining with Schiff reagent without the normal pretreatment by periodate or HCl associated with the PAS or Feulgen reactions respectively.

Tissues fixed in chromic-acid-containing fixatives will require thorough washing for the same reason as those fixed in potassium dichromate.

Picric acid ($C_6H_2(NO_2)_3OH$)

Picric acid is supplied in water and should be kept under water. When dry, it is liable to explode if heated or detonated. It is a protein precipitant, forming picrates with amino acids, including those in nucleoproteins. Although it causes shrinkage of tissues, it enhances cytoplasmic constituents, giving especially brilliant results with trichrome stains. Picric acid also dyes tissue yellow, sometimes of benefit when handling small fragments. The yellow colour is easily removed from sections. Picric acid is often employed in compound fixatives to enhance the preservation of glycogen, but may render RNA resistant to ribonuclease digestion.

It has long been suggested that the picrates formed by the reaction between basic protein and picric acid are water soluble and that tissue should be transferred directly from the fixative to alcohol. This treatment renders the picrates insoluble in water.

Osmium tetroxide (OsO_4)

Osmium tetroxide is commonly, though incorrectly, known as osmic acid.

It demonstrates lipids (e.g. myelin) but is very expensive. It gives excellent preservation of detail of single cells, or minute pieces of tissue, and for this reason it is used almost exclusively in electron microscopy (see page 607). With pieces of tissue more than 2–3 mm thick, however, it penetrates poorly and unevenly, and several routine staining methods are difficult, if not impossible, following its use.

Osmium tetroxide is supplied in sealed glass tubes containing 0.1, 0.2, 0.5 or 1 g.

To prepare the usual stock solution of 2%, the label is removed, and the tube washed several times in pure glass-distilled water. A file mark having been made, the tube is then broken and dropped into a glass-stoppered, dark bottle containing the correct amount of glass-distilled water.

Care must be taken in handling since its vapour is very irritating and can cause a conjunctivitis. It is easily reduced by light and heat and should be stored in a dark, cool place. The addition of one drop of saturated aqueous solution of mercuric chloride to every 10 ml of solution will help to check reduction. All the osmium-tetroxide-containing fixatives give very uneven fixation; the resultant sections show an over-fixed and blackened zone at the periphery, and an under-fixed zone at the centre with little cellular detail.

While there is considerable disagreement as to the actual mechanism of fixation of osmium tetroxide, it is generally agreed that it oxidizes unsaturated bonds. Saturated lipids do not react but unsaturated lipids reduce OsO_4 with the formation of black compounds.

The chemistry of the reaction between lipids and osmium tetroxide in relation to electron microscopy has been reviewed by Korn (1966). Bahr (1954) has shown that the reaction of OsO_4 with proteins depends upon their histidine, cysteine and tryptophan content; his view was supported by Hake (1965). Dallam (1957) who showed there was a 37% loss of protein during OsO_4 fixation and dehydration, and Lenard and Singer (1968) who showed that glutaraldehyde–osmium tetroxide fixation produced marked changes in the helical structure of proteins, have again indicated the need for caution in the interpretation of electron micrographs. It fixes and blackens lipids (e.g. mito-chondria and Golgi apparatus). The vapour alone can be used to fix very small pieces of tissue, or unfixed sections such as those prepared by the freeze-drying technique.

This blackening of certain elements is due to the conversion of the colourless OsO_4 to the black hydrated form, OsO_25H_2O.

Ethyl alcohol (C_2H_5OH)

Alcohol alone is of little use as a fixative except occasionally for blood films and smears. It penetrates rather slowly and tends to harden tissue after long exposure. When combined with other reagents, as in Carnoy's fluid, fixation is very rapid.

It denatures protein by precipitation, and precipitates glycogen. Denaturation of a protein may theoretically change the reactivity of its groups (Pearse, 1980) and such a possibility should be kept in mind when alcohol fixation is employed. It is used in histochemical methods for enzymes because, to some extent, it leaves them in their original state; being a fat solvent it dissolves fats and lipids.

Acetone (CH_3COCH_3)

Used cold, acetone is sometimes used as a fixative for the histochemical demonstration of tissue enzymes, notably the phosphatases and lipases. Its action as a fixative is almost identical to that of alcohol, except that glycogen is not well preserved.

Acetic acid (CH_3COOH)

Commonly called glacial acetic acid because it is solid at temperatures below 17 °C, this is never used alone because of its swelling effect on collagen fibres; but in compound fixatives it is used to counteract the shrinkage effects of other reagents.

Nucleoproteins are precipitated by acetic acid, mitochondria and Golgi apparatus are destroyed or distorted.

Trichloroacetic acid (CCl_3COOH)

Trichloroacetic acid, like acetic acid, is never used alone, but because of its swelling effect on many tissues it may be employed usefully in a compound fixative. It is a general protein precipitant, and has some slight decalcifying properties.

Fixatives

Choice of a fixative

The choice of a fixative will be governed by the type of investigation required, both immediately and in the future. There would be little point in using Carnoy's fixative because of a primary interest in chromosomes, if a need to demonstrate lipids was likely to arise later. Large pieces of tissue should be fixed in a tolerant fixative, such as formal–saline, which will allow subsequent treatment; smaller pieces can be taken from the mass either before or following formal fixation and given specialized treatment if required. It should also be remembered that museum specimens to which colour is to be restored can only be prepared from formalin-fixed tissues.

Rarely will one fixative be suitable for a variety of methods; for this reason it is convenient to divide them into three main groups: *micro-anatomical*, *cytological* and *histochemical*.

Micro-anatomical fixatives

These are used when it is desired to preserve the anatomy of the tissue, with the correct relationship of tissue layers and large aggregates of cells. It is obvious that fixatives for routine use should be drawn from this group.

Cytological fixatives

Cytological fixatives are used when the preservation of intracellular structures or inclusions is of first importance. Often these elements are preserved at the expense of even penetration, ease of cutting, and the loss of other cell structures.

Histochemical fixatives

When histochemical tests are to be applied, it is essential that the fixative employed produces minimal changes in the element that is to be demonstrated. Whilst the freeze-drying technique is probably almost ideal for this purpose it is far too troublesome and time-consuming for routine work.

While the more common fixatives employed in histochemistry are given under this heading, the fixative used should be that recommended for the specific technique to be employed.

This is not a rigid classification and it should be remembered that fixatives listed under one group may overlap in performance with those in another.

The fixatives given in this chapter are the more common and reliable. Fixatives for special techniques are given under their appropriate headings.

Micro-anatomical fixatives

Routine formalin fixatives

Although formal–saline (10% formalin in 0.9% sodium chloride) has been the routine fixative of choice for many years it has now been largely supplanted by either buffered formalin (Lillie, 1965) or neutral formal–saline. They have the same advantages and are used in the same manner as formal–saline. Since they have a near neutral pH, formalin pigment (acid formaldehyde haematin) is not formed since its occurrence is due to the interaction of formalin solutions, at an acid pH, with haemoglobin or its products; it is seen most commonly in sections of the spleen, liver, bone marrow, and so on. Should this pigment be encountered it is easily removed from sections, before staining, by treatment with picric alcohol or a 1% alcohol solution of sodium hydroxide.

The incorporation of calcium chloride in 10% formalin was designed by Baker (1944) to preserve phospholipids, but the use of calcium acetate has the added advantage of buffering the solution.

Buffered formalin, formal–calcium and neutral formal–saline, because of their tolerance are probably the most useful and most widely used fixatives. Tissue can be left in them for long periods without excessive hardening or damage, and may be sectioned easily after as long a period as one year. Other than a slight decrease in basophilia, and in the reactivity of myelin to Weigert's haematoxylin technique, those tissue elements not preserved are not destroyed, which enables most of them to be demonstrated after further treatment.

Fixation of tissue blocks, not exceeding 5 mm in thickness, is usually complete in 6–12 hours at room temperature. Fixation by formalin, and other chemical fixatives, is influenced by heat and pieces of tissue up to 3 mm in thickness can be fixed in $1\frac{1}{2}$–2 hours at 55 °C but suffer some loss of detail.

Formal–calcium

Formula

Formalin	100 ml
Calcium acetate	20 g
Water	to 1000 ml

Neutral formal–saline

Formula

Formalin	100 ml
Sodium chloride	9 g
Sat. magnesium carbonate	200 ml
Tap water	700 ml

Buffered formalin

Formula

Formalin	100 ml
Acid sodium phosphate monohydrate	4 g
Anhydrous disodium phosphate	6.5 g
Water	to 1000 ml

Buffered formal–sucrose (Holt and Hicks, 1961)

Formula

Formalin	10 ml
Sucrose	7.5 g
M/15 Phosphate buffer (pH 7.4)	to 100 ml

This fixative gives excellent preservation of fine structure, phospholipids and some enzymes. It is recommended for combined cytochemistry and electron microscopical studies. To get the best results it should be used refrigerator cold (4 °C) on fresh tissues.

Electron microscope pictures show well preserved mitochondria, endoplasmic reticulum, etc. after fixation by this method.

Alcoholic formalin

Formula

Formalin	10 ml
70–95% Alcohol	90 ml

If desired, 0.5 g of calcium acetate may be added to ensure neutrality.

Acetic–alcoholic–formalin

Formula

Formalin	5 ml
Glacial acetic acid	5 ml
70% Alcohol	90 ml

Either alcoholic–formalin or acetic–alcoholic–formalin are excellent for glycogen although not ideal as routine fixative. It is said to prevent the solution of carbohydrates before the fixation of the protein component is complete. The addition of acetic acid ensures fixation of the nuclear protein with an improved histological picture. Since both alcohol and formalin are rapidly penetrating agents, this is a reasonably rapid fixative. Tissues up to 5 mm in thickness are fixed in 4 hours.

Buffered glutaraldehyde

Formula

Glutaraldehyde stock 25% solution	16 ml
Phosphate buffer pH 7.4	84 ml

This fixative is discussed on page 31. It will, it should be remembered, give a false PAS positive reaction. The purification of the stock 25% glutaraldehyde is also discussed on page 31.

Formal–sublimate (mercuric chloride–formalin)

Formula

Saturated aqueous mercuric chloride	900 ml
Formalin	100 ml

Despite the disadvantages of causing tissue shrinkage and hardening, formal–sublimate is an excellent micro-anatomical fixative, giving often brilliant staining results with acid dyes. Metachromasia may also be enhanced. It gives less satisfactory results with silver impregnation methods for the central nervous system.

Mercuric chloride containing fixatives give rise to the formation of a black pigment in tissues. The pigment, which is seen to be randomly distributed in tissue sections, may be removed by treatment with iodine as described on page 33.

Heidenhain's Susa

Formula

Mercuric chloride	4.5 g
Sodium chloride	0.5 g
Trichloroacetic acid	2 g
Acetic acid	4 ml
Formalin	20 ml
Distilled water	to 100 ml

This is an excellent fixative for routine biopsy work, allowing brilliant staining with good cytological detail. It is well balanced and gives rapid and even penetration with a minimum of shrinkage. It is, however, an intolerant fixative, and tissues left in it over 24 hours are bleached and excessively hardened. The incorporation of trichloroacetic acid is said to give it slight decalcifying powers, but this can only be relied upon for minute calcium deposits.

Tissue must be transferred direct to 96% absolute alcohol to avoid swelling of connective tissues. Since this solution contains mercuric chloride it must not be kept in a container with a metal cap. Although it has been claimed that tissues fixed in 'Susa' do not contain mercury pigment, this is not universal experience, and the tissues should be treated with iodine to remove it (page 33).

It is doubtful whether 'Susa' has sufficient advantages over formal–sublimate to justify the extra effort involved in making up the solution.

Tissues not exceeding 7–8 mm in thickness are fixed in 12–24 hours. Small pieces, not thicker than 3 mm are fixed in 2–3 hours.

Both of these fixatives are most usefully employed as secondary fixatives (page 45). Care should be taken to observe safety rules in disposing of mercury-containing solutions.

Zenker's fluid

Formula

Mercuric chloride	5 g
Potassium dichromate	2.5 g
Sodium sulphate	1 g
Distilled water	to 100 ml
Add glacial acetic acid immediately before use	5 ml

This solution does not keep after the acetic acid has been added, but without acetic acid (Zenker's stock fluid) it keeps well and has the advantage that either acetic acid or formalin may be added immediately before use (*see below*).

Zenker's fluid is a good routine fixative giving fairly rapid and even penetration. Following its use, tissues must be washed in running water overnight to remove the excess dichromate (page 33), and mercuric chloride pigment must be removed with iodine (page 33).

Fixation is usually complete in 12 hours. Small pieces, not thicker than 3 mm are fixed in 2–3 hours.

Zenker formal (Helly's fluid)

Formula

Mercuric chloride	5 g
Potassium dichromate	2.5 g
Sodium sulphate	1 g
Distilled water	to 100 ml
Add formalin immediately before use	5 ml

This fixative is stock Zenker mixture to which formalin is added instead of acetic acid. It is irrational in that it contains potassium dichromate which is an oxidizing agent, and formaldehyde which is a reducing agent, but it is an excellent micro-anatomical fixative.

It is variously known as Helly's, Spuler's, or Maximow's fluid, although the formalin content and the amount of mercuric chloride and potassium dichromate varies.

As with Zenker–acetic the excess dichromate must be washed out, and mercuric pigment removed with iodine.

It is an excellent fixative for bone marrow and spleen, and is recommended for blood-containing organs in general.

Zenker–formal is slower than Zenker–acetic; fixation is usually complete in 6–24 hours.

Bouin's fluid

Formula

Picric acid, saturated aqueous solution	75 ml
Formalin (40% formaldehyde)	25 ml
Glacial acetic acid	5 ml

This fixative, which keeps well, penetrates rapidly and evenly and causes little shrinkage. Tissue fixed in it gives brilliant staining by the trichrome methods. The excess picric acid, to which the yellow colour of the tissue is due, may be removed from the section by treatment with alcohol or prolonged washing. This is particularly important if basic aniline dyes are to be used, as a precipitate may be formed (Drury and Wallington, 1980).

Bouin's fluid can be used to demonstrate glycogen, but Gendre's fluid is a better picric-acid fixative for this purpose. Owing to the formation of some water-soluble picrates, tissues must be transferred from the fixative direct to alcohol.

Fixation is usually complete in 24 hours, but small pieces not exceeding 2–3 mm in thickness are fixed in 2–3 hours.

Gendre's fluid

Formula

Picric acid, saturated solution in 95% alcohol	80 ml
Formalin (40% formaldehyde)	15 ml
Glacial acetic acid	5 ml

This fluid is said to give good fixation of glycogen, after 3–4 hours at room temperature; however, see the discussion on page 216.

Rossman's fluid

Formula

Formalin (neutralized)	10 ml
Absolute ethyl alcohol saturated with picric acid (approximately 8.5–9%)	90 ml

It will be seen that this is similar to Gendre's fluid but without the acetic acid. This fixative has also been recommended for carbohydrate fixation.

Cytological fixatives

For convenience, this group of fixatives is subdivided into (a) nuclear, and (b) cytoplasmic.

Nuclear fixatives

Carnoy's fluid

Formula

Absolute alcohol	60 ml
Chloroform	30 ml
Glacial acetic acid	10 ml

Carnoy's fluid penetrates very rapidly, and gives excellent nuclear fixation with preservation of Nissl substance and glycogen. This has been recommended by many workers for the fixation of carbohydrates. It causes considerable shrinkage, and destroys or dissolves most cytoplasmic elements.

Being a rapid fixative it is sometimes used when a diagnosis is urgently required.

Many lipids are also dissolved by Carnoy's fixative and this property may be used to advantage in the preparation of paraffin-wax sections of certain lipid rich tissues such as lipomas. Most fat will in any case be lost from these tissues during processing, so that removal of this material by treatment with Carnoy's fixative following conventional fixation will help penetration of processing fluids.

Fixation is usually complete in 1–2 hours; small pieces 2–3 mm in thickness are fixed in 15 minutes.

Clarke's fluid

Formula

Absolute alcohol	75 ml
Glacial acetic acid	25 ml

This fixative penetrates rapidly and gives good nuclear fixation and reasonably good preservation of cytoplasmic elements. It is excellent for smears or coverslip preparations of cell cultures for general fixation or chromosome analyses.

Sanfelice's fluid

Formula

Solution A
Formalin	128 ml
Acetic acid	16 ml

Solution B
1% Chromic acid

Mix 9 ml solution A with 16 ml solution B immediately before use.

The fixative penetrates small pieces of tissue (2–3 ml thick) in approximately 12 hours giving good nuclear detail. It is especially useful in the demonstration of mitotic figures and chromosomes. Tissues should be washed well in running water before processing.

Newcomer's fluid

Formula

Isopropanol	60 ml
Propionic acid	30 ml
Petroleum ether	10 ml
Acetone	10 ml
Dioxane	10 ml

This fixative, which penetrates rapidly, was devised for the fixation of chromosomes, and preserves the chromatin better than Carnoy's fluid, giving an improved Feulgen reaction. It was recommended by Saunders (1964) for the fixation and preservation of mucopolysaccharides.

Fixation is complete in 12–18 hours; small pieces of tissue not exceeding 3 mm in thickness are fixed in 2–3 hours.

Flemming's fluid

Formula

1% Aqueous chromic acid	15 ml
2% Aqueous osmium tetroxide	4 ml
Glacial acetic acid	1 ml

Flemming's fluid, originally a nuclear fixative, is rarely used as such because of its poor and uneven penetration. For chromosomes, the full 1 ml of acetic acid is used, but when this is omitted, the fluid is used as a cytoplasmic fixative. Unlike other fixatives the bulk need only be five to ten times that of the tissue. Following fixation tissue should be washed overnight.

In common with all the osmium tetroxide fixatives, pieces of tissue must be small (not more than 2 mm in thickness), when fixation will be complete in 12 hours.

Although introduced in the last century as a nuclear fixative, because of its uneven penetration and the blackening of the outer tissue layers by the osmium tetroxide, Flemming's fluid is rarely used as such today. The presence of acetic acid does make the fixative suitable for chromosomes. However, if the acetic acid is omitted and 0.75% sodium chloride added instead it becomes a useful cytoplasmic fixative (Baker, 1966). Drury and Wallington (1980) draw attention to the poor nuclear staining with alum haematoxylins.

In common with all osmium tetroxide fixatives, pieces of tissue must be small (<2 mm thick), when fixation will be complete in 12 hours. It must be remembered that lipids will be blackened.

Cytoplasmic fixatives

Champy's fluid

Formula

3% Potassium dichromate	7 ml
1% Chromic acid	7 ml
2% Osmium tetroxide	4 ml

This fixative does not keep and should be prepared freshly from stock solutions. It penetrates poorly and unevenly, only thin pieces of tissue should be treated.

Champy's fluid preserves mitochondria, fat, yolk and lipids, and gives results similar to those of Flemming's fluid without acetic acid, although Champy's fluid is preferred for mitochondria.

Tissue must be washed overnight after fixation which, for pieces of tissue not thicker than 2 mm will be complete in 12 hours.

Régaud's fluid

Formula

3% Potassium dichromate	80 ml
Formalin (40% formaldehyde)	20 ml

Régaud's fluid does not keep, and the solutions should only be mixed immediately before use. It penetrates evenly and fairly rapidly, but has a tendency to overharden tissue. It may be used as a routine fixative, but is particularly good for mitochondria if followed by 4–8 days' chromation in 3% potassium dichromate. Chromaffin tissue is well demonstrated by the same method, but fluids may be improved for this purpose by the addition of 5% acetic acid.

Fixation is usually complete in 24 hours, small pieces not more than 3–4 mm in thickness are fixed in 4–6 hours.

No attempt should be made to mix potassium dichromate crystals with formalin solutions as a violent oxidative reaction will occur.

Formal–saline and formal–calcium

Fixation in formal–saline, followed by post-chromatization (page 45) gives good cytoplasmic fixation in most instances, with improved preservation of the micro-anatomical features of the tissue.

Zenker–formal (Helly's fluid)

Like formal–saline it can be used with good results, both as a cytoplasmic fixative and a micro-anatomical fixative, particularly for bone marrow and the blood-forming organs.

Schaudinn's fluid

Formula

Mercuric chloride, saturated aqueous solution	2 parts
Absolute alcohol	1 part

This fixative has been popular for many years as a cytoplasmic fixative for wet smears. It is not recommended for tissue, being harsh in action and causing excessive shrinkage; probably due to the time of exposure needed for penetration.

Tissue or smears need treatment with iodine–alcohol and sodium thiosulphate to remove mercury deposit (page 33).

Wet smears are well fixed in 10–20 minutes and unless too thick they rarely become subsequently detached from the slide.

Ether/alcohol

Formula

70% Alcohol   1 part
Di-ethyl ether   1 part

This is a rapid fixative for cytological smears, although very hazardous due to the highly flammable nature of the ether. Great care should be taken in its use.

Spray fixatives

There are many alcohol-based fixatives commercially available in aerosol spray cans. They are intended for fixing cell smears on slides and usually contain a water-soluble wax which acts as a barrier against contamination by dust, etc.

Histochemical fixatives

A good histochemical fixative should:

(1) preserve the constituent to be demonstrated, preferably preserving its morphological relationships;
(2) bind or otherwise preserve the specific tissue constituent, without affecting the reactive groups to be used in its visualization;
(3) not affect the reagent to be used in the process of visualization; for example, glutaraldehyde fixation leaves the tissue proteins so fixed with a coating of free reactive aldehyde groups which give a positive Schiff or PAS reaction.

For the majority of histochemical methods it is best to use cryostat cut sections of rapidly frozen tissue (*see* page 104), or sections of frozen dried tissue. Such sections may be used unfixed or they may be fixed by a vapour fixative.

Certain broad generalizations may be made. For example, lysosomes, which contain many hydrolytic enzymes, are damaged during the freeze/thaw procedures involved in the production of cold sections. This leads to a loss of localization of the enzymes which may be prevented, to a degree, by the use of carefully controlled fixation. However, many oxidative enzymes are lost during fixation. Acrolein, in particular, has been recommended for hydrolases (Saito and Keino, 1976) and low concentrations of glutaraldehyde for certain oxidases (Asano *et al.*, 1976).

Formal–saline

As formalin is the most common fixative, it is likely that much of the material on which histochemical methods are to be applied will have been so fixed. Provided it is buffered to prevent the formation of formalin pigment, and the tissue is well washed to remove the excess fixative, many histochemical techniques are applicable.

Cold acetone

Immersion in acetone at 0–4 °C is widely used for the fixation of tissues in which it is intended to study enzymes, particularly the phosphatases.

Absolute alcohol

Fixation of sections cut from freeze-dried material may be effected by immersion in absolute alcohol for 24 hours.

It is occasionally recommended as a basic fixative, but in most histochemical techniques formalin can be used as an alternative with a consequent improvement in micro-anatomical and cytological preservation.

Post chroming and secondary fixation

Post chroming is the treatment of tissues with 3% potassium dichromate following normal fixation. Post chroming may be carried out either before processing, when the tissue should be left for 6–8 days in dichromate solution, or after processing, when sections, before staining, are immersed in dichromate solution for 12–24 hours, followed in each case by washing well in running water.

This technique is said to mordant tissues, giving improved preservation and aiding the demonstration of mitochondria and myelin.

Secondary fixation requires the sequential application of two fixatives, the rationale being that the primary fixative, whilst not being totally effective, leaves the tissue more able to withstand the action of a second, harsher fixative, bringing benefits in more brilliant staining. Wallington (1955) has investigated the effects of secondary fixation in protein precipitants, such as mercury-containing fixatives, on tissue initially fixed in formal–saline.

Post fixation is a term that has been applied to the secondary fixation of lipid-rich tissues following processing through clearing agents. The term is more properly applied to the fixation of freeze-dried tissue using the vapour phase of the fixative.

Vapour fixation

Vapour fixatives may be used to fix cryostat-cut sections of fresh tissue and sections or blocks of frozen dried tissue. Formaldehyde vapour, generated from heated paraformaldehyde, is of very high reactivity. Cryostat sections, mounted on slides may be placed in a closed vessel above the paraformaldehyde and the vessel placed in an oven at 60–70 °C for 2 hours. Using this method, we have produced sections showing excellent localization of glycogen with very good morphological detail.

Although this is a simple technique, often giving superior localization and morphology, it has not been widely used except for demonstrating those biogenic amines which exhibit formaldehyde induced fluorescence. Briefly it may be stated that condensation reactions between formaldehyde and arylethylamines lead to the formation of fluorescent quinonoids, iso-quinolines and β-carbolines. In theory, most aldehydes should behave in a similar manner. This subject is considered more fully in Chapter 26.

Amongst fixatives which have been used for vapour fixation, usually at a temperature of from 60–80 °C, are:

Formaldehyde
Glutaraldehyde
Acrolein

Osmium tetroxide
Diacetyl
Acetic acid
Glyoxylic acid
Glyoxal
Acetaldehyde (Pearse, 1980).

Freeze-drying

The preservation of tissues by freeze-drying is often discussed as a method of fixation, but it is, correctly, an alternative to fixation. It is a method of initially preserving tissue with little alteration in cell structure or chemical composition which permits embedding in wax without the normal intermediate stages of dehydration by alcohols and clearing. The resultant sections may be examined unfixed in an inert medium, by micro-incineration or after extraction with buffered solutions; or they may be fixed and normal histochemical or histological techniques applied.

The technique of freeze-drying consists of the following three stages:

(1) initial rapid freezing, known as 'quenching';
(2) drying of the frozen tissue;
(3) embedding, sectioning and mounting.

Quenching

Small pieces of tissue, not more than 1 mm in thickness, are placed on a thin strip of folded aluminium foil or copper foil and plunged into isopentane cooled to a temperature of -160 to $-180\,°C$ with liquid nitrogen; cooling should be continued until the isopentane becomes more viscous. The frozen tissue is then removed from the foil, and the isopentane poured off.

It is essential that tissues be absolutely fresh so that the initial rapid freezing not only inhibits autolysis and putrefaction, but also prevents any diffusion of substances within the cells. The low temperature used for the initial freezing is important, for unless the whole of the tissue is frozen rapidly large ice crystals are formed which will disrupt cell structure. Pieces of tissue more than 1 mm in thickness will probably show this disruption artefact at the centre, and for this reason are to be avoided.

Drying

The frozen tissue is transferred quickly to the drying apparatus, where a high vacuum is established and the ice in the tissue transferred by sublimation to a vapour trap. The rate of drying depends on the following three factors:

(1) temperature,
(2) vacuum pressure,
(3) distance of tissue from vapour trap.

Temperature

The higher the temperature at which the tissue is maintained the more rapid is the drying: for example, raising the temperature from -60 to $-40\,°C$ increases the rate of evaporation tenfold: to prevent the formation of ice crystals the temperature should theoretically be maintained below the eutectic point of the tissue (about $-55\,°C$); and noticeable deterioration of the tissue occurs if it is allowed to rise to $-20\,°C$. In practice, satisfactory results are combined with reasonable speed of drying if the temperature is maintained between -30 and $-40\,°C$.

Vacuum pressure and the distance of tissue from vapour trap

In the process of drying, water molecules sublime from the frozen tissue to form water vapour and this condenses on a vapour trap maintained at a temperature below that of the tissue; for example, liquid nitrogen $(-185\,°C)$ or an acetone–CO_2 mixture $(-70\,°C)$. This transfer of water molecules is hindered by the presence of air, or by bends or constrictions obstructing the flow of vapour: if the pressure is kept below 10^{-3} mmHg, and the vapour trap is within 5 cm of the tissue, molecules of water leaving the tissue will cross directly to the vapour trap and condense upon it, and the maximum rate of drying will be achieved. If the pressure is higher the distance must be reduced (and vice versa) to achieve the same rate of drying, for example, with a vacuum of 5×10^{-5} mm the vapour trap may be up to 30 cm distant.

The vapour trap may be a 'cold finger' type, where a small tube containing liquid nitrogen is inserted into the drying tube so that it is within 5 cm of the tissue; on the surface of this 'cold finger' the sublimed water condenses as ice, and when drying is completed the cold finger is removed.

A phosphorus pentoxide (P_2O_5) moisture trap must be placed in the pipeline close to the pump. This trap in addition to preventing backstreaming of water vapour from the pump is also used at the end of the drying operation to absorb re-vaporized ice from the walls of the drying tube while the tube is brought up to room temperature prior to the removal of the specimen. By this means the condensate is prevented from rehydrating the specimen.

There are several examples of commercially produced apparatus available for freeze-drying tissues. Among the first of these purpose-made freeze-driers was that designed by Edwards High Vacuum in conjunction with Professor A. G. E. Pearse. Temperature control depends on a thermo-electric device exploiting the Peltier effect (*see* Chapter 5). Although early models were unable to reach temperatures much below about $-45\,°C$, the newest model, the EPTD4, is said to reach $-60\,°C$.

Embedding, sectioning, mounting, fixation and storage

Embedding

The embedding of the tissue in wax may be carried out in one of two ways.

(1) The dried tissue may be transferred quickly to a vacuum embedding oven containing molten wax, with a vacuum of routine pressure. The tissue on sinking to the bottom of the wax bath will be impregnated with wax, a period of only 5–10 minutes being required.

(2) The embedding media, thoroughly degassed, may be placed at the bottom of the drying tube prior to the drying operation. When drying is complete the tube is allowed to reach room temperature and then heated slowly until the wax just melts: the dried tissue sinks and is impregnated.

While the first method will give satisfactory results, the second is obviously the better technique, since at no time is there a possibility of absorption of moisture from the air.

The embedding medium may be paraffin wax, or one of the water-soluble waxes, the latter being indicated for the demonstration or investigation of fats or fatty compounds.

Sectioning

This is generally carried out on a standard microtome, sections being cut slightly thicker than usual to facilitate handling.

The floating out of sections presents difficulties, since the use of warm water would result in disintegration. Sections may be directly affixed to warm albuminized slides (page 98) by finger pressure or light blotting.

If fixation will not interfere with the technique to be employed, sections may be floated on warm formal–saline or formal–calcium; this method may be used with success for the demonstration of fats and fatty substances in tissues embedded in water-soluble wax.

Mounting

Unfixed, unstained sections can be mounted for microscopic examination in an inert medium such as liquid paraffin which dissolves the paraffin wax and the preparations are suitable for examination by phase-contrast, fluorescent, polarized light, or ultraviolet light microscopy. For the examination of lipids by polarized light, thick Carbowax-embedded sections are taken quickly through water and mounted in Karo corn syrup.

Fixation

Fixation of sections is easily effected, either by floating on formalin, as already described, or by immersion of the mounted sections in 80% alcohol or acetone for 12–24 hours after removal of the wax.

Storage

Embedded blocks of tissue and sections of freeze-dried material must *not* be stored in the conventional manner. They may be kept in a desiccator over calcium chloride in a cold room to avoid the absorption of moisture from the air (with resultant dissolution of the tissue). Sections are best kept by fixation in alcohol, or formalin, but if such solutions must be avoided, then fixation may be effected by the vapour of osmium tetroxide, or formaldehyde, with consequent denaturing of proteins.

For a more complete discussion on the theory and practice of freeze-drying, the appropriate chapter in *Histochemistry, Theoretical and Applied*, by Everson Pearse (1980) is recommended.

Freeze substitution

Simpson (1941) described a freeze substitution technique as an inexpensive alternative to freeze-drying. While in general the results are not always as good as with the latter it does offer a method which can be employed in a routine laboratory without the purchase of expensive equipment.

This method is based on the quenching of the tissue to

(1) inhibit autolysis and putrefaction;
(2) prevent diffusion and dissolution of the substances within the tissues;
(3) prevent the formation of large ice crystals in the quenched tissues.

This is done at low temperatures in liquid dehydrating agents which are also fixatives. It has been shown that many substances which are soluble in these agents at room temperature are insoluble, and thus preserved, at the low temperatures used.

Tissues are quenched, as for freeze-drying, in either isopentane in liquid nitrogen ($-160\,^{\circ}$C) or in acetone containing, and surrounded by, dry ice. They are then transferred to Rossman's fluid or into 1% osmium tetroxide in acetone. These are kept at -60 to $-70\,^{\circ}$C in a low-temperature freezer for 1–6 days. The tissues are then allowed to reach room temperature slowly when they are processed by the normal paraffin-embedding technique.

The method has proved particularly successful in these laboratories for the study of tissue damage inflicted by the use of a cryoprobe during routine surgical procedures (Whittaker, 1978). Tissues quenched in isopentane cooled by liquid nitrogen were successfully substituted with acetone containing 2% OsO_4, ethanol with 5% glutaraldehyde and methyl cellosolve containing 5% glutaraldehyde. The substitution is temperature dependent, requiring 12 days at $-70\,^{\circ}$C, 7 days at $-50\,^{\circ}$C or three periods of 10 minutes each at $-13\,^{\circ}$C. In the above experiments, chloroform was used as an intermediate solvent prior to paraffin-wax embedding.

References

ASANO, M., KURONO, C., WAKABAYASHI, T. and KIMURA, H. (1976). Stabilization of configurational states and enzyme activities in sub-cellular fractions after fixation with extremely low concentrations of glutaraldehyde. Histochem. J., 8, 113–120

BAHR, G. F. (1954). Osmium tetroxide and ruthenium tetroxide and their reactions with biologically important substances. Exp. Cell Res., 7, 457–479

BAKER J. R. (1944). Structure and chemical composition of the Golgi element. Quart. J. Micr. Sci., 85, 1–71

BAKER, J. R. (1950). Cytological Technique. 3rd Ed. Methuen, London, p. 46

BAKER, J. R. (1956). Improvements in the Sudan Black technique. Quart. J. Micr. Sci., 97, 621–623

BOSMAN, F. T., LINDEMAN, J., KUIPER, G., VAN DER WAAL, A. and KREUNIG, J. (1977). The influence of fixation on immunoperoxidase staining of plasma cells in paraffin sections of intestinal biopsy specimens. Histochemistry, 53, 57–62

BOWES, J. H. (1963). A fundamental study of the mechanism of deterioration of leather fibres. Br. Leather Manuf. Res. Assoc. Report.

BOWES, J. A. and CATOR, C. W. (1967). The reaction of glutaraldehyde with proteins and other biological materials. J. R. Micr. Soc., 85, 193–200

CHAMBERS, R. W., BOWLING, M. C. and GRIMLEY, P. M. (1968). Glutaraldehyde fixation in routine histopathology. Arch. Pathol., 85, 18–30

DALLAM, R. D. (1957). Determination of protein and lipid lost during osmic acid fixation of tissues and cellular particulates. J. Histochem. Cytochem., 5, 178–181

DRURY, R. A. B. and WALLINGTON, E. A. (1980). Carleton's Histological Technique. 5th Ed. Oxford University Press, Oxford

HAKE, T. (1965). Studies on the reactions of OsO_4 and $KMnO_4$ with amino acids, peptides and proteins. Lab. Invest., 14, 1208–1212

HOLT, S. J. and HICKS, R. M. (1961). Studies on formalin fixation for electron microscopy and cytochemical staining purposes. J. Biophys. Biochem. Cytol., 11, 31–45

HOPWOOD, D. (1967). Some aspects of fixation with glutaraldehyde. J. Anat., 101, 83–92

HOPWOOD, D. (1968a). Fixatives and fixation: a review. Histochem. J., 1, 323–360

HOPWOOD, D. (1968b). Some aspects of fixation by glutaraldehyde and formaldehyde. J. Anat., 103, 581

HOROBIN, R. W. (1982). Histochemistry. Butterworths, London

KORN, E. D. (1966). Synthesis of bis(methyl 9,10-dihydroxystearate osmate) from methyl oleate and osmium tetroxide under conditions used for fixation of biological material. *Biochim. Biophys. Acta*, **116**, 317–324

LENARD, J. and SINGER, S. J. (1968). Alteration of the conformation of proteins in red blood cell membranes and in solution by fixatives used in electron microscopy. *J. Cell Biol.*, **37**, 117–121

LILLIE, R. D. (1965). *Histopathologic Technic and Practical Histochemistry.* 3rd Ed. Blakiston, New York

PEARSE, A. G. E. (1980). *Histochemistry, Theoretical and Applied.* Vol. 1. Churchill-Livingstone, London

SABATINI, D. D., BENSCH, K. and BARNETT, R. J. (1963). Cytochemistry and electron microscopy. The preservation of cellular ultrastructure and enzymatic activity by aldehyde fixation. *J. Cell Biol.*, **17**, 19–58.

SAITO, T. and KEINO, H. (1976). Acrolein as a fixative for enzyme cytochemistry. *J. Histochem. Cytochem.*, **24**, 1258–1269

SAUNDERS, A. M. (1964). Histochemical identification of acid mucopolysaccharides with acridine orange. *J. Histochem. Cytochem.*, **12**, 164–170

SIMPSON, W. L. (1941). Experimental analysis of Altman's technique of freeze drying. *Anat. Rec.*, **80**, 329–345.

WALLINGTON, E. A. (1955). Secondary fixation as a routine procedure. *J. Med. Lab. Technol.*, **13**, 53–67

WHITTAKER, D. K. (1978). Electron microscopy of ice crystals formed during cryosurgery. Relationship to duration of freeze. *Cryobiology*, **15**, 603–607

4
Processing

For microscopic examination, tissue specimens must be thin enough to permit the passage of transmitted light and, for detailed morphological examination, no more than one cell in thickness. To achieve this end, tissue slices need to be approximately 4–6 µm in thickness, although for highly cellular tissues, such as lymph node, 2–3 µm may be more appropriate and when examining larger cells and processes, such as those of the nervous system, 10–20 µm. This is facilitated by infiltrating and embedding the tissue in a support medium. Although there is no perfect medium for these purposes, paraffin wax has proved the most universally popular. Other media, which have particular advantages are detailed below. In the case of frozen sections, rigidity is given to the tissue by freezing it, thus eliminating the need for specialized processing techniques.

Paraffin-wax embedding

As paraffin wax is immiscible with water, tissues fixed in aqueous fixatives must be treated to remove the water. This process of dehydration is almost invariably achieved using alcohol which is itself also immiscible with paraffin wax. Paraffin-wax embedding, therefore, employs three stages:

(1) dehydration,
(2) clearing, that is, the replacement of the dehydrating fluid with a solution miscible with paraffin wax,
(3) infiltration with molten paraffin wax.

The tissue is finally cast into a block of solidified wax. Most tissues are easily sectioned following this treatment and it is the best way of storing tissue for morphological examination.

Water-soluble waxes

These waxes offer the advantage of eliminating the necessity for dehydration and clearing, thus avoiding deleterious effects of these fluids, especially the shrinkage that may be induced. Tissue may be transferred directly from aqueous fixatives to molten wax. However, there are considerable difficulties in handling the sections as they may only be 'floated out' on water with great difficulty. The blocks themselves call for carefully controlled storage in a dry atmosphere.

Celloidin (low viscosity nitrocellulose; LVN)

Delicate tissues, such as brain, and those of particularly hard consistency, such as bone, are more easily cut if the embedding medium has a certain amount of resilience. Celloidin has a rubbery consistency allowing a continuous shearing type of cutting which is beneficial for this purpose. Infiltration and embedding of tissues is achieved simply by dehydration followed by impregnation with celloidin in solution. The solvent is allowed to evaporate, producing a block of embedded tissue, avoiding completely the damaging effects of heat. The results achieved, particularly where the relationship of different tissues to one another are important (such as the eye) can be spectacular. However, the method demands more exhaustive technical expertise.

Double embedding

This method seeks to achieve the advantages of both paraffin wax and celloidin embedding. Tissue is infiltrated with celloidin and subsequently embedded in a block of paraffin wax. The procedure is more tedious than paraffin-wax embedding, but does provide added support to tissues and enables ribbons of sections to be cut more easily than celloidin alone.

Synthetic resins

Used initially for the production of ultrathin sections for electron microscopy, resin embedding has been applied with advantage to light microscopy. The extra hardness provided by various resins permits sections only 0.5–2.0 μm to be prepared. Generally, a glass knife has to be used to achieve this objective. Broadly it may be assumed that tissue is dehydrated, infiltrated with resin in monomeric form which is subsequently polymerized, either chemically or physically, to give a hard, glass clear block. Both methacrylates and epoxy resins have been used. Resin embedding is also used for embedding very hard tissues, such as undecalcified bone and teeth which are to be cut with a diamond impregnated disc and ground to a suitable thickness, or cut on a specially designed microtome at 10 μm.

Gelatin

Fragments of friable tissue to be cut on the freezing microtome or cryostat may be first embedded in gelatin. Gough and Wentworth (1949; 1960) developed a method of producing sections from whole organs, such as lung, embedded in gelatin. This method is enjoying a resurgence in popularity in the study of breasts, for example.

Freeze-drying and freeze substitution

These methods, detailed in the previous chapter, may also be considered methods of tissue processing.

Whilst each of these methods requires a separate technique, there are certain stages which are common to all, and these will be dealt with in detail only in the first technique in which they occur.

Specimen handling

Having care of a biopsy or other tissue specimen removed from a patient is a major responsibility. Not only will the patient have undergone trauma to provide the specimen but a mistake may lead to a major operation on the wrong patient, or an incorrect diagnosis which could eventually lead to the death of a patient. Correct labelling and identification are therefore first essentials of any technique of processing. It is impossible to over-emphasize the amount of care that should be given to:

(1) a foolproof system of labelling;
(2) ensuring that the correct label remains with the specimen throughout; and
(3) constant vigilance.

Ordinary ink should never be used as this is usually soluble in the reagents used in processing. Graphite pencil has proved to be most satisfactory. It should be noted that any label accompanying tissue to be treated with osmium tetroxide will be blackened. In such cases, labels should be fixed to the outside of the osmium container.

It is recommended that on receipt in the laboratory, details of the patient and specimen (including full name, date of birth, hospital record number, hospital, ward, surgeon and some description of the tissue) should be entered into a log-book and the specimen assigned a unique laboratory number. Basically it is desirable that this number identifies the specimen and the year and enables it to be differentiated from specimens logged in separate pathology departments. It is also advantageous to be able to identify each sample taken from the specimen by including an additional number as a suffix. For example, S123/83.2 would indicate a surgical specimen (S), the 123rd specimen received in 1983 (83), and the second block from that specimen.

Where specimens are to be processed in individual capsules, this number may be written on a small slip of card which accompanies the tissue right through processing and is finally attached to the solidified wax block. It is important that only one specimen and its label is handled at one time.

The introduction of the Tissue-Tek II (Miles Scientific, Stoke Poges, Bucks., England) processing cassettes has reduced the margin for error and simplified the processing system. Originally, these cassettes consisted of a small perforated plastic container with a snap-on stainless steel lid. They may now be purchased in a variety of sizes and colours and with an integral plastic lid. The edges of the cassette are roughened enabling them to be marked in pencil with the identification number. As the cassettes form a part of the final wax block, the number stays with the specimen from the time it is first put in. Automatic embossing machines which produce serial numbers on demand are presently becoming available. These systems, and similar ones introduced by other manufacturers, bring further benefits in specimen handling as identified below.

Factors affecting processing

Specimen size

To be effective, processing fluids have to impregnate the tissue. Obviously, the thicker the specimen, the longer will impregnation take. Ideally, tissue slices, or biopsy fragments should be no thicker than 3–4 mm. This will permit satisfactory processing overnight on automatic tissue processors, or in two working days if processed manually. Where thicker slices are unavoidable, the processing schedule has to be prolonged accordingly.

Agitation

The greater the surface area of the tissue in contact with the processing fluid, the more effective the fluid interchange. It therefore follows that the speed of processing is seriously impeded if tissue is allowed to sit on the bottom of a container. With manual processing the sample must be suspended in the fluid, either on a bed of cotton wool or gauze.

Agitation is a much more effective way of ensuring interchange between the saturated fluids coming out of tissue and the virgin fluid replacing it. Commercial tissue processors invariably incorporate some form of automatic agitation, either by vertical or rotary movement of the specimen containers, or by drawing and refilling the containers. Over-enthusiastic agitation carries an inherent danger of damaging friable tissues.

Heat

Heat undoubtedly increases the rate of penetration and exchange of processing fluids. Unfortunately it also hardens tissue, increases brittleness and causes shrinkage. The latest closed tissue processors enable heat to be applied at all stages, but this facility should be used with caution as our experience shows it may also interfere with subsequent staining.

Viscosity

Although this factor does not apply to dehydration, certain clearing fluids, such as cedar wood oil, and molten wax are of high viscosity and require longer immersion times to achieve impregnation. Although heating reduces viscosity, it should be avoided when using cedar wood oil (as this causes tissue hardening, thus negating the very reason for using cedar wood oil) and kept to a minimum for paraffin wax for similar reasons and to avoid denaturing the wax.

Vacuum

The use of reduced pressure to assist infiltration of molten paraffin wax has been advocated for over 100 years. It is often stated that the use of vacuum infiltration can reduce the time necessary for impregnation by one-half. This is obviously desirable, as there can be no doubt that heat hardens tissue. Reduced pressure helps remove trapped air from tissues, especially important in the treatment of lung, and has also been stated to assist in the removal of clearing agents because of increased volatility. Brain (1970) has cast doubts on these assumptions. Modern automatic closed-tissue processors provide the facility of reduced pressure for each of the processing steps, but the advantages of such procedures remain to be proven.

Ultrasonics

The use of ultrasonics has been suggested as a means of reducing the time necessary for tissue processing (Gagnon and Katyk, 1959; 1960). This application has not received widespread support and should be adopted with great caution, as it may be a source of artefact and has to be carefully controlled for heat production.

Paraffin-wax processing and embedding

Since most of the tissue fixatives employed are in aqueous solution, the water has to be removed in order to embed the tissue in paraffin wax. This is generally achieved by immersion in increasing strengths of ethyl alcohol (ethanol), and is known as dehydration. Since alcohol and wax are not miscible, the alcohol must be replaced by a wax solvent, and since the majority of wax solvents have the effect of raising the refractive index of tissue, which makes them appear clear, this stage has become known as clearing. Finally, there is the impregnation of the tissue with wax, and its casting into a solid block.

Routine paraffin-wax embedding can, therefore, be conveniently discussed under the following five headings:

(1) fixation,
(2) dehydration,
(3) clearing,
(4) impregnation,
(5) embedding or 'blocking'.

Fixation has been dealt with in the previous chapter.

Dehydration

The concentration of alcohol in the first bath depends on the fixation, size and type of tissue to be dehydrated. After fixation in aqueous solutions delicate tissue needs to be dehydrated slowly, starting in 50% ethyl alcohol, whereas most tissue specimens may be put into 70% alcohol. Tissue immersed in too great a concentration of alcohol after an aqueous fixative will usually show a high degree of shrinkage, due to the too rapid removal of the water; an exception is made in the case of Heidenhain's Susa, which must be followed directly by 96% alcohol. Tissue from alcoholic fixatives such as Carnoy's fluid, may be placed in higher grade alcohols or even in absolute alcohol, but it should be remembered in these instances that several changes are needed to remove acids.

The minimum duration of treatment in graded alcohols will depend on the size and type of tissue, but it can be accepted that long periods in dilute alcohol will not harm tissue; indeed, tissues may be stored in 70% alcohol after fixation in intolerant fixatives such as those containing mercuric chloride. Giant sections of whole organs are best dehydrated successively in 50, 70, 96 and 100% alcohol for 24–48 hours in each, depending on their thickness, using three changes of each strength. The same series of dilutions may be used for delicate tissue, or for cytological research, with a reduction in time to 2–4 hours in each, according to their size. For routine biopsy specimens and post-mortem tissue of not more than 7 mm in thickness, 70%, 90% and absolute alcohol (three changes, for 1–2 hours each) are sufficient to give reasonable results compatible with urgency (*see* page 65).

The use of copper sulphate in final alcohols

This is not uncommon in some parts of the world. A layer of anhydrous copper sulphate, $\frac{1}{4}$–$\frac{1}{2}$ inch deep, is placed at the bottom of a dehydrating bottle or beaker and is covered with two or three filter papers of an appropriate size to prevent staining of the tissue.

Anhydrous copper sulphate, which is white, removes water from the alcohol as it, in turn, removes it from the tissue. This action not only speeds the process of dehydration of the tissue, but also prolongs the life of the alcohol. The change of colour of the copper sulphate from white to blue indicates that the alcohol and copper sulphate should be changed. In the interests of economy this alcohol can be used with fresh anhydrous copper sulphate for the first and second absolute alcohol baths, but the alcohol of the final bath should be renewed as soon as a trace of blue shows in the copper sulphate.

Substitutes for absolute alcohol

Cheaper substitutes for absolute alcohol are available, such as 74° OP* spirit (which is about 99% alcohol) and isopropyl alcohol can be used in conjunction with copper sulphate. Such a substitute for alcohol should not be used to dissolve stains or reagents until they have been tested for each use by control with pure absolute alcohol. There is a school of thought that isopropyl alcohol impairs successful eosin staining.

Dioxane (diethyl dioxide), previously included because of its compatibility with water, alcohol, hydrocarbons and paraffins should not be used because of its proven toxicity.

Clearing

There are many reagents suitable for the intermediate step of clearing. Historically these have included chloroform, benzene, xylene, toluene and cedar wood oil. Benzene, because of its toxicity, and cedar wood oil, because of its viscosity are less commonly used nowadays. Although chloroform has been implicated as a carcinogen, it is still a popular clearing agent in many countries. Several commercial, so-called xylene substitutes have been introduced in recent years, including CNP30 and Inhibisol. More recently, natural food oil derivatives have been introduced bringing the benefits of nil toxicity and easy disposal. They are as yet expensive but prove perfectly satisfactory in use.

Chloroform

Chloroform is probably the commonest reagent in routine use by manual methods, because of its tolerance: tissues may be left in it overnight without rendering them unduly brittle—an advantage over xylene and toluene. A further advantage is that it is not flammable. It has the disadvantage of not affecting the refractive index of the tissue, and the end-point of clearing cannot easily be determined; the tissue must therefore be

---

* The purchase and use of absolute ethyl alcohol is subject to restrictions for customs and excise purposes: 74° OP spirit (Absolute Industrial Methylated Spirit) is not subject to these restrictions.

Proof spirit is legally defined as 'That which, at the temperature of 51°F weighs exactly twelve-thirteenth parts of an equal volume of distilled water'. At 60°F it has a specific gravity of 0.9198 and contains 57.1% v/v, or 49.2% w/w of ethyl alcohol. Spirits are described as so many degrees over-proof (OP) or under-proof (UP). Proof spirit is the standard and is referred to as 100°. A spirit stated as 70° would therefore be 30° UP (100−70°). A spirit stated simply as 160° would be 60° OP, which means that 100 volumes of this would contain as much ethyl alcohol as 166 volumes of proof spirit.

As proof spirit (100°) contains approximately 57% ethyl alcohol, 74° OP (174°) would contain

$$\frac{57 \times 174}{100}\% \text{ ethyl alcohol} = \text{approx. } 99\%$$

From *An Introduction to Medical Laboratory Technology* (1976). 5th Ed. Butterworths, London.

immersed for a rather longer period than is actually necessary to ensure complete penetration and replacement of the alcohol.

Xylene and toluene

Xylene and toluene are fairly rapid in action, small pieces of tissue being cleared in $\frac{1}{2}$–1 hour, and biopsy specimens of 5 mm thickness in 2–4 hours. They possess the advantage that the tissue becomes clearer as the alcohol is replaced, owing to the difference in the refractive index. It is then possible to determine the end-point with some accuracy and to avoid over-exposure of the tissue to the hardening effects of these reagents. Both are flammable and there is some evidence of side effects from vapour inhalation.

CNP30 and Inhibisol*

These industrial cleaning agents have been employed for histological purposes. Although they are claimed to be less toxic than xylene, toluene and chloroform, they are unfortunately more volatile resulting in a higher atmospheric concentration. Some workers find the vapours more uncomfortable than xylene. The use of these reagents has been investigated by Maxwell (1978) whose results should be read in conjunction with the comments by Reid and Young (1981).

Food oil derivatives

These are a recent innovation. Citrus essence is added to give a pleasant odour to these substances which have been graded as GRAS (Generally Regarded As Safe) by the American Federal Drug Administration. Although personal experience has shown them to be satisfactory clearing agents, recent adverse comments suggest that they may interfere with the demonstration of copper and with MGP staining. Additionally, if the material is used as a solvent for mounting media, haematoxylin staining is rapidly diminished (Anderson, 1984).

Cedar wood oil

This is the best reagent for research and treatment of delicate tissue, since it has the least hardening effects. Tissue may be left in this clearing agent for long periods, even for months, without damage. In some institutions it is used as a clearing agent for hard tissue such as skin, and dense fibrous tissue, since sections are easier to cut after such treatment. When ordering it should be specified that the cedar wood oil is for use as a clearing agent.

Even very small pieces of tissue need to be left overnight in cedar wood oil; specimens from 5–7 mm in thickness will need 2–5 days.

Cedar wood oil may be poured into a small specimen jar, and a similar quantity of absolute alcohol superimposed on it, avoiding any mixing at the junction of the two fluids; the specimen is then placed gently into the alcohol when it will float at the interface of the two fluids. As clearing takes place the specimen slowly sinks into the cedar wood oil. The alcohol is then removed by pipette or syphon, the specimen is

* Bestobell Chemical Products Ltd, Bassington Industrial Estate, Cramlington, Northumberland, England.

transferred to fresh cedar wood oil for a few hours, and is transferred finally to paraffin wax.

Following clearing in this reagent, several extra changes of paraffin wax will be required to remove the oil. Treatment of tissues with xylene for 30 minutes before paraffin-wax impregnation helps remove cedar wood oil.

Recycling processing fluids

In many countries, it is forbidden to dispose of processing fluids, especially clearing agents, via the drains or sewerage system. Apparatus is now available for recycling these fluids by distillation. It is probably more cost effective to use commercial sources for recycling, if available, than to pay for removal and disposal. Recycled processing fluids from reputable companies seem to be as efficient as virgin fluid.

Impregnation with wax

Paraffin wax is a mixture of straight-chain hydrocarbons produced by sweating and pressing the residue of vacuum-distilled crude oil. For histological purposes, paraffin wax is most commonly categorized according to the melting point. As all paraffin waxes are mixtures of hydrocarbons, each having its own particular melting point, these are not particularly accurate. As a general rule it may be stated that the higher the melting point of a paraffin wax the harder it will be at any given temperature. However, there may be exceptions as it is the plastic point of the paraffin wax that governs its behaviour. The plastic point is generally about 10 °C below the melting point and is the temperature at which a crystalline rearrangement takes place during solidification and at which the behaviour characteristics of the wax change. These may be illustrated by the way warm wax will adjust to accommodate stress whereas cold wax will break or shatter under similar strain.

In theory, a low melting point (i.e. softer) paraffin wax is most suitable for soft, friable tissue and a higher-melting-point paraffin wax (i.e. harder) for tough tissue. It is also theoretically beneficial to impregnate with a low-temperature paraffin wax and embed in a higher-temperature paraffin wax. However, the practical effects are often so limited and microtomy such a personal experience as to render such refinements superfluous.

Various substances have been added to paraffin wax, primarily to improve the performance during microtomy. Generally, these have been employed to increase the hardness of the wax and thus the support for tougher tissues; to increase the plasticity of the wax and thus improve ribboning qualities and presumably change the sectioning from point-to-point cleavage to a continuous-flow shearing; and to produce a more uniform crystalline structure to the wax. Allison (1978) has studied the effect of many of these additives on the crystalline structure of paraffin wax and found them to be minimal. Examples of additives include ceresin, microcrystalline wax, rubber, beeswax and dental wax. More recently, plastic polymers have been added to paraffin wax and these composites sold as commercial products. Their use is a matter of personal preference, although the authors' experience has been that the addition of DMSO (dimethyl sulphoxide) to Paraplast (Sherwood Medical Industries, County Oak, Crawley, England) is particularly beneficial and that Histoplast Special (Shandon Southern Products, Astmoor, Cheshire, England) and Ralwax I (Raymond A. Lamb, 6 Sunbeam Rd, London, England) compounded specially as final embedding media, are helpful in cutting tough tissues or producing thin (i.e. 2 μm) sections.

It is recommended that paraffin wax (MP 58 °C) be available for routine embedding, and Histoplast Special for tough or decalcified tissue.

Time of impregnation

The length of time and the number of changes required for thorough impregnation of the tissue with wax will largely depend on the following three factors:

(1) the size and type of the tissue;
(2) the clearing agent employed;
(3) the use of a vacuum-embedding oven.

The size and type of the tissue

The size of the specimen will, as throughout the whole process, influence the time required for complete impregnation. The thicker the tissue the longer will be the time required for wax to penetrate to the centre; moreover, thick tissue will carry over more of the clearing agent, and more changes of wax will be necessary to remove it. Even small amounts of clearing agent contaminating the wax will cause crystallization, and crumbling of the sections during cutting.

The type of tissue should also be taken into account since dense tissue, such as bone, skin and central nervous system, will require nearly twice as long as soft tissue such as liver and kidney. Tissue containing a high proportion of blood, muscle and fibrous strands has a tendency to over-harden and become brittle in the wax bath, and consequently the time of impregnation in such cases must be kept to a minimum. This reduction in time of impregnation can be achieved quite satisfactorily by using a vacuum-embedding oven, except in the case of tissue from the central nervous system. The cutting of such sections is made easier if the tissue has been left in paraffin wax overnight in the ordinary oven, with two or three changes; sections from tissue so impregnated do not curl and crack in the drying oven.

The clearing agent employed

Some clearing agents are more easily replaced and eradicated than others. Xylene, toluene, chloroform, CNP30 and food oils require two changes of wax as a safe routine. Cedar wood oil, as has been mentioned, will require several changes dependent on the size of the tissue: small pieces should be given at least three changes, and larger pieces correspondingly more.

When impregnating delicate tissue, such as embryonic tissue, it is recommended that it be transferred from the clearing agent to a mixture of clearing agent and paraffin wax. This mixture should be a nearly saturated solution of paraffin wax in the clearing agent at room temperature. This method is used as a routine in some institutions but, with the possible exception given above, it would seem to be an unnecessary and time-wasting procedure.

The use of a vacuum-embedding oven

Using the normal paraffin oven, tissues are as a routine given two changes of paraffin wax over a period of 4 hours; by the use of a vacuum-embedding oven this time may be halved.

Vacuum-embedding ovens

The apparatus consists of an airtight embedding oven attached to an exhaust pump, the degree of vacuum achieved being controlled by an attached mercury manometer or vacuum gauge. By reducing the pressure during wax impregnation air bubbles and clearing agent are more speedily removed from the tissue, resulting in more rapid impregnation.

One type of apparatus in common use is shown in *Figure 4.1*. It consists of an outer bath, normally controlled at 56 °C (or 2 °C above the melting point of the wax being used), into which the vacuum chamber fits. The vacuum chamber is a circular, flat-

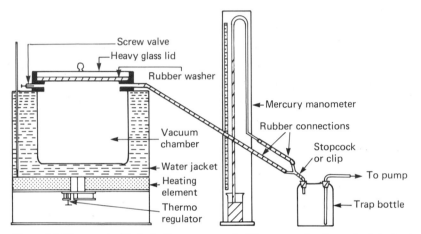

Figure 4.1 Diagram to illustrate the vacuum embedding apparatus (from *An Introduction to Medical Laboratory Technology* (1976), 5th Ed., Butterworths, London)

bottomed brass vessel, which has a thick plate-glass lid resting on a thick rubber ring. There are two valves, one being connected to the exhaust pump, the other being used to admit air to restore atmospheric pressure at the end of impregnation. To avoid contamination of the wax in the bath by the water or oil used in the vacuum pump, the pump is connected to a thick-walled vessel (flask or bottle) which acts as a trap; this in turn is connected by a 'T' or 'Y' piece to the vacuum chamber and to a mercury manometer (*Figure 4.1*).

Embedding or blocking

Tissue is finally transferred from the last wax bath to a mould filled with molten paraffin wax, inverting the tissue to free all surfaces of air bubbles and orientating the intended cutting surface so that it faces the base of the mould. The relative terms 'embedding' and 'blocking' reflect the progress that has been achieved in simplifying this task.

Leuckhart's L pieces

These represent the traditional blocking method, simple in construction and use. They consist of two L-shaped pieces of metal, usually brass, which are laid on a metal or glass plate to form an oblong. By adjusting the L pieces the relative shape and size of the mould can be modified according to the size and number of tissues. Various sizes of L pieces are available, enabling almost any piece of tissue to be blocked by this method. When the wax has set, the L pieces are easily removed, and are ready for further use with a minimum of cleaning required.

Ice trays

Ice trays of the plastic type used to produce domestic ice cubes are useful. Each tissue is blocked into its own individual compartment, thus saving on the labour involved in separating blocks. Unfortunately they are of uniform size and tend to wear out with use. Small pieces of tissue need to have a large excess of wax removed before microtomy. Similar trays are produced commercially, in various sizes, as disposables.

Paper 'boats'

Paper 'boats' make cheap and convenient alternatives, although their advantages over disposable plastic trays are now minimal. They do have the advantage that the paper need be removed only from the cutting surface and upper edges, so that the blocked tissues may be stored with the identifying number written on the projecting tag. Ordinary paper may be used, but they are best prepared from glossy paper—old catalogues are suitable.

  Another theoretical advantage of paper-boat moulds is that the wax block may be clamped directly into the microtome vice without the need of mounting on a wooden block or special holder. This is less satisfactory in practice.

Embedding cassettes

The development of a scheme whereby tissue may be processed in a single cassette which eventually forms a part of the embedding system represented a great step forward in security, simplicity and labour saving. Continuous development has overcome virtually all the disadvantages of the original system.

  A plastic cassette, which may be provided with either a metal snap-on lid, or an integral plastic one, holds the tissue during processing. A roughened surface is provided on which the reference number may be written. Embedding is performed in specially-made base mould and the cassette inverted over the tissue and filled with wax. After solidification of the wax, it is removed, complete with cassette. The cassette fits into a purpose-made microtome clamp which has the advantage of a simple one-handed spring action. After cutting, the block is stored with the cassette still in place, the identification number therefore only having to be written once and accompanying the tissue through all stages. Moulds are available in a variety of sizes and cassettes in a variety of depths and colours.

■ Technique of embedding

(1) Metal moulds should be sprayed or smeared lightly with mould release fluid.
(2) The mould is filled with the appropriate paraffin wax.
(3) The tissue is transferred rapidly to the wax-containing based mould with a pair of warm forceps. Care should be taken that the forceps are not too hot and that excessive pressure is not used. Electrically-heated forceps are ideal for this purpose.
(4) Ensure that no air bubbles are trapped and place the tissue, with the surface to be sectioned down, against the base of the mould. Allow the wax in the bottom of the

mould to solidify sufficiently to hold the tissue in place. If the cassette system is in use, place it over the base mould and top up with molten paraffin wax. Orientation is very important and some features are noted below. If several pieces of tissue are to be embedded in the same mould, this stage must be carried out rapidly, otherwise the wax in the mould will solidify. The skin which forms on the surface may be broken with the warmed forceps, but care must be taken to ensure that all fragments are, as far as possible, embedded on the same plane. With practice this operation presents no difficulty.

(5) The block should be immediately transferred to a refrigerated surface, a tray of ice or, once a skin has formed on the surface, immersed in a trough of cold water. It is often stated that this is done to promote the formation of smaller paraffin-wax crystals than would otherwise be the case. Dempster (1943) has found this not to be the case, and Allison (1978; 1979) agrees that cooling from a single surface probably helps promote the formation of unidirectional crystals and a more uniform block.

(6) Once solidification is complete—and care must be taken that it *is* complete—the block may be removed from the mould. Mould-release spray should ensure that this happens easily enough, but if it does stick, a sharp tap should release it.

Orientation

Embedding blocks of homogeneous tissue from large organs such as liver, kidney and brain usually presents no problem. There are, however, structures which require special attention.

Epithelium

Skin- or mucosa-covered tissue must be cut at right angles to the surface, so that the full thickness of the epithelium is visualized. Wedge-shaped biopsies may present special problems (*Figure 4.2a*); dermatologists and surgeons should be encouraged to remove straight-edged specimens wherever possible.

It is often advantageous to embed skin so that the epithelial surface, particularly where it has a tough surface such as that found on palms and the soles of feet, meets the blade after the softer, underlying connective tissue has been cut (*Figure 4.2c*).

Muscle biopsies

Muscle should be embedded so that both longitudinal and transverse sections are obtained.

Tubes

Tubes should be sectioned at right angles so that the lumen is clearly visible (*Figure 4.2d*).

The orientation of the specimen to the blade during microtomy should also be considered. In general, and contrary to the technique for producing cryostat sections, the longest axis of the specimen should be parallel to the blade. However, it is sometimes advantageous when cutting, particularly hard tissue, such as bone or teeth, to orientate the specimen so that the blade meets a corner of the specimen first (*Figure 4.2b*). This helps obviate the 'jump' that may occur when the blade meets the tissue.

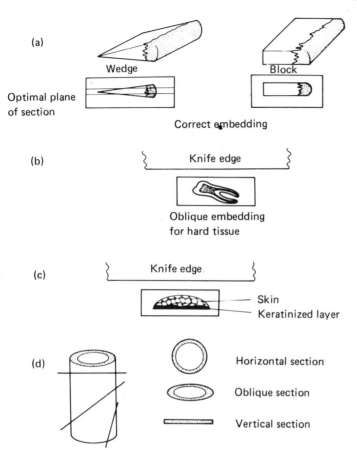

(a)

Wedge   Block

Optimal plane
of section

Correct embedding

(b)   Knife edge

Oblique embedding
for hard tissue

(c)   Knife edge

                                   Skin
                                   Keratinized layer

(d)

                         Horizontal section

                         Oblique section

                         Vertical section

Figure 4.2 Some problems that may be encountered in embedding. *See* text for details

Difficulties in recognizing the surface to be cut may be overcome in several ways. A small nick may be cut in the opposite surface, or a suture inserted. This should be removed during embedding. Alternatively indelible ink may be used, but great care should be taken to ensure it does not flow all over the specimen. If it is necessary to identify a given surface microscopically, after staining and mounting, for example, to determine the surface distal to a margin of clearance, 5% silver nitrate may be applied directly to the surface. This is reduced to black metallic silver, presumably as a result of the action of residual formalin in the tissue (*see* Chapter 6).

Instrumentation for paraffin-wax processing

Automatic tissue processors (*Figure 4.3*)

The overall length of time required to fix, dehydrate, clear and impregnate tissues with wax during a series of normal working days has long been the obstacle to more rapid diagnosis. Tissues which are laid at the bottom of a container may require up to 4–5 hours in each reagent. It follows, therefore, that only two such changes may be made

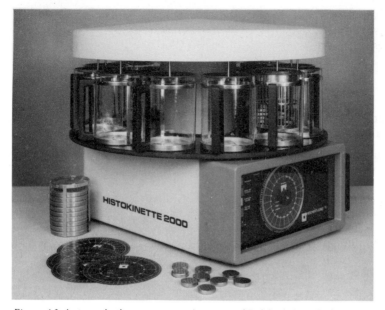

Figure 4.3 Automatic tissue processor (courtesy of Reichert–Jung Ltd)

during a normal working day; furthermore, schedules must be arranged so that tissues are not left overnight in fluids which will unduly harden them.

Automatic tissue processors have two advantages. In addition to transferring the tissues mechanically from reagent to reagent both by day and by night, they also reduce the time required in each fluid by the action of continual agitation. They are equipped with a 1-hour clock in addition to a 24-hour clock, and so can be used for rapid processing of tissue. A 7-day clock is also available for longer processes.

This method eliminates the possibility of human error and forgetfulness, and may be trusted to the most junior member of the staff.

Most machines have a 12-stage cycle with the last two usually reserved for paraffin-wax infiltration. Static beakers are provided to hold the processing fluids, and tissues, held in individual containers or cassettes in a suspended basket, are mechanically moved from one to another. Agitation is provided either by vertical or rotating movements of the basket. Facilities exist to allow for user-designed schedules. The wax baths may incorporate an optional vacuum. Using these machines, tissue may be routinely processed overnight, so that it is ready for embedding first thing in the morning.

Closed tissue processors

Of relatively recent design, closed-tissue processors offer distinct advantages over the more traditional designs. The primary advantages are in safety and capacity, although many other features introduce greater flexibility into processing schedules. The major design difference is that the tissue cassettes are held in a static 'reaction chamber' and the processing fluids pumped in and out. This allows for the potentially hazardous fluids to be housed separately from the reaction chamber, in a special cabinet reducing risks of fire and spillage. By using a single reaction chamber, it has been possible to provide facilities to process tissues with the application of heat and vacuum at all stages. Microprocessor control and memory permit a greater flexibility and variety of processing schedules. It has proved possible to process tissue in remarkably short times.

Embedding centres

These instruments are a valuable asset in work simplification. Although many models are available, they all consist of the same basic components.

(1) An area for holding cassettes containing processed tissue awaiting embedding. This is a warm area where the wax infiltrating and surrounding the tissue remains molten.
(2) An embedding area, usually well illuminated, with a wax dispenser. A warm surface is provided to maintain paraffin wax in a molten state in the embedding moulds. A cold spot may be included so that a layer of solid wax may be induced in the base of the mould to hold the tissue in position. Heated forcep wells are also a common feature.
(3) A refrigerated surface to assist in the solidification of blocks.

A storage compartment is invariably provided to hold base moulds warmed and ready for use.

Rapid processing in paraffin wax

There are occasions when it is necessary to produce paraffin sections faster than the normal overnight schedule (*Table 4.1*). This may be achieved if two important

Table 4.1 Paraffin-wax processing schedules

	Automatic processor		Closed processor	
Reagent	Routine overnight	Rapid	Routine overnight	Rapid
Formal–saline[a]				
70% alcohol	1 hour	15 minutes	1 hour	5 minutes
80% alcohol	1 hour		1 hour	5 minutes
90% alcohol	1 hour		1 hour	15 minutes
100% alcohol	1 hour	20 minutes	1 hour	15 minutes
100% alcohol	1 hour	20 minutes	1 hour	15 minutes
100% alcohol	2 hours	20 minutes	1 hour	15 minutes
Chloroform	1 hour	20 minutes	1 hour	15 minutes
Chloroform	1 hour	20 minutes	1 hour	15 minutes
Chloroform	$1\frac{1}{2}$ hours	30 minutes	1 hour	15 minutes V[b]
Paraffin wax	$1\frac{1}{2}$ hours	1 hour	$1\frac{1}{2}$ hours V	1 hour V
Paraffin wax	$1\frac{1}{2}$ hours	1 hour	$1\frac{1}{2}$ hours V	1 hour V
Paraffin wax	30 minutes V	30 minutes V		
See Note				

Note: If the automatic processor does not have vacuum facilities for paraffin-wax infiltration, a third, vacuum assisted, impregnation should be carried out in a vacuum-embedding chamber.
[a] Time in formal–saline will depend on time it is wished to terminate processing. In closed processor, this stage may be used to fix tissues at 45 °C.
[b] Heat to 45° C
V = Apply vacuum.

considerations are met. Tissue slices, or fragments, must be as thin as possible, and in any event not more than 3 mm in thickness. Secondly, the use of continuous agitation at all stages, and the use of vacuum during paraffin-wax infiltration are strongly recommended. Adequate fixation may be achieved by using formal–saline warmed to 45 °C for 30 minutes. In extreme cases, the tissue may be plunged into boiling formal–saline for 5 minutes. It is doubtful if in this event the cross-linking induced by formaldehyde is more important than the precipitation of proteins by heat. Nevertheless, on reasonably robust tissue, this protocol may be used with success. Some workers substitute Carnoy's fixative for formal–saline with good results. Whilst it should not be expected that tissue morphology will be anywhere near perfect, it should be sufficiently preserved to permit a diagnosis. Accepting these limitations, dehydrating and clearing agents are chosen for speed of action rather than gentleness. It is for this reason that graded alcohols may be omitted from the schedule, and, in some laboratories, acetone substituted for alcohol. Vacuum at stages other than paraffin-wax infiltration does not seem to help very much, although some users of modern closed tissue processors claim, with the help of heat, agitation and vacuum at all stages, to process tissue in less than 1 hour.

Ester wax

Embedding in ester wax, described by Steedman (1960), is said to combine certain advantages of both paraffin and celloidin. Ester wax is much harder than paraffin wax, although it has a lower melting point (46–48 °C). It is similar to celloidin in that it can be compressed, and is therefore less likely to crumble when one is cutting hard tissue. Cutting is very similar to that of tissue in paraffin wax: thin sections (1–2 μm) are more easily cut and ribbons present no difficulty.

Technique

Tissue should not be transferred directly from the clearing agent to ester wax, but into a mixture of clearing agent and wax where it is left for 3–6 hours according to size.

At least three changes of wax should be used during impregnation, and four or even five for large pieces of tissue. Tissue should be left in each change for 3–6 hours.

For embedding, the wax is best heated to 68–70 °C, and poured into a mould as for paraffin-wax embedding. The tissue is put in and orientated with warm forceps to ensure cutting in the correct plane. The block should be rapidly cooled in water, but since contraction occurs, and it may be necessary to fill the central depression with more wax to avoid exposure of the tissue, it is not advisable to submerge the block.

When completely solid, the block is freed from the mould and trimmed. Because of the hardness of the wax, sections from these blocks need to be cut slowly, with a very sharp knife. The microtome used should be of a heavy type, preferably one of the sledge variety, and should be rigidly secured. Failure to fulfil these conditions will result in sections of uneven thickness.

Sections should be flattened in the usual way, by floating on warm water at a temperature of 35–40 °C; they are then picked up on clean plain or albuminized slides, and dried in an oven at 37 °C. *They must not be dried at room temperature* or sections will crumble. Following de-waxing, sections are stained as are paraffin sections. Owing to the water tolerance of this wax, sections may be stained with the wax still present by floating on staining reagents, with a slight increase in staining times. The sections are then fixed to slides, de-waxed and mounted.

Ester was has secured a small place in traditional histology but newer waxes, developed to give similar advantages in sectioning hard tissues, or even producing thin sections (1–2 μm) are much easier to use in the authors' experience. Ralwax, which contains a polymer with quite dramatic properties, may be used as a final embedding medium following routine processing to give extra support to tough tissues. Histoplast Special has properties which give the block cutting characteristics theoretically similar to LVN. Used only as a final embedding medium, it facilitates the cutting of thin sections, although the temperature of the floating out bath (*see below*) must be kept below 45 °C.

Water-soluble waxes

Water-soluble waxes (e.g. Carbowax) are solid polyethylene glycols having the great advantage of not requiring the tissues to be dehydrated and cleared before infiltration. They have the additional advantage, probably due to the avoidance of dehydrating and clearing reagents, that the degree of shrinkage of tissue is considerably less than that caused by the paraffin-wax technique. Several types of water-soluble wax are available commercially.

These waxes have been used with success for the demonstration of lipids, and to preserve enzymatic activity in plants after freeze-drying or special fixation.

Miles and Linder (1952) compared the tissue shrinkage caused by a water-soluble wax (Nonex 63B) and paraffin. They found the shrinkage was 11% using paraffin wax. and only 4.7% using water-soluble wax. The technique they employed, which they now use routinely for hard tissues, is given below with slight modifications.

■ **Technique**

(1) Wash tissue well to remove all traces of fixative. If a large amount of fat is present remove it by treatment with acetone.

(2) Transfer the tissue to 50% polyethylene glycol 900 in distilled water, and leave until it sinks (about 10–15 minutes).

(3) Transfer to four successive changes of molten polyethylene glycol 900 at 28–30 °C, allowing 45 minutes in each bath.

(4) Transfer to a mixture of equal parts of polyethylene glycol 900 and Nonex 63B at 39 °C for 30–40 minutes.

(5) Transfer to a mixture of three parts of Nonex 63B and one part of polyethylene glycol 900 and leave for 15 minutes. (In stages 4 and 5 a layer of glass wool on the bottom of the containers will keep the tissue off the bottom where the polyethylene glycol 900 tends to accumulate.)

(6) Transfer the tissue to the first of three changes of Nonex 63B at 39 °C, and leave it in each change for 30–45 minutes. At the end of the third change it is ready for embedding.

(7) Embed in a paper boat as for paraffin-wax embedding (*see* page 61), or, as Miles and Linder suggest, in a paraffin-wax boat made by pouring molten paraffin wax into L pieces adjusted to a convenient size, allowing the outside layer of wax to set, and then pouring out the molten centre. This leaves a thin wax-embedding mould which, when the Nonex 63B has set, can easily be broken away.

Blocks should be stored temporarily in a desiccator, and coated with paraffin wax for permanent storage.

Cutting

Sections are cut in the usual manner. On microtomes with a tilt adjustment this should be greater than is used for cutting paraffin sections.

Fixing to slides

The floating of these sections is probably the most difficult part of the technique, since if they are floated on water violent diffusion currents are set up which cause the sections to fragment. These currents may be minimized by the addition of a trace of soap or a few drops of Teepol to the water: alternatively 10–20% polyethylene glycol 900 may be added to the water. The wax-free sections thus flattened may be floated on slides in the usual manner, and stained; or they may be treated in the manner described for frozen sections (*see* page 139).

Gelatin embedding

Gelatin embedding may be used when frozen sections of friable or partially necrotic tissue, or numbers of small fragments such as uterine curettings, are required.

Following embedding, the block may be immersed in 10% formalin to convert the gelatin to an irreversible gel.

The usual method, employing formalin to harden the gelatin, is as follows.

■ Technique

(1) Tissue is fixed in formal–saline, and then washed in running water for 6–12 hours to remove the formalin.
(2) Tissue is transferred to 10% gelatin in 1% phenol (to prevent the growth of moulds) for 24 hours at 37 °C.
(3) Tissue is transferred to 20% gelatin–phenol for 12 hours at 37 °C.
(4) Tissue should now be embedded in 20% gelatin, using a mould as for paraffin-wax embedding.
(5) Having been allowed to set, preferably in the cold, excess gelatin should be trimmed, leaving a margin of approximately 3 mm around the specimen, and as little as possible on the surface to place on the freezing microtome stage.

A minimum amount of gelatin remaining, consistent with adequate support of the specimen, is essential as the gelatin tends to inhibit freezing. For the same reason, pieces of tissue for inclusion by this technique should not exceed 2–3 mm.
(6) The trimmed block is then immersed in 10% formalin for 12–24 hours to harden.
(7) Frozen sections can now be cut in the usual way; it is preferable to cut them thin to avoid undue background staining caused by the gelatin.

The disadvantage of this method is that when staining techniques are applied the gelatin tends to hold the stain, giving an indifferent background to the section. Some workers recommend avoiding stage 6 (*above*), and after fixing sections to the slide remove the gelatin with warm water. The difficulty with the latter technique lies in floating out and fixing the section to the slide, but this may be overcome to some degree by floating out on very cold water, and transferring immediately to albuminized slides. The slides are then drained on the bench, gently heated two or three times (except when demonstrating lipids) to coagulate the albumin, and placed in warm water to remove the gelatin.

Celloidin and LVN (Low Viscosity Nitrocellulose)

Celloidin, the classic embedding medium of the neuropathologist, has lost favour to LVN, forming a less viscous fluid which penetrates tissue more easily and gives a harder block. Cox (1983) sounds a note of caution due to the difficulty of removing LVN blocks from the moulds. It is also explosive when dry and should be kept damp with butanol.

As embedding in LVN requires only that the tissue be completely dehydrated, the hazards of clearing and heating tissue are avoided with consequent benefits. In particular, shrinkage is limited, tough tissue is not made any harder, the relationship of different tissues is maintained and dense, but soft tissue is more completely impregnated and supported. Obvious applications are therefore in the study of bone and teeth, the central nervous tissue and eyes. Different mechanical forces also occur during sectioning, continuous shearing type cutting facilitating easier sections of tough tissue in particular.

Disadvantages of nitrocellulose

(1) It is very difficult to cut sections thinner than 10 μm.
(2) As it is impossible to prepare ribbons of sections, it is a tedious process to prepare serial sections.
(3) Processing is slow, impregnation and subsequent hardening of the block taking weeks to complete.
(4) Blocks and sections must be stored in 70% alcohol and, preferably, in the dark. This is both hazardous and space consuming.
(5) The reagents are highly flammable.

Preparation of solutions

Nitrocellulose is supplied rather like granules of wool dampened with alcohol. This wool is used direct from the container and dissolved in absolute ethanol, if possible taking account of the alcohol present in the wool. Celloidin is much more difficult to dissolve than LVN. Once dissolved, an equal volume of ether is added to make the working concentration. The following concentrations are used:

Thin solution   5% LVN or 2% celloidin in ethanol/ether
Medium solution   10% LVN or 4% celloidin in ethanol/ether
Thick solution   20% LVN or 8% celloidin in ethanol/ether

These solutions, particularly the thick solution, take some time to dissolve and should be made long before they are required and kept in stock. Solutions of celloidin and low viscosity nitrocellulose should be kept in well-stoppered jars, preferably of the ground-glass-stoppered variety, to avoid evaporation of the ether–alcohol solvent and to prevent contamination with water vapour. It must be remembered at all times that *ether is one of the most highly inflammable materials used in a laboratory and care should therefore be taken to ensure that naked lights are extinguished before it is used.* A fire has been started in a laboratory by an uncorked bottle of ether which was no nearer than 10 yards from a lighted Bunsen burner. The flame ignited the vapour and leapt across the 10-yard gap causing the bottle of ether to explode.

Nitrocellulose processing schedule

The times given in the following schedule are only an approximation and will obviously be dependent upon the size of the tissues being processed. These are applicable to tissue up to 10 mm thick.

(1) 70% Ethanol	Two changes 24 hours each	
(2) 95% Ethanol	Two changes 48 hours each	
(3) Absolute ethanol	Two changes over 2–5 days	
(4) Thin solution		3–5 days
(5) Medium solution		5–7 days
(6) Thick solution		5–7 days

There is no harm done by leaving tissues in the nitrocellulose solutions for considerable periods, provided it is not allowed to evaporate.

Embedding

The tissue is transferred to either 30% LVN (preferably containing 1% celloidin*) or 8% celloidin in a glass mould or paper boat. Sufficient space should be allowed to cover the tissue with nitrocellulose to a depth of 25–30 mm and leave a 10-mm margin each side. The block is hardened by evaporation of the solvents. If this is uneven a bad and uneven block will result. It is essential to prevent the formation of air bubbles, particularly from the surface to be cut. Tissue, with the surface to be cut uppermost, is placed in the mould containing nitrocellulose for 12 hours to allow the bubbles to come to the surface. During this procedure the block is kept in an air-tight container to prevent evaporation, either in a desiccator or under an air-tight bell jar. Following elimination of the air bubbles, the tissue is inverted so that the surface to be cut faces downwards. The solution is then thickened by sliding the desiccator lid to one side, or by raising one side of the bell jar. To ensure even evaporation the area of the mould directly exposed to the air is changed every 3 or 4 hours. At night it is best to close the container. This hardening process is continued until the nitrocellulose is of a rubbery consistency so that the ball of the finger no longer leaves an imprint.

Hardening of nitrocellulose may be accelerated by the use of chloroform vapour. A few drops of chloroform in a separate container under a bell jar, or in the bottom of the desiccator, will harden small blocks 2 cm square in about 12–24 hours; larger blocks take proportionately longer.

When the block is sufficiently hardened, the excess nitrocellulose is trimmed off with a sharp knife, leaving a margin of $\frac{3}{16}$–$\frac{1}{4}$ inch all round, with the exception of the surface to be cut which should not be trimmed at this stage. This nitrocellulose block is then fixed to a vulcanite fibre or hardwood (teak) block of an appropriate size to fit the microtome chuck. The surface of the wooden or vulcanite block must be roughened, or

---

* This helps to overcome a tendency of LVN to crack during handling and staining. 1% Tricresyl phosphate and 0.5% castor oil have also been recommended to increase plasticity.

serrated with a saw, followed by a liberal application of thin (2%) celloidin; the celloidin block is then pressed on and a lead weight used to hold the surfaces in close contact for about 1 hour. The block is then hardened in 70% alcohol for half an hour before cutting.

The dry celloidin method

This method was devised to overcome the disadvantages of the standard method, that is to say, that blocks must be stored in 70% alcohol and the block and knife kept wet with 70% alcohol during cutting.

Celloidin blocks are prepared as already described, but instead of being fixed to vulcanite blocks are transferred to Gilson's mixture, which is equal parts of chloroform and cedar wood oil. Cedar wood oil is added twice daily, over a period of 3–10 days, until the mixture is composed of about 90% cedar wood oil. The celloidin will gradually become quite transparent during this process, and should then be removed and exposed to the air until dry. When the block is dry it is fixed to a vulcanite block in the usual way and sections are cut dry. Blocks should be kept in air-tight bottles.

Double embedding

The preparation of serial sections of celloidin-impregnated tissue is normally a tedious procedure since the sections will not adhere to one another in the same manner as paraffin-embedded material. Double embedding is the name given to a technique whereby the tissue is first impregnated with celloidin, and subsequently blocked in paraffin wax. In this manner the advantages of both materials are, to some degree, combined.

While some workers simply transfer tissue directly from 8% celloidin, following the routine celloidin technique, to two changes of chloroform, or benzene, and subsequently embed in paraffin wax as for ordinary tissue, the method of Peterfi, as given below, is recommended.

■ Peterfi's double embedding method

(1) After dehydration of the tissue in the usual manner, the tissue is transferred to celloidin–methyl benzoate mixture, which is prepared by dissolving 1% dry celloidin in methyl benzoate in a stoppered bottle. The bottle should be shaken several times daily to assist solution of the celloidin, which may take several days.
(2) The celloidin solution is replaced daily for 2–3 days, depending on the size of the tissue. Complete impregnation is indicated by the tissue becoming transparent.
(3) The tissue is transferred to benzene and given two or three changes each of 6 hours. Should the tissue need three changes of the celloidin solution, it will require three changes of benzene.
(4) Transfer tissue to paraffin wax, and impregnate and embed in the usual manner.
(5) Sections are cut, as are ordinary paraffin sections, on any of the standard microtomes.
(6) If sections, after floating on water in the usual way, tend to curl off slides, they should be floated on 90% alcohol which will soften the celloidin without dissolving it.

Resin embedding

Resin is a much harder material than paraffin wax and these properties are exploited either to cut hard material such as undecalcified bone, or to cut thin, that is, 0.5–1.5 μm, sections. The impact of resinous embedding media has been such that many resins have been developed. For practical purposes two groups of resin may be employed.

Acrylic resins (methacrylates)

These are monomers of acrylic and methacrylic acids. A mixture of butyl and methyl methacrylates was one of the first resins to be routinely employed in histopathology, but has now been largely replaced in popular usage by 2-hydroxyethyl methacrylate (HEMA). Glycol methacrylate (GMA), it should be noted, is a synonym for HEMA. To be effective a resin must have two phases:

(1) a liquid phase with which the tissue can be infiltrated; and
(2) a solid phase which will support the tissue during microtomy.

Liquid resin is converted to a solid block by a process known as polymerization. In the liquid state, the resin is termed a monomer, molecules of the resin existing independently. Polymerization, which may occur spontaneously, by the application of gentle heat or by ultraviolet irradiation, results in the formation of repeating units held together by covalent bonds. These repeating units are the polymers, the molecular size of which may vary considerably. It is these branching and interconnecting molecules which give rigidity to the resin block. The process of polymerization is often referred to as 'curing'.

To prevent spontaneous polymerization, commercial methacrylates contain hydroquinone as an inhibitor. Although it is usually advantageous to remove this from butyl/methyl methacrylate it is rarely necessary to do so for HEMA. However, it is advisable to test new batches of resin for polymerization before use.

HEMA is a water-miscible resin and the ease with which HEMA-embedded sections may be stained with aqueous dyes has led to its popularity with light microscopists. It is beneficial to dehydrate tissue before infiltrating with the resin, although transferring tissue direct from aqueous fixatives has been successful.

Polymerization is achieved by the use of a catalyst, benzoyl peroxide, and an activator N,N-dimethylaniline. By varying the concentration of these components, the speed of polymerization may be controlled. The optimum concentration of benzoyl peroxide should be determined for each new batch of resin. To improve the cutting

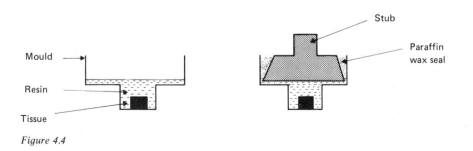

Figure 4.4

characteristics of the block, two plasticizers, 2-butoxyethanol and polyethylene glycol 400, are incorporated into the mixture. Increasing the butoxyethanol will decrease the hardness of the block. The addition of 2% polystyrene improves the constitution of the final block, especially for cutting bone. It also makes sections stable in the electron beam. Slightly acidified HEMA gives a clearer background to stained sections.

Commercial resins with many characteristics similar to HEMA are widely available under the names JB-4 and LR White.

■ Recommended method

Solutions
Resin solution. A—Monomer

2-Hydroxyethyl methacrylate	80 ml
2-Butoxyethanol	8 ml
Benzoyl peroxide	1 g

Resin solution. B—Activator

Polyethylene glycol 400	15 parts
N,N-dimethylaniline	1 part

Fix tissue in 10% neutral formal–saline	
70% ethanol	1 hour
90% ethanol	1 hour
100% ethanol—three changes	30 minutes each
Solution A—monomer	2 hours
Fresh monomer	Overnight
Embed in the following mixture	
Solution A 42 parts	
Solution B 1 part	
Mix well	

Embedding is most conveniently carried out using Sorvall moulds and block holders (*Figure 4.4*). The plastic mould should be filled to the level of the ledge with the embedding mixture and the tissue orientated in the base of the mould with the surface to be cut down. The aluminium block holder is placed on top of the resin and the mould filled through the hollow stem until overflowing. Complete polymerization only occurs under anaerobic conditions. Many workers seal the rim of the plastic block holder with paraffin wax to exclude the atmosphere. It is most important to ensure that no air bubbles are trapped in the mixture. Polymerization should be complete within a few hours if maintained at room temperature. As the reaction is exothermic, it is advisable to apply ice to the lower portion of the block, where polymerization begins.

Smaller blocks of tissue may be embedded in EM capsules, used 'upside down', that is, the lid forming the base of the mould. Reynolds (1982) recommends making two holes in the conical end of the capsule and introducing the embedding mixture through one via a hypodermic needle. The capsule may be cut away with a razor blade when polymerization is complete.

Although the finished resin block does not represent a health hazard, all the component chemicals should be handled with care. They are flammable, toxic and give rise to skin sensitization. Gloves must be worn and the materials handled in a fume cupboard.

Epoxy resins

Because of their stability in the electron beam, a property not shared by HEMA, epoxy resins are popular with electron microscopists. The high mechanical strength and, particularly, the low shrinkage together with the ease and consistency of polymerization, led to applications in light microscopy. Unfortunately, sections from epoxy-embedded tissues do not stain readily. Before staining with other than simple dyes, such as toluidine blue, the sections need to be etched in alcoholic sodium hydroxide. Another limiting factor in the use of epoxy resins has been high viscosity and consequent difficulties in impregnation. Low viscosity epoxy resins are now available, however.

Araldite was one of the first epoxy resins to be introduced as an embedding medium. As with all epoxy resins, it is a mixture of the resin, a hardener, a plasticizer and an accelerator. It is most important that all solutions are thoroughly mixed so that the various components are evenly dispersed throughout the resin. During mixing, care must be taken to avoid air bubbles.

Many formulas exist for producing blocks of resin of the required consistency. The effects of each component are obvious from the names and it is advisable to experiment to find the relative proportions which give blocks of the required consistency. It is often the case, for example, that particularly hard tissue may cut more easily if the amount of the plasticizer is reduced or omitted altogether.

Less viscous epoxy resins, introduced to overcome the long processing schedules for Araldite, include Epon and Spurr. Polymerization of the epoxy resins is usually carried out at 60 °C or more. The health hazards associated with these resins are slightly greater than with the acrylic resins, contact dermatitis being a serious problem. These comments apply particularly to Spurr resin.

Epoxy resins are an essential tool for processing tissues for electron microscopy and schedules given in that section (Chapter 34) can be applied to light microscopy by making due allowance for the larger block size.

Critical-point drying

Critical-point drying is a method for processing that seeks to avoid inducing structural artefact in the tissue. The principal application is in tissue preparation for scanning electron microscopy (SEM), although it does have some value in transmission electron microscopy. Both require that the specimen be fully dried before examination. Unfortunately, the large surface tension forces that exist where there is a liquid/gas interface will damage tissue during simple drying, because it involves conversion of the liquid infiltrating and surrounding the tissue into its gaseous form. The essential feature of critical-point drying is that no liquid/gas interface occurs (*Figure 4.5*).

If a liquid is in equilibrium with its vapour in a closed container, no matter how much pressure is applied above a particular temperature, it is impossible to liquefy the vapour. This is the *critical temperature*. However, as the pressure is increased, so the density of the vapour increases until it is equal to the density of the liquid. The point at which vapour and liquid density are equal is the *critical pressure*. Together, these constitute the *critical point* and there is no interface, and thus no surface tension, between the two phases.

Critical-point drying seeks to exploit this phenomenon by converting the liquid phase of tissue directly to the vapour phase, avoiding tissue distortion.

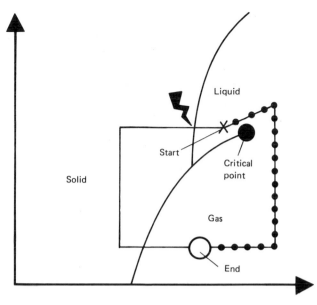

Pressure

Temperature

Figure 4.5 Diagrammatic representation of the relationship of temperature and pressure to the 'critical point'. At, or above, the critical point there is no phase interface between gas and liquid. Freeze-drying involves 'crossing the interface', whilst critical point drying avoids it

The critical point of water is very high (374 °C, 3184 lb/in^2) so that it is convenient to replace it with a liquid with a lower one. Liquid carbon dioxide (CO_2) is by far the most convenient and cheapest, although Freon 13 has also been recommended. The critical temperature of liquid CO_2 is only 31.5 °C and the critical pressure 1100 lb/in^2. 'Dry' CO_2 should always be specified when ordering, as it may be contaminated with water.

The specimen is first dehydrated, as water and liquid CO_2 are not miscible. Acetone or ethanol in graded series are recommended. With the latter, amyl acetate is commonly used as an additional intermediary as it is miscible with CO_2 and has the added advantage that its smell is easily detected. This is useful for judging whether removal is complete prior to drying. Finally, the specimen is immersed in liquid CO_2 under pressure and raised to the critical temperature at which the liquid will be converted to vapour. The gas is released and the now dry specimen is ready for examination. The complete method, in abbreviated form, is as follows:

Method

(1) Wash specimen free of surface contamination by blood, mucus, etc. with normal saline.
(2) Fix.
(3) Dehydrate in graded ethanols.
(4) Substitute ethanol with amyl acetate.
(5) Substitute amyl acetate with liquid CO_2.
(6) Heat to 10 °C above critical temperature—this allows for a small degree of specimen contamination by residual water.
(7) Release gas.

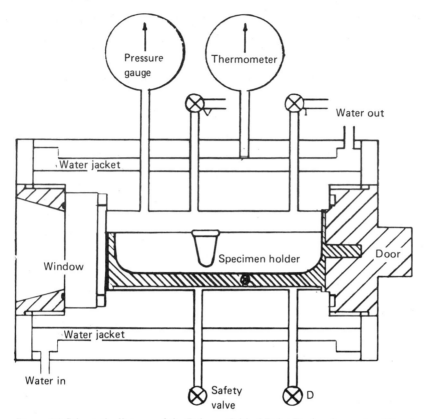

Figure 4.6 Schematic diagram of the Polaron Critical Point Drying Apparatus. (Courtesy of Polaron Equipment Ltd)

As such high pressures are reached during the procedure, a specially constructed pressure vessel is required. This is fitted with an inlet valve for the liquid gas, a vent to control pressure and allow the escape of vapour after drying and a safety valve. A water jacket is the usual way of controlling temperature. Ideally, the specimens should be visible through a porthole and the apparatus fitted with pressure and temperature gauges.

A schematic diagram is given in *Figure 4.6*.

References

ALLISON, R. T. (1978). The crystalline nature of histology waxes: a preliminary communication. *Med. Lab. Sci.*, **35**, 355–363

ALLISON, R. T. (1979). The crystalline nature of histology waxes: the effects of microtomy on the microstructure of paraffin wax sections. *Med. Lab. Sci.*, **36**, 359–372

ANDERSON, G. (1984). Tissue clearing agent. *Gazette*, **xxviii**, No. 1, p. 8. Institute of Medical Laboratory Sciences, 12 Queen Anne Street, London W1M 0AU

BRAIN, E. B. (1970). Infiltrating histological specimens with paraffin wax under vacuum. *Br. Dent. J.*, **128**, 71–78

COX, G. (1983). Neuropathological techniques. In *Theory and Practice of Histological Techniques*. Ed. Bancroft, J. D. and Stevens, A. 2nd Ed. Churchill-Livingstone, Edinburgh

DEMPSTER, W. T. (1943). Properties of paraffin relating to microtechnique. *Michigan Acad. Sci. Arts Lett.*, **29**, 251–264

GAGNON, J. and KATYK, N. (1959). Preliminary results in the use of ultrasonics in histological technique. *Rev. Can. Biol.*, **18**, 346–357

GAGNON, J. and KATYK, N. (1960). Les ultra-sons en technique histologique. *Arch. Anat. Pathol.*, **8**, A203–A208

GOUGH, J. and WENTWORTH, J. E. (1949). The use of thin sections of entire organs in morbid anatomical studies. *J. R. Micr. Soc.*, **69**, 231–235

GOUGH, J. and WENTWORTH, J. E. (1960). Thin sections of entire organs mounted on paper. In *Recent Advances in Pathology*. 7th Ed. Ed. Harrison, C. V. Churchill, London

MAXWELL, M. H. (1978). Safer substitutes for xylene and propylene oxide in histology, haematology and electron microscopy. *Med. Lab. Sci.*, **35**, 401–403.

MILES, A. E. W. and LINDER, J. E. (1952). Polyethylene glycols as histological embedding media with a note on the dimensional change of tissue during embedding in various media. *J. R. Micr. Soc.*, **72**, 199–213

REID, K. J. and YOUNG, F. J. (1981). Are trichloroethane-based substitutes safer than xylene? *Med. Lab. Sci.*, **38**, 145–146

REYNOLDS, G. (1982). *Lymphoid Tissue*. Wright, Bristol

STEEDMAN, H. F. (1960). *Section Cutting in Microscopy*. Blackwell, Oxford, England

5

Microtomy

Introduction

The production of thin sections of tissue for examination with the microscope is not a subject that can be taught by written instructions. However, as good quality sections depend on (a) a thorough knowledge of the equipment used, its maintenance and use, and (b) practical experience, guidance can be given to the student who must then practice this art, which calls for great manual dexterity. It is prudent to learn how to cut paraffin-wax sections of soft tissue, such as liver or kidney, until long ribbons of thin sections (4–5 µm) can be cut. Tougher tissue such as uterus, skin or decalcified bone will be found to be more demanding. Once the skill has been acquired, it will never be lost. Inadequate training will reflect for years afterwards, but a high standard achieved during training will be maintained throughout. Speed in itself must never be a primary object, it leads to poorly cut and badly mounted sections. Conscientious training will produce good quality sections in a far shorter time than training that has always aimed primarily at speed. The need for blemish-free sections of the appropriate thickness is not purely aesthetic as poorly-cut sections may give rise to artefacts serious enough to interfere with interpretation. Pride in the quality of sections obtained should be a guiding principle.

Sections are produced on an instrument called a microtome. Although the mechanical design may differ, all microtomes are of rigid construction with facilities to firmly clamp the tissue block and blade, together with some means of accurate advance of the tissue in relation to the blade, measurable in µm. In the case of paraffin-wax embedded tissue, sections are normally cut at a thickness of 4–5 µm. On occasions thicker sections (10–20 µm) are called for, for example, when attempting to demonstrate certain features of the central nervous system, and on others, thin sections (1–2 µm), especially when examining highly cellular tissue such as lymph nodes.

Microtome knives

Central to the production of good sections is the microtome knife. Microtomy virtually begins and ends with a sharp, blemish-free cutting edge. Ideally, each worker should have a personal knife, jealously guarded. The introduction of disposable blades has made easier the production of good quality, thin sections, but they are often unsatisfactory for sectioning harder tissues, especially bone. As these tissues constitute the greatest challenge to the microtomist, the necessity for maintaining a sharp knife has not been diminished.

Microtome knives for sectioning paraffin-wax embedded tissues are made of steel, and it is with these that we are primarily concerned in this section. Resin-embedded tissue is normally cut using glass knives. The quality and hardness of the steel affects the quality and longevity of the edge obtained. It is possible to buy knives of guaranteed hardness according to the Vicker's scale. The Vicker's Hardness Test (VHN) measures the stress needed to produce plastic flow in brittle materials. The method involves pushing a diamond point into the surface under a standard load. The VHN is calculated by reference to the size of the diamond indentation made in the surface of the material under test. The length, d, of a diagonal between the corners of the rectangular indentation determines the hardness number for a given standard load, P, through the formula

$$VHN = \frac{1.72P}{d^2}$$

Knives are classified according to their shape when viewed in profile, as follows (*Figure 5.1*):

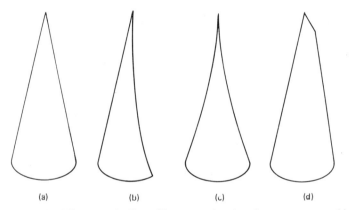

(a)   (b)   (c)   (d)

Figure 5.1 Microtome knife profiles: a=wedge; b=plano-concave; c=biconcave; d=tool edge or D-profile

Wedge

This shape, originally designed for cutting frozen sections, gives great rigidity to the knife and has led to its popular adoption for cutting all types of section on any microtome.

Plano-concave

These knives are used primarily for cutting nitrocellulose-embedded tissues, although even for these purposes they have largely been supplanted by the wedge. Plano-concave knives are available with varying degrees of concavity.

Tool-edge (D-profile)

This design, not dissimilar to a woodworker's chisel (and sometimes called a 'chisel-edge'), is used primarily to section exceptionally hard tissue, such as decalcified dense cortical bone, undecalcified bone and even materials outside the pathology field, such as plastic and wood. These knives are usually stouter than conventional knives to give added rigidity, and the edge may be coated with tungsten-carbide for increased life. They are not particularly suitable for tissue sectioning due to constraints on the angle at which the knife may be set.

Biconcave

This is the classical knife shape introduced by Heiffor and used with the rocking microtome. With the gradual adoption of more substantial microtomes, this knife design has lost popularity. Although relatively easy to sharpen, it is less rigid and prone to more vibration than other knives.

Disposable blades

After repeated attempts over the years, the manufacture of disposable blades has become a reality. Although relatively expensive, disposable blades are available which are at least the equal of a well-sharpened knife. The blade is held in a special holder resembling a microtome knife which is in turn clamped in the microtome in the conventional manner (*Figure 5.2*).

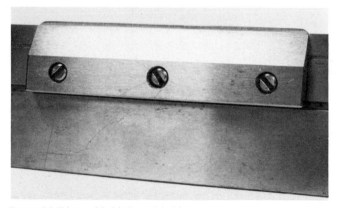

Figure 5.2 Disposable blade and holder

Sharpening microtome knives

Theoretical considerations

Ideally, the cutting edge of a knife would be the straight line formed by the convergence of two planes, the cutting facets, or bevels (*Figure 5.3*). Unfortunately, the internal crystal structure of the metal does not allow this, and the edge is, inevitably, slightly rounded. This feature is defined in terms of the average radius of curvature of the real edge. It should be obvious that the smaller the average radius of curvature, the closer it is to an exact mathematical bevel and therefore the sharper the edge. Using measurements based on the reflection of light by the knife edge when viewed under the microscope, figures of 0.3 and 0.1 µm have been defined as necessary for maximal acuity or sharpness (Kisser, 1927; Von Ardenne, 1939). Such dimensions are close to the limits

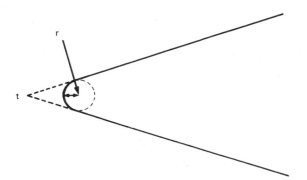

Figure 5.3 Theoretical edge (t, broken line) and actual edge measured by the average radius of curvature (r)

of resolution in the microscope and it is therefore suggested that the knife edge be viewed, edge on, using reflected light at a magnification of × 100. Under these conditions, a barely perceptible and even line of reflected light represents minimal edge curvature.

The production of a fine edge and its durability will depend on the hardness of the metal used, and the angles of the facets (bevels) which meet to form the edge. Carbon or tool steel is usually employed, the cutting edge being tempered for greater strength. For this reason, heat should never be applied to microtome knives. It is widely known that the hardness of the steel in microtome knives varies not only from manufacturers, but also between knives from the same manufacturer. As measured on the Vicker's hardness scale, figures up to at least 900 are attainable for steel knives, 750–800 being most desirable. Softer steel will not maintain an edge and harder steel has a tendency to become more brittle.

Facet bevels have been somewhat arbitrarily fixed and may be found to vary between perhaps 18 and 35 degrees. The width of the two facets which make the cutting edge of the knife may vary and has an influence on sectioning. The angle of bevel is not related to either the rake or clearance angles, as may be seen from *Figure 5.4*. It may be expected that longer facets and a smaller bevel would give rise to a keener edge. However, this thinness of the bevel permits a greater degree of edge 'displacement'. This is a term given to the properties of elastic distortion inherent in the metal and which may be exaggerated in knife edges having narrowly bevelled edges. The consequences of this property are that as the knife is forced through tissue, the edge may be deflected by resistant forces until the limits of its elastic distortion have been reached, whereupon it will return to its original position (*Figure 5.5*).

The rake angle is directly related to the clearance angle (*Figure 5.4*). In practice, a high rake angle gives rise to less compression of the tissue block during sectioning. This may be visualized as a knife laying 'flatter' to the block surface. The largest rake angles obviously require thinly bevelled knives and a very low clearance angle. The constraints of thinly bevelled knives have already been given and low clearance angles demand that the facet opposing the tissue block be kept clean and not allowed to accumulate paraffin-wax debris.

A further consideration is the effect of frictional resistance occuring between the inner facet and the block surface, and the outer facet and the section being cut. It is axiomatic that the facets should be kept well polished to reduce the frictional resistance which would result in compressive strains ahead of the knife edge.

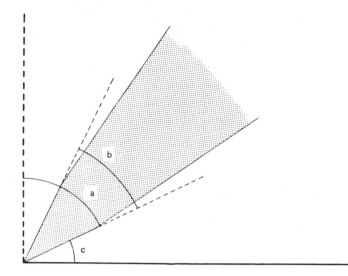

Figure 5.4 Angles associated with the knife edge. (a) rake; (b) bevel; (c) clearance

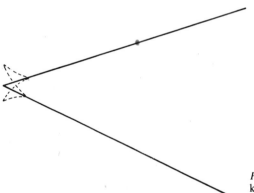

Figure 5.5 Elastic distortion (broken line) at knife edge

Dempster (1942) suggests that there are five factors associated with the use of microtome knives which should concern the user: bevel angle, sharpness or acuity, facet polish, clearance angle and rake angle.

Microtome knife sharpening

The production of a sharp edge may be achieved by manual or automatic procedures. In each case, two stages are involved—abrasive grinding of the facets followed by polishing. Traditionally, the first process is referred to as honing and the second as stropping.

Honing

Naturally occurring slabs of stone with varying abrasive properties and, later, composite slabs of abrasive materials have been used to grind the knife edge. Glass, copper or bronze plates, to which abrasive is added as a superficial slurry, have become increasingly popular in recent years. Stones which have proved suitable include Belgian Black Vein and Arkansas; Aloxite and Carborundum of various grades are examples of composites. In each case they should be lubricated with soapy water or light oil during use.

Glass plates have proved to be most popular for hand sharpening, being readily available, cheap and eminently suitable. To be effective, the surface needs to be roughened so that particles of abrasive adhere to the glass and effect their action on the underside of the knife. After use they are easily cleaned.

Copper and bronze plates are more expensive, but have superior properties. Care has to be taken that the surface, softer than glass, does not become scored by excessively coarse abrasives. They have become almost universally adopted in automatic knife sharpening machines.

Abrasives

The choice of abrasives available is considerable but certain basic principles should be applied to selecting a suitable one. The larger and coarser the particles, the swifter will be the sharpening process. However, large coarse particles are liable to cause nicks in the edge. A compromise has to be reached, therefore, between reasonable speed and a well-polished facet. This is most often achieved by the use of a coarse and fine abrasive in sequence.

Aluminium oxide (alumina)

This is not a particularly hard abrasive, available in a range of particle sizes. The so-called alpha and gamma aluminas are especially suited to final polishing. Aluminium oxide is often graded on a two-figure system, for example, 3/50 or 5/20. The first figure indicates that there are not more than 5% particles present exceeding that size in μm. The second figure indicates the percentage of particles present which are finer than 1 μm. For example, 3/50 indicates less than 5% of the particles are coarser than 3 μm, and that at least 50% are finer than 1 μm. This would be considered a polishing alumina.

Iron oxide (jeweller's rouge)

This is a fine abrasive used in optical grinding. It is only really suitable for polishing.

Silicon carbide

Silicon carbide, available in a wide range of particle sizes, may, with judicious selection of grades, be used for both coarse grinding and polishing. Light oil is the lubricant of choice.

Diamond

Diamond, generally used in paste form, is an exceptionally fine if expensive abrasive. The particles retain their outline better than any other abrasive, and therefore may be used over longer periods. Copper and bronze plates used in automatic sharpeners are deliberately superficially impregnated with diamond particles. The rigidity with which the particles are held in the soft metal surface ensures rapid grinding of the knife facets.

(a)

(b)

Retaining spring

Knife back

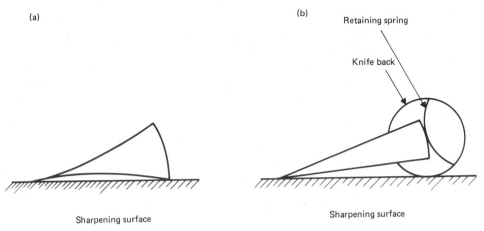

Sharpening surface

Sharpening surface

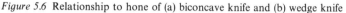

Figure 5.6 Relationship to hone of (a) biconcave knife and (b) wedge knife

Manual method

If a biconcave knife is placed flat on a hone, a natural facet will be formed (*Figure 5.6*). However, wedge profile knives will not produce a facet. For this purpose they are fitted with a 'back' which effectively raises the non-cutting edge up off the hone (*Figure 5.6*). As the back will be ground simultaneously with the edge, it should be reserved for use only with that particular knife. It is useful to mark each knife and its matching back. Chisel-edge knives, though sharpened on one side only, also require a back. It should be noted here that the non-ground edge will require a light polish to remove any metal burrs.

The original Heiffor knife was designed with an integral handle. All other knives have detachable handles that are fitted, via a screw thread, for sharpening purposes only.

■ Method

(1) The home is placed on the bench on a non-skid surface (a damp cloth laid on a shiny bench will usually suffice) since it is essential that it does not move during honing.
(2) A small quantity of light oil or soapy water is applied to the hone and smeared over the surface. If using a glass or metal plate, a sloppy slurry of abrasive is similarly applied.
(3) The knife, complete with handle and backing sheath, is laid on the hone with the cutting edge facing away from the operator (*Figure 5.7a*), and the heel roughly in the centre of the nearest end of the hone.

Correct positioning of the fingers is important during honing to ensure an easy flowing movement, and this is achieved by holding the handle of the knife between the thumb and forefinger with the cutting edge facing away from the operator (so that the thumb is on the back). When the knife is on the hone the tips of the finger and thumb of the other hand (which placed together form a V) rest on the other end of the knife, ensuring an even pressure along the whole edge of the knife during honing. The V prevents the fingers from slipping on the knife when it becomes greasy with the oil; only light pressure is applied during both honing and stropping.

(4) The knife is pushed forward diagonally from heel to toe (*Figure 5.7b*), turned over on its back and moved across the hone until the heel is in the centre with the cutting

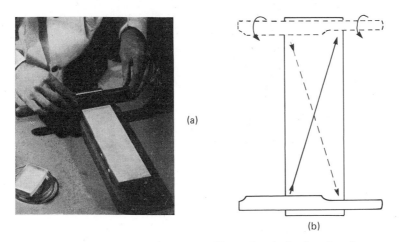

Figure 5.7 Photograph (a) and diagram (b), illustrating the honing of a microtome knife (from *An Introduction to Medical Laboratory Technology*, 2nd Ed. Butterworths, London)

edge leading, and then brought back diagonally. It is then turned over on its back and moved across the hone to its original position, thus completing a figure-of-eight movement. Practice will bring speed of action and a sharp knife, but to aim at speed too early will result in a blunt knife and cut fingers.

(5) The process is continued until all jagged edges have been removed; in the case of a very badly damaged knife both a coarse and fine hone should be used, the larger nicks being removed on the coarse hone and the remainder on the fine hone. The knife is then ready for stropping.

A knife well looked after, never laid on a bench when it should be placed in its box, not used for cutting obviously calcified tissue, will last a competent user for months without honing.

Stropping

Stropping is the process of polishing an already fairly sharp edge; a really blunt knife cannot be sharpened on a strop.

Types of strop   The best strops are made from hide from the rump of the horse, and are usually marked 'shell horse'. Such a strop, properly cared for, will give many years of wear. They may be either flexible (hanging), or rigid.

The type of strop used will depend on personal preference; it is claimed by those who prefer the rigid strop that the hanging strop imparts a rounded edge to the knife, but this fault is generally due to the strop not being held sufficiently taut. The back of the strop is made of canvas and is intended to support the leather during stropping, although most users strop their knives on the back for a dozen or so strokes before using the leather. Strops should be kept soft by working a small quantity of vegetable oil into the back of the leather, and, like hones, they should be kept free from grit and dust. Strop dressings are available which incorporate jeweller's rouge and other mild abrasives, but if used they should be applied sparingly and the surface should not approach the sticky mess that has been observed in laboratories from time to time.

The rigid type may be either a single leather strop stretched over a wooden frame, to give a standard tension, or a block of wood about $12 \times 2 \times 2$ inches in size having a handle at one end, with four grades of leather, or even a soft stone, cemented on each side. The sides of these strops are numbered, and the knife is first stropped on No. 1, then No. 2, and so on, finishing on the finest leather.

Technique   The knife is laid on the near end of the strop with the cutting edge towards the operator (that is to say, in the opposite direction to that used in honing). The knife is held mainly with the forefinger and thumb (as for honing) to facilitate easy rotation at the each of each stroke. The action is the exact opposite to that used in honing, trying to make use of the full length of the strop and stropping evenly the whole of the blade. Care must be exercised in turning the knife over on its back at the end of each stroke to avoid cutting the strop.

Stropping may be necessary between the cutting of each block, or only once or twice a day, depending on the type of tissue being cut.

Automatic knife sharpeners

Completely automatic knife sharpeners have reached the stage of development that they fully justify the capital expense necessary. Two basic designs are available. The most rapid clamps the knife in a vertical position with revolving sharpening wheels grinding the cutting edge. The angle of the bevel may be preset and is reproducible. Although knives may be sharpened very quickly, it requires a little more practice to use successfully than the alternative design. This seeks to simulate the mechanics of hand sharpening, the knife being held horizontally against the surface of a slowly rotating flat plate. After a predetermined number of strokes, the knife is turned over so that the opposite bevel is sharpened. It is possible to accurately preset the bevel angle and the downward pressure exerted on the knife. The plates may be of glass, copper or bronze construction and charged with abrasive as described above. Glass plates need to be roughened or lapped before use and at infrequent intervals thereafter. This roughens the surface and allows the abrasive particles to be held more easily in place. Copper and bronze plates are usually used in conjunction with diamond paste, 6 µm particle size being most appropriate for rough sharpening and 1.0 µm for final polishing. If knives are finally polished on a clean plate using lubricant only, it will often be found that stropping is unnecessary.

Microtomes

Microtomes are mechanical devices for cutting thin uniform slices of tissue—sections. The tissue is supported in its embedding medium—usually paraffin wax, but possibly resin or nitrocellulose—and is normally moved, one step at a time between cuts, by an automatic advance towards the knife. In certain designs, the knife is moved towards the tissue block. In both cases, the amount of the advance is operator determined, most commonly in graduated 1 µm stages. When cutting paraffin-wax embedded tissue, the properties of the wax causes each section to adhere by its edge to the previous one forming a ribbon of sections.

Excluding ultramicrotomes there are five basic types, named according to the mechanism—rocking, rotary, base sledge, sliding and freezing microtomes. Occasionally a microtome may be referred to as a retracting microtome, referring to the withdrawal of the block from the back of the knife on the return stroke. It is essential for the production of resin sections, and usually a feature of rotary microtomes.

The rocking microtome

This instrument is one of the oldest in design, cheap and simple to use. It is also extremely reliable, requiring the very minimum of maintenance (*Figure 5.8*). The knife

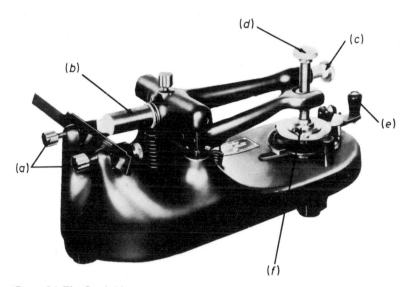

Figure 5.8 The Cambridge rocking microtome: (a) knife clamps; (b) blockholder; (c) tension adjustment; (d) micrometer screw; (e) operating handle; (f) feed mechanism

is fixed and the block of tissue moves through an arc to strike the knife; between strokes the block is moved towards the knife for the required thickness of the sections, by means of a ratchet operated micrometer thread. The name of the microtome derives from the rocking action of the cross-arm.

A disadvantage is that the size of block that can be cut is limited, although designs have been introduced to overcome this. Moreover, since the block moves through an arc when cutting, the sections are cut in a curved plane. This is more of a theoretical than a practical disadvantage unless the block is subsequently to be cut on a different type of microtome. However, rocking microtomes designed to cut perfectly flat sections, the block moving through an arc at right angles to the knife edge, are available.

In view of the lightness of this type of microtome it is advisable either to fit it into a tray which is screwed to the bench, or to place it on a damp cloth to avoid movement during cutting. The movement of the cutting arm should depend on the type of tissue to be cut; normally a steady forward and backward movement of the handle will give ribbons of good sections, but with difficult tissues there are two alternative movements worth trying:

(1) pulling the handle forward and releasing it from this position, allowing the spring to pull it back sharply, or, if this does not produce a good section, or,
(2) pulling the handle forward and letting it back very slowly. One of these methods will usually result in a ribbon of good sections.

The rotary microtome

The rotary microtome is so called because a rotary action of the hand-wheel actuates the cutting movement. The block-holder is mounted on a steel carriage which moves up and down in grooves, and is advanced by a micrometer screw; it therefore cuts perfectly flat sections (*Figure 5.9*).

It has the advantage of being heavier and therefore more stable than the rocking type, and is ideal for cutting serial sections; consequently it is more often used in teaching establishments for cutting large numbers of sections from each block. Larger blocks of tissue may be cut on this machine, and the cutting angle of the knife (tilt of knife) is adjustable. Since a heavier and larger knife is used with this type of microtome there is less likelihood of vibration when cutting exceptionally hard tissue. The first

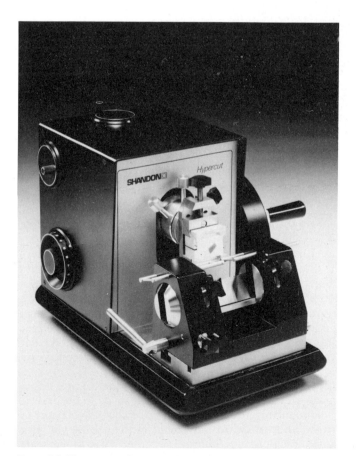

Figure 5.9 The rotary microtome (by courtesy of Shandon Southern Products Ltd)

machine of this type was designed by Professor Minot, and is sometimes known as the Minot Rotary. By using a special holder to set the knife obliquely it may be used for cutting celloidin-embedded sections.

The sledge microtome

Originally designed for cutting sections of very large blocks of tissue (e.g. whole brains), the sledge microtome has become a popular machine for routine use since the Second World War. Within very wide limits the size of the block is of no account. The block-holder is mounted on a steel carriage which slides backwards and forwards on guides against a fixed horizontal knife (*Figure 5.10*). This microtome is heavy and

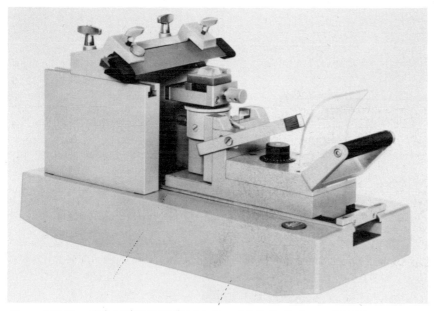

Figure 5.10 Base sledge microtome (by courtesy of E. Leitz (Instruments) Ltd)

consequently very stable and not subject to vibration; the knife used is a large one (24 cm in length) and usually wedge-shaped, which again reduces the possibility of vibration and requires less honing. The knife-holding clamps are adjustable and allow the tilt and the angle (slant) of the knife to the block to be easily set.

A variety of stages is obtainable for use with blocks of various sizes.

A criticism often heard about the routine use of this instrument is that it is very much slower in use than a rocker or rotary microtome: this is true only when a change from one instrument to another is first made for, with practice, sections from routine paraffin blocks can be cut as quickly on the sledge as on any other type of microtome. Moreover, there is no restriction on size when selecting pieces of tissue for sectioning.

Because of the adjustable knife holder, this machine may be used for cutting celloidin sections by setting the knife obliquely, and in some laboratories the knife is left permanently in this position because it is felt that even paraffin-wax embedded sections are more easily cut in this manner.

A freezing stage is available on this machine.

The sliding microtome

In this type, the knife is moved horizontally against a fixed block which is advanced against it up an inclined plane.

The sliding microtome was designed for cutting celloidin-embedded sections, and is probably the best type if sufficient celloidin sections are cut to justify its purchase. It can also be used for paraffin-wax embedded sections.

The freezing microtome

Although other microtomes can be modified for cutting frozen sections, this type (*Figure 5.11*) will give the best results and is used almost universally.

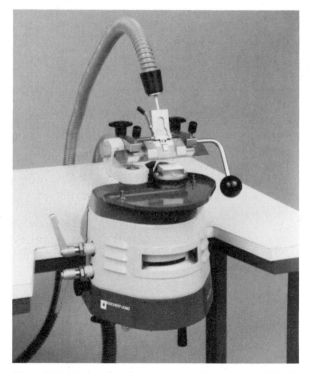

Figure 5.11 Modern freezing microtome (by courtesy of Reichert–Jung (UK) Ltd)

The machine is clamped to the edge of a bench and is connected to a cylinder of CO_2 by means of a specially strengthened flexible metal tube. Some care is necessary with regard to the position of the cylinder for this work: liquid CO_2 must reach the valve in the chuck, therefore ordinary cylinders must be held upside down in a special holder, or blocks placed under them to ensure that

(1) the cylinder valve is the lowest point of the cylinder; and
(2) that the cylinder valve is above the level of the chuck of the microtome.

A special cylinder fitted with a central tube is available and this type may be used in a floor-stand with the valve uppermost, since the pressure inside the cylinder (about 1000 lb/in^2) will force liquid CO_2 up the tube from the bottom of the cylinder. At one time it was advised that a very short tube be used between the cylinder and the microtome, but with the type now available this is not important and the normal length supplied may be used with complete safety. Serious accidents can happen if connexions are made hurriedly, or the machine is dismantled before closing the valve on the cylinder. In practice, the connexions between the cylinder and the machine should be checked before turning on the gas, and the cylinder valve should be opened only during the time of actual cutting.

A knife-freezing attachment is supplied with most machines; that is to say, a separately controlled flow of CO_2 on to the edge of the knife. This is not generally used, but is intended to delay the thawing of the sections on the knife and make it possible to transfer them directly from the knife to slides.

The feed mechanism is similar to that of the other types except that the section thickness gauge is graduated in units of 5 μm instead of 1 μm.

The 'Peltier' effect—freezing tissue with a thermoelectric module

This device enables tissue to be frozen without the necessity of solid carbon dioxide or liquid nitrogen. The method was acquiring popularity before the cryostat became widely used for frozen sections (*see* page 104), and is still usefully employed during freeze-drying (*see* page 46).

If two dissimilar metals are placed in apposition and a direct electric current passed through them, heat is generated on one surface and lost from the other. This is the 'Peltier' effect. The thermomodules used consist of bismuth telluride and copper, laid side by side and connected in series. Direct current applied in one direction generates heat on one surface and it is lost from the other. If the current is reversed, so is the effect. Running water is used to conduct heat away from the warm side. As the temperature achieved is directly related to the current applied, it is possible to regulate it accurately down to at least $-25\,°C$, and much lower with 'cascade' type thermomodules.

In microtomy, water is used to freeze the tissue onto a piece of tissue paper or blotting paper which is in turn placed on the surface of the thermomodule clamped into the microtome block holder.

Vibrating microtome

This instrument has been designed to cut tissue which has not been fixed, processed or frozen. It finds its greatest application in enzyme histochemistry and ultrastructural histochemistry. In the latter case, the sections are subjected to histochemical methods before being further processed for ultramicrotomy.

During sectioning, the tissue is immersed in either water, saline or fixative. It is cut by a vibrating razor blade, at thicknesses generally greater than used for paraffin wax. Generally, tissues are cut at a very slow speed to avoid disintegration.

Microtomy

Paraffin wax

Introduction

There are many factors involved in producing good paraffin-wax sections apart from the inherent characteristics of the tissue. For example, the temperature of the block, knife and atmosphere, humidity, sharpness of the knife, the angles at which it is set and speed of cutting.

Sections of wax which are cut at a relatively high temperature—which will be dependent upon the characteristics of the paraffin wax used—behave in a manner different to those cut at a lower temperature. The knife cuts smoothly through the block, smooth continuous shearing 'flowing' through the wax ahead of the knife, the resultant sections being narrower, or more compressed than cold sections. At the lower temperature, discontinuous shearing occurs. However, as thinner sections are cut, the effect of locally generated heat of friction becomes greater, the relatively poor conductivity of paraffin wax being less critical.

To a large extent, tissues infiltrated with paraffin wax behave in a similar fashion, differences being essentially in the degree of response to the forces applied. Cleavages which may occur in paraffin wax, occur less readily in tissue unless it is particularly brittle, too cold or the rake angle of the knife too small (*see below*). Homogeneous tissue, such as cartilage, does not give rise to cleavages, or tears, the cutting forces being more akin to the smooth plastic shearing. Tough connective tissue may tear, however, and this effect is most noticeable on the block surface. Subsequent sections are difficult to obtain as the underlying tissue is less well supported.

It is possible to minimize some of these less desirable effects. It has already been suggested that infiltrating with a 'soft' wax and embedding in a harder one may bring benefits to the cutting process.

Temperature

In general, blocks of tissue are more easily sectioned if at a lower temperature than that of the atmosphere. Lowering the temperature has the effect of bringing tissues of differing composition to a more uniform consistency, that is, degree of hardness. This in turn helps ensure a uniform cutting process. Most commonly, blocks are cooled by being kept, prior to sectioning, face down on an ice-tray. Although 2–3 minutes should suffice, it is common practice to keep all the blocks to be cut at one session lined up on the ice-tray. It should be remembered that, once removed from the ice, expansion of the block will occur and sections may therefore be somewhat thicker than determined by the microtome setting.

There is a school of thought that moistening the block surface, by pressing a wet tissue against it, facilitates sectioning. There is no doubt that certain tissues, even after paraffin-wax infiltration and embedding, will absorb water. However, laying the blocks on ice, at room temperature, combines both possible benefits.

Particularly difficult blocks may be cooled once in place in the microtome by holding an ice-cube against the surface, or by spraying with an aerosol freezing compound. In the latter instance, the block should be allowed to warm a little before resuming sectioning—expansion may be even greater than usual.

Very occasionally the reverse problem may occur, that is, the surrounding atmosphere may be so cold as to inhibit successful sections. In such cases it may be possible to warm the atmosphere locally, with the aid of a strategically placed Bunsen burner, for example.

Knife angles

Consideration has already been given to the bevel angles of the knife. The other important angles can be set individually on the microtome. Unfortunately, some confusion arises over the terminology of these angles. The authors prefer the terms *rake* and *clearance*. Clearance, sometimes called tilt, refers to the angle formed by a line drawn along the block surface and the lower bevel of the knife. Rake is the angle between the upper bevel of the knife and a line at 90 degrees to the block surface (*see Figure 5.4*). Most microtomes are fitted with a scale to identify one or other of these angles.

In general terms it is true to say that the greater the angle of rake (i.e. the flatter the knife) the more likely is a smooth plastic flow type cutting action. It follows, therefore, that high rake angles are more suitable to softer tissues, and this may need to be reduced to cut tougher or harder tissues.

Slant

This term was commonly used to refer to the relationship of the knife edge to the block when cutting nitrocellulose-embedded tissue on a sliding microtome. Most modern base sledge microtomes have the facility to vary the angle of slant. The advantages of the block meeting the cutting edge of the knife at an angle are that a larger area of the edge is employed and, more importantly, that the resistance to the cutting force is applied more gently. In the authors' experience, the same benefits may be achieved by embedding known hard tissue obliquely in the wax mould (*see Figure 5.12*). In this way, ribbons of sections may still be produced.

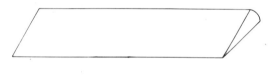

Figure 5.12 Method of embedding tissue (shaded area) to meet knife edge at an angle

Speed of cutting

The optimum speed for cutting sections will vary with the type of tissue being cut. Only experience can show the appropriate rate for a given piece of tissue. However, it is true that soft tissues are usually cut more easily at a slow speed and hard ones a little faster. If sections are cut at too fast a speed, compression will become more marked. If cut too slowly, it is difficult to maintain the rhythmic action required.

Cutting technique

(1) Insert the appropriate knife in the knife-holder and screw it tightly in position; check that the adjustable knife angles are correctly set.
(2) Fix the block in the block-holder of the microtome and ensure it is secure.
(3) Move the block-holder forward or upward, or adjust the feed mechanism until the paraffin wax is almost touching the knife edge. Ensure that the whole surface of the block will move parallel to the edge of the knife, and that the leading edge of the block is parallel to the edge of the knife in order to ensure a straight ribbon of sections.

(4) To trim the excess wax from the block surface and expose the tissue, advance the block either by setting the thickness to about 15 μm or by using the coarse trimming device if fitted. This operation should be performed using an old knife, or one end of a large knife should be kept for trimming. Trimming knives should not be allowed to become too blunt or nicked. Similarly, care should be taken not to trim too coarsely because (a) small biopsies may be lost, (b) the tissue in the block may be torn, giving rise to considerable artefact, (c) unsuspected small foci of calcification may cause tears in the tissue and nicks in the knife.

(5) Once the surface of the tissue has been revealed, return the block to the ice-tray and proceed to trim the next block.

(6) Replace the trimming edge by a sharp one and check it is tightly secured. Reset the thickness gauge. For routine work 4 or 5 μm is recommended. Retract the block-holder.

(7) Insert the block to be cut and tighten securely. Lack of rigidity is one of the most common faults in producing inadequate sections. Bring the block face up until it nearly touches the knife edge.

(8) Begin cutting. When the first section comes off it should be held gently with a fine, moistened brush, or with a pair of fine forceps. Holding the ribbons with the finger is to be discouraged, as not only the section, but also the water-bath may become contaminated with the operator's exfoliated squames.

Between each section it will be found an advantage to breathe on the block, particularly if the tissue is difficult to cut. Successful section cutting is really a set of reflex actions with the breathing regulated to the speed of cutting. If difficulty is experienced in forming a ribbon, it is sometimes overcome by rubbing the leading edge of the block with a finger.

Floating out and mounting sections

During cutting, paraffin-wax embedded sections become slightly compressed and creased. Before being attached to slides these creases must be removed and the section flattened. This is achieved by floating them on warm water.

Water-bath method

Thermostatically-controlled water-baths with the inside coloured black are most popular. Square or rectangular baths are most suitable, especially if serial sections are to be mounted in ribbons on a single slide. The bath should be filled with distilled water, to lessen the formation of air bubbles, and set to a temperature about 10 °C below the melting point of the wax employed.

The ribbon of sections should be gently transferred from the microtome, the free end allowed to touch the water and the remainder of the ribbon dragged slightly across the surface as the whole ribbon is laid down. The number of sections in the ribbon will obviously depend upon the size of the block and dimensions of the water-bath. Individual sections are separated by touching the junction between sections with the end of a pair of flat forceps and allowing them to spring open. This should be done with a kind of pecking motion. Creases in sections may be flattened by a similar movement.

Some workers prefer to lay the ribbon of sections on a piece of black card, cut individual sections from the ribbon with a sharp scalpel blade and float them on the water-bath singly.

Air bubbles which may appear under sections that cannot be discarded, may be removed, with practice, by the following procedure. During trimming, thick sections of wax are cut which curl into a roll. Hold one of these vertically in the end of a pair of forceps and bring the end of the wax roll up under the section to touch the air bubble. The bubble will adhere to the wax roll and come away with it when removed.

Sections which are curled will flatten on the warm water, but they do not flatten with the same plastic change which causes the curl. Cracks occur in the section and are seen especially in tissues such as lymph node, colloid and blood clots. Special effort should be made to prepare sections as flat as possible of these tissues. A useful analogy is to imagine flattening a wood shaving from a plane.

To mount the section, a clean slide is half submerged in the water and brought into contact with one edge of the section. The section should be approached from the side, as a straight on approach will merely push the section away. Once the slide has touched the section, the slide is gently withdrawn, bringing the flattened section with it. The section may be orientated on the wet slide using the edge of the forceps or a dissecting needle. With practice it will be found possible to have the section correctly orientated and positioned on the slide as it is withdrawn from the water. If more than one slide is required, it will be equally possible to have the section on each of identical position and orientation.

The slide should be immediately identified by inscribing the appropriate number on the slide with a diamond pencil. Normal practice is to position the section centrally on the slide; room must always be left for the necessary labels after staining.

The slide should be set either upright or on its side to drain. It is often convenient to place the slides direct into a staining rack. The mounted sections may then be placed in an oven at 50 °C for 1 hour to dry. This ensures the section adheres to the slide, although certain tissues will require the use of a section adhesive (*see below*). The sections are then ready for staining.

In the case of staining machines designed to accept slides singly rather than in batches, special slide holders are provided into which the slides are affixed straight from the water-bath. These staining machines include a special rapid drying area.

Hot-plates

Hot-plates may be used in one of two ways. The slide, complete with section, may be transferred directly to the surface of the hot-plate maintained at a temperature of 55–60 °C and left for 15 minutes. The section should be left face up until the water has evaporated and then turned over to prevent dust settling. Small creases will disappear as the section warms up. Alternatively, a slide is placed on the hot-plate, flooded with distilled water and the section floated directly onto it. When the section is completely flat, the excess water is drained off and the section orientated into the correct position. It is then returned to the hot-plate face down.

Cutting difficult tissue

The vast majority of tissues will cut reasonably well provided they are properly fixed, decalcified if necessary, completely dehydrated, cleared and impregnated with paraffin wax, and if a sharp knife is rigidly held in a properly adjusted microtome. There are rare occasions, however, when in spite of correct technique it will prove difficult, if not impossible, to produce good sections from a piece of tissue such as skin, bone, uterus or tendon. The problems usually occur as alternate sections being thick and thin, only part of the tissue being cut, or the sections being extremely compressed.

These difficulties may be divided into two groups:

(1) where the tissue is exceptionally hard or tough; and
(2) where fragmentation of the tissue occurs as it is cut.

The following techniques may help to overcome these difficulties.

Hard tissue

If ice treatment, resharpening the knife, or decreasing the rake angle fails to overcome the difficulty, the block may be soaked in a softening agent. A solution of 4% phenol may be effective, but Mollifex (British Drug Houses Ltd) has proved most useful in the authors' hands. It is usually sufficient to soak the block for 30–60 minutes, and although the surface will have a soapy consistency after this treatment, sections cut reasonably and stain quite well.

Fragmentation of tissue

If sections tend to break down in spite of the application of ice to the surface of the block—this is most likely to happen when there is a large amount of blood in the tissue—the block should be coated with celloidin between sections. The surface of the block should be wiped dry, and painted with a camel-hair brush which has been dipped in 1% celloidin. After allowing a few seconds for the celloidin to dry a section is cut in the usual way. The process must be repeated for each section.

It must be remembered that when floating the sections to remove the creases, the celloidin layer must be uppermost, and the water should be a little hotter than usual to counteract the effect of the celloidin. The sections are floated on the slides and dried in the usual way. Following drying, the celloidin is removed with equal parts of ether and alcohol before removing the wax with xylol.

Problems with blood clots or lymphoid tissue may be eased by cutting sections at room temperature (i.e. no ice treatment) and by increasing the rake angle.

Serial sections

On special occasions, it is necessary to cut and preserve every section from a piece of tissue, or from a specific area of it. These are called serial sections and meticulous care is required in their preparation. Serial sections may be called for when trying to identify a small ulcer, the presence of malignant cells tracking along a lymphatic or neural sheath, scarce organisms, such as acid-fast bacilli which would make definitive an otherwise equivocal diagnosis, in embryology and in reconstruction studies, to give just a few examples.

Most frequently it is small blocks of tissue that require serial sections in diagnostic pathology. This is fortuitous, as it is possible to mount many sections on the same slide. A 3-mm thick block will produce 750 sections at 4 µm.

Sections are cut in the normal manner, but careful organization is required. Ribbons of sections of a number that will fit on a microscope slide are cut and carefully transferred to a water-bath. When determining the length of the ribbon, remember the size of coverslip available, and that room must be left for a label. If long coverslips are not available, it is possible, with care and practice to use two smaller coverslips laid next to each other. The ribbon of sections should be mounted, in its entirety, onto a single slide from the water-bath. Convention dictates that the first section be at the top of the slide. If the tissue block is small enough, it is often possible to mount two ribbons on a slide, side by side. In such cases, the first cut section should be at the top left of the slide and the last at bottom right. Lifting sections from the water-bath is a slightly different operation, and it is here that the benefit of a straight-walled water-bath is appreciated. The slide should be held, not by the top, but by one edge and the ribbon pushed against the side of the water-bath, the slide brought into contact with the ribbon lengthways, and slowly withdrawn from the water. With the first ribbon safely mounted, along one side, the second ribbon may now be cut and mounted on the free side, remembering that the last section be at the bottom right-hand corner. The slides should be identified chronologically.

The block should be withdrawn slightly from the knife edge to avoid a thick section, due to expansion, being cut at the beginning of the next ribbon. It may be necessary to apply an ice-cube to the block face for 1 minute or so between ribbons.

Some workers prefer to cut many ribbons and arrange them on black paper before separating the appropriate number with a scalpel blade, floating out and mounting. The inherent dangers of a draught disrupting the arrangement does not commend it. If mounting two ribbons on a single slide, however, it should be possible to cut a ribbon twice the desired length, float on water and separate into two equal ribbons. Great concentration is required to ensure that these are then correctly mounted. Sometimes the term serial section is used when serial sections are cut but only perhaps every tenth section stained, the rest being kept either in ribbons in boxes or mounted unstained on slides.

In clinical practice it is sometimes possible to avoid the tedious preparation of serial sections and provide what have been variously called semi-serial, step, cut down or

Table 5.1 Faults in paraffin section cutting

Fault	Reason and remedy
(1) Sections scored (or cut) vertically.	(a) Knife edge is damaged (has small nicks in it) and needs sharpening.
	(b) Knife is dirty and needs cleaning.
	(c) Calcium salts in tissue.
(2) Sections curl or 'roll up'.	(a) Knife is blunt.
	(b) Tilt of knife is too great.
(3) Sections are alternately thick and thin, or each have thick and thin zones ('chatters').	(a) Microtome adjusting screws need tightening.
	(b) Tissue is very hard and needs treatment with a softening agent.
	(c) Tilt of knife is too great.
(4) Sections crumble on cutting.	(a) Knife is blunt.
	(b) Wax is too soft and needs ice applied to its cutting surface.
	(c) Wax is crystallized due to slow cooling, or contamination with water or clearing agent.
(5) Ribbon of sections curved.	(a) Block edges are not parallel to each other.
	(b) Block edges are not parallel to the knife edge.
(6) The breadth of sections is less than the breadth of the block and, consequently, creases cannot be removed without splitting the surrounding wax.	Caused by compression of the block; this is due to:
	(a) loss of bevel on the knife which needs to be honed to restore it;
	(b) wax too soft;
	(c) blunt knife.

Note: Almost all the faults encountered in cutting paraffin sections are due to either: (a) a blunt or damaged knife edge; or (b) the block or knife are not being held sufficiently firm by the adjusting or locking screws. An experienced microtomist therefore avoids most of these faults by double checking both (a) and (b) before commencing the cutting of sections.

levels. This is in effect a compromise, various amounts of tissue—say 50 or 100 μm—being discarded between the sections that are mounted. It is advantageous to keep a single section on a slide from random levels in such cases; these may be used for special stains if required. Unstained paraffin-wax sections may be kept indefinitely without deterioration provided they are protected from surface damage, and heat.

Section adhesives

Provided the sections have been thoroughly dried on the slides an adhesive is not necessary in the case of routine haematoxylin and eosin and many other stains; it is essential, however, for techniques which employ strongly alkaline solutions such as ammonia, for tissue that has been in chrome salts for long periods, for central nervous tissue and for decalcified tissue. Brain (1974, personal communication) has suggested that sections from decalcified tissue remain on the slide if particular care is taken to ensure the final absolute alcohol used in processing the tissue is totally water free.

For sections from ester or polyester-wax embedded tissue, adhesives are virtually mandatory.

Albumen

Widely available commercially, egg albumen adhesive is simple to prepare. Equal parts of glycerin, distilled water and the white of an egg are mixed and filtered through coarse filter paper. A crystal of thymol is added to inhibit the growth of moulds, and the solution kept in a refrigerator. In use, a small quantity of the solution is lightly smeared over the surface of the slide immediately before mounting sections from the water-bath. Sections are dried in the usual manner. If the albumen is clear and free of growth, there should be little background staining.

Gelatin

This may be used as a 0.5% solution in distilled water in the same way as glycerin albumen. It also is liable to contamination by moulds and needs to be melted with gentle heat before use.

Drury and Wallington (1980) recommend the addition of 0.002% gelatin and 0.002% potassium dichromate to the floating out bath. Fresh adhesive and water should be used daily and the water surface cleaned frequently in use.

Chrome gelatin is a more satisfactory adhesive, but may take up slightly more stain. Clean slides, and chromic acid cleaning may be necessary*, are dipped in a solution of 0.1% chrome alum in 1% aqueous gelatin, drained and allowed to dry in a dust-free atmosphere. They are then used as required.

Araldite

This epoxy resin is perhaps the most successful adhesive. Clean slides are coated with a 1 in 10 dilution of the resin in acetone immediately before use. As the section dries the resin polymerizes forming a rigid bond between tissue and slide. Many dyes give more intense staining when this adhesive is used.

* Chromic acid: dissolve 100 g potassium dichromate in 1000 ml distilled water and very slowly add 100 ml concentrated sulphuric acid. Stir continuously whilst adding the acid. Leave slides in this solution overnight then wash well in running water. Rinse in distilled water.

Starch

Although a successful adhesive, starch has lost popularity due to its staining reactivity with many dyes. As it is a carbohydrate, its use in many techniques, for example, the PAS reaction, is precluded.

The finger should never be used to smear adhesive on slides; contamination with squames is a common result.

Cutting of celloidin-embedded sections

The wet method

The vast majority of celloidin-embedded sections are cut by the wet method and it should therefore be regarded as the standard technique. The sections are best cut on a sliding microtome, but the ordinary sledge microtome does almost as well, and a rotary microtome may be used, with a special attachment to hold the knife obliquely.

The block, knife and sections have to be kept 'wet' throughout with 70% alcohol. A camel-hair brush dipped in the alcohol is used to wet the knife and block between each section and to remove sections from the knife. If they are not to be stained immediately they should be put into a glass-stoppered or screw-capped bottle containing 70% alcohol.

Technique

(1) The block together with the embedded tissue is fixed in the block-holder of the microtome.
(2) The feed mechanism on the microtome should be turned back as far as possible.
(3) A plano-concave knife is fixed in the knife-holders with only a very slight tilt and set obliquely to the edge of the block (an angle of 30–40 degrees). The screws holding the knife are tightened to clamp it securely.
(4) Move the block-holder, or knife, depending on the type of microtome used, and adjust the feed mechanism until the celloidin block is almost touching the knife. With the adjustments on the microtome, ensure that the whole surface of the block will move parallel to the cutting edge of the knife; thoroughly tighten the adjustments.
(5) Set the section-thickness gauge at about 15 µm. By means of the camel-hair brush flood the surface of the block and the knife with 70% alcohol and operate the microtome until complete sections of the tissue are being cut.
(6) Adjust the section-thickness gauge to an appropriate thickness; celloidin-embedded sections cannot be cut as thinly as paraffin-wax embedded sections, and although with care sections of 8–10 µm can be cut, for routine work the gauge should be set at 12–15 µm.
(7) Flood the surface of the block and the knife with 70% alcohol and operate the microtome slowly; the section so cut will slide up on the knife blade. Some workers prefer to use a jerking action to cut celloidin-embedded sections, while others find that better sections are produced by cutting halfway through the block, moving the knife or block back a little, then going forward to complete the cutting of the section. A slow smooth action is better, but if any difficulty is encountered either or both of the other techniques are employed.
(8) The section is removed from the knife either with the brush or with a pair of fine forceps, and placed in 70% alcohol in the prepared container. An alternative

method, particularly useful for serial sections, is to prepare beforehand small squares or oblongs of tissue paper a little larger than the sections, numbered with Indian ink if serial sections are required (every tenth piece numbered will suffice); when such a piece of paper is dropped on to the wet section it will adhere to it, and the paper is placed with forceps in the container where subsequent sections will form a pile, all in order. The sections are easily detached from the paper in 70% alcohol.

The dry method (*see* page 71)

Sections are cut as described in the previous section, but without keeping the block and the knife wet with alcohol. The sections must, however, be stored in 70% alcohol.

Serial sections

Ribbons of celloidin-embedded sections cannot be cut, therefore successive sections must be cut and stored in order of cutting; this is best done as detailed above using tissue paper; an alternative method is to mark the number of the section each time on the face of the block with Indian ink, after wiping it free of alcohol. The method of staining celloidin serial sections is given on page 141.

Fixing celloidin-embedded sections on slides

Celloidin-embedded sections are generally, and more satisfactorily, stained by carrying them loose through the staining reagents, and attaching them to slides immediately before mounting. Should a method of staining on the slide be preferred a section may be attached in the following manner:

(1) Transfer the section from 70 to 95% alcohol for 1–2 minutes.
(2) Float it on a slide, and orientate in the correct position, allowing to drain for a few seconds to remove the excess alcohol; if necessary blot lightly to flatten the section, but do not let the section dry.
(3) Pour ether vapour over the sections, taking care that only vapour is poured and not the liquid ether. This will partially dissolve the celloidin and cause it to adhere to the slide.
(4) Place the slide in 80% alcohol for 5 minutes to harden the celloidin, and finally in running tap-water for 10 minutes. The section is now ready for staining.

Frozen sections

Tissue may be frozen and sections cut on a freezing microtome. This technique is useful for two special purposes:

(1) the demonstration of fats, lipids and special tissue components; and
(2) for the rapid preparation of sections for diagnostic purposes.

Fats are removed from tissue during the normal process of paraffin or celloidin embedding, but not by the frozen section technique. There is usually no urgency for either paraffin- or celloidin-embedded sections and tissue may be fixed for the optimal time.

The preparation of a routine paraffin- or celloidin-embedded section (using an automatic tissue processor) takes about 24 hours, and the shortest time in which it can possibly be prepared is about $1\frac{1}{2}$–2 hours. If the tissue is sectioned while frozen, sections may be cut and stained and ready for examination within 5–15 minutes of receipt in the laboratory. These sections are not as satisfactory as paraffin-embedded sections for critical examination, but when examined by an experienced observer they enable a rapid diagnosis to be made.

Fixation

Formal–saline

If the utmost speed is required it is possible to cut sections of frozen unfixed tissue, and in some institutes biopsies from the operating theatre for immediate diagnosis are cut unfixed as a routine. A short period of fixation before freezing, however, makes section cutting easier and usually yields better sections; this is particularly so in the case of tissue containing much fat or mucin, of which it is difficult to cut good frozen sections even when properly fixed.

Small pieces of such tissue should be immersed into preheated 10% formal–saline for 10 minutes at 60 °C, which will have a hardening and stabilizing effect on them. Another technique which has been used with success is to drop small pieces of tissue in boiling formal–saline, leave for 5 minutes, then section in the usual way. The former technique is preferred for any rapid frozen section if time will allow.

The fixative of choice for frozen sections is 10% formal–saline; it gives a consistency to the tissue which is ideal for this technique, and does not interfere with its rapid freezing. Some textbooks advocate the washing of formalin-fixed tissue in running water before sectioning, but the writer has not found this to be necessary; there appears to be no difference between comparable sections from washed and unwashed formalin-fixed tissue. Tissue which has been fixed routinely in formal–saline may be transferred directly to the stage of a freezing microtome.

Fixatives containing mercuric chloride

These tend to make sectioning difficult because of their over-hardening effect. Thin tissue so fixed should be put into iodine alcohol for 30 minutes, followed by sodium thiosulphate for 15 minutes, then washed in running water for several hours.

Chrome–osmium fixatives

These tend to over-harden the tissue, and generally make sectioning almost impossible. Such tissue should be washed overnight in water, and soaked in gum syrup solution for 2–3 hours before sectioning.

Alcohol-containing fixatives

Alcohol inhibits freezing and tissue so fixed must, therefore, be well washed—overnight if possible—before sectioning.

Friable sections

Friable material should be embedded in gelatin (page 68).

Gum syrup

Immersing the tissue in a thick aqueous solution of gum arabic or gum syrup for 1–2 hours prior to cutting is thought by some workers to make sectioning easier; when such tissue is frozen, instead of solid ice forming in and around the tissue, the gum imparts a hard, rubbery consistency. It is recommended that tissue be pretreated with gum syrup for 1 minute, and that it be used on the microtome stage to support the tissue; the tissue is slightly easier to cut than when using water. It should be remembered, however, that many institutes use water routinely to get first-class results.

Cutting of sections

(1) Set up the microtome and CO_2 cylinder as described on page 90.
(2) Check the connexions between the CO_2 cylinder and the microtome, and ensure that there is no leak. Open the cylinder valve and lift the CO_2 operating lever on the microtome to ensure the gas is flowing freely.
(3) If gum syrup is to be used, apply a coating with a brush to the microtome stage and place the tissue in the desired position; some workers prefer the knife edge to cut obliquely (from one corner of the tissue), but unless the tissue is difficult to cut this is not of as much importance as in celloidin section cutting. A piece of filter paper, soaked in water, should be laid on the stage to hold the tissue in position during cutting.
(4) Clamp the knife in position and rack up the stage by means of the coarse adjustment at the bottom of the microtome until the upper surface of the tissue is almost level with the edge of the knife.
(5) Lift the CO_2 control lever for short bursts of 1–2 seconds with a pause of 3–4 seconds between each; when the gum or water on the stage is frozen (it turns white) apply more gum or water with the brush and build it up around the side of the tissue. Using gum syrup, this building-up process is continued until the tissue is completely surrounded to a thickness of $\frac{1}{8}$ inch, but with water it is advisable only to build a base to support the tissue during cutting. The brush should not be allowed to touch the frozen material or it will adhere. Continue freezing until the tissue is quite hard.
(6) Ensuring that the knife is well clear, rub the top surface of the tissue with the finger until it has a firm rubbery consistency—this must be judged in the light of experience. Set the section-thickness gauge at 20 μm and operate the microtome until complete sections are being cut.
(7) Set the section-thickness gauge at the appropriate mark; for routine diagnosis sections may be cut at 8–10 μm, while for fat staining 15 μm is the normal setting.
(8) In operating the microtome some workers prefer to catapult the sections forward with a jerky cutting action, and to catch them in a bowl of water held down on the front left of the microtome; others, with the tissue a little softer, collect the sections from the blade of the knife with a wet brush, or finger, and put them into a jar of water.

Fixing sections on slides

While many techniques are carried out by floating frozen sections through the various reagents and floating on slides immediately before mounting for rapid diagnosis and routine haematoxylin and eosin staining, the mounting of sections on slides before staining is recommended.

Floating on slides

Floating on slides may be done by orientating the section in a dish of clean water, inserting a slide beneath it and slowly withdrawing the slide even if a few creases are present (the section must not be twisted). Allow the excess water to drain off, then put the slide back in the water so that only one half of the section is submerged or floating; the creases are then easily removed and the slide taken out. The excess water is drained off, the slide reversed and the other half of the section is freed of creases.

An alternative method is to transfer sections with a glass hockey stick (a thin glass rod, the last 2 cm of which have been bent at right angles) to a small container of 70% alcohol for a few seconds, and then transfer them to the dish of water. The difference in surface tension between the two fluids will cause the section to flatten on the surface of the water for a few seconds (after which it slowly sinks), when it may be quickly transferred to the surface of a clean slide.

A method of floating and fixing frozen sections on slides for rapid diagnosis has been devised by J. F. Wilson (unpublished) and is as follows:

(1) Pieces of fine filter paper are cut slightly larger than the sections to be mounted.
(2) The sections are placed in 70% alcohol for a few seconds and then transferred to a dish of clean water. The dish must be at least 9 inches in diameter otherwise the filter paper will sink.
(3) The sections will flatten on the surface of the water, and if any creases are present they should be put back to the 70% alcohol for a few seconds and then returned to the water.
(4) With a pair of fine forceps lightly place a filter paper square or oblong on the section, and hold a starched or albuminized slide (page 98) in the water close to the section. By a gentle pushing motion the section with its filter paper covering is brought in contact with the slide, which is then withdrawn. The filter paper and the section should, of course, be in the centre of the slide. Ensure that the section is beneath the paper, it occasionally sinks while the paper is still floating.
(5) The slide is then blotted firmly between filter paper and held over a Bunsen flame for a second; when the filter paper becomes white it is easily removed from the slide without damaging the section. Although such heating is theoretically bad it has not, using formal-fixed tissue, produced any gross artefacts. Sections so fixed to slides are very secure and will withstand quite rigorous treatment.

Attachment to slides

There are three basic methods of fixing frozen sections to slides in addition to the one described above. These involve using:

(1) albuminized slides;
(2) gelatinized slides; and
(3) celloidinization.

Albuminized slides

Sections are floated on to prepared slides and the excess water is drained off without allowing the section to dry. It is then blotted gently but firmly with fine filter paper and a mixture of equal parts of clove and aniline oil is poured on the slide and allowed to remain for 3 minutes to coagulate the albumin. Xylol is then poured on the slide, followed by alcohol, and the section may be stained in the usual way.

Gelatinized slides

These are clean, grease-free slides having a thin layer of glycerin jelly spread on the surface; the jelly is melted in hot water, a drop placed on one end of the slide and spread over the whole surface with the edge of another slide. Such slides should be dried in an incubator and stored in a dust-free container. In use the section is floated on to a prepared slide and the excess water is drained off before being placed into a covered glass container (Coplin jar), at the bottom of which is put a piece of cotton-wool soaked in formalin. The formalin converts the gelatin to an irreversible gel which holds the section in position. After 30 minutes the section is washed in running water for 10 minutes and is then ready for staining.

Celloidinization

The section, having been floated on to a clean, grease-free slide, is drained of excess water and blotted gently but firmly with fine filter paper. Fresh filter paper is then laid on the section to which is added a few drops of alcohol, and the section blotted with the alcohol-soaked paper. The slide is then transferred to a container of 1% celloidin, left for 5 minutes and, after wiping the back, transferred to 70% alcohol for 10 minutes to harden the celloidin.

   The section is then ready for staining, the times of which should be increased slightly. After staining, the celloidin should be removed by immersion in equal parts of alcohol and ether, or by blotting with alcohol-soaked filter paper. The latter is more rapid, but there is a risk in that the section may adhere to the blotting paper.

Cryostat-cut sections

The introduction of fluorescent antibody staining techniques by Coons, Creech and Jones in 1941 led to a need for thin sections (3–5 μm) of fresh frozen tissue free of ice crystal defects.

   To satisfy these criteria such tissue must be quick frozen at a very low temperature (Quenching *see* page 46), and sections cut without allowing the tissue to thaw.

   In addition to being suitable for fluorescent antibody staining, such sections are ideal for many histochemical techniques, particularly enzyme methods.

   Indeed, the appeal and potential application of cryostat sections led to the widespread acquisition of cryostats by the majority of pathology laboratories. The easy production of 'frozen' sections using this apparatus quickly led to its adoption for whenever these were required, including rapid diagnosis. The cryostat has largely been responsible for the demise of the freezing microtome except, perhaps, in some areas of neuropathology. This in turn has led to a modification of the staining reactions subsequently applied.

   Linderstrom-Lang and Mogensen designed the first cryostat in 1938. Coons and his colleagues redesigned it in 1951 when it was produced commercially by the Harris Refrigeration Company. It consists of a microtome of any type but preferably rustproof, which is enclosed and operated within a deep freeze cabinet. The cabinet is fitted with a double glass window, and a door through which material may be passed in and out.

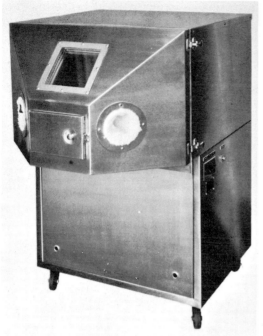

Figure 5.13 Harris Microtome Cryostat

The cabinet is equipped with a fluorescent light and a fan to ensure the circulation of cold air, the latter being controlled by a foot switch to disengage it during the actual cutting of sections.

The temperature may be regulated between -10 and $-40\,°C$.

Later models permit operation of the microtome through an open top giving direct control over the cutting procedure. This unit operates on the 'open top–cold box' principle, and the temperature remains constant with the cover open or closed.

The microtome supplied with the unit is an International Minot rotary which is completely rust proof. It is mounted at an angle of 45 degrees which makes for easy manipulation of sections during cutting.

Any cryostat can be used as an alternative to a freezing microtome for rapid sectioning. Some have been designed for this purpose by incorporating an internal Freon quick freeze stage. This stage holds four block-holders which, after the tissue is frozen on them, are transferred to the microtome. Because the sections adhere firmly to warm slides, staining and mounting may be carried out more rapidly.

The cabinet temperature may be varied between -10 and $-20\,°C$. The microtome may be adjusted to cut sections from 2–16 µm, in 2-µm steps.

Cryostat development has now proceeded to a stage where there are machines incorporating large base sledge microtomes capable of cutting frozen sections of whole breasts, rats and even larger animals (*Figure 5.14*). All types of microtome are available in cryostats and facilities exist in many for controlling knife and block temperature individually. Motor drive is a common optional extra and microprocessor control is becoming the norm.

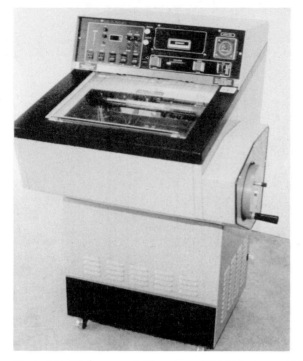

Figure 5.14 Modern cryostat (courtesy of Bright Instrument Co. Ltd)

Operation of the cryostat

The operation of a cryostat calls for only a little practice by a competent microtomist. It is most important that a very sharp knife is used, as the majority of difficulties encountered in cutting are due to the knife not being sufficiently sharp. Disposable blade-holders are becoming available.

Attachment of tissues

Tissues for rapid diagnosis are usually frozen directly on to a metal chuck-holder. Unattached frozen tissue is attached as follows: a small piece of filter paper is placed on the surface of the chuck-holder, a drop of water placed on it with a Pasteur pipette, followed by the tissue. The water freezes almost instantly holding the tissue firmly in place.

Better results can be obtained with some of the commercial solutions, such as OCT (Miles Scientific). These syrupy liquids freeze easily, fix the tissues well to the chuck and may be used to support the tissue by surrounding it with the solution before freezing. OCT is easily cut and does not interfere with the section on the slide or subsequent staining. If a cork disc is used between the tissue and the metal chuck, this may be removed with the tissue intact for storage. Orientation is then easier if the block has to be recut. OCT may be used as the adhesive.

Temperature of cabinet

For the cutting of thin sections of most tissues this should be kept at -15 and -20 °C. Thick sections (30–40 μm) of brain, and so on, will tend to crumble unless the temperature is raised to -5 °C.

Cutting

Ideally, a knife should be reserved exclusively for cryotomy, and kept permanently in the cabinet. Otherwise, the knife must be cooled to the working temperature of the cryostat.

An essential feature of the cryostat is the antiroll plate. This device prevents the section from rolling up on the knife edge as it is cut. With the antiroll plate in position, the section slides between it and the knife, remaining flat. Made of glass or plastic, the adjustment of the antiroll plate is critical. The space between plate and knife must be set within narrow limits, achieved by fixing adhesive tape to either edge of the plate and then positioning the plate against the face of the knife (*Figure 5.15*). The top of the plate should project about 0.5 mm above the cutting edge of the knife and parallel to it. Until this device is correctly positioned, successful cryotomy is impossible.

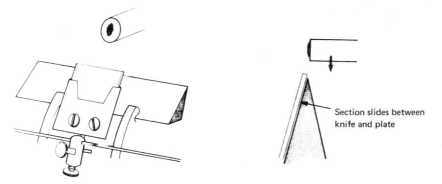

Section slides between knife and plate

Figure 5.15 Diagrammatic representation to show position and function of the cryostat anti-roll plate

When the section is cut the antiroll plate is swung back and the section picked up. The edge of the knife and corresponding edge of the plate should be kept scrupulously clean; a long-handled bristle brush is ideal for this purpose.

As with conventional microtomy, the optimum cutting speed will be determined by experience. It is generally true to say that with the cryostat, a faster stroke is better. The tissue should be orientated so that its shortest axis meets the knife first and it is cut along its length rather than breadth.

Handling of sections

Sections may be attached directly to warm slides or coverslips (at room temperature) by simply touching the slide (or coverslip) against the section. When the section is air-dried, it will remain on the slide throughout most staining techniques. Coverslips may be held by a suction device, a rubber suction disc connected through a metal or plastic tube with a rubber bulb; a light touch on the bulb being sufficient to pick up or release the coverslip.

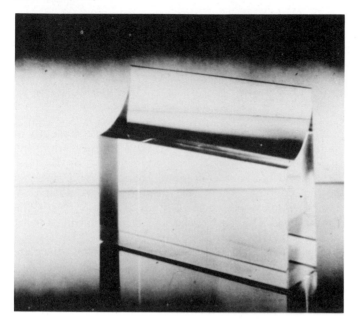

Figure 5.16 Glass 'Ralph' knife. The curve leading up to the cutting edge is exaggerated for the purpose of this illustration

Sections should be air-dried for 5 minutes before being placed directly into a substrate, or into a fixative. Slides with attached sections may be fixed either before or after air-drying.

For rapid diagnosis, sections are usually air-dried, fixed for 1 minute in acetic alcohol and stained with Polychrome methylene blue or any of the techniques detailed on page 144. This technique results in a section which is superior in most respects to that produced by the standard freezing technique.

For fluorescent antibody techniques sections are used either directly after air-drying on slides or following post-fixation in 95% alcohol after air-drying.

Notes

(1) Blocks of tissue should not be left in the cryostat cabinet for more than a few hours. With longer periods, the tissue is liable to 'freeze-dry' and become impossible to cut. They should be stored in an air-tight container with an ice-cube included.
(2) It is difficult to affix formal-fixed tissue to the chuck. It may be a little easier if the tissue is *well* washed in running water first. Remember the possible effects of water on tissue constituents. The methylene bridges formed between formalin and protein are to some extent reversible, and other constituents may not have been fixed.

Cutting resin sections

In the previous chapter it was indicated that resin sections fall into three groups:

(1) approximately 50 nm for electron microscopy;
(2) 0.5–2.0 μm for fine detail with the light microscope;
(3) 10 μm for the study of undecalcified bone.

This section is concerned only with 0.5–2.0 µm sections, referred to as semithin or plastic sections: the others are dealt with in the appropriate chapters.

Semithin sections may be cut on conventional microtomes using conventional knives. However, such an achievement will be marked by considerable patience and no little skill. Owing much to the development of methods applied to ultramicrotomy, special microtomes and knives have made the production of semithin resin sections much easier. Foremost amongst these was the 'Ralph' knife (Bennett *et al.*, 1976), the fractured edge of a strip of plate glass being used for cutting (*Figure 5.16*). The favoured microtomes are of the rotary type, the block being retracted from the back of the knife face on the return stroke.

A slow, steady cutting stroke is essential and best provided via a variable speed motor. As the section is cut, it is held by a pair of fine forceps and dropped onto a bowl of cold water, whereupon it will flatten. The section may then be picked up on a microscope slide in a manner similar to paraffin-wax sections. The section should be dried in an oven or on a hot-plate prior to staining.

References

BENNETT, H. S., WYRICH, A. D., LEE, S. W. and McNEIL, J. H. (1976). Science and art in preparing tissues embedded in plastic for light microscopy, with special reference to glycol methacrylate, glass knives and simple stains. *Stain Technol.*, **51**, 71–97

COONS, A. H., CREECH, H. J. and JONES, R. N. (1941). Immunological properties of an antibody containing a fluorescent group. *Proc. Soc. Exp. Biol. NY*, **47**, 200–202

DEMPSTER, W. T. (1942). The mechanics of paraffin sectioning by the microtome. *Anat. Rec.*, **84**, 241–267

DRURY, R. A. B. and WALLINGTON, E. A. (1980). *Carleton's Histological Technique*. Oxford University Press, Oxford, England

KISSER, J. (1927). Methoden zur Bestimmung der Winkelgrössen an Mikrotommessern. *Ztschr. Wiss. Mikrosk.*, **44**, 452–459

VON ARDENNE, M. (1939). Die Kielschnittmethode ein Weg zur Herstellung von Mikrotomschnitten mit weniger als 10^{-8} mm Stärke für elektronenmikroskopische Zweche. *Ztschr. Wiss. Mikr.*, **56**, 8–23

Part III

Staining and impregnation

6

Theoretical

Staining

Biological stains have been used to visualize and identify tissue and cell components for over a century. By and large this practice has been adopted in virtual ignorance of the mechanisms involved. Only when stains have been used as strictly histochemical reagents has any attempt been made to understand the physicochemical reactions between tissue and dye. Perhaps fortunately, this is of little significance when employing stains merely to enhance morphological characteristics. However, some understanding of the principles involved will help the user to employ stains more scientifically and to investigate failures with a degree of wisdom. A full account of biological staining is outside the scope of this book; the enquiring mind is referred to the comprehensive text by Horobin (1982) and to the fertile grounds of the textile industry.

Basic structure of dyes

The early microscopists had available to them only the *natural dyes* extracted from plants and animals. Only carmine and, especially, haematoxylin still have a useful role in the armamentarium of the modern histologist.

 Synthetic dyes are a product of the modern petrochemical industry, although the oft-quoted term 'coal-tar' dyes denotes an origin in the coal-gas industry. All of these dyes have the aromatic hydrocarbon benzene as a central component.

 Benzene has a ring structure that gives it great flexibility (*Figure 6.1a*). As the double bonds are not static, and because of the complexity of many benzene-containing compounds, the structural formula is commonly abbreviated (*Figure 6.1b*). Benzene is not itself coloured, although in ultraviolet light it does have a specific absorption band. Certain chemical groups, if introduced into the benzene ring by substitution, induce a colour to the compound. The groupings are referred to as *chromophores* and the resultant structure as a *chromogen*.

 If two oxygen atoms replace two hydrogen atoms of the benzene ring, the laws of valency are satisfied and a new compound is formed. This is quinone, containing the active chromophore group, —C=C— (*Figure 6.1c*). Other important chromogens are those containing the nitro grouping, —NO$_2$, and the azo coupling, N=N.

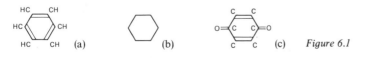

Figure 6.1

113

To turn coloured compounds, chromogens, into stains, it is necessary to introduce ionizing groups, termed *auxochromes*. Only then will the coloured compound stain tissue and be resistant to simple washing.

Production of colour

Colour is seen as a result of the effect of specific electromagnetic waves on the eye. These waves, which have a varying length, will determine the colour that is seen, 'white' light being composed of, or the sum of, all colours of the visible spectrum. This ranges from about 400 to about 700 nm. Ultraviolet light has a wavelength shorter than 400 nm and a higher frequency, whereas infrared light is in excess of 700 nm and of lower frequency. Whilst these two extremes are invisible to the naked eye, both have a role in laboratory medicine (*see*, for example, fluorescent microscopy Chapter 33).

Light rays may be considered as a source of radiant energy, and if a particular wavelength of white light is removed, or absorbed, by a structure, the remaining radiant energy, that is, that transmitted, or reflected, will no longer possess the sum of the visible spectrum and will appear coloured. For example, if white light is allowed to strike a material which absorbs red light, the resultant light, which is seen by the eye, will appear green. The reverse applies, so that if red and green light rays are recombined, in the appropriate proportions, white light will be created. The production of complementary colours should not be confused with monochromatic light, that is, light of a narrow specified wavelength. In this case, a substance is inserted in the light path that will absorb virtually the entire spectrum, permitting only a small, selected wavelength to pass through.

It was stated above that the double valency bonds of the benzene ring are not static; light waves provide the energy necessary to excite the electrons in the molecule, and the bonds to change position. This property is referred to as *resonance*, and the ease with which this can occur in the cyclic configuration of the benzene molecule is the property that makes it the central component of virtually all biologically useful dyes. As the excitement of benzene takes place in the invisible ultraviolet range of the spectrum, special groupings are needed to push the absorption bands into the higher, visible, wavelengths. This is the special property of the chromophores, and it is by the chromophore groupings that dyes are usually classified.

Staining mechanisms

Biological staining is the union between a coloured dye and a tissue substrate which resists simple washing. The union is not usually particularly tenacious, although it may be avid. By appropriate means, dyes may be recovered unadulterated by the union. It is usually agreed that the dyes become adsorbed by the tissue, the mechanisms of which are many, varied and often simultaneous. For this reason, it is unlikely that a single physicochemical reaction can be implicated as the *modus operandi* of biological staining. Certain procedures, such as metallic impregnation, do not fall within the above description and they are discussed at the end of the chapter.

Let us now consider some of the reactions that may occur between dye and tissue.

Electrostatic bonding

Most authors consider the affinity between opposite ionic groups of dye and tissue to play a major role in staining. It is for this reason that dyes are often classified as *acid* or *basic*, reflecting an affinity for basic or acid tissue groupings respectively. For example, eosin is an acid dye with an affinity for the basic protein of cytoplasm whereas methyl green is a basic dye which has an affinity for the phosphate groups of deoxyribonucleic acid of the nucleus. Salt linkage and ionic binding are alternative terms to electrostatic binding; the correct name for the forces involved is *Coulombic attraction*.

Some simple reminders about acids and bases are as follows:

Acids have a negative charge$^{(-)}$. They attach to positive charges$^{(+)}$, especially hydrogen (H^+). In an electrical field they migrate to the anode. They are anions. Tissues carrying a positive charge will attract dyes with a negative charge (i.e. acid dyes); such tissue is therefore referred to as being acidophilic.

Bases have a positive charge$^{(+)}$. They attach to negative charges$^{(-)}$, especially hydroxyl groups (OH^-). They migrate to the cathode. They are cations. Tissues carrying a negative charge will attract dyes of positive charge and are termed basophilic.

Examples of anions (i.e. negatively charged) groups are the phosphates of nucleic acids and the sulphate groups of acid mucopolysaccharides. Cations (i.e. positively charged) include most amino acids such as lysine and arginine.

Although these terms have no direct relevance to pH, increasing the pH of a solution favours the dissociation of negative ionic groups, and hinders the dissociation of cationic or positively charged groups. Decreasing the pH has the opposite effect. They are in balance at the isoelectric point.

Auxochromes which, it will be remembered, give dyes their 'bite', are in fact salts, which, by definition also carry an electrostatic charge. Dyes, therefore, carry an organic, charged moiety and an inorganic salt with an opposite charge. Two further points must be understood to appreciate how tissue staining results from electrostatic binding.

First, when dyes go into solution they ionize or dissociate. Acid dyes provide available anionic or negatively charged ions representing the chromogen, or coloured component, and cationic, or positively charged ions representing the auxochrome, or salt. Similarly, basic dyes have a cationic chromogen and anionic auxochrome. The degree of dissociation is pH dependent.

Second, the reactive tissue groupings will consist of a bound moiety of one charge and an available, or mobile moiety of opposite charge. The tissue dissociates when immersed in the dye bath.

Staining occurs when a chromogen of one charge attracts to the bound tissue moiety of opposite charge. For this concept, Horobin (1982) prefers the more explicit term 'ion exchange'.

In simplistic terms, the reaction may be represented in the staining of basic cytoplasmic protein by the acid dye eosin, as follows:

Tissue		Eosin		Stained tissue		Free salt

$$NH_2^{\oplus}Cl^{\ominus} + Chromogen^{\ominus}Na^{\oplus} = NH_2^{\oplus}Chromogen^{\ominus} + Na^{\oplus}Cl^{\ominus}$$

In other words, an acid dye has a coloured acid radical which attaches to a basic tissue component.

Hydrogen bonding

Strictly speaking, hydrogen, being of single valency, can only bond to one other atom. It can, however, form weak bonds, or at least attractions, to other atoms, usually those of strong electronegative charge. Such bonding occurs naturally in water, the weak bonds being formed between hydrogen and oxygen of adjacent molecules. This characteristic gives water its non-homogeneous molecular structure, with many molecular aggregates present. It has been suggested that hydrogen bonding may be of importance in tissue staining. However, as these bonds are (a) weak, (b) occur readily in water, (c) will occur between the dye and the water it is dissolved in, and (d) the water will also be in competition for hydrogen bonding sites on the tissue, there appears little chance that they are of any significance in aqueous staining.

Hydrogen bonding may be of consequence where alcoholic dye solutions are used. It has, for example, been suggested that Best's carmine stain depends upon hydrogen bonding between carminic acid and hydroxyl groups (which are conspicuously involved in hydrogen bonding) present in glycogen (Horobin and Murgatroyd, 1971). A decrease in staining intensity with increasing water concentration provided the principal evidence for this conclusion.

Van der Waal's forces

These intermolecular forces are polar attractions. They are weak and are effective over a very short distance. As they act over such short distances, the presence of water molecules (e.g. from the dye solvent, or from hydrophilic tissue) may prevent the close contact necessary for van der Waal's forces to be effective.

The attractions are between dipoles, that is, molecules possessing separated positive and negative charges, behaving in a manner similar to magnets. There are, therefore, attractions between positive and negative charges, and a strong dipole may induce a dipole in a neighbouring molecule, provided it is polarizable. Non-symmetrical molecules, if polarizable, will possess stronger dipoles than symmetrical ones.

Although a degree of van der Waal's attractions are to be expected with most dye–tissue interactions, if certain conditions are met these forces may be dominant. Dyes of large, asymmetrical molecular structure in non-aqueous solution will attract to poorly hydrated, strongly polarizable tissue groups.

One example is the staining of elastic fibres by orcein. Orcein is a large molecular weight dye with strong dipoles and used in alcoholic solution. Elastin is a hydrophobic protein with many polarizable amino acids. Although the criteria for effective van der Waal's attractions have been met, it may be noted that these are similar to the prerequisites for hydrogen bonding. Furthermore, if urea, known to be strongly competitive for hydrogen bonding, is included in the dye bath, diminished staining results. Unfortunately, this conflicting sort of evidence is not unusual in biological staining but serves to indicate that in most procedures, a mixture of reactions is involved.

Covalent bonding

In ionic bonding, one element donates an electron from its outer shell to that of another (*Figure 6.2*). The element losing an electron acquires a positive charge as a result and the element gaining an electron, a negative charge. In contrast, covalent bonding involves sharing electrons. As a simple example, in water each of two hydrogen atoms shares an electron with oxygen, and the oxygen atom likewise shares the two hydrogen electrons (*Figure 6.3*).

This type of reaction is a common one, the possibility existing for two atoms to share two, three or more electron pairs, leading to multiple covalent bonds. It would seem, however, that it is in mordant dying processes that it is of greatest significance.

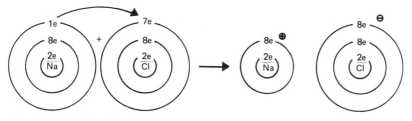

Figure 6.2 Ionic bonding

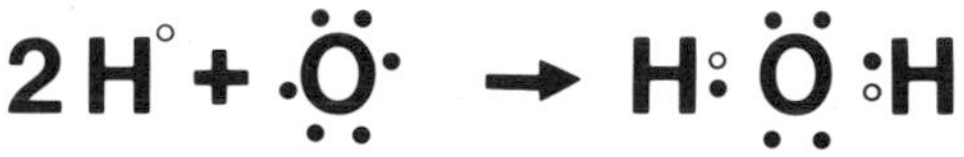

$$2H° + \cdot\ddot{O}\cdot \rightarrow H\colon\ddot{O}\colon H$$

Figure 6.3 Covalent bonding

Each of the four types of reaction outlined above relates to attractions that may occur between the dye in solution and reactive tissue groups. Other influences on staining are *hydrophobic bonding, dye aggregation* and *tissue permeability.*

Hydrophobic bonding

In an attempt to isolate themselves from surrounding water molecules, reactive hydrophobic dye molecules will become bound to reactive hydrophobic tissue groups. Water may be considered to be a structured liquid, hydrophobic dye molecules in the dye bath contributing to this organization by stabilizing groups of water molecules (*see* hydrogen bonding *above*). Spontaneous thermodynamic change towards dis-organization leads to the attraction between dye molecules and tissue groups. This reaction is only possible between dyes in aqueous solution—alcohol in the water will form hydrogen bonds with the water, thus inhibiting hydrophobic effects—and poorly hydrated tissue groups.

Dye aggregation

Dye molecules may have an affinity for each other, often a result of some of the attractive forces outlined above. Dyes which aggregate in solution penetrate or permeate tissues less easily than dispersed dye molecules. However, dyes which aggregate once bound to tissue may bring advantages, as in the case of metachromasia described below, or by becoming resistant to removal from tissue spaces. Factors which increase dye aggregation include large dye molecular size, high concentration and ionic strength and low temperature. Substances which inhibit attractive forces, such as alcohol or urea, will diminish dye aggregation. It is possible to reverse aggregation by dilution or by raising the temperature of the dye bath, or, as in the case of metachromasia, by treatment with alcohol.

Tissue permeability

The physical structure of tissue and consequent effect on the uptake of dyes is amongst the most poorly understood of all the factors known to influence biological staining. Rarely is the biologist confronted with a tissue of homogeneous structure. Some of the purely physical factors which may influence the microscopic appearance of stained tissue sections follow, usually as little more than descriptive fact.

Thick sections will obviously appear more densely stained than thin ones. However, the very term 'density' gives a clue to further variability. Dense tissue, that is, that in which available tissue macromolecules are closely packed, will give rise to more intense staining than loose tissue, where similar molecules are less frequent. The dye tissue bond is more rapidly broken in less dense tissue.

Dye penetration into the tissue is easier with smaller dye molecules than with large ones. However, staining is itself a barrier to further penetration. The degree of penetration will depend also on the permeability or porosity of the tissue. Highly permeable tissues are more easily stained and decolorized than poorly permeable tissue. It is possible to exploit such factors. For example, if two dyes, one of large molecular size and therefore slowly diffusing and the other small and fast diffusing, are applied simultaneously they may stain two tissue components selectively. In van Gieson's stain, both acid fuchsin and picric acid are anionic dyes which selectively differentiate collagen, which is cationic, from other cationic connective tissues. This is because the slowly staining, large molecular dye, acid fuchsin, will, in the time available, react only with collagen fibres, whilst the smaller picric acid will rapidly react with all available tissue sites. Another example is the differential staining of nucleic acids by simultaneous application of methyl green and pyronin. The smaller dye molecules of pyronin more easily penetrates the RNA rich sites in the cytoplasm and nucleoli, leaving methyl green to bind to the more readily available DNA of the nuclear chromatin. The attractive forces responsible for staining with both dyes are ionic bonds.

It is through an understanding of the factors involved in physical dye staining and a knowledge of the tissue structure that dyes suitable for selective demonstration are chosen, rather than by a blind trial with a battery of dyes.

In relatively few specific staining reactions is the mechanism of affinity between dye and tissue group fully understood. Still less frequently is a single attractive force responsible. Usually a mixture of physical and chemical factors are involved, although one may predominate.

Metachromasia

A dye which has the ability to change its colour without changing its chemical structure is said to be metachromatic. A simple indication of this property is to dissolve such a dye in water at low concentration. If the concentration is increased, a colour change occurs. Adding more water reverses the colour change.

The physical changes that bring about this colour change are a specialized, orderly form of dye aggregation. Principally, van der Waal's forces hold dye molecules together to form dimers, trimers or polymers. Other forces implicated are hydrogen bonding and hydrophobic bonding.

The dyes most commonly exhibiting metachromatic properties are those of the thiazine group—thionin, toluidine blue, azur A and azur B. Certain dyes of other groups are also known to be metachromatic, including methyl violet—especially useful for demonstrating amyloid metachromatically—and safranin. Using as an example the thiazine dyes, as they polymerize they undergo a colour shift from blue (monomeric form, absorption maxima 620–630 nm) through purple (dimeric and trimeric, 590 nm) to red (polymeric, 550 nm).

Since metachromasia is enhanced as intermolecular distances are reduced, factors which favour metachromasia are:

(1) increasing concentration of the dye;
(2) decreasing temperature;
(3) aqueous solvent. Water, a polar solvent, contributes to the efficiency of van der Waal's forces by which the molecules are held together;
(4) pH.

Although metachromatic dyes may polymerize in solution, the presence of high charge densities at tissue sites facilitates this process. In tissue groupings where there is a high concentration or density of anions (e.g. SO_4^- in sulphated mucopolysaccharides), cationic dye molecules may be held in such close proximity to one another that van der Waal's forces can exert their influence and cause the dye to polymerize. The consequent colour change from blue to red, discussed above, may now occur. Somewhat confusingly, the term 'metachromatic' may also be applied to the tissue.

If there are small numbers of anionic groups amongst a more widely dispersed area of isolated anions, partial metachromasia may occur, exhibiting a purple coloration. There are two explanations for this phenomenon:

(1) a mixture of blue monomeric dye and red polymerized dye are present, giving a purple coloration; and
(2) the cationic groups are not large enough to permit full polymerization, only dimers and trimers of the dye being formed.

Thus there are three types of metachromasia, which may be tabulated as follows:

Type	Colour	Structure
α alpha (orthochromatic)	Blue	Monomeric (single molecules)
β beta	Purple	Di- and trimeric (aggregates of two and three molecules—or a mixture of α and β);
γ gamma (metachromatic)	Red	Polymeric (long-chain aggregates of molecules)

These colours refer only to the thiazine dyes. Others, such as safranin O, an azine dye, will have different spectral characteristics. There are also useful fluorescent dyes (*see below*) which exhibit metachromasia, the most interesting of which is acridine orange. The orthochromatic form of this dye fluoresces green and the metachromatic form red. Unfortunately, increasing metachromasia is accompanied by decreasing fluorescence as the emission spectrum moves towards the longer wavelengths (Pearse, 1980). Nevertheless this dye has proved popular in the differentiation between DNA, which stains orthochromatically, and RNA, which stains metachromatically.

It has been estimated by Sylven (1954) that the interchange distance necessary for metachromasia (i.e. the distance between anionic tissue groups) is 0.5 nm or less. It is therefore possible for water molecules—dimensions approximately 0.4 nm—to be intercalated between dye molecules. Indeed, water enhances metachromasia, being a polar solvent, and it is generally accepted that, in practical terms, dehydration abolishes most metachromasia. Strongly hydrated tissues, such as cartilage (chondroitin sulphate) and mast cells (heparin) retain metachromasia better than less hydrated tissues such as non-sulphated acid mucopolysaccharides.

Metachromatic staining is sometimes referred to as being dye–dye interaction. This is a somewhat misleading term, suggesting that more than one dye is involved. Dye intermolecular attractions may be more apt.

Leucocompounds

Leuco dyes

Certain chromophore groups have unsatisfied affinities for hydrogen. On reduction, the double carbon bonds of the dye molecule are broken so that it becomes colourless. The prefix *leuco* is then applied. Subsequent oxidation restores the molecule to its former structure and colour. This property has limited value in biological staining. Leuco-methylene blue has proved of value in muscle pathology and leuco-patent blue is useful for the demonstration of haemoglobin peroxidase.

The reaction, using basic fuchsin as an example, is as follows:

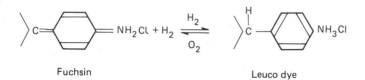

Fuchsin   Leuco dye

Leuco base

These are included because of the confusion that may occur in terminology. A reaction different to that above occurs if the dye is neutralized, that is, if hydroxyl groups replace hydrogen in the reaction. Once again, a reversible reaction occurs, this time producing a compound termed *carbinol*. Although this reaction is of interest as it represents an indicator of pH change, carbinols are of greater interest to dye chemists in that upon dehydration, an anhydride is produced which is a true dye base. Again, basic fuchsin is used as the example:

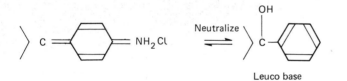

Leuco base

Schiff's reagent

It was for many years believed that dialdehydes were able to recolorize Schiff's reagent. In fact the reaction is more complex, and the coloured reaction product is not simply the result of a reversible action with leuco-fuchsin. The chromophore grouping is broken by sulphurous acid. In the presence of excess SO_2 the aldehydes combine with the colourless derivative to give an unstable aldehyde condensation product. This in turn undergoes molecular rearrangement during hydration to give a coloured end product (*Figure 6.4*).

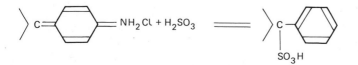

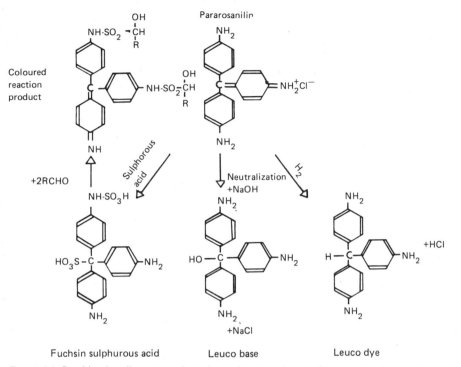

Figure 6.4 Combination diagram to show the various reactions leading to colourless products of basic fuchsin and the coloured reaction product resulting from Schiff's reaction

Fluorescent dyes

When dyes absorb light they are absorbing a form of energy and this excites them, that is, causes vibrational movement. This energy is duly released by the dye molecules, either within itself causing a photochemical reaction which may modify the molecule, or as a form of radiant energy; or as heat. The first alternative may be the cause of colour fading, but it is the second that is the useful property in biological staining.

If light of short wavelength is absorbed, a small amount of energy may be used or lost within the molecule and the remainder emitted as light of longer wavelength. This phenomenon is known as fluorescence. This term is reserved for dyes which absorb in the ultraviolet, or blue violet part of the spectrum (i.e. around 400 nm) and emit above about 500 nm. Dyes which possess this property are termed *fluorochromes.*

There are many dyes which exhibit this characteristic, most of which appear coloured in visible light, for example, eosin, congo red and basic fuchsin. Their fluorescence is of little advantage because they are readily identified, at the same location, in visible light. Other dyes, such as thioflavine T, have little visible colour under normal light, but fluoresce brightly when illuminated by ultraviolet light.

A major advantage of fluorescent dyes is their apparent high sensitivity. This is, in fact, due to the high contrast achieved against the dark background, a feature of fluorescence microscopy. Thus much smaller deposits of stained material are easily seen.

Effects of fixation

In general terms it may be stated that fixation enhances staining. Formaldehyde, for example, reveals reactive tissue groups that may otherwise be buried and inaccessible in the molecular structure of protein. Glutaraldehyde and mercuric chloride have similar effects. As most fixatives employed react with protein, it is the staining of these tissues that is most affected. An illustration of this effect may be demonstrated by comparing fresh frozen sections with mercuric chloride fixed tissue sections following Sudan Black B staining. Lipids present bound to protein, lipoproteins, will be unstained in fresh frozen sections, but modification of the protein groups exposes the lipid to react after fixation.

On occasions, a fixative may be chosen for its particular effect on subsequent staining. Potassium dichromate, for example, is the fixative of choice when myelin is to be demonstrated in central nervous tissue by haematoxylin staining. On the other hand, there are fixatives whose use is contraindicated for the demonstration of certain tissue structures. Formaldehyde blocks or destroys reactive cationic amino groups in nucleic acids which results in reduced staining. Carnoy's fixative is more suitable.

Other fixatives may be chosen for their reactivity with specific substrates resulting in direct visualization. Examples include chromium which forms coloured products by oxidizing catecholamines, osmium tetroxide which blackens lipids and formaldehyde in the vapour form which induces fluorescence in certain amine groups.

Finally, fixatives may enhance, or reduce, the ionic strength of reactive groups, that is, make the tissue more strongly acidic or basic in nature.

Progressive and regressive staining. Differentiation

It should be clear from the above that different tissue groupings will have different affinities for dyes. These differences may be expressed either by the degree to which the dye is taken up by the tissue, that is, stained, by the speed at which this occurs or by the avidity with which the dye is held by the tissue after it has stained.

Progressive staining

Progressive staining exploits the first two characteristics. A tissue section is immersed in a dye bath until such time as only the desired structures are stained. This may be a difficult process to control, especially if possible variables are not kept to a minimum, for example, temperature, section thickness, dye concentration, pH, fixation, etc. It has, however, proved a popular method, particularly if dyes with a reasonable degree of selectivity are used. Mayer's haematoxylin, used for staining cell nuclei, is one example.

Regressive staining

Regressive staining involves overstaining of all tissue structures and then exploiting the different avidities of various tissue groups for the dye. The dye is selectively removed from unwanted tissue groups, either by simple solution, or by reversing some of the factors involved in dye/tissue affinity. This process is termed *differentiation* and it should be noted that the simple reversal of progressive staining is not the only method of differentiation. Oxidizing agents may be employed to decolorize the dye, a mordant (*see below*) may cause a break up of the dye–mordant–tissue complex, acid or alkali may depress or reverse ionic bonding or one dye may be used to replace another of lesser affinity.

Mordants

Strictly, mordant means 'to bite', but the term has also been applied to the method by which goldleaf is affixed to underlying material. In biological staining, the term refers to a substance which acts as an intermediary between dye and tissue. The mordant enters into a chemical combination with the dye and irrespective of whether the original dye is anionic, cationic, amphoteric or uncharged, the resultant combination—*a lake*—is invariably basic in action. One advantage of the dye–mordant–tissue complex is that it is virtually insoluble in most fluids ordinarily used in biological staining, and therefore is little altered by subsequent treatment of the tissue section. The dye and mordant are usually applied simultaneously, although occasionally, as in Heidenhain's haematoxylin method, the mordant may be applied first (*Figure 6.5*). The mordant may be used to differentiate overstained structures.

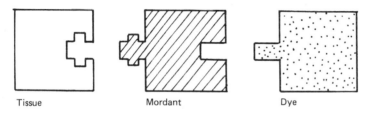

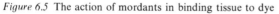

Tissue   Mordant   Dye

Figure 6.5 The action of mordants in binding tissue to dye

The mordants are alums; that is, they are double sulphates with an active, usually trivalent metal such as iron, aluminium or chromium, together with potassium or ammonium as a second cation.

Most frequently, mordants are used with haematoxylins, without which the active derivative, haematein, may be regarded as merely a poor colouring agent, not a dye. Combination with the mordant converts it into a strong, basic dye, the cationic metal binding to both dye and tissue.

Accentuators

Accentuators and accelerators were the names given to a group of substances which, while not acting as mordants and forming lakes with the dyes, or taking part in any obvious chemical union, increase the selectivity or staining power of the dyes which were already capable of staining without the accelerators. Common examples of accentuators are potassium hydroxide in Loeffler's methylene blue, and phenol in carbol thionin and carbol fuchsin. It will be obvious that the effect on staining of this group is due to the change in pH of the staining solution.

Accentuators when used in the impregnation of the nervous system with metallic salts have been called *accelerators*. These are generally hypnotics but the reasons why this should be so is not understood; examples are veronal in Cajal's method for axis cylinders, and chloral hydrate in Cajal's method for motor end-plates.

Direct colour production

One method of identifying tissue groups which does not involve biological staining results from a chemical reaction which produces a coloured end product. The most well known is the Perls reaction in which almost colourless potassium ferrocyanide combines with ferric ions, released from protein by the action of hydrochloric acid, to form the coloured compound potassium ferric ferrocyanide. There are very few such reactions available to the histologist, but this principle is widely utilized to visualize the site of enzyme activity in histochemistry. Here the product of enzymic activity is allowed to react with a substance that produces a coloured precipitate, usually by reduction.

Controls in biological staining

It should be appreciated that many variables can occur in staining, and that the mechanism of staining is a complex one. For these reasons, methods should be standardized as much as possible. Even so many factors over which the laboratory has little control can thwart such good intentions. These include fixation, variation in dye batches and solvents, especially tap-water. Other variables, over which there is control, include temperature, processing procedures, section thickness, pH, dye concentration, etc. It is axiomatic that these latter factors receive meticulous attention. It is not satisfactory to use tap-water if distilled is specified, or to estimate dye concentrations because they are 'only counterstains'.

Since the beginning of biological staining, the value of control sections has been appreciated. Only if sections of known reactivity are stained simultaneously with 'test' sections can any faith be held in the efficacy of the procedure applied. This is particularly so if the presence or absence of some specific component is being determined, for example, haemosiderin, micro-organisms. Every laboratory should strive to maintain a stock of control sections.

It is often possible, particularly with so-called histochemical techniques, to specifically remove and modify chemical groups or tissue components present in sections by chemical or enzymic action. For example, diastase removes glycogen; ribonuclease removes ribonucleic acid; methylation esterifies carboxyl groups making them non-reactive to methods employed for their demonstration and removes sulphate groups; acetylation renders 1:2 glycols non-reactive in the PAS reaction.

It must be remembered that test and control section should be treated as near as possible in an identical manner. If control sections are to be treated with enzymes, for example, the test section should be incubated in the appropriate buffer solution and the remainder of the procedure carried out simultaneously on both sections.

Classification of dyes

The system of dye classification that has found common acceptance is based on the type of chromophore present. Thus whether dyes are natural or synthetic, acid or basic, blue or red becomes a property and not a basis for classification.

Unfortunately, there is still sufficient uncertainty about the purity, total dye content and structural formulas to make biological staining an often capricious science. It is good practice to evaluate the performance of each batch of new dye against controls held by the user's laboratory. Apart from purely visual testing, there are straight-forward investigative techniques that may be useful. Spectrophotometry of dilute alcoholic solutions will establish that the dye under test absorbs at the predicted wavelength, and by comparison with known controls, its relative concentration may be judged. Thin layer chromatography will help detect contamination of the dye with other coloured compounds. The testing procedures of the Biological Stain Commission and the IMLS Dye Approval Scheme encourages confidence in the user of certified dyes that they are satisfactory.

Because dyes are synthesized primarily for the textile industry, a highly competitive and commercial field, confusion has arisen over the nomenclature of dyes. Thus many dyes have been marketed with trade names and with a variety of suffixes. The *Colour Index*, published jointly by the Society of Dyers and Colourists and the American Association of Textile Chemists and Colorists has helped to avoid much of this confusion by publishing preferred names and synonyms as well as assigning a unique number to each dye.

The system of classifying dyes according to the chromophore present has the advantage of grouping together dyes of similar chemical structure. One interesting aspect of this classification is that although all dyes of a group may not be of the same colour, generally, as the dye molecule increases in complexity, so the colour is of a deeper shade. These colours may vary from yellow, through red, to blue and green. For a fuller description of dye classification and testing, the reader is referred to *Conn's Biological Stains* (Lillie, 1977), from which *Table 6.1* is abbreviated.

Table 6.1

Classification			*Examples*
Nitro			Picrid acid. Martius yellow
Azo	Mono azo		Orange G. Chromotrope 2R
	Diazo		Sudan IV. Congo red
Tetrazolium			Auramine O
Aryl methane		Diphenyl methane	Pararosanalin. Crystal violet
		Triaminotriphenyl methane	Pyronin. Rhodamine B
Xanthene	Aminoxanthene		Eosin. Phloxine
	Hydroxymethane		Acridine orange
Acridine			Pinacyanol
Quinoline			Thioflavine T
Thiazol			Neutral red. Safranin
Quinoneimine	Azin		Cresyl violet. Celestin blue
	Oxazin		Thionin. Methylene blue
	Thiazine		Alizarin red S
Anthraquinone			Alcian blue. Luxol fast blue
Phthalocyanins			

Impregnation

Gold, and silver, in particular, may be deposited in the metallic state on certain tissue structures. The techniques are often historical and have been subject to numerous modifications, but still carry the names of early pioneers in microscopy. Most commonly, the salts used are ammoniacal silver nitrate and silver proteinate (protargol S).

Silver is easily reduced by reactive tissue groups, although to a variable degree. In the case of melanin or Kultschitzky cells, for example, the reduction is sufficient to produce visible deposits of metallic silver. Such a reaction is said to be *argentaffin*. Other cells, much of the central nervous system and reticulin fibres, although binding the silver, are not sufficiently reactive to fully reduce the silver to its metallic state. It is believed that submicroscopic silver nuclei, similar to those present on an exposed but undeveloped photographic film, are formed. A second stage of development or reduction is required to help these nuclei grow. Cells and tissue which require the use of an extraneous reducer are termed *argyrophil*.

Although these techniques cannot be considered to be staining—there are no chromophore groups in the reagents—the affinity between the salts and tissue is probably electrostatic. Because of the growth of the silver nuclei during development, structures to which the silver salt has bound often appear larger than they really are. This is particularly useful in identifying fine structures, such as spirochaetes, which are otherwise difficult to visualize.

References

HOROBIN, R. W. (1982). *Histochemistry*. Butterworths, London

HOROBIN, R. W. and MURGATROYD, L. B. (1971). The staining of glycogen with Best's Carmine and similar hydrogen bonding dyes. A mechanistic study. *Histochem. J.*, **3**, 1–9

LILLIE, R. D. (1977). *Conn's Biological Stains*. 9th Ed. Williams and Wilkins, Baltimore

PEARSE, A. G. E. (1980). *Histochemistry, Theoretical and Applied*. 3rd Ed. Vol. 1. Churchill-Livingstone, Edinburgh

SYLVÉN, B. (1954). Metachromatic dye-substrate interactions. *Quart. J. Micr. Sci.*, **95**, 327–358

7

Staining procedure

Preparation of stains

The preparation of stains is a very important basic procedure in histological technique and therefore should not always be left to the most junior member of the staff. Careless preparation, such as inaccurate weighing, the absence of chemical cleanliness, and the use of tap-water instead of distilled water may all lead to great confusion at a later stage; and in those laboratories where a control section is not stained by each new batch of stain as a routine, it may lead to incorrect negative or even positive reactions. During the preparation of any stain or staining reagent the following basic rules should be rigidly adhered to.

(1) All glassware should be thoroughly cleaned and well rinsed in distilled water (of neutral pH) and dried. After drying, a clean cottonwool plug should be inserted to prevent contamination by dust if the receptacle is not to be used immediately.
(2) The correct solvent should be used. Distilled water should be used unless tap-water is specified.
(3) Silver and osmic acid solutions should always be kept in dark bottles, preferably in a cool dark place.
(4) Dilute ammonia used for staining solutions should preferably be freshly prepared, the stock of ammonia being kept in a refrigerator.
(5) Constituents of stains should be dissolved in the order given in the formulas; for example, haematoxylin should always be dissolved in alcohol before the remainder of the constituents are added.
(6) Alcoholic solutions of stains should be kept in glass-stoppered bottles or containers to avoid evaporation of the alcohol and consequent precipitation of the stain.
(7) All dyes used for the demonstration of bacteria should be filtered immediately before use.

Solvents

Water

Water is the most common solvent for stains and, as noted above, distilled water should always be used unless the formula specifies tap-water. The distilled water should be checked periodically to ensure that it is at pH 7.

Table 7.1 Solubility chart

Stain	Water	Alcohol	Stain	Water	Alcohol
Acid fuchsin	18.0	0.3	Methyl orange	0.05	0.01
Alizarin	nil	0.125	Methyl violet 6B	4.2	6.2
Alizarin red S	5.3	0.15	Methylene blue	2.5	1.5
Auramine	0.35	7.0	Night blue	2.25	2.35
Aurantia	1.3	0.3	Nile blue sulphate	1.0	1.0
Azo black	0.3	0.25	Neutral red	3.2	2.0
Basic fuchsin	0.4	7.6	Oil red O[a]		
Bismarck brown	1.2	1.1	Orange G	7.1	0.3
Brilliant cresyl blue	2.2	0.5	Phloxine	39.4	8.0
Brilliant green	3.0	3.3	Picric acid	1.1	8.5
Carminic acid	8.3		Pyronin	11.0	
Congo red	4.5	0.8	Purpurin	nil	0.76
Crystal violet	1.5	7.0	Safranin	6.0	2.5
Eosin–water soluble	40.5	3.5	Scarlet R	nil	0.2
Eosin–alcohol soluble	nil	0.45	Sudan black B	nil	0.23
Erythrosin	11.0	2.0	Sudan II	nil	0.3
Fluorescein	nil	2.1	Sudan III	nil	0.15
Gallamine blue	0.07		Sudan III[b]		
Haematoxylin	1.75	60.0	Sudan IV	nil	0.08
Indigo carmine	1.1		Tartrazine	11.0	0.13
Janus green	5.3	1.1	Tartrazine[c]		
Jenner's stain		1.3	Thionin	0.22	0.23
Light green	18.5	0.85	Toluidine blue	3.1	0.5
Martius yellow (Na)	4.7	0.16	Trypan blue	10.4	
Methyl green	9.2		Uranin (sodium fluorescein)	50	6.0
Methyl blue	10.4		Victoria blue 4R	2.0	18.4

Solubilities, expressed as g/100 ml of solvent, of the more common histological stains in water and ethyl alcohol at room temperature.
[a] Oil red O: 0.1% in isopropyl alcohol.
[b] Sudan III: 0.2% in propylene glycol.
[c] Tartrazine: 2.3% in Cellosolve.
Note: The above figures can only be a guide since batches of stain vary slightly in solubility; room temperature, which varies between 19 and 25 °C, also affects the solubility.

Ethyl alcohol (ethanol)

Alcohol in varying concentrations is a commonly used solvent. When 'alcohol' is specified it should be understood to mean absolute ethyl alcohol unless the context indicates otherwise. Substitutes for alcohol should not be used as a solvent for stains unless experiment has shown that they have no effect on the subsequent staining reaction.

Methyl alcohol (methanol)

Methyl alcohol, usually absolute, is used principally as a solvent for Romanowsky stains for which purpose, it is said, it must be free of acetone.

Acetone

Acetone is used alone or in combination with other fluids.

Phenol

Phenol is used as a 0.5–5.0% aqueous solution.

Buffer tables

The use of buffers as solvents, differentiators or controls is increasingly important in the histological laboratory. A complete range of such buffers is outside the scope of a work such as this, and students who wish to study the subject more deeply, or who want a special buffer, are referred to a standard chemical textbook. In the following pages details are given of the more useful and commonly used buffers. *Table 7.2* lists the chemicals used in their preparation.

Table 7.2 Molecular weights of reagents commonly used in buffer solutions

Reagent	Molecular weight
Acetic acid—$CH_3.COOH$	60.03
Borax (sodium tetraborate)—$Na_2B_7O_7.10 H_2O$	381.43
Boric acid—$B(OH)_3$	61.84
Citric acid (anhydrous)—$C_3H_4(OH)(COOH)_3$	192.12
Citric acid crystals—$C_3H_4(OH)(COOH)_3.H_2O$	210.14
Glycine—NH_2CH_2COOH	75.07
Hydrochloric acid—HCl	36.465
Potassium acid phosphate (potassium dihydrogen phosphate)—KH_2PO_4	136.09
Potassium hydroxide—KOH	56.104
Sodium acetate (anhydrous)—CH_3COONa	82.04
Sodium acetate crystals—$CH_3COONa.3 H_2O$	136.09
Sodium acid phosphate (sodium dihydrogen phosphate)—$NaH_2PO_4.H_2O$	138.01
Sodium citrate crystals—$C_3H_4OH(COONa)_3.5\frac{1}{2} H_2O$	357.18
Sodium citrate, granular—$C_3H_4OH(COONa)_3.2 H_2O$	294.12
Sodium chloride—$NaCl$	58.46
Sodium hydroxide—$NaOH$	40.0
Sodium phosphate, dibasic—Na_2HPO_4	141.98
Sulphuric acid—H_2SO_4	98.082

Walpole's sodium acetate–hydrochloric acid buffer (pH range 0.65–5.2)

Solutions required

M/1 *Sodium acetate*, prepared by dissolving 82.04 g (anhydrous), or 136.09 g crystals in distilled water, and making up to 1 litre in a measuring flask.

M/1 *Hydrochloric acid*, prepared by diluting concentrated hydrochloric acid which is approximately 10 M, and titrating against a normal alkali.

Method

To prepare buffer solution, take the appropriate amount of each solution (*Table 7.3*) and make up with distilled water to 500 ml.

Table 7.3

pH	M/1 Sodium acetate (ml)	M/1 Hydrochloric acid (ml)
0.65	100	200
0.91	100	160
1.09	100	140
1.24	100	130
1.42	100	120

Table 7.3 (*continued*)

pH	M/1 Sodium acetate (ml)	M/1 Hydrochloric acid (ml)
1.71	100	110
1.99	100	105
2.32	100	102
2.72	100	99.5
3.09	100	97
3.29	100	95
3.5	100	92.5
3.79	100	85
3.95	100	80
4.19	100	70
4.58	100	50
4.76	100	40
4.92	100	30
5.2	100	20

Sodium citrate–hydrochloric acid buffer (pH range 1.1–7.5)

Solutions required

0.1 M Sodium citrate, prepared by dissolving 35.718 g (crystals) or 29.412 g (granular) in distilled water, and making up to 1 litre.

0.1 M Hydrochloric acid, prepared by diluting concentrated acid (approximately 10 M), and titrating against a normal alkali (*Table 7.4*).

Table 7.4

pH	0.1 M Hydrochloric acid	0.1 M Sodium citrate
1.1	100	0
1.35	90	10
1.85	80	20
2.5	76	24
3.6	70	30
4.51	60	40
5.1	50	50
5.49	40	60
5.75	30	70
6.0	20	80
6.4	10	90
6.73	4	96
6.99	2	98
7.5	0	100

Walpole's acetic acid–sodium acetate buffer (pH range 3.6–6.8)

Solutions required

0.1 N Acetic acid, prepared by diluting glacial acetic acid (mol. wt 60.03) and titrating against 0.1 N alkali.

0.1 N Sodium acetate, prepared by dissolving 8.204 g (or 13.6 g of crystals) in distilled water, and making up to 1 litre in a measuring flask.

Method

To prepare buffer solution take the appropriate amount of acetic acid and sodium acetate solutions (*Table 7.5*).

Table 7.5

pH	0.1 N Acetic acid (ml)	0.1 N Sodium acetate (ml)
3.6	185	15
3.8	176	24
4.0	164	36
4.2	147	53
4.4	126	74
4.6	102	98
4.8	80	120
5.0	59	141
5.2	42	158
5.4	29	171
5.6	19	181
6.0	10	190
6.3	5	195
6.8	0	200

Sörensen's phosphate buffer (pH range 5.3–8)

Solutions required

M/15 Sodium phosphate dibasic (Na_2HPO_4), prepared by dissolving 9.465 g of the salt in distilled water and making up to 1 litre in a measuring flask.

M/15 Potassium acid phosphate (KH_2PO_4), prepared by dissolving 9.07 g in distilled water, and making up to 1 litre.

Method

To prepare M/15 buffer solution take the appropriate amount of each solution in millilitres, as given below in *Table 7.6*. The resulting 100 ml of buffer solution may be diluted with distilled water to 1000 ml for certain staining techniques.

Table 7.6

pH	M/15 Sodium phosphate dibasic (ml)	M/15 Potassium acid phosphate (ml)
5.3	2.5	97.5
5.6	5.0	95
5.91	10	90
6.24	20	80
6.47	30	70
6.64	40	60
6.8	49.6	50.4
6.98	60	40
7.2	72	28
7.38	80	20
7.73	90	10
8.04	95	5

Michaelis's veronal–hydrochloric acid buffer (pH range 4.5–9.2)

Solutions required

Veronal acetate solution

Sodium acetate	1.943 g
Veronal (sodium barbiturate)	2.943 g
Distilled water	to 100 ml

Method

To prepare a buffer solution add to 5 ml of the veronal acetate solution the amount of M/10 hydrochloric acid and distilled water given in *Table 7.7*.

Table 7.7

pH	Veronal acetate solution (ml)	M/10 Hydrochloric acid (ml)	Distilled water (ml)
4.5	5	11	9
4.95	5	9	11
5.3	5	8	12
6.1	5	7	13
6.75	5	6.5	13.5
7	5	6	14
7.25	5	5.5	14.5
7.4	5	5	15
7.66	5	4	16
7.9	5	3	17
8.2	5	2	18
8.6	5	1	19
8.7	5	0.75	19.25
8.9	5	0.5	19.5
9.2	5	0.25	19.75

Tris(hydroxymethyl)aminomethane maleic acid (Gomori's buffer) (pH range 5.08–8.45)

Solutions required

$M/1$ *Maleic acid* $(C_4H_4O_4)$. Dissolve 116 g in distilled water and make up to 1 litre in a measuring flask.

$M/1$ *Tris(hydroxymethyl)aminomethane* $(CH_2OH)_3C—NH_2$. Dissolve 121 g in distilled water and make up to 1 litre in a measuring flask.

$M/2$ *Sodium hydroxide* (NaOH). Dissolve a little over 20 g in 1 litre of distilled water and titrate against a normal acid.

Method

To prepare the buffer solution take the appropriate amounts of each solution in millilitres as given in *Table 7.8*. The resulting 50 ml of buffer solution may be diluted up to 250 or 500 ml for certain techniques.

Table 7.8

pH	M/1 Maleic acid (ml)	M/1 Tris(hydroxy-methyl)aminomethane (ml)	M/2 Sodium hydroxide (ml)	Distilled water (ml)
5.08	5	5	1	39
5.30	5	5	2	38
5.52	5	5	3	37
5.70	5	5	4	36
5.88	5	5	5	35
6.05	5	5	6	34
6.27	5	5	7	33
6.5	5	5	8	32
6.86	5	5	9	31
7.20	5	5	10	30
7.5	5	5	11	29
7.75	5	5	12	28
7.97	5	5	13	27
8.15	5	5	14	26
8.30	5	5	15	25
8.45	5	5	16	24

Gormori's 0.2 M 'Tris' buffer (pH range 7.2–9.1)

Solutions required

0.2 M Tris(hydroxymethyl)aminomethane (mol. wt 121.14)
0.1 N Hydrochloric acid

Method

To prepare buffer solution take the appropriate amount of each solution and make up with distilled water to 100 ml (*Table 7.9*).

Table 7.9

pH	0.2 M Tris (ml)	0.1 N Hydrochloric acid (ml)
7.19	25	45.0
7.36	25	42.5
7.54	25	40.0
7.66	25	37.5
7.77	25	35.0
7.87	25	32.5
7.96	25	30.0
8.05	25	27.5
8.14	25	25.0
8.23	25	22.5
8.32	25	20.0
8.41	25	17.5
8.51	25	15.0
8.62	25	12.5
8.74	25	10.0
8.92	25	7.5
9.10	25	5.0

Holmes's boric acid–borax buffer (pH range 7.4–9.1)

Solutions required

$M/5$ Boric acid, prepared by dissolving 12.368 g of boric acid in distilled water in a 1 litre measuring flask, and making up to 1 litre with distilled water.

$M/20$ Borax (sodium tetraborate), prepared by dissolving 19.071 g of borax in distilled water in a 1 litre measuring flask, and making up to 1 litre with distilled water.

Method

To prepare buffer solution mix the appropriate amounts of each solution, as given in Table 7.10.

Table 7.10

pH	$M/5$ Boric acid (ml)	$M/20$ Borax (ml)
7.4	90	10
7.6	85	15
7.8	80	20
8.0	70	30
8.2	65	35
8.4	55	45
8.7	40	60
9.0	20	80

Sörensen and Walbum's glycine–sodium chloride–sodium hydroxide buffer (pH range 8.45–12.77)

Solutions required

0.1 M Glycine in 0.1 M NaCl, prepared by dissolving 5.846 g of NaCl in a quantity of distilled water in a 1 litre measuring flask. Add 7.507 g of glycine and more distilled water to dissolve it; make the resultant solution up to 1 litre with distilled water.

0.1 M NaOH, prepared by dissolving 4 g of NaOH in distilled water, and making up to 1 litre with distilled water. This solution should be checked by titrating against a decimolar acid.

Method

To prepare a 0.1 M buffer solution mix the appropriate amounts of each solution as given in Table 7.11.

Table 7.11

pH	0.1 M Glycine in 0.1 M NaCl (ml)	0.1 M NaOH (ml)
8.45	95	5
8.79	90	10
9.22	80	20
9.56	70	30
9.98	60	40
10.32	55	45
10.9	51	49
11.14	50	50

Table 7.11 (*continued*)

pH	0.1 M Glycine in 0.1 M NaCl (ml)	0.1 M NaOH (ml)
11.39	49	51
11.92	45	55
12.21	40	60
12.48	30	70
12.66	20	80
12.77	10	90

Basic staining and mounting procedures

Equipment

The most satisfactory layout of equipment in a histological laboratory is one that allows for an easy flow of work from one procedure to another without too much crossover. Logically, this should run as follows: cutting up of specimens, processing, embedding, staining, mounting and microscopy. Constraints will be the position of fume cupboards, sinks and doors.

Preferably, the staining bench should face the windows and be well illuminated by fluorescent warm white tubes. At least two sinks should be available, one for routine staining, the other for special stains. Each should be fitted with at least two cold water taps.

An adequate supply of distilled water is essential, stored in 5 or 10 litre polythene aspirator jars and in polythene wash-bottles. A simple staining microscope, equipped with × 4 and × 25 objectives and, if possible, a × 50 water immersion lens, is essential. Since this is to be used for examining wet slides the stage should permit easy and rapid cleaning: for this reason a mechanical stage may well prove to be a hindrance.

Stock stains and reagents should be kept in glass or polypropylene stoppered bottles. Reagents which require protection from light should be kept in amber bottles— preferably in a cupboard. They should be well labelled, and when the strain or reagent is poured, it should always be poured from the side of the bottle opposite the label so that drips do not run down and obliterate it.

Stains and reagents in frequent use are best kept in polythene wash-bottles or drop-bottles. Glass or polythene Coplin jars are also useful. The choice of containers for particular stains depends on their speed of evaporation, the frequency of use, the length of exposure of sections to their action, the need for speedy access and whether the staining is to be carried out at an elevated temperature.

Large batches of stains may be processed manually or on an automatic staining machine. For manual methods, glass troughs are available which will take racks of 12, 25 or even 50 slides. These troughs should be arranged sequentially, so that there is a natural progression through the reagents. Xylene, in which the staining procedure begins and ends, should be situated in a position where the fumes may be extracted. The sink should be fitted with some device whereby racks of slides may be efficiently washed in running water. It is usually sufficient to attach one end of a length of tubing to the tap and submerse the other end at the bottom of a large glass trough, although there are more sophisticated slide-washing trays available commercially.

Coverslips may be stored in 70% alcohol and wiped clean with a dust-free cloth immediately before use, or stored in Perspex boxes. A variety of sizes should be available and it is good practice to use No. 1 thickness as a routine as these permit oil immersion examination of the section.

Dissecting needles should be available to adjust coverslips during and after mounting. The mountants in routine use are kept in covered pots with glass applicators—those which are specially made commercially for this purpose are recommended.

Heat during staining

A reduction in the staining times of certain procedures may be effected by the application of heat; sometimes it is mandatory. This is usually achieved by immersing the sections or smears in stain—for example, Heidenhain's haematoxylin—in a Coplin jar. It should be remembered that a jar of stain will heat up to the required temperature more quickly if it is placed in a water-bath than if in an oven. It is good practice to have the stain at the required temperature before commencing the staining procedure.

Where the technique requires boiling, or near boiling, stain to be applied, such as in the Ziehl–Neelsen technique, the stain may be boiled in a test-tube and poured onto the slide. It has been a popular alternative technique to flood the slide with stain and heat it to steaming by applying direct heat below the slide. Neither of these methods are recommended, naked flames should be avoided as much as possible. It is quite adequate for this technique to stain in a Coplin jar at 60 °C for 30 minutes.

Paraffin sections

The basic steps in staining and mounting paraffin sections are as follows:

(1) removal of wax with xylene;
(2) hydration through alcohols;
(3) staining;
(4) dehydration with alcohol;
(5) clearing in xylene;
(6) mounting under a coverslip.

The steps given in this technique are the routine ones for haematoxylin and eosin and will apply (apart from the actual staining) to all methods given in this book, unless an alternative method is specifically given.

■ Technique

(1) *Removal of wax.* Sections are placed in xylene for 3–5 minutes to dissolve the wax.
(2) *Hydration.* The section is removed from xylene, drained and transferred to absolute alcohol for 1–2 minutes, when it will become opaque. It helps to agitate the sections. If all the wax has not been removed, clear patches will be seen, and such sections should be returned to the xylene for a further minute.
(3) The section is rinsed in a second bath of absolute alcohol, drained and taken to water. If the water becomes cloudy, the second alcohol bath is contaminated with xylene and should be changed.

If the sections were fixed in a mercury-containing fixative, the deposit should be removed at this stage with the iodine–sodium thiosulphate treatment.

(a) The section is placed in Lugol's iodine for 3 minutes.
(b) The slide, after draining and rinsing in water, is transferred to 3% sodium thiosulphate for 3 minutes and then well washed in water.

If sections are known to contain formalin pigment, they are treated as follows.

(a) The section is taken directly from alcohol and placed in picric alcohol (saturated solution of picric acid in alcohol) for 5–10 minutes.
(b) Wash in running water for 10 minutes.

(4) *Staining.* Slides are immersed in haematoxylin for the appropriate time (e.g. Mayer's haemalum 12 minutes, Gill's $3 \times$ haematoxylin 2 minutes). These are progressive stains (*see* Chapter 6). If a regressive stain is used, a longer time is required to overstain the tissue (e.g. Ehrlich's for 30 minutes) before the stain is selectively removed in acid alcohol (1% hydrochloric acid in 70% ethanol). This is differentiation and has the advantage that the degree of staining is controlled and a perfectly clear cytoplasm and background can be obtained.

(4a) *Differentiation.* Sections are dipped into acid alcohol where they are agitated for a few seconds and then washed in tap-water. They should be examined under the low power of the staining microscope to ensure they are sufficiently differentiated. With practice this microscopic control may be omitted. If the section is underdifferentiated it is returned to the acid alcohol and if overdifferentiated it may be returned to the haematoxylin for a further 10–15 minutes, after which it must be differentiated again.

(5) Slides, after draining off excess haematoxylin (or washing off the acid alcohol) are transferred to the sink washing trough and left in running water for about 10 minutes. When sections are first removed from the haematoxylin, or the acid alcohol, they are pink. Washing turns them blue, a change which has led to this step being universally known as 'blueing'. To expedite this stage, or when tap-water is not alkaline, alkaline 'tap-water substitute' of Scott (potassium bicarbonate 2 g, magnesium sulphate 20 g, distilled water 1000 ml) or dilute lithium carbonate may be used for 2–3 minutes. Sections must be briefly washed in water after this treatment, or the slides may be coated with a white deposit.

(6) Transfer slides to 1% aqueous eosin for 2 minutes to counterstain them. Wash in running water for 2–3 minutes to differentiate the eosin. Some workers prefer to use alcoholic eosin, in which case slides, once blued, should be immersed briefly in 95% ethanol and then stained in the alcoholic eosin for $1\frac{1}{2}$–2 minutes. They are then differentiated for 2–3 minutes in fresh 95% alcohol.

This stage has not been correctly carried out unless muscle fibres, keratin, cytoplasm, connective tissue and red blood cells are easily identified by varying shades of pink and red.

(7) *Dehydration.* Take slides through three changes of absolute ethanol sequentially, agitating for about 30 seconds in each.

(8) *Clearing.* Sections should be transferred from absolute alcohol to the first of two xylene baths and left until completely clear. This should take about 15 seconds, and they may be tested for clarity by being held against a dark background with the light striking them, when any patches containing water will have an opaque appearance. Such sections should be returned to the last alcohol and agitated for a further 15 seconds before being placed back in the xylene. If the xylene turns milky, the first alcohol should be discarded, the next two moved along and fresh alcohol used for the third bath.

(9) Sections are transferred to a second xylene bath from which they may be mounted.

(10) *Mounting.* A sufficient number of coverslips for the sections to be mounted are wiped clean of dust with a soft, fluffless cloth. If the coverslips are dirty or greasy, they should be cleaned from 70% alcohol. Cleaned coverslips may be conveniently laid in rows on a piece of filter paper folded like a concertina which allows them to be picked up by the edges. Alternatively they may be laid flat on blotting paper. If not used immediately they should be covered to prevent dust settling on them and care must be taken in handling to ensure they never acquire fingermarks.

A coverslip is laid on clean blotting paper: the stained section is removed from the xylene, surplus xylene is wiped from the back of the slide and around the section, leaving a margin of about 3 mm—this stage should be completed quickly to avoid the section drying. One or two drops of mountant—depending on the size of coverslip used—are placed on the section. This should be laid along the middle of the section to minimize the likelihood of trapping air bubbles.

The slide is quickly inverted over the coverslip and then brought down horizontally until the mountant makes contact. The mountant quickly spreads under the coverslip, and the slide, with the coverslip attached, is again quickly inverted. If necessary, the coverslip may be guided into place with a dissecting needle. This whole operation will, with practice, be complete in 5–10 seconds.

The quantity and quality of mountant can only be assessed with experience; too little will cause air bubbles, and too much a messy slide. Similarly, mountant that is too thin will dry back away from the edges of the coverslip and if too thick will take an inordinate time to dry.

Air bubbles. While an odd air bubble may be expressed by gentle pressure on the coverslip with a dissecting needle, the practice of chasing air bubbles under a coverslip is a time-wasting procedure, and will almost certainly damage the section. When there is more than one air bubble in the mountant it is quicker to put the slide back into xylene (which will remove the coverslip) and remount the section. Such a practice will soon lead to the mounting of sections without bubbles every time.

Frozen sections

Frozen sections may be stained by either of the two following methods.

(1) *Attached to slides.* After frozen sections have been attached to slides by one of the methods described on page 103, they are stained by the method given for paraffin sections above. Obviously there will be no need to go through the steps for the removal of paraffin wax and hydration and lipids will be removed by the xylene at the final stages.

(2) *Floating through reagents.* This entails the transference of loose sections from one reagent to the next by means of a 'hockey stick', the section being mounted on a slide after staining. This method is detailed below.

Equipment

Small glass dishes with covers. Glass embryo blocks are most useful. For reasonable sized sections, the lids of glass Coplin jars may be used.

Glass beakers, at least 5 cm in depth. These are used for washing sections and for final mounting of the sections onto slides.

It is good practice to lay the glassware on blotting paper in an organized fashion, with the name of each reagent written on paper beneath each dish. Occasionally it is helpful to use a piece of dark coloured card as a background to help identify the section.

Hockey sticks are conveniently made from glass rod 3–4 mm in diameter. A 10-cm length of rod, rounded at both ends in a Bunsen flame, is heated about 2–5 cm from the end. When softened, the short end is allowed to fall down at right angles (90 degrees) to the remainder of the rod.

■ Floating through technique

The steps given in this technique are for haematoxylin and eosin staining, and will apply (apart from the actual staining process) to any staining method described in this book, unless an alternative method is specified (e.g. fat staining). Frozen sections, which are not attached to slides, stain much more rapidly than those which are attached, and therefore diluted stains are used, or the time of staining reduced.

It must be remembered that frozen sections are very fragile, and careless handling in staining and processing will result in a poor section. To pick up a section, put the bent end of the hockey stick into the dish and gently agitate the fluid above the section, causing it to float off the bottom. Slide the end of the hockey stick under the middle of the section and lift it out; the section should be draped over the glass rod evenly and without creases. The section should now be lowered into the next reagent, and the hockey stick gently slid out from underneath it. Care must be taken to ensure that sections lie absolutely flat in reagents, as creases will result in uneven staining.

The numbers in the following description refer to *Figure 7.1* which shows the layout of the bench.

(1) The sections, which will have been received in distilled water after cutting, are transferred to a dish of fresh distilled water (1). Sections which have been stored in formal–saline are washed in tap-water (two changes) and then transferred to the distilled water

Note: Occasionally it is necessary to remove fatty material, which would otherwise interfere with staining, by a preliminary dehydration and clearing (stages 2–8).

Stages 2–8 are optional.
(2) Transfer sections to 70% alcohol (2) for a few seconds.
(3) Transfer to 90% alcohol (3) for a few seconds.
(4) Transfer to absolute alcohol (4) for a few seconds.
(5) Transfer to xylene (5) for a few seconds.
(6) Transfer to absolute alcohol (6) for a few seconds.
(7) Transfer to 90% alcohol (7) for a few seconds.
(8) Transfer to 70% alcohol (8) for a few seconds.
(9) Transfer to haematoxylin diluted 50% in distilled water (9) for 15 minutes.
(10) Wash in tap-water (10).
(11) Transfer to 1% acid alcohol (11) for a few seconds, gently agitate the fluid.
(12) Transfer to fresh tap-water (12) (with lithium carbonate added) until blue. Staining may be controlled by floating the section on to a slide (page 103), and examining to ensure that only nuclei are stained. If sections are not sufficiently differentiated, they should be returned to acid alcohol for a few seconds, blued and re-examined under the microscope.

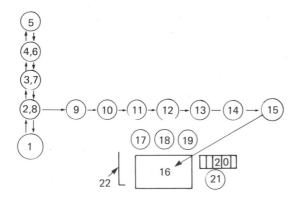

(1) Distilled water in a large container (8 inches in diameter).	(13) 1% eosin in water, in a small Petri dish.
(2) and (8) 70% alcohol in a small Petri dish.	(14) Tap-water in a large Petri dish. Sections may be mounted from this dish, or from the next, but a better eosin differentiation is possible from 70% alcohol.
(3) and (7) 90% alcohol in a small Petri dish.	
(4) and (6) Absolute alcohol in a small Petri dish.	
(5) Xylol in a small Petri dish.	(15) 70% alcohol in a large container (6 inches in diameter).
(6) (7) and (8) *(see above)*.	(16) Pad of blotting paper or filter paper.
(9) Haematoxylin (diluted equal parts with distilled water) in a small Petri dish.	(17) 90% alcohol in a drop bottle.
	(18) Absolute alcohol in a drop bottle.
	(19) Xylol in a drop bottle.
(10) Tap-water, to which a few drops of lithium carbonate have been added, in a large Petri dish.	(20) Coverslips, which may be kept dry in a container, or in various sizes in pots of acid alcohol.
(11) 1% acid alcohol (1% HCl in 96% alcohol) in a small Petri dish.	(21) HSR or DPX (glycerin jelly would be used to mount the section direct from water).
(12) Tap-water, with a few drops of lithium carbonate added, in a large Petri dish.	(22) Glass 'hockey stick'.

Figure 7.1 Layout of bench for routine haematoxylin and eosin staining of frozen sections

(13) Transfer sections to 1% eosin (13) for 1 minute.

(14) Transfer to tap-water (14) for 2 minutes, gently agitating the fluid periodically.

(15) Transfer to a large dish of 70% alcohol (15), from which section should be attached to a clean, grease-free slide.

Although some workers prefer to mount from alcohol, or even xylene, it is in these reagents that gross shrinkage of the section is likely to take place, and it is therefore better to attach them to slides from dilute alcohol or water.

(16) The section is now drained, but not allowed to dry, laid on the pad of blotting paper (16), and blotted firmly with fine filter paper.

(17) Without removing the slide from the pad of blotting paper, pour 90% alcohol (17) from a drop bottle on to the section, leave for a second or two, and blot with filter paper.

(18) Repeat the above stage but with the use of absolute alcohol (18).

(19) Without moving the slide, pour on xylene from a drop bottle (19), leave for a second or two, blot with fresh filter paper, and pour on more xylene. The section should now be completely clear. If any milky patches are present, they may usually

be removed by blotting once more, followed by fresh xylene. Should patches still persist, stages 18 and 19 should be repeated.

(20) Wipe excess xylene from the back of the slide and around the section, and mount as described for paraffin sections on page 138.

Celloidin sections

Celloidin sections are stained in a manner very similar to that used for frozen sections in that they must be floated through reagents and are only attached to a slide after staining is completed. They have an advantage over frozen sections in that they are not so fragile, but it is still important to remember that damage done to sections while staining cannot be repaired.

Since the tissues are impregnated with celloidin, which decreases the rate of penetration by reagents, the times of staining should be increased. Sections when stained are mounted without removing the celloidin, and this factor makes them more difficult to clear (*see* stage 11, page 142). Mounting is also made more difficult because the celloidin surrounding the section tends to corrugate, and unless care is taken these corrugations may trap air bubbles.

■ *Technique*

The equipment listed for frozen section staining is also suitable for celloidin section staining, including the glass hockey stick.

The steps given below are those used routinely for haematoxylin and eosin, but they will apply (apart from the actual staining technique) to all methods described in the book unless an alternative technique is specifically given.

The numbers in the following description refer to the key in *Figure 7.2*.

(1) Transfer the sections from the container of 70% alcohol, into which they have been received after cutting, or in which they have been stored, to the large dish of 70% alcohol (1). Leave in this dish for 2–3 minutes.

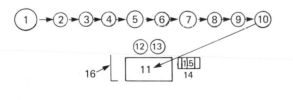

(1)	70% alcohol in a large container (6–8 inches in diameter).	(10)	Absolute alcohol in a large Petri dish (96% alcohol may be used to float section on slide at this stage, and the previous stage of 90% alcohol omitted).
(2)	Haematoxylin in a small Petri dish.		
(3)	Tap-water in a small Petri dish.		
(4)	1% acid alcohol (1% HCl in 70% alcohol) in a small Petri dish.		
(5)	Tap-water in a large Petri dish.	(11)	Pad of blotting or filter paper.
(6)	1% aqueous eosin, in a small Petri dish.	(12)	Carbol-xylol (or carbol-cresol-xylol) in a drop bottle.
(7)	Tap-water in a large Petri dish.	(13)	Xylol in a drop bottle.
(8)	70% alcohol in a small Petri dish.	(14)	Mountant (HSR or DPX).
(9)	90% alcohol in a small Petri dish.	(15)	Coverslips.
		(16)	Glass 'hockey stick'.

Figure 7.2 Layout of bench for routine method of staining celloidin sections with haematoxylin and eosin

(2) Transfer to haematoxylin in a small Petri dish (2) for 40 minutes.
(3) Transfer to tap-water in a large Petri dish (3) with several changes of water.
(4) Transfer to acid alcohol (1% HCl in 70% alcohol) in a small Petri dish (4) for a few seconds to differentiate, gently agitating the fluid.
(5) Transfer to fresh tap-water in a large Petri dish (5) (to which a few drops of saturated aqueous lithium carbonate may be added). Examine the sections to ensure that they are correctly differentiated.
(6) Transfer to 1% aqueous eosin in a small Petri dish for 2 minutes (6).
(7) Transfer to a large dish of tap-water (7), gently agitating the fluid occasionally until the eosin is differentiated, usually about 4–5 minutes, or longer.
(8) Transfer to 70% alcohol in a small Petri dish for 1–2 minutes (8).
(9) Transfer to 90% alcohol in a small Petri dish for 1–2 minutes (9).
(10) Transfer to absolute alcohol in a large Petri dish (10), from which the sections are attached to clean, grease-free slides (as described for frozen sections on page 103).

> *Note:* Sections may be mounted from 96% alcohol (methylated spirit) if preferred; when this is done the previous step of 90% is omitted. The reason for mounting from absolute alcohol is that the celloidin is softened in this reagent, and therefore is less likely to corrugate. Beginners are advised to mount from 96% alcohol, and only when they are reasonably proficient with this reagent, to mount from absolute alcohol.

(11) Flood the slides with carbol–xylene (12) (saturated solution of phenol in xylene) to clear the section, and then blot again, this process being repeated until the section is clear.
     The reason for using an intermediate between alcohol and xylene is because of the difficulty of clearing sections by the routine method.
(12) Flood the sections with xylene (13), blot, flood again and blot with fresh filter paper to remove the phenol.
(13) Place the mountant of choice (14) on to the sections, a generous amount being used, and lay one end of a clean coverslip of an appropriate size on the slide about one-eighth of an inch from the section. Place the point of a dissecting needle under the other end, and slowly lower it on to the section. The trapping of air bubbles should be avoided as the coverslip is lowered, but any that are trapped may be expressed from the sides of the coverslip by pressure with the dissecting needle on the centre of the coverslip. The use of thicker balsam for mounting celloidin sections will make mounting easier. When the coverslip has set (the following morning) the excess balsam is wiped away and the slide cleaned with a cloth which has been moistened with xylene.

Rapid frozen sections for emergency diagnoses

Demand will occasionally be made for a very rapid section, usually in a case of suspected malignancy. The patient may be in the operating theatre under an anaesthetic, and the operation may be suspended until a diagnosis on a biopsy specimen is given by the pathologist.

These emergency diagnoses may sometimes be made from a Terry slice: a thin slice of tissue (0.5–1 mm) is cut with a sharp scalpel, laid on a slide and the upper surface painted with a polychrome methylene blue or Field's stain 'A' which will stain the top layer of cells. The stain is washed off, a coverslip laid on the upper surface, and it is then examined under the microscope. While the author has seen this technique used with success by one pathologist it demands a great deal of experience and generally a frozen section is preferred; in the case quoted, a frozen section was always cut to confirm the findings of the Terry slice.

Sections may be cut in a cryostat as described on page 107, or by the frozen section technique (page 102).

Technique

Fixation

Tissue may be frozen unfixed or fixed. The choice is a matter of whether a cryostat or freezing microtome is used. Fresh unfixed tissue is more easily cut with a cryostat than fixed tissue, and presents a slightly different appearance under the microscope. Fixation prolongs the processing, but a tube of boiling formalin may be at hand into which the tissue is immersed for 1 or 2 minutes before sectioning.

Cutting

Sections are cut as already described on page 102 or 107.

Attachment of sections to slides

Although some technologists prefer to carry sections through solutions, as described on page 139, it is recommended that the sections be attached to slides immediately after cutting, and then stained. Any of the methods given on page 103 may be used, but Wilson's technique, which was devised for rapid work, is probably the most efficient. Three sections should be attached to slides to guard against damage to one of them during staining.

Choice of staining technique

The stain or stains to be employed are again a matter of personal preference, and will depend largely upon the experience of the pathologist. A single stain will quite often suffice to show malignancy, and simple toluidine blue is often used first as a routine because of its speed of action. Further sections may be stained by a double stain such as haematoxylin and eosin, or the phloxine–methylene blue method. The latter is exceptionally good for staining sections of unfixed tissue which occasionally gives a hazy picture with haematoxylin and eosin; it is also quicker and gives a better nuclear definition than a rapid haematoxylin and eosin. A toluidine blue stain is recommended, followed by phloxine–methylene blue for rapid frozen section staining.

■ Toluidine blue staining

Method

(1) Slides should be placed in 90% alcohol for a second or two.
(2) Transfer to absolute alcohol for a second or two.
(3) Transfer to xylene and agitate the slide until the section is clear (about 2 seconds).
(4) Transfer to absolute alcohol for a second or two.
(5) Transfer to 90% alcohol for a second of two.
(6) Transfer to the slide rack, flood with 1% toluidine blue, and leave for $\frac{1}{2}$–1 minute.
(7) Rinse rapidly in water, transfer to a pad of filter paper, and blot firmly.

(8) Flood with 90% alcohol and blot firmly.

(9) Flood with absolute alcohol and blot firmly.

(10) Flood with xylene, blot firmly and, if the section is clear, mount under a coverslip with balsam or DPX. If the section is not completely clear after the first application of xylene, flood the slide with xylene and blot a second time, and repeat until the section is clear, when it is mounted.

The whole staining process should take 3–4 minutes.

■ Phloxine–methylene blue

Solutions required

A	Phloxine	0.5 g
	Acetic acid	0.2 ml
	Distilled water	to 100 ml
B	Methylene blue	0.25 g
	Azure B	0.25 g
	Borax	0.25 g
	Distilled water	to 100 ml

Method

Stages 1–5 are as described above for toluidine blue staining.

(6) Transfer the slide to the slide rack, flood with water and drain.

(7) Flood with solution A for 1 minute.

(8) Wash in water for 10 seconds, and drain.

(9) Flood with solution B, and leave for half a minute.

(10) Wash with 0.2% acetic acid in distilled water until clouds of excess stain cease to flow from the section (about 20–30 seconds).

(11) Give three washes with 96% alcohol to differentiate the section.

(12) Flood with absolute alcohol and blot firmly.

(13) Flood with xylene, blot firmly and, if the section is clear, mount in balsam or synthetic resin.

Results

Nuclei and bacteria	Blue
Collagen and muscle	Bright red
Erythrocytes	Bright scarlet

The staining process should be completed in 3–4 minutes.

■ Rapid haematoxylin and eosin

Method

Stages 1–5 are as described for toluidine blue staining.

(6) Transfer the slide to a Coplin jar of haematoxylin for 2 minutes.

(7) Rinse in tap-water and dip in 1% acid alcohol; wash immediately in tap-water to which a few drops of saturated aqueous solution of lithium carbonate have been

added, and leave in this solution until the section is blue (about 20–30 seconds).
(8) Transfer the slide to a Coplin jar containing 1% eosin, leave for 10–15 seconds and
then rinse in water.

Stages (8), (9) and (10), as described for toluidine blue staining, are carried out to
dehydrate, clear and mount the section.

The time taken to complete the staining process is approximately 5 minutes.

Table 7.12 Recommended demonstration methods

Element	Recommended method
Adrenalin	Dichromate fixation—Giemsa
Amyloid	Alkaline Congo red
	Thioflavine T
Argentaffin cells	Masson–Fontana
Basement membrane	Methenamine silver
Calcium	Von Kossa
Collagen	Celestin blue haematoxylin—Van Gieson
Deoxyribonucleic acid (DNA)	Feulgen reaction
Elastic tissue	Hart–Weigert
Endocrine granules	Grimelius
Eosinophils	Carbol chromotrope
Fibrin	MSB
Glycogen	Diastase/PAS
Haematoidin (Bilirubin)	Gmelin's
Haemosiderin	Perls' Prussian blue
Keratin	Phloxine tartrazine
Lipofuscin	Schmorl's ferric-ferricyanide
	Long Zn
Mast cells	AB pH 2.5/safranin
Micro-organisms	Gram
Inclusion bodies	Macchiavello
	Phloxine tartrazine
Australia antigen	Shikata
Fungi	Methenamine silver
Tubercle bacilli	Ziehl–Neelsen
Mucin	
Neutral	PAS
Acidic	Alcian blue
Sulphated	High iron diamine
Muscle	
Types	ATPase
Striations	PTAH
Myelin	
Normal	Luxol fast blue
Degenerate	Swank Davenport
Nerve cells and axons	Bielschowsky
Neutral fats	Oil red O
Neuroglia	PTAH
Nissl substance	Toluidine blue
Paneth cell granules	Phloxine tartrazine
Pituitary	PAS/orange G
Plasma cells	Methyl green pyronin
Reticulin	Gordon and Sweet

Mountants

Sections are mounted under coverslips to maintain the high refractive index necessary for critical microscopy and to protect the section during storage. Attempts have been made to develop spray-on resins to achieve these objectives but they have not received any degree of acceptance. Occasionally, when there is much unstained tissue to be examined, it may be advantageous to view the section with a lower refractive index.

Mounting media fall into two main classes:

(1) aqueous media, used for material which is unstained, stained for fat, meta-chromatically stained or following immunofluorescent and certain enzyme histo-chemical methods—in summary, those methods where the action of alcohol or xylene would be detrimental to the stained preparation; and

(2) resinous media for routine staining techniques where the section is mounted from xylene.

For many years, the resinous Canada balsam was the universally accepted mountant of choice despite its well-known disadvantages. Many synthetic mountants have been developed, designed to overcome these disadvantages, but there has been a justifiable caution over their adoption. It may be years before the effects of storage on mounted sections become apparent and the user should adopt a new medium only after becoming satisfied that there will be no long-term deterioration in valuable stored slides.

It is inevitable that a degree of bleaching will occur with all mounting media if the sections are exposed to light (Drury and Wallington, 1980), a feature that has been critically evaluated by Barr (1970). In those experiments, Dammar xylene showed least bleaching amongst the natural media and Cristalite (E. Gurr, no longer available) and Permount (Fisher Scientific Co., 711 Forbes Ave, Pittsburgh, PA 15219, USA) were the best of the synthetic media. There is a variety of synthetic media available from commercial sources including many marketed since the evaluation quoted above was completed.

Aqueous mounting media

Most of these media have a low refractive index (1.4–1.42), although higher levels are obtainable with certain of the syrups. Occasionally single reagents, such as pure or dilute glycerin, are used, but generally these media are of three types: (a) the syrups; (b) gelatin media; and (c) gum arabic media. In the last two media glycerin is usually incorporated to prevent cracking and splitting on drying; all three are best preserved by coating with a ringing medium (*see below*).

Some of the metachromatic stains tend to diffuse from the section into the mounting media shortly after mounting: this may be prevented by using a fructose syrup, or by mounting in potassium acetate gum syrup. About 20% by weight of potassium acetate, or 50% by weight of sugar, is necessary (Report of the Committee on Histological Mounting Media, 1953).

The setting qualities of simple syrups may be improved by the addition of 12% gelatin.

All aqueous mounting media should contain a bacteriostatic agent such as a crystal of thymol, 0.25% phenol or sodium merthiolate, 0.025%, to prevent the growth of moulds.

Glycerin jelly (refractive index 1.47)

This is usually regarded as the standard mountant for fat stains.

Formula

Gelatin	10 g
Distilled water	60 ml
Glycerin	70 ml
Phenol	0.25 g

Dissolve the gelatin in the distilled water in a conical flask in a water-bath, using just sufficient heat to melt the gelatin; add the glycerin and phenol, mix well and transfer to containers. One ounce screw-capped bottles make suitable containers for all the aqueous mounting media, one of the caps (which can be changed to the bottle in use) being drilled to take a piece of glass rod which has been rounded at each end to serve as an applicator.

For use melt in a water-bath, hot water or wax oven; avoid shaking to speed this process otherwise the mountant will be full of air bubbles; 0.025% sodium merthiolate may be substituted for phenol as a preservative.

Apathy's medium (refractive index 1.52)

This medium is used when an aqueous medium of higher refractive index is required. It is a useful aqueous mountant for fluorescent microscopy, being virtually non-fluorescent.

Formula

Gum arabic	50 g
Cane sugar	50 g
Distilled water	50 ml
Thymol	0.05 g

Dissolve the ingredients with the aid of gentle heat. As this mountant sets by evaporation it must be kept in a well-stoppered bottle, or screw-capped container.

Highman's modification of Apathy's medium (refractive index 1.52)

This medium is recommended for use with metachromatic stains.

Formula

Gum arabic	20 g
Cane sugar	20 g
Potassium acetate	20 g
Sodium merthiolate	10 ml
Distilled water	40 ml

Dissolve the ingredients with the aid of gentle heat, and keep in an air-tight container.

Farrant's medium (refractive index 1.43)

This medium, being liquid, is more convenient than glycerin jelly for mounting, but has the disadvantage that it takes much longer to set, and air bubbles sometimes form during the setting process.

Formula

Gum arabic	50 g
Distilled water	50 ml
Glycerin	50 ml
Arsenic trioxide	1 g

Dissolve the gum arabic in the distilled water with gentle heat, add glycerin and arsenic trioxide.

The addition of 50 g of potassium acetate will give a neutral medium (pH 7.2) instead of an acid one (pH 4.4), and raises the refractive index to 1.44. Sodium merthiolate (0.025%) may be substituted with advantage for the arsenic trioxide as a preservative.

Fructose (laevulose) syrup (refractive index 1.47)

This syrup is useful as a temporary or special mountant, but is not recommended for routine use.

Formula

Fructose (laevulose)	75 g
Distilled water	25 ml

A high concentration of sugar such as this will require some time to dissolve in the 60 °C oven or water-bath, and unless the high refractive index and more viscid solution is required Mallory's formula of 30 g of fructose with 20 ml of distilled water is easier to prepare. Gelatin (10 g) may be added so that it sets; alternatively, it may be used as a permanent mount by using a ringing medium (page 150). The advantage of fructose over the other sugars used in mounting media is that it does not crystallize in the preparation.

Resinous mounting media

At one time the great majority of stained preparations were mounted in Canada balsam as a routine. Today there is available a wide range of natural and synthetic resins which are used both routinely and for special purposes.

In general these media are composed of a resin (natural or synthetic) either in its natural solvent, or dissolved in a solvent such as xylene until sufficiently liquid to allow easy mounting compatible with fairly rapid drying and hardening. The ideal viscosity of these media will vary according to personal preference; they should be sufficiently liquid to allow trapped air-bubbles to be removed easily, and to flow freely between coverslip and section, yet sufficiently viscid to avoid the formation of air spaces under the coverslip during drying.

Selection of a resinous mounting medium

A mounting medium should be chosen that will not fade the particular stains used; for example, basic aniline dyes should be mounted in non-acid-containing mountants; preparations showing the Prussian blue reaction should be mounted in non-reducing media. The medium should have the correct refractive index; unstained tissue shows best in a medium having a very low or very high refractive index, while stained preparations are most transparent when the mounting media has a refractive index of 1.54.

Canada balsam (refractive index 1.52)

Canada balsam, from the Canadian fir tree (*Abies balsamea*), is a solid resin and is composed of terpenes, carboxylic acids and their esters; it is usually dissolved in xylene. Haematoxylin and eosin stained slides are fairly well preserved, but basic aniline dyes tend to fade, and Prussian blue is slowly bleached.

Canada balsam is dissolved in xylene to 55–70% by weight; the actual amount used will vary according to personal preference and a 55% solution is a suitable strength for routine use. This is a very messy reagent to prepare, since it must be ground in a pestle and mortar with the solvent until free of lumps, and it is more economical to purchase the ready-made mountant.

Dammar balsam

Dammar balsam is similar to Canada balsam. It is rarely used today because of the dirt and impurities usually present, and the difficulty of filtering prepared mountant.

Colophonium resin

This is occasionally used as a mountant, when it is dissolved in xylene. In alcoholic solution it may be used as a differentiating agent. As a mountant, it has a tendency to crystallize.

Terpene resin

In our hands this has proved to be a suitable replacement for Canada balsam, being less acid and considerably cheaper.

Synthetic resins

There are a great number of synthetic resins either made in the laboratory or prepared commercially; those in most common use are the polystyrenes, such as Kirkpatrick and Lendrum's DPX.

Plasticizers, such as tricresyl phosphate or dibutylphthalate, should be incorporated with the solution of polystyrene in xylene, otherwise air spaces appear under the coverslip as the preparation dries; alternatively, higher boiling solvents, such as technical dimethylbenzene, or technical diethylbenzene, may be used. The report mentioned on page 146 recommends a polystyrene dimethylbenzene as the best mountant for preserving the Prussian blue reaction.

Kirkpatrick and Lendrum's DPX (refractive index 1.52)

Distrene 80	10 g
Dibutylphthalate	5 ml
Xylene	35 ml

This is the most commonly used routine mountant preserving, as it does, most routine stains. It has the great advantage over balsam that slides can be cleaned of excess mountant simply by stripping it off after cutting around the edge of the coverslip.

Other mounting media

Euparal (refractive index 1.48)

Euparal is a semisynthetic mountant composed of sandarac resin dissolved in a mixture of eucalyptus, paraldehyde and camsal (a liquid composed of camphor and phenyl salicylate). It is of use when a lower refractive index is required, and has the advantage that sections may be mounted from xylene, or from graded alcohol of 90% upwards. There is a green variety containing copper salt which is said to preserve haematoxylin stains.

Other mountants

While there are many more mountants available commercially, the range given above will suffice for all routine work, and the majority of special techniques.

Ringing media

Mounting media which dry back from the edges or develop air bubbles should be coated at the edges of the coverslip with a non-porous ringing medium. The term 'ringing' originated because round coverslips were then used and the coating applied in the form of a circle or 'ring'. Any of the three methods given below may be easily and neatly applied with very little practice.

Paraffin wax

The end of a glass microscope slide is gently heated in a warm Bunsen flame—too much heat will crack the glass—and the warm end touched onto a block of solid paraffin wax. The molten wax is applied by touching the edge of the coverslip with the slide so that the wax solidifies at the junction. Of course, a messy coverslip, with mountant projecting from beneath it, will prevent a good seal.

Cement

Any type of plastic adhesive (such as Durofix) may be applied as a ringing medium direct from the collapsible tube in which it is supplied. These types of cement make more permanent mounts than paraffin wax.

Nail polish

Clear nail polish may be applied with a brush to the edge of the coverslip.

References

BARR, W. T. (1970). Effects of sunlight on stained sections mounted in various media. *Stain Technol.*, **45**, 9–14

DRURY, R. A. B. and WALLINGTON, E. A. (1980). *Carleton's Histological Technique*. Oxford University Press, Oxford, England

Part IV

Demonstration methods

8

Haematoxylin and its counterstains

Haematoxylin is probably the single most important dye employed in histological staining. A period of uncertainty over supplies during the 1970s led to a frantic search for suitable substitutes with which to stain cell nuclei. This dye forms a cornerstone of general oversight methods and acts as a morphological reference in many specialized histochemical methods. The value of haematoxylin is not limited to nuclear staining as it may be used in the demonstration of intracellular substances (e.g. chromosomes, keratohyaline), extracellular substances (e.g. elastin), ground substance (e.g. cement lines in bone), minerals (e.g. calcium, copper, etc.) and the central nervous system (e.g. myelin, neuroglia fibres, etc.).

However, it is as a general morphological stain, particularly in combination with eosin, that haematoxylin is virtually indispensable. Although there are advocates of alternative methods (e.g. azure-eosin, Lillie, 1965), most microscopists favour a well-stained haematoxylin and eosin (H & E) section in which the nuclei stain blue with cytoplasm and connective tissue fibres in varying shades of pink. In exfoliative cytology, haematoxylin-stained nuclei are the most important diagnostic features of Papanicolaou stained smears.

Haematoxylin is extracted from the logwood of the tree *Haematoxylon campechianum*. Oxidation of this extract produces a coloured substance *haematein*, which is itself a poor dye, but which, in the presence of a metallic mordant, forms a most powerful stain.

The structure of haematoxylin and haematein is given in *Figure 8.1*. Oxidation of haematoxylin gives rise to the paraquinoid structure

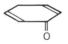

which is responsible for the staining properties of haematein.

Baker (1960, 1962) investigated the dye/mordant/tissue complex and discussed the possible attachments of aluminium–haematein complexes to nuclear DNA and cytoplasmic RNA. The close proximity of phosphoric acid groups in DNA was held responsible for the stronger staining of nuclear chromatin as against almost unstained less dense carboxyl side groups of dicarboxylic acids in cytoplasmic RNA (*Figure 8.2*). Although the tissue attachment is shown only at positions 9 and 10, similar attachment is thought to form at positions 3 and 4. As haematoxylin is used at acid pH, these bonds are incomplete due to competition by hydrogen ions. The hydrogen ions are displaced

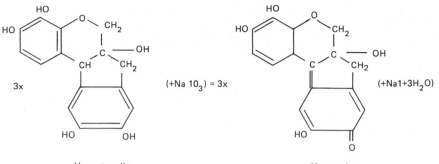

Haematoxylin   Haematein

Figure 8.1 Structural formula of haematoxylin and its oxidation product haematein. (After Gill, Frost and Miller, 1974)

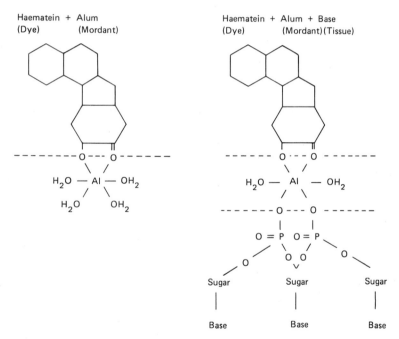

Figure 8.2 The progressive attachment of mordant to dye and tissue to dye/mordant. See text for explanation. (After Baker, 1960)

by 'blueing' (i.e. treating with weak alkali), which stabilizes the bonds and forces a colour shift from red to blue.

Oxidation may be achieved by either natural or chemical methods. The advantage of natural oxidation is that once oxidation has reached an acceptable level, the staining solution may be used, and although the stock will continue to oxidize, it is unlikely to proceed too far. The disadvantage lies in the planning and organization required to ensure that a usable solution is always available. Chemically oxidized haematoxylin may be used as soon as it is made up, but has a shorter shelf-life.

Natural oxidation involves the exposure of solutions of haematoxylin to sunlight and air. Usually, though not invariably, alcoholic solutions are used. Oxidation is achieved by leaving a flask of alcoholic haematoxylin, loosely stoppered with cotton wool, on the laboratory window sill for 6–8 weeks. Not surprisingly, this process is often referred to as *ripening*. Alternatively, oxygen, or even air, may be bubbled through the solution for 3–4 weeks.

Chemical oxidation is achieved by the addition of oxidizing agents such as mercuric oxide, sodium iodate and potassium permanganate. Sodium iodate is the preferred oxidizing agent according to some workers (e.g. Gill, Frost and Miller, 1974), because it does not require boiling to release its oxygen as does mercuric oxide. This may contribute to an increased shelf-life. Oxidation is instantaneous and the solution ready for immediate use. However, the possibility of over-oxidation has been clearly established by Marshall and Horobin (1972), who concur with Lillie (1965) that the production of oxyhaematein inhibits successful staining. It is also well known that commercial samples of haematoxylin contain variable quantities of haematein, a factor that should lead to caution in chemical oxidation, careful evaluation of subsequent staining and confidence in tested and approved dyes (i.e. those certified by the Biological Stain Commission or the IMLS Dye Approval Scheme). Natural oxidation has the advantage of being a more gradual procedure which may prolong the useful life of haematoxylin solutions, although 'ripened' solutions still remain popular.

Glycerol has been incorporated into many formulas for its value in preventing over-oxidation and reducing evaporation. It is commonly referred to as a stabilizer, improving the keeping qualities of the staining solution.

The staining of tissue sections may be divided into three broad groups depending upon the choice of metallic mordant and the way in which they are employed.

(1) Oversight methods: These employ alum mordants incorporated into the staining solution.
(2) Selective methods for specific structures: Metallic mordants other than alums are either applied simultaneously with the haematoxylin or as a preliminary step.
(3) Demonstration of metals: Metals or their salts present in tissue sections act as mordants to form direct chelates (or lakes) with applied haematoxylin.

Although Lillie (1965) does not consider the order in which the various ingredients are added and the nature of the oxidizing agents employed to be critical, the authors have insufficient experimental data to endorse this view.

Haematoxylins

Mayer's haemalum

Formula

Haematoxylin	1 g
Distilled water	1000 ml
Ammonium alum	50 g
Sodium iodate	0.2 g
Citric acid	1 g
Chloral hydrate	50 g

Dissolve the haematoxylin in distilled water using gentle heat. Add the alum, shaking to dissolve, followed by the sodium iodate. Continue heating whilst adding the citric acid and chloral hydrate. The stain is ready for immediate use when cool.

Chloral hydrate is believed to act as a preservative, and citric acid used to acidify the stain, a property commonly agreed to sharpen nuclear staining.

Mayer's haemalum is most useful as a progressive stain, making it especially suited to automated procedures. The optimum staining time will usually be found to be 5–6 minutes. The progressive nature of Mayer's haemalum, makes it a popular counterstain to procedures such as PAS, mucicarmine and many enzyme histochemical procedures.

Harris's haematoxylin

Formula

Haematoxylin	2.5 g
Absolute alcohol	50 ml
Ammonium alum	50 g
Distilled water	500 ml
Mercuric oxide	1.5 g
Glacial acetic acid	20 ml

Dissolve the haematoxylin in the alcohol and the alum (potassium alum may be substituted) in hot water. Mix the two solutions together and heat to boiling. Add the mercuric oxide and cool rapidly by plunging the flask into cold water. The solution is ready for immediate use. Glacial acetic acid, added after cooling gives more precise nuclear staining. Beware of excessive bubbling when mercuric oxide is added.

This is a good stain for routine use, although it requires differentiation in acid alcohol (1% hydrochloric acid in 70% absolute alcohol). The selectivity and speed of staining of this haematoxylin diminishes on storage. Any precipitate which may form should be filtered off and taken as an indication that the stain is deteriorating. Staining time 10 minutes.

Ehrlich's haematoxylin

Formula

Haematoxylin	6 g
Absolute alcohol	300 ml
Distilled water	300 ml
Glycerol	300 ml
Glacial acetic acid	30 ml
Potassium alum—to saturation	10–14 g

The haematoxylin should be fully dissolved in the alcohol before the other ingredients are added. Finally, potassium alum is added until there is a deposit of alum crystals on the bottom of the stock container. The incorporation of glycerol is said to give more even and precise staining; it certainly stabilizes the stain against over-oxidation and reduces evaporation.

Whilst natural oxidation or ripening was originally recommended, the addition of 0.9 g of sodium iodate to the above solution allows the stain to be used immediately.

Ehrlich's haematoxylin is a good, strong stain, especially useful for demonstrating the structure of decalcified bone sections. It also stains mucin in salivary glands and goblet cells and the ground substance of cartilage. It is used regressively; that is, requires differentiation. Staining time 20–30 minutes.

Cole's haematoxylin

Formula

Haematoxylin	1.5 g
Saturated aqueous potassium alum (ammonium alum is as good)	700 ml
1% iodine in absolute ethanol	50 ml
Distilled water	250 ml

Add haematoxylin to distilled water and heat gently to dissolve. Add the iodine solution followed by the alum, bring to boil and cool rapidly. Filter. The haematoxylin is ready for immediate use.

This solution has good keeping qualities, but will require filtering before use. Staining time 30 minutes (regressive).

Delafield's haematoxylin

Formula

Solution A
Ammonium alum	55 g
Distilled water	600 ml

Solution B
Haematoxylin	6 g
Absolute ethanol	50 ml

Solution C
Glycerol	150 ml
Absolute ethanol	150 ml

Mix solutions A and B together, leave to stand overnight then filter. Add solution C. Leave to ripen naturally for 6–8 weeks. The solution will keep almost indefinitely.

Gill's haematoxylin (Gill, Frost and Miller, 1974)

Formula

Distilled water	730 ml
Ethylene glycol	250 ml
Haematoxylin	2.0 g
Sodium iodate	0.2 g
Aluminium sulphate ($Al_2(SO_4)_3 . 18 H_2O$)	17.6 g
Glacial acetic acid	20 ml

The reagents are added in the order given and the mixture stirred for 1 hour at room temperature. Filter. The solution is ready for immediate use.

Notes

(1) Gill, Frost and Miller (1974) stress that anhydrous haematoxylin should be used; if crystalline haematoxylin is used (i.e. $C_{16}H_{14}O_6 . 3 H_2O$) the amount present in the above formula should be increased to 2.36 g.

(2) Sodium iodate must be added with an accuracy of ± 0.01 g.

(3) If the aluminium sulphate used does not contain 18 H_2O, the quantity should be suitably adjusted for differences in molecular weight.

(4) Double strength haematoxylin solution can be prepared by doubling the amount of haematoxylin and sodium iodate, and quadrupling the aluminium sulphate. Appropriate adjustments can be made to produce triple strength stain. Single strength haematoxylin is preferred for cytology, smears being adequately stained in 2 minutes. On deparaffinized 5 μm sections optimum staining is achieved at 3 minutes, using double strength and in $1-1\frac{1}{2}$ minutes using triple strength. These times apply to haematoxylin used progressively.

(5) Ethylene glycol is employed because it is a particularly good solvent for haematoxylin.

The advantages claimed for these solutions are that they are fast in action, stable for at least 12 months, produce little or no surface precipitate, and their preparation does not involve boiling the solution. The concept of half-oxidized haematoxylin, introduced by Baker and Jordan (1953), is the probable explanation for the extended shelf-life of these solutions.

Counterstains

Eosin

Of the many forms available commercially, water soluble eosin Y is most commonly employed, although alcoholic solutions are preferred by some workers, especially in the USA.

Eosin, a xanthene dye, is tetrabromofluorescein which may be contaminated with mono- and dibromo derivatives, affecting the shade of the dye. Until recently this contamination led to unsatisfactory staining, but the pure dye is now available from many suppliers. Because of these difficulties, phloxine and phloxine/eosin mixtures achieved brief popularity. Calcium chloride and acetic acid have been added to simple eosin solutions in an attempt to improve poor performance.

Aqueous eosin is used as a 1% solution with a crystal of thymol added to inhibit the growth of moulds.

Alcoholic eosin is employed as a 0.5% solution in alcohol. In use, sections should be treated with 95% alcohol before staining with alcoholic eosin, and the excess stain washed out in the same solvent.

■ *Method—haematoxylin and eosin*

  (1) Remove paraffin wax with xylene, 5 minutes.
  (2) Treat with absolute alcohol, two changes, 1 minute each.
  (3) Wash in water.
  (4) Stain in haematoxylin. *10 mm. Harris*
  (5) Wash in water.
  (6) If a regressive stain is used, differentiate in acid/alcohol until only nuclei remain blue.
  (7) Wash in water.
  (8) Blue in running water or Scott's tap-water substitute.
  (9) Rinse in water.
 (10) Stain in 1% aqueous eosin Y for 3 minutes.

(11) Wash in running water for 1 minute.
(12) Dehydrate in three changes absolute alcohol.
(13) Clear in two changes xylene.
(14) Mount in suitable synthetic resin.

Results

Nuclei, RNA rich cytoplasm, calcium	Blue
Muscle, fibrin, keratin	Bright red
Collagen	Pink
Red blood cells	Orange/red

Specialized haematoxylins

Included under this heading are those haematoxylins mordanted to metals other than aluminium and which are not used as general oversight methods.

Weigert's haematoxylin

Van Gieson stain (*see* Chapter 9) contains sufficient picric acid to effectively remove alum haematoxylin from cell nuclei. Weigert's haematoxylin, which is mordanted to an iron salt, has sufficient avidity to withstand this treatment and has, for many years, been the nuclear stain of choice in this procedure. More recently, the Celestin blue/Mayer's haemalum sequence has found favour. It is the procedure we recommend (but *see below*).

Formula

Solution A
   Haematoxylin   1 g
   Absolute alcohol   100 ml
Use gentle heat to dissolve
Solution B
   30% aqueous ferric chloride   4 ml
   Concentrated hydrochloric acid   1 ml
   Distilled water   100 ml

Mix equal quantities of A and B immediately before use.

Celestin blue

Formula

Celestin blue B	2.5 g
Ferric ammonium sulphate	25 g
Glycerol	70 ml
Distilled water	500 ml

Dissolve the ferric ammonium sulphate (iron alum) in cold distilled water. Add celestin blue B and boil solution for 3 minutes. When cool, filter and add glycerol. The solution keeps for up to 6 months.

Celestin blue B, which is an oxazine dye, has little useful colouring property of its own. However, it forms an additional strong mordant with certain haematoxylins which make it especially useful when acid counterstains are to be used. Celestin blue B is used as a preliminary to alum haematoxylin staining and has, for example, largely replaced Weigert's haematoxylin in the Van Gieson method (*see* page 168). It should be noted that nitrocellulose may be strongly stained by the dye.

We believe that the ferric ammonium sulphate is the major active ingredient, and equally good results may be obtained simply by using this salt as a 5% solution.

■ Heidenhain's iron haematoxylin

The most intense of haematoxylins, Heidenhain's is used as a regressive stain, careful differentiation revealing many cellular details. Counterstains are unnecessary and the results lend themselves admirably to photomicrography. Nuclear detail and muscle striations are beautifully demonstrated and the stain is of sufficient intensity to be successful on very thin sections.

Solution A—haematoxylin
Haematoxylin   0.5 g
Absolute alcohol   10 ml
Distilled water   90 ml

Dissolve the haematoxylin in the alcohol before adding distilled water. The solution should be ripened for 3–4 weeks before use.

Solution B—iron alum
Ferric ammonium sulphate   5 g
Distilled water   100 ml

Clear, violet crystals must be used, not those that have become opaque, yellow-green.

Method

(1) Take sections to water.
(2) Treat with iron alum (mordant) for 1 hour. Following fixation in dichromate containing solutions, this time may need to be extended up to 12–24 hours.
(3) Rinse in distilled water.
(4) Place in haematoxylin solution for the same time as the mordant treatment.
(5) Wash in tap-water.
(6) Differentiate in the iron alum solution. This is the crucial step of the procedure and should be carefully controlled microscopically. It helps if the mordant is diluted with an equal quantity of distilled water, and the section should be rinsed in distilled water before examining.
(7) Wash well in running tap-water, to remove all traces of iron alum.
(8) Dehydrate, clear and mount in synthetic resin.

Results

Mitochondria, chromosomes, myelin, muscle striations, nuclei, black.

Note: The times may be greatly reduced if mordanted and stained at 60 °C.

Verhoeff's haematoxylin

This is a useful stain for elastic fibres. Although it may be difficult to demonstrate the finest fibres, careful differentiation being required, in combination with Van Gieson stain, it gives spectacularly beautiful results (*see* Chapter 9).

Loyez iron haematoxylin

Ferric alum is the mordant used in this haematoxylin designed specifically for the demonstration of myelin. Full details are given in Chapter 20.

Phosphotungstic acid haematoxylin (PTAH)

Originally devised as a technique for central nervous tissue, PTAH has been popularly adopted as a connective tissue stain, particularly useful for the demonstration of muscle striations and fibrin. An unusual feature is the concomitant staining of various structures in two colours—shades of red and blue. Tungsten, as phosphotungstic acid, is the mordant used. The technique is given in Chapter 9.

References

BAKER, J. R. (1960). Experiments on the action of mordants. 1. 'Single bath' mordant dyeing. *Quart. J. Micr. Sci.*, **101**, 255–272

BAKER, J. R. (1962). Experiments on the action of mordants. 2. Aluminium-haematein. *Quart. J. Micr. Sci.*, **103**, 493–517

BAKER, J. R. and JORDAN, B. R. (1953). Miscellaneous contributions to microtechnique. *Quart. J. Micr. Sci.*, **94**, 237–252

GILL, G. W., FROST, J. K. and MILLER, K. A. (1974). A new formula for a half-oxidised haematoxylin solution that neither overstains nor requires differentiation. *Acta Cytol.*, **18**, 300–311.

LILLIE, R. D. (1965). *Histopathologic Technic and Practical Histochemistry.* McGraw-Hill, New York

MARSHALL, P. N. and HOROBIN, R. W. (1972). The chemical nature of the gallocyanin-chrome alum staining complex. *Stain Technol.*, **47**, 155–161.

9

Connective tissue

Connective tissue consists of three elements: fibres; cells; and ground substance.

The historical term ground substance is less fashionable than the more catholic term matrix, which is used not only to describe the material filling intercellular and interfibrillar spaces, but also to describe the fibrous network (e.g. collagenous matrix), the basement membrane (cell-associated matrix) and the entire complex (connective tissue matrix). It is composed of mucopolysaccharide, essentially acidic in character and dealt with in Chapter 12.

The most important connective tissue cell is the fibroblast. It is responsible for the production of collagen and most probably reticulin, secreting a ground substance which, with the addition of further metabolites, polymerizes to give these characteristic fibres. It is believed that specific cells of mesenchymal origin give rise to elastin.

Histiocytes, or macrophages, are commonly found in normal connective tissue. These are phagocytic, scavenger cells. As with fibroblasts, there is no specific stain for histiocytes, recognition depending upon the characteristic appearance in haematoxylin and eosin-stained sections, or immunoenzyme methods (Chapter 19).

Plasma cells and mast cells are frequently seen in connective tissue and may be identified with the help of selective staining procedures (Chapter 24).

The classification of connective tissue fibres is not absolute. For example, muscle may be considered to be a connective tissue or an organ in its own right with specific function. Similarly, basement membrane, which is not fibrillar, may be considered a part of epithelial tissue, or a connective tissue. In this chapter, the following structures are discussed as connective tissues.

Collagen
Reticulin
Elastin
Basement membrane
Muscle
Oxytalan

Neuroglia, the specialized connective tissue of the nervous system, is discussed in Chapter 20. It should be remembered that adipose tissue, including fat cells, is a type of connective tissue.

Collagen

An acellular product of the fibroblasts, collagen fibres may occur singly or in bundles. The work of Miller, Epstein and Piez (1971) led to the recognition that collagen may exist in several different forms. Of the five forms currently recognized, three are concerned with classical connective tissue, one is peculiar to the basement membranes and the fifth limited to certain specialized sites.

Collagen types I, II and III are termed 'interstitial' to differentiate them from basement membrane collagen.

The basic structure of collagen is a fibril, up to 0.4 μm in diameter, embedded in a hyaluronic acid containing matrix. Each fibril is composed of microfibrils, 40 nm in diameter, with crossbanding at a frequency of 64 nm. This is the characteristic feature of most collagens viewed in the electron microscope.

Bundles of collagen fibres frequently branch, although individual fibres never do. The material exhibits positive birefringence.

Collagen I is composed of large fibres of the usual periodicity. It is the common collagen present in large amounts in skin, bone, tendon and blood vessels.

Collagen II is found in hyaline cartilage and the cornea. It is composed of fine fibrils, 10–20 nm in diameter and does not usually exhibit any cross striations.

Except in young animals, collagen III is invariably present in association with type I. It is also present independent of I in relation to the basement membrane and the parenchyma of organs. It is very similar to reticulin, except that reticulin is rich in carbohydrate. Type III collagen is associated with glycoprotein.

Differentiation of these three types of collagen is most easily achieved by the use of monoclonal antibodies.

Collagen IV is the collagen associated with basement membranes, first isolated from glomerular basement membrane of the kidney. A particular characteristic of type IV collagen is that it is sensitive to pepsin digestion, unlike other types. It is also devoid of any fibrillar organization, appearing as an amorphous matrix.

Collagen V is similar to interstitial collagen but occurs in rather specialized sites, including the placenta and some atherosclerotic plaques.

Reticulin

These fibres are found as a network supporting dense, cellular organs such as liver and lymph nodes. They are less readily detected in loose connective tissue, and are in any case difficult to visualize in haematoxylin and eosin-stained sections. Reticulin fibres are delicate and frequently branch, yet have been found to have a banded periodicity identical to collagen. A difference in the quantity of interfibrillar substance between reticulin (4.2% w/w) and collagen (0.5% w/w) is thought to account for differing staining reactions between the two.

Elastin

Elastin is a protein, occurring either as branching fibres or as sheets, as in the walls of blood vessels. Mature elastin has two components, a glycoprotein containing microfibrils and an amorphous protein. Catchpole (1982) has suggested that the microfibrillar glycoprotein network associated with elastic fibres may be fibronectin (*see below*).

The molecular structure of elastin allows it to stretch and subsequently return to its relaxed configuration, behaving in a manner very similar to natural rubber. In addition to blood vessels, elastin is an important component of the dermis. With age, the fibres split and become fragmented, a feature giving rise to the characteristic 'age changes' in skin. Calcification occurring in the elastin of blood vessels leads to a loss of elastic function.

Elastin may be recognized in haematoxylin and eosin preparations as being eosinophilic, refractile and characteristically undulating in artery walls. It also exhibits autofluorescence.

Basement membrane

At the level of the light microscope, the basement membrane appears to be a homogeneous layer forming the interface between epithelial cells and connective tissue. It is also present around endothelial cells in capillaries and between epithelial cells and endothelial cells in kidney glomeruli.

The membrane not only acts as a physical support for overlying epithelium, but also acts as a barrier, allowing only water and small molecules to pass through.

Ultrastructurally, four zones of basement membrane have been recognized in skin (Yaoita, Foidart and Katz, 1978).

(1) Basal cell plasma membrane containing hemidesmosomes by which the epithelial cells are attached.
(2) Lamina lucida, an electron-lucent layer beneath the plasma membrane containing anchoring filaments.
(3) Basal lamina, or lamina densa, the most conspicuous layer and the unique site of type IV collagen.
(4) Sub-basal lamina adjacent to the connective tissue matrix and containing anchoring fibrils, dermal microfibrillar bundles and collagen fibres.

Fibronectin   Fibronectin is a glycoprotein component of extracellular matrix and of basement membrane. It is secreted by fibroblasts and is thought to combine with type I and type III collagen. Its role is associated with supporting and connecting cells and with cell adhesion—allowing cells to be organized into sheets of multiple layers, or cords, and to adhere to the basement membrane. It has been recognized primarily by immunofluorescence using antisera raised against a cold insoluble globulin thought to be the plasma homologue of fibronectin. The interest in this substance centres on its possible role in cell transformation, tumour invasion and the metastasis of tumour cells.

Laminin   Laminin is a basement membrane glycoprotein present in the matrix. It differs from fibronectin in amino acid content and immunological reactivity, failing also to cross react with type IV collagen. It is universal to basement membrane, making it a most useful marker using, for example, immunoperoxidase methods. Although the role of laminin is not established it is believed to act with type IV collagen, basement membrane proteoglycan and fibronectin to form basement membrane and to help with the selective permeability of the basement membrane.

Three methods are particularly useful for the demonstration of basement membrane.

The periodic acid–Schiff method demonstrates the glycoprotein moiety of this structure well; the method is given in Chapter 12. Methenamine–silver techniques provide particularly high contrast and are indispensible to the study of renal glomeruli (*see* Chapter 22). Of more recent origin, immunoenzyme methods using antisera raised against laminin, are proving most helpful in identifying basement membrane and establishing its integrity.

Muscle

Muscle differs from other connective tissues outlined in this chapter in that it is composed not of fibres (although it is common practice to refer to 'muscle fibres') but of greatly elongated cells. A considerable amount of true connective tissue is present in muscle bundles, forming a sheath through which the muscle extends its action and carrying blood and nervous tissue. The interpretation of muscle biopsies has become of such importance since the last edition, that the subject now merits individual attention (Chapter 23). It is included briefly in this chapter because it often features in the tinctorial methods used to differentiate connective tissues.

Oxytalan fibres

These specialized fibres have been found in tendon, ligaments, the adventitia of blood vessels, surrounding skin appendages and the periodontium. Oxytalan fibres appear to be closely related to elastic fibres, possibly representing immature or modified elastin. This assumption is based on similarities in the electron microscopic appearance of the two tissues and positive staining of oxytalan fibres with certain elastic tissue stains (resorcin fuchsin, aldehyde fuchsin and orcein) although this only occurs following peracetic or performic acid oxidation. First described by Fullmer and Lillie (1958), oxytalan fibres have been more fully reviewed by Fullmer, Sheetz and Narkates (1974).

Methods

General oversight methods—the trichromes

The most classical of the tinctorial methods, the trichromes are so-called for their ability to differentiate tissue elements into three colours. Collagen, muscle, fibrin and red blood cells are selectively demonstrated, together with cell nuclei.

Most authors agree that the factors controlling trichrome staining are the porosity or permeability of tissues and the size of the dye molecule. These arguments hold true whether dyes are applied sequentially or in combination. In these methods acid dyes are used at a low pH, but the electrostatic bonding between dye and tissue is of less importance than factors given above.

Thus if we consider the differential staining of collagen, which is relatively permeable, and muscle, which is far less so, by simultaneous exposure to dyes of different molecular size, say acid fuchsin and picric acid, we would expect collagen to be coloured by the larger molecule. This is, in fact, exactly what happens in the Van Gieson technique, collagen staining red with acid fuchsin and muscle yellow with the much smaller dye picric acid. If acid fuchsin and methyl blue were combined, collagen would now stain blue with the larger methyl blue molecule.

If the dyes are used sequentially, the first dye applied will be retained in sites slow to stain and therefore to destain; generally those with the lowest permeability. Thus acid fuchsin may be retained by red blood cells, whilst collagen would release the acid fuchsin to be replaced by a larger dye molecule such as aniline blue. Those tissue structures which are intermediary between these two extremes show evidence of staining either by both dyes, or by a third dye of intermediate molecular size.

Finally, so-called 'colourless dyes' may be used to differentiate trichrome techniques. Phosphomolybdic and phosphotungstic acids are most commonly used; the main advantage of using this intermediate step is that it allows a more precise microscopical control over the two colour staining.

Fixation is of importance in achieving the best results. Unfortunately, formal–saline is less than satisfactory for this purpose although improved results may be obtained by pretreating sections with more satisfactory fixative solutions. Generally, mercuric chloride or dichromate containing fixatives are preferred. Sections should be treated for at least 1 hour but preferably overnight.

Lendrum *et al.* (1962) have stressed the value of treating sections with trichlorethylene for 24–48 hours immediately they have been dewaxed, this treatment leading to more brilliant results. The process is known as 'degreasing'.

■ Van Gieson's stain

Reagent

Saturated aqueous picric acid	100 ml
1% acid fuchsin	10 ml

Method

(1) Dewax sections and bring to water.
(2) *Either* stain in Weigert's haematoxylin for 40 minutes
    or stain with celestin blue for 5 minutes, rinse in water and stain with Mayer's haemalum for 5 minutes.
(3) Wash in tap-water.
(4) Differentiate in 1% hydrochloric acid in 70% alcohol.
(5) Wash in running water for 5 minutes.
(6) Stain in Van Gieson's stain for 3 minutes.
(7) Rinse briefly in distilled water.
(8) Dehydrate rapidly, clear and mount in synthetic resin.

Results

Nuclei	Black
Collagen	Red
Other tissues, including muscle and RBCs	Yellow

Notes

The acid nature of Van Gieson's stain will lead to overdifferentiation if alum haematoxylin is substituted for the iron haematoxylin or celestin blue sequence recommended.

Attempts have been made to increase the crispness of collagen staining by including hydrochloric acid or nitric acid in the staining solution. They should be used cautiously if overdifferentiation is to be avoided.

Acid fuchsin may be easily lost if step 7 and dehydration is not completed rapidly.

■ **Masson's trichrome**

Method

(1) Bring sections to water.
(2) Treat with celestin blue–haemalum sequence.
(3) Differentiate in 1% acid alcohol.
(4) Wash in running tap-water for 5 minutes.
(5) Stain in 1% acid fuchsin in 1% acetic acid for 5 minutes.
(6) Rinse in distilled water.
(7) Treat with 1% aqueous phosphomolybdic acid for 5 minutes.
(8) Treat with *either* 1% methyl blue in 1% acetic acid for 2–3 minutes, *or* 1% light green in 1% acetic acid.
(9) Rinse in 1% acetic acid (to clear background), $\frac{1}{2}$–1 minute.
(10) Dehydrate clear and mount in synthetic resin.

Results

Nuclei	Blue-black
Muscle, RBCs, cytoplasm	Red
Collagen, cartilage, mucin	Blue *or* green

Notes

The red component of the stain may be improved by combining 2 parts of 1% ponceau 2R in 1% acetic acid with 1 part 1% acid fuchsin in 1% acetic acid.

Stage 7 should be monitored carefully—it may be regarded as a stage of differentiation (*see above*).

It is a matter of personal choice whether a blue or green stain is employed to demonstrate the collagen. It is easy to overstain and swamp other colours at this stage.

Collagen may not stain uniformly—dye uptake will depend upon the physical state of the fibres prior to fixation. For example, collagen that is under tension may be expected to be less permeable, and does indeed tend to retain the red dye preferentially.

The staining time may need to be prolonged at step 5 for formal–saline fixed material. Results will be improved by pretreating sections in Zenker's fluid overnight.

■ **Mallory's trichrome**

There have been many variations of this technique, including those made by Mallory himself. However, he eventually returned to his original method, a decision endorsed by Cook (1974). Save for the introduction of a nuclear stain, it is the method we recommend.

Reagent

Aniline blue–orange G solution

Aniline blue	0.5 g
Orange G	2.0 g
Phosphomolybdic acid	1.0 g
Distilled water	100 ml

First dissolve the phosphomolybdic acid in distilled water, then add the dyes. Filter before use.

Method

(1) Bring sections to water.
(2) Treat with celestin blue–haemalum sequence.
(3) Differentiate in 1% acid alcohol.
(4) Wash in running tap-water for 5 minutes.
(5) Stain in 0.5% aqueous acid fuchsin for 5 minutes.
(6) Drain slides. Stain in aniline blue–orange blue solution for 15–20 minutes.
(7) Wash in 95% alcohol. Some differentiation will occur at this stage.
(8) Dehydrate, clear and mount in synthetic resin.

Results

Nuclei	Blue
Collagen	Deep blue
Cartilage, bone, mucin	Light blue
Muscle, fibrin	Red
RBCs, myelin	Yellow

There have been many attempts both to expand, modify and simplify trichrome methods for connective tissue differentiation. Heidenhain's Azan stain, Lillie's Allochrome and Gomori's rapid one-step trichrome are all examples. Most trichrome stains require a degree of experience to produce the best results. For reproducible results, easily obtained from unskilled hands, we recommend the one-step method of Sweat, Meloan and Puchtler (1968).

■ One-step trichrome

Reagents

Trichrome solution

Chromotrope 2R	0.6 g
Aniline blue	0.6 g
Phosphomolybdic acid	1.0 g
Distilled water	100 ml
Conc. hydrochloric acid	1.0 ml

Dissolve in the order given. Add the HCl last. Allow to stand for 24 hours in the refrigerator before use. Store at 4 °C. Do not filter before use.

Method

(1) Bring sections to water.
(2) Place in Bouin's fixative (page 40) at 56 °C for 1 hour.
(3) Wash in running water to remove picric acid for 3–4 minutes.
(4) Stain in trichrome solution for 1 minute.
(5) Rinse in 1% acetic acid for 30 seconds.
(6) Dehydrate rapidly in one change 95% alcohol and three changes of absolute alcohol.
(7) Clear and mount in synthetic resin.

Results

Nuclei, cytoplasm, muscle, fibrin and elastin	Red
Collagen, reticulin, basement membrane, cartilage	Blue

Notes

A celestin blue–haemalum sequence is only partially successful. The strongly acidic trichrome stain is a powerful differentiator. Iron–haematoxylin, such as Weigert's, tends to interfere with chromotrope 2R staining.

Pretreatment with Bouin's fixative helps to equilibrate the effects of various fixatives and produces increased affinity for chromotrope 2R.

Methods for the demonstration of fibrin, which are similar in principle to the trichrome methods, are given in Chapter 25.

The acid picro–Mallory method, although valued primarily for the demonstration of fibrin, is a useful trichrome type method for staining connective tissues.

■ Acid picro–Mallory (Lendrum, 1949)

Reagents

(1) Celestin blue. Dissolve 2.5 g of iron alum in 50 ml of distilled water overnight at room temperature, and to this add 0.25 g of celestin blue. Boil for 3 minutes, and filter when cool into a staining jar; add 7 ml of glycerin. This staining solution will keep for several months.
(2) Mayer's haemalum. Refer to page 157.
(3) Picro-orange. Dissolve 0.2 g of orange G in 100 ml of 80% alcohol which has been saturated with picric acid.
(4) Acid fuchsin. One per cent acid fuchsin in 3% trichloracetic acid.

Method

(1) Bring sections to water.
(2) Stain with celestin blue in a Coplin jar for 3–5 minutes.
(3) Rinse in tap-water.
(4) Stain with Mayer's haemalum for 5 minutes (longer if the solution is not fresh).
(5) Wash in tap-water for 3 minutes, then rinse in 95% alcohol.
(6) Stain with picro-orange for 2 minutes.
(7) Stain with acid fuchsin for 5 minutes, then rinse in water.
(8) Dip sections into equal parts of picro-orange and 80% alcohol for a few seconds.
(9) Differentiate in 1% phosphotungstic acid until colours are clear (5–10 minutes), then rinse in water.
(10) Stain with 2% soluble blue in 2% aqueous acetic acid for 2–10 minutes, then rinse in water.
(11) Dehydrate, clear and mount in synthetic resin.

Results

Fibrin	Clear red
Muscle	Paler red
Red blood cells	Orange
Collagen	Blue
Nuclei	Blue-black

Methods for reticulin

Silver impregnation is necessary for the truly successful demonstration of reticulin fibres. There have been many published methods and modifications, all of which have origins in Bielschowsky's method for nerve fibres. All follow a common sequence.

Pre-oxidation with potassium permanganate, followed by bleaching in oxalic acid probably inhibits the argyrophilia of nerve fibres (Cook, 1974). However, omission of this step may result in a failure to impregnate successfully (Lillie, 1965).

Sensitization increases the affinity of reticulin fibres for silver, although it is only in the silver oxide and not the silver carbonate methods that this step is included. Iron alum is the commonest sensitizing agent, although ferric chloride, silver nitrate and uranyl nitrate are also used.

Impregnation is carried out in an ammoniacal silver solution. Silver nitrate is precipitated with either sodium or potassium hydroxide or with sodium carbonate and the precipitate redissolved in ammonium hydroxide by the addition of concentrated ammonia. The accurate preparation of the impregnating solution is crucial to all methods. It is preferably to incompletely dissolve the deposit than to add too much ammonia.

Reduction—with formaldehyde solutions—results in the deposition of metallic silver on the reticulin fibres.

Toning is an optional step wherein some substitution of metallic gold from yellow gold chloride solution occurs with a resultant increase in contrast of the 'stained' section.

Fixing in sodium thiosulphate removes unreduced silver which may subsequently reduce on exposure to light, giving a 'dirty' background. The possibility is more theoretical than real.

Counterstaining is optional. Haematoxylin, Van Gieson, light green or neutral red may be useful.

Silver impregnation techniques are often capricious unless careful attention is paid to detail. Glassware should be chemically cleaned, reagents should be pure, accuracy in weighing and measuring may be critical. Ammonia should be fresh and metal forceps should not come into contact with ammoniacal silver solutions.

It is worth repeating the advice of Wallington (1965) who, warning of the explosive hazards of ammoniacal silver solutions, advises that 'silvered glassware' is dangerous, that solutions should not be exposed to sunlight and that unused reagent should be inactivated by the addition of dilute hydrochloric acid or sodium chloride solution.

Strongly alkaline solutions have a marked tendency to lift sections off slides. Paraffin-wax sections for reticulin staining should be mounted on gelatin coated slides. Alternatively, the section may be protected by coating the slide, immediately after dewaxing, with 1% celloidin in equal parts of ether and absolute alcohol. After draining, the celloidin is hardened in 70% alcohol. After staining, the celloidin may be removed by lengthy immersion in absolute alcohol or, more rapidly, by flooding briefly with ether/alcohol or acetone following dehydration.

Of the many published methods for reticulin demonstration, we prefer the method of Gordon and Sweets (1936). It should not impregnate cell nuclei, and gives a nice clear background. As an alternative, Gomori's method is given. It is simple and reliable. A fuller review of methods is given by Lillie (1965).

■ **Gordon and Sweets' reticulin method**

Reagents

Acidified potassium permanganate
   0.5% aqueous potassium permanganate   95 ml
   3.0% sulphuric acid   5 ml

Silver solution

To 5 ml of 10.2% aqueous silver nitrate add fresh, strong ammonia (sp.gr. 0.88) drop by drop until the precipitate which is first formed just dissolves. Agitate constantly. Add 5 ml of 3.1% sodium hydroxide. Again add strong ammonia until the precipitate just dissolves. At this stage the solution should not be *completely* clear. Make the volume up to 50 ml with distilled water. Make fresh before use.

Method

(1) Bring sections to water.
(2) Oxidize in acidified potassium permanganate for 3 minutes.
(3) Wash in tap-water.
(4) Bleach in 1% oxalic acid for 2 minutes.
(5) Wash well in running tap-water then rinse in distilled water.
(6) Sensitize in 2.5% iron alum (ferric ammonium sulphate) for 10 minutes.
(7) Rinse well in distilled water.
(8) Impregnate with ammoniacal silver solution for 15–30 seconds. This stage should be performed in a Coplin jar using constant agitation: 15 seconds will suffice, but up to 2 minutes should not cause over-impregnation.
(9) Wash well in several changes of distilled water.
(10) Reduce in 10% aqueous formalin—with agitation for 1 minute.
(11) Wash well in tap-water.
(12) *Optional.* Tone in 0.1% gold chloride for 1 minute.
(13) Wash in tap-water.
(14) Fix in 5% sodium thiosulphate (hypo) for 5 minutes.
(15) Wash well, counterstain if desired.
(16) Dehydrate clear and mount in synthetic resin.

Results

Reticulin fibres only   Black
Collagen (if untoned)   Yellow-brown
Collagen (if toned)   Purple-black

■ **Gomori's reticulin method**

Silver solution

To 4 parts of 10% aqueous silver nitrate add 1 part of 10% potassium hydroxide. Allow the deposit to settle, remove the supernatant and wash the deposit twice with distilled water. Make up to original volume with distilled water. This step helps to give a cleaner background. Add fresh, strong ammonia (sp.gr. 0.88) drop by drop until the deposit is just dissolved. Carefully add 10% silver nitrate, drop by drop, until the solution takes on a faint sheen. Make solution up to twice its original volume.

Method

(1) Bring sections to water.
(2) Oxidize in 1% potassium permanganate for 2 minutes.
(3) Rinse in tap-water.
(4) Bleach in 5% oxalic acid for 2 minutes.
(5) Rinse in tap-water.
(6) Sensitize in 2.5% iron alum for 1 minute.
(7) Wash well in tap-water; rinse in distilled water.
(8) Impregnate in silver solution for 3 minutes.
(9) Rinse rapidly in distilled water.
(10) Reduce in 10% aqueous formalin for 3 minutes.
(11) Wash well in tap-water; rinse in distilled water.
(12) *Optional*. Tone in 0.1% aqueous gold chloride for 1 minute.
(13) Rinse in distilled water.
(14) Fix in 5% thiosulphate (hypo) for 5 minutes.
(15) Wash well—optional counterstain.
(16) Dehydrate, clear and mount in synthetic medium.

Results

Reticulin fibres	Black
Collagen	
Cells, including nuclei	} Purple-grey if toned.

Methods for elastin

Elastic fibres are brightly autofluorescent and often easily identified in the walls of blood vessels. They are much less obvious in the dermis where they may be present as very fine fibres. However, there are a variety of methods showing remarkable selectivity for elastic fibres, none of which show absolute specificity. We recommend Hart's modification of Weigert's resorcin–fuchsin as the most sensitive, Verhoeff's as providing the greatest contrast and orcein as the simplest. We have also found Miller's technique (1971) to be simple, reliable and selective.

■ Weigert's resorcin–fuchsin method

Reagent

Basic fuchsin	2 g
Resorcin	4 g
Distilled water to	200 ml

Basic fuchsin recommended for Schiff reagent tends not to give the best results. The above ingredients should be brought to the boil in a glass or porcelain container. Whilst still boiling, slowly add 25 ml of 30% ferric chloride and continue boiling for a further 5 minutes. Taking care to retain all the precipitate, filter when cool. Discard the filtrate and place the filter paper (with precipitate) into the original (unwashed) flask which should have been dried. Add 200 ml of 95% alcohol and heat gently in a water-bath or on a hot-plate until the precipitate has dissolved. Remove filter paper, add 4 ml of concentrated hydrochloric acid and filter. Make volume up to 200 ml by pouring fresh 95% alcohol through the used filter paper. Store at 4 °C for up to 2 months.

Method

(1) Bring sections to water.
(2) Stain for 20–60 minutes. This time has to be established by trial and error. It will depend upon the batch of basic fuchsin used and the age of the solution.
(3) Wash in 95% alcohol.
(4) Differentiate in 1% hydrochloric acid in 70% alcohol.
(5) Wash in tap-water.
(6) Counterstain as desired, e.g. haematoxylin or Van Gieson.
(7) Dehydrate clear and mount in synthetic resin.

Results

Elastic fibres   Blue-black

■ **Hart's modification of Weigert**

Reagent

Dilute Weigert's resorcin–fuchsin, prepared as above, 1 part plus 9 parts of 1% acid alcohol. This solution is more stable than Weigert's original formula.

Method

(1) Bring sections to water.
(2) Stain 18 hours at room temperature.
(3) Differentiate in acid alcohol.
(4) Counterstain with Van Gieson for 3 minutes.
(5) Dehydrate rapidly, clear and mount in synthetic resin.

Results

Elastic fibres   Blue-black

■ **Verhoeff's iron haematoxylin for elastic fibres**

Although providing excellent contrast, this method requires careful differentiation if staining is not to be lost from the finest fibres. It should be remembered than Van Gieson, the most commonly applied counterstain, will continue to differentiate the haematoxylin.

Reagent

5% Haematoxylin in absolute alcohol. This does not have to   20 ml
  have been ripened

10% Ferric chloride	8 ml
Verhoeff's iodine (iodine 2 g, potassium iodide 4 g,	
distilled water, 100 ml)	8 ml

Mix a fresh solution, in the order given, for each usage.

Method

(1) Bring sections to water.
(2) Stain in Verhoeff's iron haematoxylin for 20 minutes.
(3) Differentiate in 2% ferric chloride. This stage *must* be controlled microscopically. Differentiation should be halted when nuclei and fine fibres are still black, and the background still weakly stained. If overdifferentiated return to the Verhoeff's solution.
(4) Wash in water, then in 95% alcohol to remove iodine coloration.
(5) Wash in water then counterstain in Van Gieson's stain for 3 minutes.
(6) Dehydrate rapidly, clear and mount in synthetic resin.

Results

Elastic fibres	Black
Collagen	Red
Muscle	Yellow
Nuclei	Black

■ Orcein method for elastic fibres

Although occasional batches of orcein are reported to give indifferent results, synthetic orcein invariably provides a simple method of remarkable selectivity for elastic fibres.

Formula

Orcein (synthetic)	1 g
Hydrochloric acid	1 ml
70% Alcohol	100 ml

The orcein should be dissolved in the alcohol with the aid of gentle heat, the solution filtered and the hydrochloric acid added.

Method

(1) Bring sections to water.
(2) Stain in orcein solution at 56–60 °C for 30 minutes.
(3) Rinse in 70% alcohol.
(4) Differentiate—briefly—in acid alcohol.
(5) Wash in water.
(6) Counterstain if desired. Methylene blue or Mayer's haemalum are suitable.
(7) Dehydrate, clear and mount in synthetic resin.

Results

Elastin	Dark brown

■ **Miller's stain for elastic (1971)**

Formula

Victoria blue 4R	1 g
New fuchsin	1 g
Crystal violet	1 g

Dissolve in 200 ml of hot distilled water, then add, in the order given:

Resorcin	4 g
Dextrin	1 g
30% Ferric chloride (fresh)	50 ml

Boil for 5 minutes then filter while hot. Transfer precipitate plus filter paper to original beaker and redissolve in 200 ml of 95% alcohol. Boil on a hot-plate, or water-bath, for 15–20 minutes. Filter and make up to 200 ml with 95% alcohol. Finally add 2 ml of concentrated hydrochloric acid.

Method

(1) Bring sections to water.
(2) Then 0.5% aqueous potassium permanganate for 5 minutes.
(3) Rinse in tap-water.
(4) 1% Aqueous oxalic acid for 2–3 minutes.
(5) Rinse in distilled water, followed by 95% alcohol.
(6) Place in stain in a Coplin jar for 1–3 hours.
(7) Wash in 95% alcohol to remove excess stain.
(8) Wash in water.
(9) Van Gieson for 3 minutes.
(10) Dehydrate rapidly, clear and mount in synthetic resin.

Results

Elastic fibres and mast cell granules   Black

Note: At step 6, the stain may be diluted with an equal quantity of 95% alcohol, and the section stained overnight.

■ **Gomori's aldehyde fuchsin method for elastic fibres**

Although less selective than other methods, aldehyde fuchsin is a reliable method for staining elastic fibres strongly. Other tissue elements that may be stained include sulphated mucopolysaccharides, beta cells of the pancreas and pituitary and mast cells. However, these are easily distinguished from elastic fibres on morphologic grounds.

Reagent

Basic fuchsin	1 g
70% Alcohol	200 ml
Concentrated hydrochloric acid	2 ml
Fresh paraldehyde	2 ml

Dissolve the basic fuchsin in the alcohol before adding hydrochloric acid and paraldehyde. Shake well then leave for 2–3 days at room temperature until a deep purple colour develops. Store at 4 °C and be prepared to extend staining times as the stain ages. Schiff grade basic fuchsin is suitable.

Method

(1) Bring sections to water.
(2) Stain in aldehyde fuchsin solution. Optimal time will depend upon the batch and age of stain. A control section of skin should be used to determine the optimum which should lie between 5 and 20 minutes.
(3) Rinse in 70% alcohol.
(4) Counterstain as desired, for example, 0.2% light green, 0.2% methylene blue, Mayer's haemalum.
(5) Dehydrate, clear and mount.

Results

Elastic tissue   Deep purple

■ Elastase digestion

Although elastin is remarkably resistant to autolytic changes, it is possible to digest most deposits of human elastin with porcine elastase. The method recommended by Cook (1974) is suitable for use on formalin fixed paraffin sections. The incubation solution consists of two to three units of elastase/ml of pH 8.8 Sörensen's glycine–sodium hydroxide buffer. Digestion times of 6–8 hours at 37 °C are necessary. A control section should always be treated with buffer alone in parallel with the test section.

Methods for muscle

Methods used specifically in the interpretation of muscle biopsies are given in Chapter 23. Here are given only those methods which help identify muscle fibres within connective tissue.

■ Lendrum's Lissamine fast red method for muscle fibres

Method

(1) Bring sections to water.
(2) Stain nuclei with the celestin blue–haemalum sequence (page 171).
(3) Differentiate in 1% acid alcohol, wash in water.
(4) Stain in 1% Lissamine fast red in 1% acetic acid for 10 minutes.
(5) Rinse in distilled water.
(6) Differentiate in 1% phosphomolybdic acid, until the collagen is de-stained. Differentiation may be hastened by using warm phosphomolybdic acid solution. The time required should be in the region of 5 minutes.
(7) Rinse in tap-water.
(8) Counterstain in 1.5% tartrazine in 1.5% acetic acid for 5 minutes.

(9) Rinse briefly in 95% alcohol.
(10) Dehydrate, clear and mount.

Results

Muscle (and red blood cells)   Red
Nuclei   Blue/black
Connective tissue   Yellow

Note: The Lissamine fast red solution keeps only for a few days.

■ Phosphotungstic acid haematoxylin (PTAH)

This is a simple technique, giving often beautiful results. There have been numerous modifications to the technique since it was introduced by Mallory in 1897.

Reagent

Haematein   1 g
Phosphotungstic acid 20 g
Distilled water   1000 ml

Dissolve the haematein and the phosphotungstic acid separately in distilled water, using gentle heat. When cool, combine the solutions and make up to 1 litre. Ripening is accomplished immediately by adding 0.177 g of potassium permanganate. Alternatively, it may be achieved by exposing to sunlight for 5–6 weeks.

Method

(1) Bring section to water.
(2) Then 0.25% potassium permanganate for 5 minutes.
(3) Wash in water, then 5% oxalic acid for 2 minutes.
(4) Rinse in distilled water.
(5) Stain in PTAH solution for 16–18 hours.
(6) Dehydrate rapidly through 95% and absolute alcohol.
(7) Clear and mount in synthetic resin.

Results

Nuclei, fibrin, muscle striations, RBCs, fibroglia, neuroglia   Blue
Collagen, bone   Brick red or paler shade

Note: If the solution does not perform satisfactorily, the phosphotungstic acid should be investigated. We have found general purpose reagent grade to be more reliable than analytical grade.

References

CATCHPOLE, H. R. (1982). Connective tissue, basement membrane, extracellular matrix. In *Pathobiology Annual 1982*. Ed. Ioachim, H. L. Raven Press, New York
COOK, H. C. (1974). *Manual of Histological Demonstration Techniques*. Butterworths, London

DRURY, R. A. B. and WALLINGTON, E. A. (1980). *Carleton's Histological Technique*. Oxford University Press, Oxford, England

FULLMER, H. M. and LILLIE, R. D. (1958). The oxytalan fiber. A previously undescribed connective tissue fiber. *J. Histochem. Cytochem.*, **6**, 425–430

FULLMER, H. M., SHEETZ, J. H. and NARKATES, A. J. (1974). Oxytalan connective tissue fibres: A review. *J. Oral Pathol.*, **3**, 291–316

GORDON, H. and SWEETS, H. H. (1936). A simple method for the silver impregnation of reticulum. *Am. J. Pathol.*, **12**, 545–551

LENDRUM, A. C. (1949). The staining of erythrocytes in tissue sections. *J. Pathol. Bacteriol.*, **61**, 443–448

LENDRUM, A. C., FRASER, D. S., SLIDDERS, W. and HENDERSON, R. (1962). Studies on the character and staining of fibrin. *J. Clin. Pathol.*, **15**, 401–413

LILLIE, R. D. (1965). *Histopathologic Technic and Practical Histochemistry*. McGraw-Hill, New York

MILLER, P. J. (1971). An elastin stain. *Med. Lab. Technol.*, **28**, 148–149

MILLER, E. J., EPSTEIN, E. H. JR and PIEZ, K. A. (1971). Identification of three genetically distinct collagens by cyanogen bromide cleavage of insoluble skin and cartilage collagen. *Biochem. Biophys. Res. Commun.*, **42**, 1024–1029

STEVENS, A. (1982). In *Theory and Practice of Histological Techniques*. Eds Bancroft, J. D. and Stevens, A. 2nd Ed. Churchill-Livingstone, London

SWEAT, F., MELOAN, S. N. and PUCHTLER, H. (1968). A modified one-step trichrome stain for demonstration of fine connective tissue fibres. *Stain Technol.*, **43**, 227–231

WALLINGTON, E. A. (1965). The explosive properties of ammoniacal-silver solutions. *J. Med. Lab. Technol.*, **22**, 220–223

YAOITA, H., FOIDART, J-M. and KATZ, S. I. (1978). Localisation of the collagenous component in skin basement membrane. *J. Invest. Derm.*, **70**, 191–193

10

Nucleic acids

Nucleoproteins are combinations of basic protein with nucleic acids. In the nucleus we find mostly deoxyribonucleic acid, with some ribonucleic acid: in the cytoplasm of most cells there is abundant ribonucleic acid concentrated mainly in the ribosomes.

Deoxyribonucleic acid (DNA)

Friedrich Miescher in 1869 isolated a substance from the nuclei of cells which he called nuclein. We now know nuclein to be deoxyribonucleic acid (DNA). Robert Feulgen in 1914 first demonstrated his colour test for DNA in a test tube, but not until 1924 did he describe his method of staining cells to demonstrate that DNA is located in the chromosomes in the nucleus. The work of innumerable biochemists, biologists and biophysicists, particularly in the past 30 years, has shown that all genetic information is carried in the DNA, and it may now be postulated how this could be achieved. Chemists have shown that the molecule consists of a long, unbranched chain, the backbone of which is made up of alternate five-carbon sugar (deoxyribose) and phosphate groups; a nitrogenous base being attached to each sugar group. There are four nitrogenous bases found in most DNAs: the purines (adenine and guanine) and the pyrimidines (thymine and cytosine). The chain may be subdivided into units, or nucleotides, each consisting of a phosphate–sugar–base: polynucleotide chain is the term used to describe a series of such units.

The work of Watson and Crick (1953), using X-ray crystallography, enabled a model to be constructed of the DNA molecule. They showed that it consists, not of a single polynucleotide chain, but of two chains intertwined into a double helix, held together by hydrogen bonds (*Figure 10.1*). Some idea of its structure may be gained by thinking of it as a ladder structure, the cross-struts being the sugars and nitrogenous bases, which has been twisted into a spiral (*Figure 10.1*). Although the bases on the cross-struts are never identical, they are specifically complementary with adenine always linked to thymine and guanine to cytosine. This base pairing accounts for the ability of DNA to be self-replicating, since when DNA primes the making of more DNA the double helix uncoils and separates, and the sequence of bases on each chain will select an exact counterpart of the chain from which it has separated (e.g. adenine to thymine and guanine to cytosine). It has been shown experimentally that a single synthetic polynucleotide made up of only thymine bases will only bind a complementary chain made up exclusively of adenine bases. Kornberg and colleagues (*see* Kornberg, 1957–58) have since shown that in a cell-free substrate containing the four nucleotides

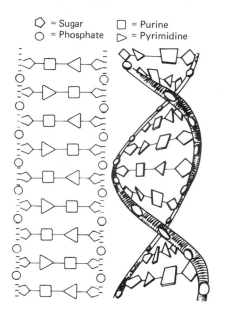

○ = Sugar   □ = Purine
○ = Phosphate ▷ = Pyrimidine

Figure 10.1 Diagram to illustrate the schematic structure of DNA

and the enzyme polymerase, together with some DNA to prime the reaction, synthetic DNA could be prepared. He has shown that some DNA has to be used to prime the reaction, and furthermore that the synthetic DNA so prepared replicates the DNA used as a primer. Using the same substrate with a number of different DNAs (from bacterial, virus and animal sources) the synthetic DNA was always identical to that used to prime the reaction.

The variation that could be achieved, by differential grouping of base pairs, is almost infinite, and is believed to function as a genetic code. Inherited DNA, being self-replicating, is eventually passed on to the next generation, genetic information is passed from cell to cell, each gene being derived from a pre-existing gene.

Ribonucleic acid (RNA)

In RNA the sugar is ribose instead of deoxyribose, and the bases, adenine, guanine, cytosine and uracil (instead of thymine), they are also linked by phosphate groups to form a polynucleotide chain. It can be seen therefore how DNA in addition to being self-replicating can in a similar manner form RNA having the same genetic information, which can pass from the nucleus to the cytoplasm. Nuclear RNA is present in the nucleolus. Cells which are actively synthesizing protein are known to be rich in RNA, this RNA is concentrated in the ribosomes of the endoplasmic reticulum. The DNA in this way predetermines the complete function of the cell.

Demonstration of nucleic acids

The demonstration of nucleic acids is dependent on the nucleotide structure consisting of phosphate radical, sugar (deoxyribose or ribose) and the nitrogenous bases (*see above*).

Phosphate radical

This being acid will combine with basic dyes, and is thought to be the mechanism of nuclear staining by basic dyes.

Deoxyribose, ribose

Backler and Alexander (1952) have described a modification of the Turchini reaction (Turchini, Castel and Kien, 1944) but in view of the excellent Feulgen methods for DNA and other methods for RNA it is not generally used. DNA and RNA can be differentiated using acridine orange techniques. Both are demonstrated by the Gallocyanin–chrome alum technique.

Nitrogenous bases

There is no reliable histochemical technique available for these groups.

Routine staining

Simple staining of the nucleus and nucleoli may be effected by any of the routine stains described in Chapter 7.

The regressive technique with haematoxylin, particularly with iron haematoxylin, may be employed to demonstrate chromosomes during mitosis, and is selective for chromatin in a resting nucleus when properly differentiated. The basic coal-tar dyes, such as toluidine blue, thionin in aqueous solution, or safranin and neutral red employed in a 0.5–1.0% aqueous acetic acid, may be employed in a similar manner.

Staining of the nuclei of living cells is generally regarded as impossible, but de Bruyn (1953) describes their staining with fluorescent dyes.

Techniques for deoxyribonucleic acid

■ **The Feulgen reaction**

The reaction, introduced by Feulgen and Rossenbeck (1924), is based upon the cleavage of the purine–deoxyribose bond by mild acid hydrolysis to expose a reactive aldehyde group. The aldehydes may then be detected by the use of a Schiff reagent, owing to the formation of a quinoid compound. In practice, those structures in a section which contain DNA are stained red by this technique.

Acid hydrolysis

The time of hydrolysis is important. Increasing the time at first results in a stronger reaction, but there is an optimum time beyond which the reaction may weaken and even become negative. As hydrolysis proceeds the DNA is depolymerized and lost through diffusion. The final result depends on the speed of the aldehyde-producing reactions and the depolymerization aldehyde-removing reactions (Kjellstrand, 1980). The type of material may occasionally affect the time of hydrolysis, but the most important single factor is the method of fixation.

Table 10.1

Fixative	Minutes
Champy	25
Chrome–acetic	14
Flemming	16
Helly	8
Regaud	14
Zenker	5
Susa	18
Zenker–formal	5
Formalin	8
Carnoy	8
Clark	6

Bauer (1932) gives the following as optimum times of hydrolysis after various fixatives (*Table 10.1*).

Immersion in cold N/1 hydrochloric acid before and after treatment at 60 °C is sometimes advised, but this has no apparent advantage.

Fixation

Provided the correct time of hydrolysis is given (*see above*), most fixatives will give reasonable results with this technique. It is obviously preferable to use a nuclear fixative, such as Carnoy, if only the nuclei are to be studied, but perfectly good results are obtainable after formal–saline fixation. For smears of tissues the use of methyl alcohol, or Clarke's fixative (page 41) is preferred.

Schiff reagents

The conventional Schiff reagent is prepared by treating basic fuchsin with sulphurous acid (aqueous SO_2), this results in the loss of the quinoid structure with the consequent loss of colour; in the presence of an aldehyde the quinoid structure (and colour) is restored.

Ornstein and colleagues (1957), Kasten (1958, 1959) and Culling and Vassar (1961) have shown that many dyes other than basic fuchsin can be utilized as Schiff reagents.

Kasten has shown that any basic dye, lacking acid groups, with at least one primary amine group can be utilized as a Schiff-type reagent after treatment with sulphurous acid. There are many such dyes, *Table 10.2* containing those recommended by him.

All the dyes listed below are not decolorized and sections may need to be treated with acid–alcohol to remove unreacted dye; similarly they are not all stable when prepared. Their usefulness may lie in the variety of colours available for the histochemical demonstration of DNA and PAS positive material in double staining methods. Culling and Vassar utilized an acriflavine–Schiff as a fluorescent reagent for the demonstration of DNA, carbohydrates and the LE cell phenomenon (*Figure 10.2*).

Preparation of Schiff reagents

Although the method of de Tomasi (1936) was formerly recommended, using sodium metabisulphite, the reagent of Barger and De Lamater (1948) is found to be simple to

Table 10.2

Dye	CI No.	Colour in nucleus after Feulgen-type reaction
Acid fuchsin	42685	Violet
Acridine yellow	46025	Yellow-green
Acriflavine hydrochloride	46000	Yellow-green
Azure A		Blue
Azure C		Blue
Bismark brown R	21010	Yellow-brown
Bismark brown Y	21000	Yellow-brown
Brilliant cresyl blue	51010	Blue-grey
Celestine blue B	51050	Blue-green
Chrysoidine 3R	11320	Yellow
Chrysoidine Y extra	11270	Yellow
Cresyl violet		Blue-violet
Crystal violet	42555	Blue-violet
Gentian violet (methyl violet)	42535	Violet
Methylene blue	52015	Blue-green to blue
Neutral red	50040	Yellow-brown
Neutral violet	50030	Red-violet
Phenosafranin	50200	Red-violet
Phosphine GN	46045	Yellow-green
Proflavine	46000	Yellow
Safranin O	50240	Red-violet to red
Thionin	52000	Blue
Toluidine blue O	52040	Blue
Toluylene blue	49410	Rust-brown

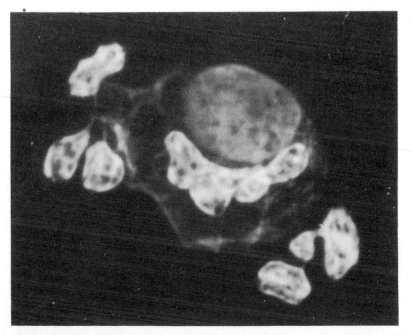

Figure 10.2 Fluorescent Feulgen staining of LE cells showing the lighter staining of the phagocytosed DNA in the cytoplasm

prepare, reliable and more stable. Equally good is the reagent of Itikawa and Oguru (1954) who simply bubble SO_2 gas slowly through a solution of 0.5% basic fuchsin. It is simpler to be able to add a reagent (thionyl chloride) to a solution than to set up the apparatus for the SO_2 gas technique. Batches of basic fuchsin may prove to be unsatisfactory for the production of Schiff reagent. We have found consistent results using pararosanilin (Sigma).

Reagents

de Tomasi Schiff reagent (1936)

(1) Dissolve 1 g of basic fuchsin or pararosanilin in 200 ml of boiling distilled water in a stoppered 1 litre flask.
(2) Shake for 5 minutes.
(3) Cool to exactly 50 °C, filter and add 20 ml of N/1 hydrochloric acid to the filtrate.
(4) Cool further to 25 °C, and add 1 g of sodium (or potassium) metabisulphite.
(5) Store for 18–24 hours in the dark, add 2 g of activated charcoal and shake the mixture for 1 minute.
(6) Remove the charcoal by filtration and store the solution in the dark at 0–4 °C.

Lillie's 'cold' Schiff reagent

(1) Dissolve 1 g basic fuchsin and 1.9 g sodium metabisulphite in 100 ml of 0.15 N hydrochloric acid.
(2) Shake the solution at intervals or on a mechanical shaker for 2 hours.
(3) Add 0.5 g activated charcoal and shake for 1–2 minutes.
(4) Filter into graduated cylinder, washing the residue with a little distilled water to restore the original 100 ml volume.

The solution should be water white. Store in the refrigerator.

Barger and De Lamater Schiff reagent (1948)

(1) Dissolve 1 g of basic fuchsin in 400 ml of boiling distilled water, cool to 50 °C and filter.
(2) Add 1 ml of thionyl chloride ($SOCl_2$), stopper the flask and, after shaking, allow to stand for 12 hours.
(3) Add 2 g activated charcoal, shake and immediately filter.

This will keep several months in a well-stoppered dark bottle in the refrigerator.

Sulphite rinses

Sulphite rinses must be freshly prepared each day by adding 7.5 ml of 10% potassium metabisulphite, and 7.5 ml of N/1 hydrochloric acid to 135 ml of distilled water; these amounts will amply fill three Coplin jars.

Method

(1) Bring sections to water.
(2) Rinse in cold N/1 hydrochloric acid.

(3) Transfer to N/1 hydrochloric acid at 60 °C and leave for optimal time of hydrolysis (*see above*). As a routine, with all but Susa and chrome–osmic fixatives, a period of 10 minutes will suffice.

Note: The hydrochloric acid must be pre-heated to 60 °C.

(4) Rinse in cold N/1 hydrochloric acid and rinse briefly in distilled water.
(5) Transfer section to Schiff's reagent for 30–90 minutes.
(6) Transfer to the first of three sulphite rinses, leave for 1 minute.
(7) Transfer to the second sulphite rinse, leave for 2 minutes.
(8) Transfer to the third sulphite rinse, leave for 2 minutes.
(9) Rinse well in distilled water.
(10) Counterstain, if desired, with 1% aqueous light green or tartrazine in Cellosolve.
(11) Dehydrate, clear and mount in Canada balsam or synthetic resin.

Results

DNA   Red–reddish purple
Other constituents   Green or yellow, depending on the counterstain used

■ Naphthoic acid hydrazine reaction (Feulgen NAH) (Pearse, 1951)

Although the Feulgen reaction is used routinely as a specific method of demonstrating DNA, doubts as to its absolute specificity have been raised in recent years on the grounds that the aldehyde–fuchsin sulphurous acid compound which is formed, being diffusible, may become attached to other protein components. This objection may be overcome by the use of the Feulgen and the Feulgen NAH reaction, since the latter utilizes a different reaction to demonstrate the aldehyde groups released by acid hydrolysis; material giving a positive reaction by both techniques may therefore be certainly described as DNA. The use of both techniques should be confined to those occasions when a critical assessment of DNA content is to be made.

Reagents

(1) NAH solution

2-Hydroxy-3-naphthoic acid hydrazine	0.1 g
Ethyl alcohol	95 ml
Acetic acid	5 ml

(2) Fast blue B salt solution

Fast blue B salt	0.1 g
Veronal acetate buffer (pH 7.4)	100 ml

Method

(1) Bring sections to water, and rinse in cold N/1 hydrochloric acid.
(2) Transfer to N/1 hydrochloric acid at 60 °C (pre-heated) and leave for the same time as for Feulgen reaction.
(3) Rinse in cold N/1 hydrochloric acid.
(4) Rinse in 50% alcohol.

(5) Transfer to NAH solution in a Coplin jar at a temperature of about 22 °C for 3–6 hours.
(6) Rinse in three changes of 50% alcohol, leaving sections for 10 minutes in each change.
(7) Rinse in water.
(8) Transfer to fast blue B salt solution at 0 °C (which has been pre-cooled) for 1–3 minutes.
(9) Wash in water.
(10) Counterstain if desired.
(11) Dehydrate, clear and mount in synthetic resin.

Results

DNA	Bluish-purple
Cytoplasmic and other proteins	Pinkish-red

■ Fluorescent Feulgen reaction (Culling and Vassar, 1961)

This technique utilizes a fluorescent Schiff reagent. It is simple in operation and, because of the intense brilliance of the fluorescence against a dark background, gives results superior to the conventional Feulgen reaction.

Control sections, treated with deoxyribonuclease (DNAse) to remove DNA, or bisulphite to block aldehyde groups, fail to stain by this technique which may be accepted as proof of specificity.

In addition to its use for the demonstration of DNA and nuclear patterns (including chromosomes), it has been utilized for the demonstration of the LE cell phenomena (Wignall, Culling and Vassar, 1962). The altered DNA of the inclusion body, which is thought to consist of DNA and histone in salt linkage, fluoresces a lighter yellow than nuclear DNA and is thus easily seen even with high dry objectives (*Figure 10.2*). Cytomegalic inclusions may also be seen.

Fixation

Carnoy or formalin-fixed paraffin sections give excellent results, as do methyl alcohol fixed smears, other fixatives may require different times of hydrolysis as for conventional Feulgen reaction.

Reagents

Fluorescent Schiff reagent

Acriflavine hydrochloride	1 g
Potassium metabisulphite	2 g
Distilled water	200 ml
N/1 Hydrochloric acid	20 ml

Dissolve the acriflavine and metabisulphite in the distilled water, then add the hydrochloric acid. This should be kept overnight before use. This reagent is reasonably stable.

Method

(1) Bring sections to water.
(2) Treat sections (or smears) in preheated N/1 hydrochloric acid at 60 °C for 10 minutes (depending on fixation, *see above*).
(3) Wash briefly in distilled water.
(4) Transfer to fluorescent Schiff reagent for 20 minutes.
(5) Wash in acid–alcohol (1% HCl in 95% alcohol) and leave for 5 minutes; this removes unreacted Schiff reagent and takes the place of sulphite rinses in the conventional method.
(6) Transfer to fresh acid alcohol for a further 10 minutes.
(7) Wash in absolute alcohol, a few changes to remove traces of acid.
(8) Clear in xylene and mount in synthetic resin.

Results

DNA   Fluoresces a bright golden yellow
Other tissue components   Green

Examine using BG 12 exciter filter and yellow (OG 4) and/or orange (OG 5) barrier filters.

Techniques for ribonucleic acid

■ **Acridine orange technique for RNA**

This method is to be preferred for the demonstration of RNA in smears or alcohol fixed tissues. It has, however, the great disadvantage of not being permanent. The method, introduced by von Bertalanffy, Masin and Masin (1956), for the quick detection of malignant cells in cervical smears is given on page 493. DNA fluoresces green and RNA fluoresces orange-red. Proof of the presence of DNA or RNA must be confirmed by their removal by the appropriate enzymes, that is, deoxyribonuclease or ribonuclease.

■ **The Unna–Pappenheim methyl green–pyronin stain (Pappenheim, 1899; Unna, 1902)**

Following treatment of the methyl green component with chloroform, and the use of buffered solutions, this stain has regained its popularity. Methyl green is regarded by many as being specific for DNA and the pyronin, if controlled by ribonuclease extraction, specifically demonstrates RNA. The type of fixative employed is important, and the best results with the methods given below are obtainable after formal–saline, formal–alcohol, Carnoy or Zenker fixation.

Each batch of stain should be tested by staining known positives, and, if possible, a section which has been treated with ribonuclease, before being used for routine purposes.

The methods preferred are those of Trevan and Sharrock for formalin-fixed material, and that of Jordan and Baker for tissues fixed in Zenker's fluid. A 2% aqueous solution of methyl green is washed with chloroform in a separating funnel to extract methyl violet (a breakdown product of methyl green). The extraction is continued until the washings are colourless; methyl green should then stay reasonably pure for 6–9 months.

Pyronin Y gives more selective staining than pyronin B. Contaminants in the pyronin should be extracted by chloroform to give less non-specific background staining.

Differentiation in *tert*-butanol gives the most consistent results (Stowell, 1942).

Reagents

(1) Trevan and Sharrock's methyl green–pyronin (1951)

		Final concentration of stain (%)
5% Aqueous pyronin Y	17.5 ml	0.16
2% Aqueous methyl green (washed)	10 ml	0.036
Distilled water	250 ml	

Dilute with an equal quantity of acetate buffer pH 4.8 (page 130) before use. (In the original technique orange G was added.)

(2) Jordan and Baker's methyl green–pyronin (1955)

		Final concentration of stain (%)
0.5% Aqueous pyronin Y	37 ml	0.185
0.5% Aqueous methyl green (washed)	13 ml	0.065
Acetate buffer (pH 4.8)	50 ml	

The prepared stains are said to have a life of 2–4 months, but smaller amounts, made up from the stock solutions weekly, appear to give more precise staining.

The same staining technique may be used with either of the above solutions.

Method

(1) Bring section to water.
(2) Pour on prepared staining solution and leave for 15–60 minutes (15 minutes will usually suffice). If several sections are to be stained a Coplin jar should be used.
(3) Rinse quickly in distilled water, and blot on non-fluffy filter paper.
(4) Flood slide with ethanol/*tert*-butanol (1/3) and leave for 3 minutes.
(5) Flood slide with two changes of *tert*-butanol leaving each for 2 minutes.
(6) Flood with xylene; leave until clear. Should this take unduly long, the section may be blotted and fresh xylene poured on.
(7) Mount in neutral mountant or synthetic resin.

Results

Deoxyribonucleic acid (DNA)	Green
Ribonucleic acid (RNA)	Red

■ **Gallocyanin–chrome alum technique**

This method stains both types of nucleic acid but may be used in conjunction with deoxyribonuclease or ribonuclease extraction for the specific demonstration of either acid.

Reagent

Einarson's gallocyanin–chrome alum (1951)

(1) To 100 ml of a 5% aqueous solution of chrome alum $(K_2SO_4Cr_2SO_4)_3$ 24 H_2O is added 0.15 g of gallocyanin.
(2) Shake well, bring slowly to the boil and allow to boil for 5 minutes.
(3) Cool, filter and make up the volume of filtrate to 100 ml by pouring distilled water through the filter paper.

Note: This staining solution will have a pH of 1.64, and will keep for 4–5 weeks.

Method

(1) Bring sections to water.
(2) Stain in gallocyanin–chrome alum in a Coplin jar for 48 hours at room temperature.
(3) Wash in water for a few seconds.
(4) Dehydrate, clear and mount in synthetic resin.

Results

Nucleic acid   Deep blue
Cartilage   Red (at pH 1.64)

Note: The non-specific staining of structures other than nucleic acids varies with the pH of the staining solution. It is very slight at low pH values (0.83), and increases with the pH reaching a maximum value of 3.3–3.5. The staining of the nucleic acids does not vary with the pH. The addition of up to 10 ml of N/1 hydrochloric acid (for pH levels 0.33–1.64), and up to 5 ml of N/1 sodium hydroxide (for pH levels 1.64–3.76) may be employed to eliminate or accentuate non-specific staining.

Enzyme extraction of nucleic acids

Deoxyribonuclease extraction

Deoxyribonuclease, a very expensive reagent, should be used to positively identify deoxyribonucleic acid. One of a pair of duplicate sections is treated with deoxyribonuclease (*see below*), and the two sections are then stained. Any structure which is coloured in the control section, but is not coloured in the enzyme-treated section, is composed of deoxyribonucleic acid.

The method described by Kurnick (1952) has been employed with success. The enzyme is used in a concentration of 2 mg/100 ml of Gomori's tris(hydroxymethyl)-aminomethane buffer at pH 7.6 which has been diluted 1:5 with distilled water. Alcohol-fixed or Carnoy-fixed material was used, and sections were treated at 37 °C for 3 hours (Kurnick recommends 2 hours at 37 °C or 24 hours at 21 °C). As with all enzyme extractions, a buffer control section which has been treated in the buffer solution alone at 37 °C for 3 hours together with one fresh untreated section, should be stained and examined in parallel; these two controls should give identical results.

The Feulgen reaction or the methyl green–pyronin stain may be used to stain the extracted sections.

Ribonuclease extraction

Ribonuclease, which is thermostable, is usually prepared from pancreas; it is available commercially in crystalline form, or boiled acid extract of fresh pancreas may be used. It can also be prepared by heating saliva at 80 °C for 10 minutes (Bradbury, 1956).

The dilutions at which the crystalline form should be used are variously given from 1:100 000 to 1:1000 in glass-distilled water. Better results were obtained with the latter dilution, in formal–saline, formal–alcohol and alcohol fixed smears and sections.

A section is treated at 37 °C for 1 hour, a control section being placed in distilled water at the same temperature and for the same time; in addition, a fresh uncontrolled section is also stained.

Following extraction, all three sections are stained by one of the methods given above. The ribonuclease-treated section is compared with the two controls: the absence of a structure which is present in the controls indicates that this structure was composed of ribonucleic acid.

Chemical extraction of nucleic acids

Perchloric acid

Perchloric acid (Erickson, Sax and Ogur, 1949) may be used to extract either RNA alone, or RNA and DNA by varying the time and temperature of exposure. To remove RNA alone, sections are treated with 10% perchloric acid in distilled water at 4 °C for 12–18 hours. To remove both nucleic acids, sections are treated with 5% perchloric acid in distilled water at 60 °C for 20–30 minutes.

Following extraction, sections are neutralized in 1% sodium carbonate for 1–5 minutes, washed in running tap-water and stained with appropriate techniques. We have used perchloric acid routinely and find it a reliable technique.

Bile salts

Bile salts (Foster and Wilson, 1952) are the only chemical compounds that have been described as selectively removing RNA alone. Continual oxygenation during extraction is essential for good results, and is best achieved by using a small aerator pump such as is used in small fish tanks.

The sections are immersed in 2% aqueous sodium tauroglycocholate for 24–48 hours, the solution being constantly aerated during the whole process.

Following extraction, sections are washed, and stained with 1% toluidine blue, Gram's stain or methyl green–pyronin.

Trichloroacetic acid

Treatment with 4% trichloroacetic acid (Schneider, 1945) at exactly 90 °C for 15 minutes will remove both types of nucleic acid (RNA and DNA). After exposure to the acid, sections are washed in distilled water and stained with methyl green–pyronin or toluidine blue.

References

BACKLER, B. S. and ALEXANDER, W. F. (1952). A modified Turchini technique for the differential staining of nucleic acids. *Stain Technol.*, **27**, 147–152

BARGER, J. D. and DE LAMATER, E. D. (1948). The use of thionyl chloride in the preparation of Schiff's reagent. *Science*, **108**, 121–122

BAUER, H. (1932). Die Feulgensche Nuklealfärbung in ihrer Anwendung auf cytologische Untersuchungen. *Ztschr. Zell Mikr. Anat.*, **15**, 225–247

BRADBURY, S. (1956). Human saliva: A convenient source of ribonuclease. *Quart. J. Micr. Sci.*, **97**, 323–327

CULLING, C. F. A. and VASSAR, P. S. (1961). Desoxyribose nucleic acid, a fluorescent histochemical technique. *Arch. Pathol.*, **71**, 76–80

DE BRUYN, P. P. H., FARR, R. S., BANKS, HILDA and MORTHLAND, F. W. (1952). *In vivo* and *in vitro* affinity of diaminoacridines for nucleoproteins. *Exp. Cell. Res.*, **4**, 174–180

DE TOMASI, J. A. (1936). Improving the technique of the Feulgen stain. *Stain Technol.*, **11**, 137–144

EINARSON, L. (1951). On the theory of gallocyanin–chromalum staining and its application for quantitative estimation of basophilia. Selective staining of exquisite progressivity. *Acta Pathol. Microbiol. Scand.*, **28**, 82–102

ERICKSEN, R. O., SAX, K. B. and OGUR, M. (1949). Perchloric acid in the cytochemistry of pentose nucleic acid. *Science*, **110**, 472–473

FEULGEN, R. and ROSSENBECK, H. (1924). Mikroskopisch-chemischer Nachweis einer Nucleinsäure von Typus der Thymonucleinsäure und die darauf berhende elektive Farbung von Zellkernen in mikroskopischen Preparäten. *Zeit. Phys. Chem.*, **135**, 203–248

FOSTER, C. E. and WILSON, R. R. (1952). Studies upon the Gram reaction of the basophil cells of the anterior pituitary: I. Some preliminary observations upon the basophil cells of the human pituitary. *Quart. J. Micr. Sci.*, **93**, 147–155

ITIKAWA, O. and OGURA, Y. (1954). Simplified manufacture and histochemical use of the Schiff reagent. *Stain Technol.*, **29**, 9–11

JORDAN, B. M. and BAKER, J. R. (1955). A simple pyronin/methyl green technique. *Quart. J. Micr. Sci.*, **96**, 177–179

KASTEN, F. H. (1958). Additional Schiff-type reagents for use in cytochemistry. *Stain Technol.*, **33**, 39–45.

KASTEN, F. H. (1959). Schiff-type reagents in cytochemistry. 1. Theoretical and practical considerations. *Histochemie*, **1**, 466–509

KJELLSTRAND, P. (1980). Mechanisms of the Feulgen acid hydrolysis. *J. Microscopy*, **119**, 391–396

KORNBERG, A. (1957–58). Enzymatic synthesis of deoxyribonucleic acid. *Harvey Lect.*, **53**, 83–112

KURNICK, N. B. (1952). Histological staining with methyl-green pyronin. *Stain Technol.*, **27**, 233–242

ORNSTEIN, L., MAUTNER, W., DAVIS, B. J. and TAMURA, R. (1957). New horizons in fluorescence microscopy. *J. Mt Sinai Hosp.*, **24**, 1066–1078

PAPPENHEIM, A. (1899). Vergleichende Untersuchungen über die elementäre Zusammensetzung des Rothen Knochenmarkes einiger Säugetriere. *Virchow Arch. Pathol. Anat. Physiol.*, **157**, 19–76

PEARSE, A. G. E. (1951). A review of modern methods in histochemistry. *J. Clin. Pathol.*, **4**, 1–36

SCHNEIDER, W. C. (1945). Phosphorus compounds in animal tissues; extraction and estimation of desoxypentose nucleic acid and of pentose nucleic acid. *J. Biol. Chem.*, **161**, 293–303

STOWELL, R. E. (1942). The use of tertiary butyl alcohol in microtechnique. *Science*, **96**, 165

TREVAN, D. J. and SHARROCK, A. (1951). Methyl green–pyronin–orange G stain for formalin fixed tissues. *J. Pathol. Bacteriol.*, **63**, 326–329

TURCHINI, J., CASTEL, P. and KIEN, K. V. (1944). *Bull. Technol. Histol. Micr.*, **21**, 124

UNNA, P. G. (1902). Eine Modifikation der Pappenheimschen Färbung auf Granoplasma. *Manat. Prakt. Derm.*, **35**, 76.

VON BERTALANFFY, L., MASIN, F. and MASIN, M. (1956). The use of acridine orange fluorescence technique in exfoliative cytology. *Science*, **124**, 1024–1025

WATSON, J. D. and CRICK, F. H. C. (1953). Molecular structure of nucleic acids. A structure for deoxyribose nucleic acid. *Nature (Lond.)*, **171**, 737–738

WIGNALL, N., CULLING, C. F. A. and VASSAR, P. S. (1962). A fluorescent histochemical method for lupus erythematosus (LE) cells. *Am. J. Pathol.*, **36**, 469–470

11

Proteins

Introduction

The histochemical differentiation of proteins requires a knowledge of their characteristics, as well as the types and reactive groups of the amino acids. The time spent on this aspect will enable the student of histochemistry to utilize the right technique, and the appropriate blocking methods.

The proteins are a group of complex organic nitrogenous compounds, widely distributed in plants and animals, which form the principal constituents of the cell protoplasm. They are essentially combinations of α-amino acids and their derivatives. It is perhaps appropriate that the word 'protein' is derived from the Greek word *proteios* meaning 'of first importance'.

Chemistry

Proteins are macromolecules and, like nearly all biological macromolecules, are polymers. There is no definitive number of monomeric units required to make a protein. The lower boundary for the molecular weight of proteins is about 5000, but those commonly occurring in living material have molecular weights very much higher.

The peptide bond

Proteins have been likened to strings of beads, each bead being an amino acid, the amino acids being held together by the peptide bond.

In 1902, Fischer and Hofmeister independently suggested that proteins were formed by the splitting out of water (H_2O) from the α-amine (or α-imino) group (NH_2) of one amino acid and the terminal carboxyl (COOH) of the adjacent amino acid (*see Figure 11.1*), the resulting linkage is called 'the peptide bond'. Experimental evidence over the past 60 years has confirmed the theory of the peptide bond which is now considered to be the principal type of linkage.

Proteins may be classified into *simple proteins*, yielding only α-amino acids on hydrolysis, and conjugated proteins which yield α-amino acids and one or more groups of a non-protein nature. The latter are known as prosthetic groups (Gr. *prosthesis*, an addition).

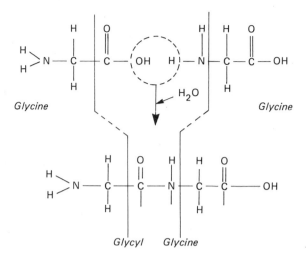

Figure 11.1 The peptide bond

Simple proteins

Albumens

These are very soluble proteins which can be precipitated from an aqueous solution by saturating with an acid salt such as ammonium sulphate, or by saturating with a neutral salt such as sodium sulphate in slightly acid solution.

Globulins

These are insoluble in water but soluble in dilute salt solutions, for example, 5% sodium chloride solution, and are precipitated by half saturation with ammonium sulphate. They occur in serum and tissue; antibodies are found in the globulin fraction of serum.

Scleroproteins (albuminoids)

These are the fibrous proteins having a supporting or protective function in the animal organism. Submembers are the *collagen* of the skin, tendons and bones, the *elastins* of elastic tissue, and the *keratins* from hair, nail and horn.

Histones

These are soluble proteins which are basic and are precipitated by the addition of ammonium hydroxide. Very few examples of this class of proteins are known; they are probably limited to the nuclei of cells. Thymus histone is a classic example.

Protamines

These are water-soluble proteins which are very basic in nature and are not coagulated by heat. Protamines form crystalline salts with mineral acids, and insoluble salts with other more acidic proteins. An example of a protein salt is the commonly used drug, protamine–insulin. Protamines are the simplest proteins.

Conjugated proteins

Nucleoproteins

These are proteins combined with nucleic acids.

Glycoproteins

These are proteins combined with carbohydrates, for example, mucin.

Lipoproteins

These are proteins combined with lipids, for example, serum lipoprotein.

Chromoproteins

These are proteins combined with pigments, for example, haemoglobin.

Phosphoproteins

These are proteins combined with phosphoric acid, for example, casein of milk.

Amino acids

The most commonly occurring 22 amino acids are listed in *Table 11.1* with their isoelectric points, and have been grouped as neutral, basic or acidic; the subgroups indicating structural differences, and so on.

A protein with a high proportion of amino acids with two carboxyl radicals (e.g. aspartic) will be an acid protein and one that has a high proportion of basic amino groups (e.g. histidine) will be a basic protein. Those that are mainly composed of amino acids with one amino and one carboxyl radical, or have balanced amounts of acid and basic amino groups will be neutral proteins.

Identification of proteins

In view of the fact that tissue sections are composed mainly of proteins and that there are many commonly used stains (both acid and basic) which will stain a section in its entirety, it follows that proteins will stain with relative ease. However, when the conditions of staining are carefully controlled proteins can be shown to be either acid, basic or neutral. Their ability to bind each stain is due to the fact that they are amphoteric in nature; that is, they have the capacity to ionize as acids or bases, depending upon the medium immediately surrounding them. An acid protein will therefore stain with an acid dye if the dye solvent is sufficiently acid and vice versa.

Proteins are ubiquitous components of all living tissue and, because of their complexity, the infinite nature of their variety and the fact that their constituent molecular chains may fold, spiral or crosslink with other chains, complete histochemical identification is extremely difficult, if not completely impossible. This is true because the multiplicity of reactive groups available to us for identification (*Table 11.2*) are not specific for any one amino acid, much less for any one type of protein. Some of them, however, do have certain features which, when combined with available blocking

Table 11.1

	Isoelectric point
Neutral amino acids	
(1) Glycine	5.97
(2) Alanine	6.02
(3) Valine	5.97
(4) Leucine	5.98
(5) Isoleucine	6.02
(6) Serine	5.68
(7) Threonine	6.53
Sulphur-containing	
(8) Cysteine	5.02
(9) Cystine	5.06
(10) Methionine	5.75
Aromatics	
(11) Phenylalanine	5.98
(12) Tyrosine	5.65
(13) Thyroxine	
(14) Tryptophan	5.88
Imino acids	
(15) Proline	6.10
(16) Hydroxyproline	5.83
Basic amino acids	
(17) Lysine	9.74
(18) Hydroxylysine	9.15
(19) Arginine	10.76
(20) Histidine	7.58
Acidic amino acids	
(21) Aspartic acid	2.87
(22) Glutamic acid	3.22

Table 11.2 Reactive groups in amino acids

Group	Formula	Chemical nature	Distribution
Amino	$-NH_2$	Primary amine	All amino acids except the prolines
Imino	$-N-H-$	Secondary amine	Proline, hydroxyproline
Carboxyl	$-COOH$	Acid carboxyl	Aspartic, glutamic acids
Hydroxyl	OH	Alcoholic hydroxyl	Serine, threonine, hydroxyproline
β-Thio	$-S-S-$	Disulphide	Cystine
β-Thiol	$-S-H$	Sulph-hydryl	Cysteine
δ-Guanidine	$\begin{array}{c} NH \\ \parallel \\ H_2N-C-N \\ \mid \\ H \end{array}$	Strongly basic group	Arginine
β-Hydroxyphenyl	HO—⬡	Phenol (aromatic —OH) derivative	Tyrosine
Indole	(indole ring structure)	Aromatic heterocycle	Tryptophan

procedures and micro-anatomical localization, will enable group and occasionally individual identification. It should be remembered that immunocytochemical methods can be used to give specific information as to the nature of individual proteins. Enzymes are also a special group of proteins which can be identified specifically. They are considered separately in Chapter 16.

In spite of the foregoing, it is often of importance to identify material as being proteinaceous in nature and to demonstrate increases in certain types of amino acids in particular areas.

Fixation

The type of fixative used will depend upon the reactive groups involved in the method to be employed; obviously, methods for amino groups (NH_2) are unlikely to be positive after fixation with aldehydes, since they interact; similarly, mercuric chloride containing fixatives are to be avoided when sulph-hydryl (SH, thiol) groups are to be demonstrated. The recommended method of fixation is given for each technique.

General methods for protein

■ **Determination of proteins by insolubility at their isoelectric points (Catchpole, 1949; Pearse, 1968)**

This method is based upon the fact that a protein will be least soluble at its isoelectric point. Freeze-dried sections are treated in a selected buffer solution at room temperature for 1–2 hours. Sections are then fixed in alcohol (general proteins), formalin (mucoproteins) or Carnoy's fluid for nucleoproteins for 4–12 hours. They are then stained by an appropriate method.

■ **Millon reaction (modified by Baker, 1956)**

This reaction for tyrosine may be used as an oversight method for most proteins (but not collagen). It depends upon the hydroxyphenyl group (only found in tyrosine in tissue) being converted into a nitrosophenol by the sodium nitrite to which the mercury links to form a red compound.

Fixation

Fixation is not critical—formalin, alcohol and so on, may be used.

Reagents

(1) Mercuric sulphate solution

Sulphuric acid (conc.)	10 ml
Distilled water	90 ml
Mercuric sulphate	10 g

Add acid to water, then add mercuric sulphate. Stir and heat to dissolve. Allow to cool and make up to 200 ml.

(2) 0.25% Aqueous solution of sodium nitrate.

Method

(1) Bring paraffin sections to water.
(2) Place the sections in a small beaker containing 30 ml of mercuric sulphate solution and 3 ml of sodium nitrate solution. Heat beaker gently until solution boils and leave sections for 30 seconds.
(3) Remove sections and rinse in three changes of distilled water (1–2 minutes each).
(4) Dehydrate, clear and mount in a synthetic resin.

Results

Tyrosine containing proteins (most proteins) are stained red, pink or yellow-red.

■ Oxidized tannin-azo technique (OTA) (Dixon, 1959, 1962)

This method is dependent upon the attachment of tannic acid to the tissue proteins; it is thought to react with the amino groups since there is a marked diminution of staining after deamination in nitrous acid (page 211). Following the reaction of the tannic acid with protein, it is oxidized by periodic acid to a 1:2-quinone, which is coupled with diazotized O-dianisidine to produce a salmon-red azo dye (azoquinone).

Fixation

Carnoy's fluid gives excellent results (Dixon, 1962).

Reagents

(1) Tannic-HCl

Tannic acid	10 g
Distilled water	225 ml
N/1 Hydrochloric acid	25 ml

(2) 0.5% aqueous periodic acid (pH 4.0)
(3) Buffered diazotized O-dianisidine (pH 4.0) (ice-cold solutions should be used in preparation)

Fast blue **B**	100 mg
0.2 M Acetic acid	82 ml
0.2 M Sodium acetate	18 ml

Method

(1) Bring sections to distilled water.
(2) Transfer sections to Coplin jar of tannic-HCl and leave for 10 minutes.
(3) Wash well in distilled water (three changes).
(4) Oxidize with periodic acid for 5 minutes (sections darken).
(5) Wash well in distilled water (three changes).
(6) Transfer to ice-cold distilled water for 2 minutes.
(7) Place in ice-cold buffered diazotized O-dianisidine solution in the refrigerator and leave for 20 minutes.

(8) Wash in running tap-water.
(9) Dehydrate, clear and mount in a neutral synthetic resin.

Results

Tannophilic proteins are salmon pink.

Control sections

Stain an extra section omitting steps (4) and (5); this section should be either colourless or a faint pink colour.

■ Oxidized tannin-oxazine technique (OTO) (Dixon, 1962)

This is a variant of the above (OTA) method and differs in that the 1:2 quinone is reacted with freshly prepared 6-amino 3-dimethylaminophenol into a blue-grey oxazine.

Reagents

(1) Tannic-HCl solution (as above).
(2) 0.5% Aqueous periodic acid.
(3) Freshly prepared aminophenol solution

6-Nitroso-3-dimethyl aminophenol	500 mg
Glacial acetic acid	50 ml

Dissolve 500 mg of 6-nitroso-3-dimethyl aminophenol in 50 ml of glacial acetic acid. This dark orange solution is cooled until crystals begin to form and then an excess of zinc dust is added. The orange colour disappears and the mixture is filtered free of zinc dust into a 100 ml cylinder, until 34 ml of filtrate is obtained; this is made up to 100 ml with glacial acetic acid. In contact with air, the solution becomes blue. It should be used immediately.

Method

(1) Steps (1) to (5) as for OTA above.
(6) Wash with three changes of glacial acetic acid.
(7) Place in aminophenol solution at 37 °C for 20 minutes.
(8) Wash in glacial acetic acid.
(9) Dehydrate in alcohol, clear in xylene and mount.

Results

Tannophilic proteins are stained blue-grey (including nuclear chromatin and what appears to be mitochondria).

■ Acrolein–Schiff technique

According to van Duijn (1961) the double bond of acrolein will react with SH, NH_2,

NH and imidazoles leaving a free aldehyde to react with Schiff reagent. Acrolein is toxic and lachrymatory and should be handled in a fume hood.

Fixation

Fixation is not critical.

Reagents

(1) 5% Acrolein in 95% ethanol in screw-capped Coplin jar. The acrolein must be fresh and should not be discoloured.
(2) Schiff reagent.

Method

(1) Bring sections to 95% alcohol.
(2) Place in 5% acrolein for 15–60 minutes (usually 15 minutes).
(3) Wash in three changes of 95% ethanol.
(4) Wash in distilled water.
(5) Place in Schiff reagent for 10–30 minutes.
(6) Wash in running water for 1 minute.
(7) Dehydrate, clear and mount.

Result

Sites of protein reactive groups (*see above*) are coloured red.

■ **Dinitro-fluoro-benzene technique (DNFB) (Danielli, 1953; Tranzer and Pearse, 1964)**

This technique is dependent upon the reaction of the aromatic hydroxyl of tyrosine, SH, free α-amino groups (and possibly the imidazole of histidine) with DNFB to give a colourless product; this product is reduced with titanous chloride, diazotized and then coupled with 'H-acid' to give a red-purple colour.

Fixation

Fixation in Carnoy, alcohol and so on.

Reagents

(1) Alkaline DNFB solution

DNFB	1 ml
Absolute ethanol	99 ml
N/1 Sodium hydroxide	0.2 ml

(2) Titanous chloride solution

15% Titanous chloride	2 ml
0.5 M Sodium citrate buffer (pH 4.5)	8 ml

(3) Freshly prepared nitrous acid

5% Sodium nitrite	8 parts
N/1 Sulphuric acid	1 part

(4) 'H-acid' solution

Saturated solution of 'H-acid' (8-amino-1-naphthol-3-6-disulphonic acid) in veronal acetate–HCl buffer at pH 9.0.

Method

(1) Remove wax with light petroleum.
(2) Wash sections with absolute ethanol.
(3) Incubate in alkaline DNFB (at 22 °C) for 2–20 hours (usually 2–4 hours).
(4) Wash four times in 90% alcohol, and rinse in distilled water.
(5) Reduce in titanous chloride solution at 37 °C for 15–30 minutes.
(6) Wash in 0.5 M sodium citrate buffer (pH 4.5), followed by distilled water.
(7) Diazotize in fresh nitrous acid at 4 °C (in refrigerator) for 5 minutes.
(8) Wash in distilled water.
(9) Couple in 'H-acid' solution (pH 9.0) in refrigerator at 4 °C for 5 minutes.
(10) Wash in running water.
(11) Dehydrate, clear and mount in a synthetic resin.

Result

Proteins (*see above*) will be coloured red-purple. Appropriate blocking methods can be used to make reaction specific for tyrosine.

■ **Biebrich scarlet technique for basic protein (Spicer and Lillie, 1961; Lillie, 1965)**

This method is based upon the principle of selective dye uptake at various pH levels (*see above*).

Fixation

Buffered mercuric chloride (6% $HgCl_2$ in 1.25% sodium acetate), Carnoy, alcohol, but *not aldehydes* are used for fixation.

Reagents

Spicer and Lillie (1961) used 0.01% Biebrich scarlet in glycine NaOH buffers at pH 8, 9.5 and 10.5. Lillie prefers using 1 ml of 1% Biebrich scarlet in 49 ml of each of the appropriate buffer solutions (0.02%) for a shorter period.

Method

(1) Bring sections to water, treat with iodine–hypo sequence if mercury fixative is used.
(2) Stain for 30–90 minutes in each of the 0.01% staining solutions, or stain for 20 minutes in Lillie's 0.02% solutions.
(3) Without rinsing in water, dehydrate with 95% then 100% alcohol.
(4) Clear in xylene, and mount in synthetic resin.

Results

At pH 9.5 basic proteins stain strongly, above and below this pH the staining is appreciably lighter.

Methods for specific groups of amino acids

It should be remembered that very few of these methods are specific alone, they must always be controlled by the appropriate blocking methods.

Tyrosine

The Millon reaction (page 198) is probably the best and most reliable, almost equally so is this diazotization coupling technique. The technique is based upon the fact that tyrosine bearing proteins develop a yellow colour on treatment with nitrous acid (diazotization), this compound is then coupled with 'S-acid' to give a red compound. The urea (Lillie) or ammonium sulphamate (Glenner) is added to the coupling reagent to decompose excess HNO_2.

Fixation

Neutral formalin, Carnoy and so on, are used for fixation.

■ **Diazotization—coupling technique (Glenner and Lillie, 1959)**

Reagents

(1) Diazotizing agent

Sodium nitrite	4 g
Distilled water	56 ml
Dissolve the nitrite in the water, then add: glacial acetic acid	3.4 ml

(2) Alkaline coupling reagent

70% Alcohol	50 ml
8-Amino-1-naphthol-5-sulphonic acid (S-acid)	500 mg
Potassium hydroxide	500 mg
Either urea	1 g
Or ammonium sulphamate	500 mg

Dissolve in order and chill to 3 °C in refrigerator.

Method

(1) Bring sections to water.
(2) (Optional) Geyer (1962) recommends pretreatment of sections in 10% iodine in alcohol for 1–6 hours to accelerate and intensify the reaction.
(3) Diazotize overnight at 3 °C in strict darkness (or for 1–6 hours after iodine treatment).
(4) Rinse in four changes of distilled water at 3 °C for 5 seconds each.
(5) Place in alkaline coupling reagent for 1 hour at 3 °C also in the dark.

(6) Wash in three changes of 0.1 N hydrochloric acid for 5 minutes in each.
(7) Wash in running water for 10 minutes.
(8) Dehydrate, clear and mount.

Results

Tyrosine sites are coloured red-purple to pink. Hair cortex, soft keratin, the inner sheath cells and medulla of the root zone of hairs show a strong reaction.

Tryptophan

■ **DMAB–nitrite method (Adams, 1957)**

This method is based upon the reaction of the DMAB (dimethylaminobenzaldehyde) with the indole to form a β-carboline, which is converted to a blue pigment by nitrate oxidation. The structure of the pigment (carboline blue) is unknown.

Fixation

Short formalin (6–12 hours), 70% methanol, 10% aqueous sulphosalicylic acid.

Reagents

(1) DMAB solution 5% p-dimethylaminobenzaldehyde in concentrated hydrochloric acid (sp.gr. 1.18).
(2) 1% sodium nitrite in concentrated hydrochloric acid.

Method

(1) Sections should be firmly affixed to slides (albuminized or coated with chromate gelatin), dry in 37 °C oven for 2–3 days.
(2) Bring slides to alcohol, and coat with celloidin if there is doubt about their ability to withstand treatment.
(3) Immerse sections in DMAB solution for 1 minute.
(4) Transfer to 1% sodium nitrite–HCl solution for 1 minute.
(5) Wash in water for 30 seconds.
(6) Rinse in 1% acid–alcohol.
(7) Dehydrate, clear and mount.

Results

Tryptophan containing proteins are coloured deep blue, for example, fibrin, Paneth cell granules and so on.

Arginine

■ **Sakaguchi dichloronaphthol hypochlorite technique (Deitch, 1961)**

This method is based upon the linking of the dichloro-α-naphthol to the guanidine group of arginine; colour is produced by alkaline hypochlorite treatment.

Fixation

Carnoy's fluid, acetic ethanol are used for fixation.

Reagents

(1) Reaction mixture

Prepare and mix the following solutions in order, immediately before use:

(a) 4% Aqueous barium hydroxide (filtered)   25 ml
(b) 1% Sodium hypochlorite in distilled water   5 ml
(c) Dissolve 75 mg 2,4-dichloro-α-naphthol in 5 ml *tert*-butanol   5 ml

(2) Dehydrant

5% Tributylamine in *tert*-butanol (aniline in place of tributylamine is almost as good (Lillie, 1965).

(3) Clearing agent

5% Tributylamine in xylene (or 5% aniline).

(4) Mountant

Shillaber's oil plus 10% tributylamine *or* cellulose caprate (resin 50 g: xylene 50 ml) to which is added 10% tributylamine (or aniline) (Lillie, 1965).

Method

(1) Bring slides to distilled water, blot dry.
(2) Place sections in freshly mixed reactant solution in Coplin jar for 10 minutes at room temperature (22 °C).
(3) Take sections through three changes of dehydrant of 5 seconds each change, agitating vigorously in each change.
(4) Clear in two changes (30 seconds each) of clearing agent.
(5) Drain and mount in Shillaber's oil or cellulose caprate (above).

Results

An orange-red colour at sites containing arginine (this colour will fade in 7 days to 1–2 months, depending upon the mountant).

Sulph-hydryl groups

It is most important to remember that —SH *groups* are sensitive to oxidation, and oxidation of undeparaffinized sections or of previously cut paraffin blocks of tissue can take place in atmospheric air which in days and/or weeks can make a previously positive section negative, it is obviously of similar importance to avoid oxidant fixatives. *Disulphide groups (—SS—) can be reduced to sulph-hydryl (—SH) with alkaline reagents* (Lillie, 1965).

■ **Dihydroxy-dinaphthyl-disulphide (DDD) technique (Barnett and Seligman, 1954; Pearse, 1968)**

In this method the reagent splits and forms a protein–naphthyl disulphide by combining with the protein SH. After washing in acid distilled water to convert the reagent and the other reaction product to free naphthols they are then removed by washing first in alcohols then ether. The sections are then treated with a diazonium salt (fast blue B salt); this combines with the naphthol to form an azo dye.

Fixation

Use Carnoy, formalin and so on.

Reagents

(1) DDD reagent

Dihydroxy-dinaphthyl-disulphide (DDD)	25 mg
Absolute alcohol	15 ml

Dissolve DDD in alcohol, and add to 35 ml of 0.1 M veronal–acetate buffer (pH 8.5).

(2) Fast blue B salt solution

Fast blue B salt	50 mg
0.1 M Phosphate buffer (pH 7.4)	50 ml

This must be *freshly prepared*.

Method

(1) Bring sections to water.
(2) Incubate in DDD reagent for 1 hour at 50 °C.
(3) Cool to room temperature, and rinse in distilled water.
(4) Wash for 10 minutes in two changes of distilled water acidified to pH 4 with acetic acid.
(5) Remove the free naphthols by washing in 70, 80, 95 and 100% alcohol, followed by two washes in absolute ether for 5 minutes each.
(6) Rinse in distilled water.
(7) Immerse for two minutes (at room temperature) in fast blue B salt solution.
(8) Wash in running tap-water.
(9) Dehydrate, clear and mount.

Results

Blue staining indicates a high concentration of SH groups; red staining may indicate areas of lower concentration although elastic tissue (which may non-specifically bind free naphthols) and collagen may stain pink.

Note: If the reaction is intended to demonstrate —SS— and —SH groups together, then pretreat sections with thioglycollate (*see* page 212).

■ Mercury orange technique (Bennett and Watts, 1958; Pearse, 1968)

This technique uses the ability of mercurials to 'block' or react specifically with sulph-hydryl groups. The mercury is attached to an azo dye and therefore acts as a marker for SH groups. This method rarely gives a strong reaction.

Fixation

Use Carnoy's, 1% trichloroacetic in 80% alcohol or formalin. Pearse (1968) recommends unfixed cryostat sections.

Reagents

Mercury orange solution

Mercury orange saturated in butanol, propanol, toluene or dimethylformamide.

Method

(1) Bring sections to alcohol.
(2) Immerse in mercury orange solution for 1–3 hours in alcoholic solution, overnight in toluene, or 16–48 hours in dimethylformamide.
(3) Dehydrate, clear and mount.

Results

Orange-red indicates the presence of sulph-hydryl groups.

■ Ferric–ferricyanide reaction

This reaction is considered by some to be the most sensitive for —SH groups, the method will be found on page 286, as Schmorl's technique. It will be seen that it is not specific and must be used in combination with a sulph-hydryl (—SH) blocking method.

Disulphide groups

The disulphide (—SS—) groups in cystine may be demonstrated directly by use of the performic acid–Alcian blue which is very specific, but not very sensitive; or indirectly with the DDD method by first blocking the —SH groups (*see* page 212), then reducing the —SS— groups to — SH by treatment with potassium cyanide. Pearse's performic acid–Schiff (*see* page 274) may also be used with appropriate controls.

■ Performic acid–Alcian blue technique (Adams and Sloper, 1956)

This method is based upon the conversion of cystine to cysteic acid by oxidation with performic acid (or peracetic acid). The cysteic acid is then stained preferentially by Alcian blue in 2 N sulphuric acid (pH 0.2); sections should be well affixed to slides for this method.

Fixation

Use formalin, Carnoy and so on.

Reagents

(1) Performic acid (*see* page 274)
(2) Alcian blue solution

Alcian blue 8 GS	3 g
2 N Sulphuric acid (approximately 5.4% conc. H_2SO_4)	100 ml

Heat to 70 °C to dissolve dye and filter when cool. This solution has an approximate pH of 0.2.

Method

(1) Bring sections to water, remove excess water by blotting lightly.
(2) Immerse in fresh performic acid reagent for 5 minutes.
(3) Wash gently in several changes of distilled water for 5–10 minutes.
(4) Stain in Alcian blue solution for 1 hour.
(5) Wash in water for 5 minutes.
(6) Counterstain if preferred (with tartrazine, and so on).
(7) Dehydrate, clear and mount.

Results

Structures containing 4% or more of cystine appear as a dark steely blue, lesser amounts are pale blue (Pearse, 1968). Neurosecretory substance and hair keratin stain bright blue. Nuclei may stain faintly.

Carboxyl groups

■ Mixed anhydride method for protein-bound side chain COOH (Barnett and Seligman, 1958)

This method is based upon conversion of the COOH groups into amido ketones by treatment with acetic anhydride in pyridine. The ketones condense with 2-hydroxy-3-naphthoic acid hydrazide (NAH), this compound is coupled with fast blue B to give a highly coloured product.

Fixation

Use formalin, Carnoy and so on.

Reagent

NAH reagent

2-Hydroxy-3-naphthoic acid hydrazide	50 mg
Glacial acetic acid	2.5 ml
50% Alcohol	47.5 ml

Dissolve the hydrazide in warm glacial acetic acid, then add the alcohol.

Method

(1) Remove wax from sections with light petroleum.
(2) Allow to dry, and immerse in glacial acetic acid for 2 minutes.
(3) Incubate in equal parts of acetic anhydride and anhydrous pyridine (redistilled over barium oxide) for 1 hour at 60 °C.
(4) Rinse in glacial acetic acid and wash in absolute alcohol.
(6) Incubate in NAH reagent for 2 hours at room temperature.
(6) Wash in three changes of 50% alcohol, 10 minutes each.
(7) Immerse in 0.5 N hydrochloric acid for 30 minutes.
(8) Rinse in distilled water and then in three changes of 1% sodium bicarbonate.
(9) Rinse in several changes of distilled water.
(10) Transfer to equal parts of absolute ethanol and 0.06 M phosphate buffer (pH 7.6) containing 1 mg/ml fast blue B salt for 5–6 minutes.
(11) Rinse in distilled water.
(12) Dehydrate, clear and mount in resinous mountant.

Result

Protein-bound side chain COOH groups—red-purple.

■ **C-terminal carboxyl (COOH) groups (Stoward and Burns, 1967)**

This method is based upon the conversion of the COOH groups to amido-ketones by treatment with acetic anhydride in pyridine. These ketones interact with salicyloyl hydrazide to give an intense blue fluorescence. Treatment with zinc acetate quenches the fluorescence of mucosubstances. This method appears to be specific.

Fixation

Use formalin, alcohol and so on.

Reagents

(1) Acetic anhydride–pyridine

Equal parts of acetic anhydride and anhydrous pyridine (redistilled over barium oxide).

(2) 1% Salicyloyl hydrazide in 5% glacial acetic acid

(3) PAF solution

A fresh dilute solution of pentacyano-amine-ferroate (tri-sodium salt).

(4) 1% Aqueous zinc acetate solution

Method

(1) Remove wax from sections with light petroleum.
(2) Allow to dry, wash in glacial acetic acid for 2 minutes.
(3) Treat with acetic anhydride–pyridine in a Coplin jar at 60 °C for 1 hour.
(4) Wash in two changes of 95% alcohol, then water.

(5) Transfer to salicyloyl hydrazide in a Coplin jar, and leave at room temperature for 30–40 minutes.
(6) Rinse in distilled water.
(7) Treat for 2 minutes in PAF solution to remove excess hydrazine.
(8) Rinse well in distilled water.
(9) Treat with zinc acetate solution for 5–10 minutes.
(10) Rinse in distilled water, dehydrate and clear in xylene.
(11) Mount in non-fluorescent mountant such as Unimount or Fluormount.

Result

C-terminal COOH groups give an intense blue fluorescence.

Amino groups

Both alloxan and ninhydrin react with amino acids to yield an aldehyde and pale red or pale blue products respectively. The colour produced is not sufficiently intense for histochemical purposes. However, the aldehyde can be demonstrated using Schiff reagent.

ε-Amino groups of lysine and hydroxylysine and the α-amino groups of terminal γ-glutamyl and β-aspartyl peptides are likely to react (Glenner, 1963) whilst the α-amino groups of proline and hydroxyproline will not react (Kasten, 1962).

■ Ninhydrin–Schiff method (Yasuma and Ichikawa, 1953)

Fixative

Various fixatives can be used.

Method

(1) Bring sections to ethanol.
(2) Treat with 0.5% ninhydrin in ethanol overnight at 37 °C.
(3) Wash in water.
(4) Treat with Schiff reagent for 30 minutes.
(5) Wash in running water.
(6) Counterstain in haematoxylin and blue.
(7) Wash, dehydrate, clear and mount in synthetic resin.

Result

Proteins containing a sufficient number of reactive amino groups stain pink to magenta.

Blocking methods for proteins

While the specific demonstration of many proteins is not yet possible with the methods available, a greater degree of specificity may be conferred by the use of appropriate blocking methods for specific groups. It should be remembered that while many of these are not universally accepted as being completely specific, in combination with the above methods many proteins can be identified with a degree of certainty.

Amino group blockade

■ **Deamination**

This has been achieved by treatment with nitrous acid alone, but Stoward (1963) showed that the following deamination method is much more specific.

Method

(1) Bring sections to water.
(2) Immerse in fresh nitrous acid (1 g of sodium nitrite in 30 ml of 3% sulphuric acid) for 48 hours at the refrigerator at 0–5 °C in the dark.
(3) Wash in distilled water.
(4) Treat for 4 hours at 60 °C in either (a) water, or (b) alcohol.
(5) Stain sections by the appropriate method for the protein in question, absence of staining after treatment in a previously stained area is a reliable indication *of the presence of amino groups before treatment.*

Carboxyl group (COOH) blockade

■ **Methylation technique**

Method

(1) Bring sections to alcohol.
(2) Treat with 0.1 N hydrochloric acid in absolute methanol at 37 °C for 4–48 hours (*mild methylation*), or at 60 °C for 4–24 hours (normal methylation). Four hours at 60 °C with a control section to ensure that methylation is complete is recommended.
(3) Rinse in alcohol.
(4) Stain by appropriate method.

'Mild methylation' is said to block protein carboxyls, but not primary amines (Pearse, 1968). Normal methylation desulphates in addition to its methylating action. Methylation is reversed by treatment with KOH/alcohol (saponification), *the loss of sulphate groups is, of course, irreversible.*

Tryptophan blockade

■ **Persulphate block**

The persulphate is thought to block reactions for tryptophan by breaking the pyrrole ring.

Method

Sections are brought to water, then incubated in 2.5% potassium persulphate in 0.5 N potassium hydroxide, for 16–18 hours (overnight) at room temperature.

Tyrosine and tryptophan blockade

■ **N-haloamide bromination block**

Proteins containing tyrosine and tryptophan are split by N-haloamide bromination and this can be regarded as a specific method for tyrosine provided that it is not required that tryptophan remains reactive (Pearse, 1968).

Method

Sections are brought to absolute alcohol and then transferred to 0.02% N-bromo-succinimide in 50% alcohol at pH 4.0.

Sulph-hydryl group blockade

These may be blocked by the iodoacetate or maleimide methods.

■ **Iodoacetate method**

Bring sections to water and treat with 0.1 M (approximately 2%) aqueous sodium iodoacetate at pH 8.0 (with NaOH) for 20 hours at 37 °C.

■ **Maleimide method**

(1) Bring sections to water.
(2) Treat in 0.1 M (1.25%) N-ethyl maleimide in 0.1 M phosphate buffer at pH 7.4 for 4 hours at 37 °C.
(3) Rinse at 1% acetic acid then with tap-water.

Disulphide reduction method (—SS to SH)

Lillie (1965) recommends the use of a freshly prepared 10% sodium thioglycolate solution, adjusted with sodium hydroxide to pH 9.5, for 10 minutes at room temperature. Pearse (1968) specifies a freshly prepared 0.5 M thioglycollic acid solution at pH 8.0 (with 0.1 N NaOH) for 4 hours at 37 °C. In spite of precelloidinization, the latter is much more likely to remove sections.

References

ADAMS, C. W. M. (1957). A p-dimethylaminobenzaldehyde–nitrite method for the histochemical demonstration of tryptophan and related compounds. *J. Clin. Pathol.*, **10**, 56–62

ADAMS, C. W. M. and SLOPER, J. C. (1956). The hypothalamic elaboration of posterior pituitary principles in man, the rat and dog: histochemical evidence derived from a performic acid–Alcian blue reaction for cystine. *J. Endocrinol.*, **13**, 221–228

BAKER, J. R. (1956). The histochemical recognition of phenyls especially tyrosines. *Quart. J. Micr. Sci.*, **97**, 161–164

BARNETT, R. J. and SELIGMAN, A. M. (1954). Histochemical demonstration of sulphydryl and disulphide groups of protein. *J. Nat. Cancer Inst.*, **14**, 769–804

BARNETT, R. J. and SELIGMAN, A. M. (1958). Histochemical demonstration of protein bound alpha-acylamido carboxyl groups. *J. Biophys. Biochem. Cytol.*, **4**, 169–176

BENNETT, H. S. and WATTS, R. M. (1958). In *General Cytochemical Methods.* Ed. Danielli, J. F. Academic Press, London

CATCHPOLE, H. R. (1949). Distribution of glycoprotein hormones in anterior pituitary gland of rat. *J. Endocrinol.*, **6**, 218–225

DANIELLI, J. F. (1953). In *Cytochemistry. A Critical Approach.* Chapman-Hall, London

DEITCH, A. D. (1961). An improved Sakaguchi reaction for microspectrophotometer use. *J. Histochem. Cytochem.*, **9**, 477–483

DIXON, K. C. (1959). Oxidized tannin–azo method for protein in tissue. *Am. J. Clin. Pathol.*, **35**, 199–211

DIXON, K. C. (1962). Hepatic protein located by the oxidised tannin–azo method. *Quart. J. Exp. Physiol.*, **47**, 1–6

FISCHER, E. (1902). *Ber. Dtsch. Chem. Ges.*, **35**, 1095

GEYER, G. (1962). A modification of the Morel–Sisley reaction for tyrosine. *Acta Histochem. (Jena)*, **13**, 355–356

GLENNER, G. G. (1963). A re-evaluation of the ninhydrin–Schiff reaction. *J. Histochem. Cytochem.*, **11**, 285–286

GLENNER, G. G. and LILLIE, R. D. (1959). Observations on the diazotisation–coupling reaction for the histochemical demonstration of tyrosine: metal chelation and formazan variants. *J. Histochem. Cytochem.*, **7**, 416–422

HOFMEISTER, F. (1902). *Ergebn. Physiol.*, **1**, 759

KASTEN, F. H. (1962). Some comments on a recent criticism of the ninhydrin–Schiff reaction. *J. Histochem. Cytochem.*, **10**, 769–770

LILLIE, R. D. (1965). In *Histopathologic Technic and Practical Histochemistry.* 3rd Ed. Blakiston, New York

PEARSE, A. G. E. (1968). In *Histochemistry, Theoretical and Applied.* 3rd Ed. Vol. 1. Churchill, London

SPICER, S. S. and LILLIE, R. D. (1961). Histochemical identification of basic proteins with Biebrich scarlet at alkaline pH. *Stain Technol.*, **36**, 365–370

STOWARD, P. J. (1963). DPhil. Thesis, University of Oxford

STOWARD, P. J. and BURNS, J. (1967). Studies in fluorescence histochemistry. The demonstration of the C-terminal carboxyl groups of protein. *Histochemie*, **10**, 230–233

TRANZER, J. P. and PEARSE, A. G. E. (1964). Titanous chloride as a reducing agent in the dinitrofluorobenzene reaction for protein. *J. Histochem. Cytochem.*, **12**, 325–326

VAN DUIJN, P. (1961). Acrolein–Schiff, a new staining method for protein. *J. Histochem. Cytochem.*, **9**, 234–241

YASUMA, A. and ICHIKAWA, T. (1953). Ninhydrin–Schiff and alloxan–Schiff staining. *J. Lab. Clin. Med.*, **41**, 296–299

12

Carbohydrates

The histochemical differentiation of polysaccharide–protein complexes in normal and pathological tissue is of ever increasing importance in the investigation of normal and disease processes.

Although this chapter is entitled Carbohydrates, it is concerned with the study of polymers of carbohydrates, most of which are linked covalently to protein. The protein moiety may constitute a majority or a minority of the residues present and this factor has, at times, been used as one basis for their classification. To the histochemist such a classification has no meaning, since even the demonstration of both protein and carbohydrate at the same site is no proof that they are part of the same molecule.

Whether a reaction is given by a series of long-chain carbohydrate polymers attached to a small core of protein (e.g. nucleus pulposa in intervertebral discs), or a series of short-chain carbohydrate polymers attached to a large protein core (e.g. salivary glycoproteins), cannot be determined histochemically. The only information that can be derived is based upon the reactive groups that are demonstrable in carbohydrates, namely 1:2 glycols (vicinal diols), carboxyl (COOH) and ester sulphate, with information gained from enzyme hydrolysis with diastase, hyaluronidase, sialidase (neuraminidase) and various chemical procedures (blocking, and so on).

It is for this reason that, in spite of the many (and complex) classifications of carbohydrates that are currently in use, the following has been adopted because it is based upon their histochemical differentiation and can easily be interpreted within the scope of any of the other existing chemical classifications (Meyer, 1953; Jeanloz, 1960; Spicer, Leppi and Stoward, 1965; Pearse, 1968; Zugibe, 1970).

Classification of naturally occurring polysaccharides (*Figure 12.1*)

Group I: neutral polysaccharides (non-ionic homoglycans)

(1) Glucose-containing; glycogen (starch, cellulose).
(2) *N*-acetyl-glucosamine-containing (chitin).

Group II: acid mucopolysaccharides (anionic heteroglycans)

All in this group are thought to be attached to protein, even though the word protein is not embodied in their name. These are found in connective tissues and are PAS negative.

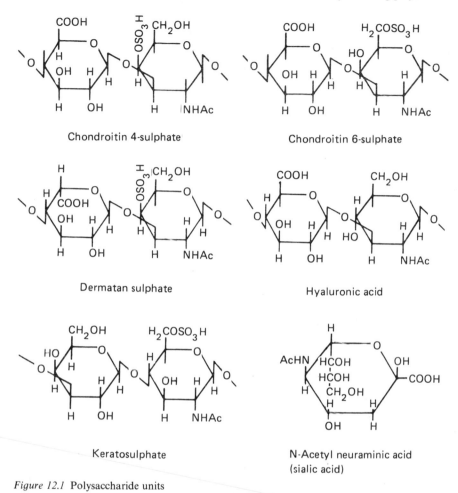

Figure 12.1 Polysaccharide units

(1) Carboxylated; hyaluronic acid—connective tissues, umbilical cord.
(2) Sulphated (OSO_3H)
   (a) Containing hexuronic acid (COOH)
      (i) Chondroitin sulphate A (chondroitin-4-sulphate).
      (ii) Chondroitin sulphate C (chondroitin-6-sulphate), found in cartilage, chondrosarcomas, cornea and blood vessels.
      (iii) Chondroitin sulphate B (dermatan sulphate), found principally in skin, also in connective tissue, aorta and lung.
      (iv) Heparin, found in mast cells, and intima of arteries.
   (b) Not containing hexuronic acid (COOH-free).
      (i) Keratosulphate, in human aorta and bovine cornea.

Group III: glycoproteins (mucins, mucoids, mucoproteins)

These are found in epithelial mucins, but some may occur in connective tissue. They are potentially, but not necessarily, PAS positive. Group 2 (containing sialic acid) is potentially sialidase labile, but for reasons not completely understood, may show no loss of alcianophilia after sialidase (*see* page 251).

(1) Neutral; ovimucoid (egg white), mucin in stomach, Paneth cell granules.
(2) Carboxylated; sialoglycoproteins (containing sialic acid, but no sulphate).
   (i) Sialomucins, found in submaxillary gland mucins, small intestine mucins, fetal mucins, upper part of colonic crypts and human sublingual gland (PAS positive, sialidase-resistant even after KOH).
   (ii) Serum glycoproteins.
   (iii) Blood group substances.
(3) Sulphated; sulphated sialoglycoproteins (containing sialic acid and sulphate). Colonic mucins.

Group IV: glycolipids

The members of this group have a fatty residue bound to a carbohydrate structure.
   Cerebrosides, in central nervous system and other tissues.
   Phosphatides are a group of non-carbohydrate-containing lipids, which include lecithin, cephalin and sphingomyelin, which are only mentioned in this chapter because of their PAS positivity (*see* page 261).

Fixation of carbohydrates

The object of fixation of carbohydrates in tissue is to ensure their total preservation, without diffusion. The main obstacle is that most carbohydrates are water soluble, and for this reason aqueous fixatives have not been recommended. It has been shown, however, that many carbohydrates are covalently bound to protein (Engfeldt and Hjertquist, 1967) and that the fixation of the protein will in turn bind the polysaccharides. Even in the case of glycogen, which is not protein bound, it is thought that the fixation of the tissue proteins forms a lattice around the glycogen, with its consequent preservation. There is little agreement on which method of fixation is ideal, with the possible exception of formaldehyde vapour fixation of freeze-dried tissue. Even this method, however ideal it may be histochemically, can hardly be utilized in a routine laboratory.

For glycogen, Best (1906) specified celloidin embedding following alcohol fixation. The celloidin was thought to be essential to prevent diffusion of the glycogen from the tissues, but Lillie (1947) has shown that tissues may, after fixation, be washed in running water for 24 hours without any appreciable loss of glycogen. Fixatives containing a high concentration of picric acid are thought by some to give the best results.

It has been shown by Vallance-Owen (1948) that glycogen is as adequately fixed by formal–saline as by alcohol and alcohol–picric acid fixatives. Glycogen studies may be carried out on formalin-fixed tissue if fixation is initiated as quickly as possible, preferably at 4 °C to minimize streaming artefact. Rossman's fluid (10% formalin in saturated alcoholic picric acid) is preferred by Cook (1974), especially when abnormal carbohydrates present in the glycogenoses and mucopolysaccharidoses are to be demonstrated.

For most routine purposes formal–saline will give satisfactory results with mucopolysaccharides (Cook, 1959; Allison, 1973). The use of cetylpyridinium chloride in 10% formalin, while recommended by many workers, was thought by Sochor (1965) to interfere with staining, presumably by binding with reactive groups.

When the presence of hyaluronic acid is suspected formal–sublimate or formal–alcohol are the recommended fixatives.

Identification of carbohydrates

Table 12.1 is intended as an aid to the identification of carbohydrates in tissues. It will be seen that differentiation between neutral mucopolysaccharides and muco- or glycoproteins is not possible histochemically although quite often histological localization will permit an 'informed guess'. It must also be remembered that almost invariably polysaccharides occur in the body as a mixture.

Because sialic acid contains a carboxyl (COOH) group in addition to adjacent 1:2 glycol groups, it will react with the PAS technique and also give a positive reaction for acid mucopolysaccharides.

Periodic acid–Schiff procedures

The histochemistry of carbohydrates was for a long time largely based on the PAS technique and it remains today, if properly controlled, the most useful single technique.

The use of Schiff reagent for the demonstration of aldehydes produced after hydrolysis with hydrochloric acid (the Feulgen reaction) has been dealt with on page 183. McManus (1946) described a periodic acid oxidation–Schiff (PAS) method for the demonstration of mucin, and later extended its use to the demonstration of reticulin and glycogen.

Other oxidation -Schiff procedures using chromic acid, potassium permanganate or lead tetra-acetate have been described. Although they are positive with most PAS positive material, they are not usually employed since the reaction is not as intense and may even be negative. The use of performic or peracetic acid with Schiff reagent for the demonstration of unsaturated lipids is dealt with on page 274.

The PAS reaction is now accepted as a routine method. It is used with various controls, block procedures, and supplementary staining techniques, which are necessary to distinguish between the wide variety of tissue elements that are demonstrated.

The reaction is based on the fact that certain tissue elements are oxidized by the periodic acid (or other oxidant), one of the reaction products being an aldehyde; such aldehydes are then demonstrated with a Schiff reagent.

The chemical basis of the reaction is that periodic acid will cleave the carbon–carbon bonds where these carbon atoms have adjacent hydroxyl (—OH) groups (1:2 glycol groups) (*Figure 12.2a*), or adjacent hydroxyl and amino (—NH$_2$) groups (1:2 amino, hydroxy groups) (*Figure 12.2b*).

Any substance that satisfies the following criteria will give a positive result with the PAS reaction (Hotchkiss, 1948).

(1) The substance must contain the 1:2 glycol grouping, or the equivalent amino or alkyl-amino derivative, or the oxidation product CHOH—CO.
(2) It must not diffuse away in the course of fixation.
(3) It must given an oxidation product which is not diffusible.
(4) Sufficient concentration must be present to give a detectable final colour.

The acid mucopolysaccharides (hyaluronic acid, the chondroitin sulphates, and so on) all contain 1:2 glycol groups (vicinal diols) but have been shown to be PAS negative

Table 12.1 Identification chart

Classification class	Type and reactive groups	Substance	Schiff reaction	PAS	Acetyl/PAS	Diastase/PAS	Alcian blue pH 2.5	Hale	Alcian blue pH 1	HID	Aldehyde fuchsin	M/S AB pH 2.5	T Hyal/AB pH 2.5	T Hyal/AB pH 1	S Hyal/AB pH 2.5	S Hyal/AB pH 1	Sial/AB pH 2.5	Sial/AB pH 1	Sudan black	Bromine PAS
I	Neutral (1:2 glycol)	Glycogen	−	+	−	−	−	−	−	−	−	−	−	−	−	−	−	−	−	+
	Carboxylated (COOH)	Hyaluronic acid	−	−	−	−	+	+	−	−	−	+	−	−	−	−	+	−	−	−
		Chondroitin S (A and C)	−	−	−	−	+	+	−	−	−	+R	−	−	+	−	+	−	−	−
II	Sulphated (COOH and OSO$_3$H)	Chondroitin S (B)	−	−	−	−	+	+	+	+	+	+R	+	+	+	+	+	+	−	−
	Sulphated (OSO$_3$H)	Heparin	−	−	−	−	+	+	+	+	+	+R	+	+	+	+	+	+	−	−
		Keratosulphate	−	−	−	−	+	+	+	+	+	−	+	+	+	+	+	+	−	−
III	Neutral (1:2 glycol)	Mucins	−	+*	+R	+*	−	−	−	−	−	−	−	−	−	−	−	−	−	+*
	Carboxylated (COOH, 1:2 glycol)	Sialomucins	−	+*	−*	+*	+	+	−	−	−	+†	+	−	+	−	−	−	−	+*
	Sulphated (COOH, 1:2 glycol, OSO$_3$H)	Sulphated sialomucins	−	+*	−*	+*	+	+	+	+	+	+†	+	+	+	+	+	+	−	+*
IV	Glycolipids (1:2 glycol, lipid)	Cerebrosides	+	+	+R	+	−	−	−	−	−	−	−	−	−	−	−	−	+	+R
—	Unsaturated lipids (double bonds)	Unsaturated lipids	−	+	+	+	−	−	−	−	−	−	−	−	−	−	−	−	+	−
—	Aldehyde groups	Aldehyde groups	+	(+)	(+)	+	−	−	−	−	−	−	−	−	−	−	−	−	−	+

Abbreviations:

R	Positive reaction is reduced.
*	These mucins may occasionally be PAS negative.
†	Methylation may remove sialic acids resulting in a negative reaction.
Acetyl	Acetylation.
M/S	Methylation/saponification.
T/Hyal	Testicular hyaluronidase.
S/Hyal	Streptococcal hyaluronidase.
Sial	Sialidase (neuraminidase).
AB	Alcian blue.
HID	High iron diamine.

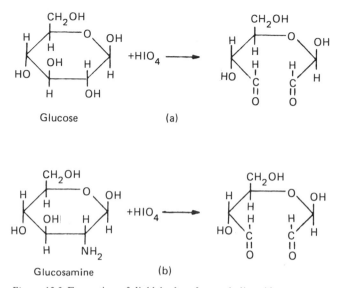

Figure 12.2 Formation of dialdehydes after periodic acid treatment

(Braden, 1955; Hoogh Winkel and Smits, 1957). These groups are known to oxidize only slowly (7–16 hours, Zugibe, 1970). It is presumed that this is due to the presence of a highly charged group in the molecule ($COOH$ or OSO_3H) which interferes with the periodic acid oxidation. That this is probably true was shown by Scott and Harbinson (1968) who suppressed the electrostatic field of the COOH groups of hyaluronic acid, by increasing the ionic strength of the periodate solution, when it became PAS positive.

Sialic acids, however, in spite of their COOH groups were shown by Montreuil and colleagues (1959) and Montreuil and Biserte (1959) to be oxidized by periodic acid (in 20 minutes) and to be PAS positive.

PAS technique

Oxidation

Sections must be oxidized with periodic acid to convert 1:2 glycol groups to dialdehydes in order that they will react with Schiff reagent to produce a coloured end product. Hotchkiss (1948) recommends an alcoholic buffered periodic acid whenever there is the possibility that the substances to be demonstrated are soluble in water (e.g. glycogen). However, we find a simple aqueous solution of periodic acid to give equally good, if not better, results. The time of exposure to periodic acid must be kept to a minimum and should not exceed 15–20 minutes at room temperature; heat should never be used because of the chemical changes that may occur.

It should be realized that the specificity of the PAS technique is dependent upon its short oxidation time. Longer exposure to periodic acid will cause proteins and (with times of 7–24 hours) the acid mucopolysaccharides to become PAS reactive.

Choice of Schiff reagent

Most of the accepted Schiff formulas give equally good results.

Reducing rinses

Sulphite rinses were recommended for the purpose of removing uncombined Schiff reagent. Most laboratories have found that simple washing in running water does not result in section staining with recoloured fuchsin, therefore the sulphite rinses have been omitted from the recommended method. Hotchkiss suggested using a reducing rinse between periodic acid and Schiff reagent to remove iodate or periodate remaining combined in the tissues, since these restore the colour of the Schiff reagent. This has also been found to be unnecessary.

■ Recommended technique

Method

(1) Bring sections to water.
(2) Oxidize for 5 minutes in 1% aqueous periodic acid.
(3) Wash in running water for 5 minutes, and rinse in distilled water.
(4) Treat with Schiff reagent for 15 minutes.
(5) Wash for 10 minutes in running water.
(6) Counterstain with haematoxylin and, if desired, tartrazine in Cellosolve.
(7) Dehydrate, clear and mount in synthetic resin.

Results

PAS positive substances	Bright red
Nuclei	Blue
Other tissue constituents	Yellow

■ Hotchkiss' buffered alcoholic PAS technique (1948)

Certain of the cheaper substitutes for alcohol cannot be used in this technique since they give false positive results.

Reagents

(1) Alcoholic periodic acid

Periodic acid	0.8 g
Distilled water	20 ml
M/5 Sodium acetate solution (2.72%)	10 ml
Pure ethyl alcohol	70 ml

(2) Acid-reducing rinse

Potassium iodide	2 g
Sodium thiosulphate	2 g
Distilled water	40 ml
Pure ethyl alcohol	60 ml
N/1 Hydrochloric acid	2 ml

(3) Schiff reagent (*see* page 186).

Method

(1) Bring sections to 70% alcohol.
(2) Treat with alcoholic periodic acid for 5–10 minutes.
(3) Rinse in 70% alcohol.
(4) Treat with acid-reducing rinse for 1 minute.
(5) Rinse in 70% alcohol.
(6) Wash in running water until free of alcohol.
(7) Treat with Schiff reagent for 10–30 minutes.
(8) Wash in running tap-water for 10 minutes.
(9) Counterstain if desired as in the preceding method.

A section for histochemical assessment should be examined without counterstaining.

(10) Dehydrate, clear and mount in synthetic resin.

Results

PAS positive material   Bright red
Other tissue constituents   Dependent on counterstain

■ **Periodic acid–methenamine silver technique (Gomori, 1946; Grocott, 1955)**

Gomori utilized a silver solution to demonstrate aldehydes exposed by periodate treatment, subsequently modified by Grocott; the method cannot, however, be used in a Feulgen technique.

While it is not generally recommended as a substitute for Schiff reagent, it does give very good results with basement membranes (particularly in kidney) and with fungi in tissue sections. This modification, in which the stock silver methenamine solution is diluted in equal parts with distilled water, avoids the grossly overstained sections which sometimes resulted with the original method.

Technique

Sections should be as thin as possible, preferably 2–3 μm.

Reagents

(1) Gomori's silver methenamine solution

Add 5 ml of 5% silver nitrate to 100 ml of 3% methenamine (hexamethylene tetramine) to prepare stock solution. For use add 3 ml of 5% borax to 25 ml of stock silver and 25 ml of distilled water.

(2) Differentiator

0.5% Sulphuric acid in 0.2% ferric sulphate.

Method

(1) Bring sections to water.
(2) Oxidize in 5% chromic acid for 1 hour.

(3) Wash in running water for 1–2 minutes.
(4) Treat with 2% sodium bisulphite for 1 minute to remove chromic acid.
(5) Wash in running water for 5 minutes.
(6) Place in preheated methenamine–silver solution at 60 °C for 1–3 hours. Examine sections microscopically at 10-minute intervals after the first 30 minutes. Do not use metal forceps. Sections should be rinsed in distilled water and if stain is too light may, after a further rinse in distilled water, be returned to the silver solution. If they are too dark they may be treated briefly in differentiator.
(7) Wash well in distilled water.
(8) Toning in 0.2% gold chloride for 2 minutes may be carried out, but in our opinion is best omitted.
(9) Place in 3% sodium thiosulphate for 2 minutes, then wash in running water for 2–3 minutes.
(10) Sections may be counterstained if desired with haematoxylin or with 0.2% light green in 0.2% acetic acid.
(11) Dehydrate, clear and mount in synthetic resin.

Results

PAS-positive structures, basement membranes, fungi, mucin, etc.	Black-brown
Background	Light yellow or green

■ **Light and electron microscopic demonstration of PAS-positive substances with thiosemicarbazide (Stastna and Travnic, 1971)**

The principle of this method is the oxidation of tissue to convert 1:2 glycols to dialdehydes; these are reacted with thiosemicarbazide, which binds to them by its hydrazine group to give a thiosemicarbazone. This is treated with osmium tetroxide which binds with the thiocarbamyl groups to yield a final product which can be seen equally well by light (semithin sections) or electron microscopy (ultrathin sections). Controls are not oxidized in periodic acid.

Method A (semithin sections)

(1) Tissues are fixed in the usual manner in glutaraldehyde and osmium tetroxide (OsO_4), and after dehydration, embedded in Epon 812. Semithin sections are cut and placed upon slides.
(2) Oxidize in fresh 1% periodic acid for 45 minutes.
(3) Rinse in water.
(4) React in 2.5% thiosemicarbazide in 5% acetic acid for 3 hours.
(5) Rinse well in water.
(6) Treat with 1% aqueous OsO_4 for 90 minutes.
(7) Rinse in distilled water.
(8) Dehydrate, clear and mount in synthetic resin.

Results

PAS-positive substances   Dark brown/black

Method B (ultrathin sections)

(1) Fix tissues in formaldehyde in 0.15 M phosphate buffer at pH 7.4 in a refrigerator for 4 hours (glutaraldehyde is not recommended by the authors). Tissues must not exceed 1 mm^3.
(2) Wash tissues in 0.5 M glucose in 0.15 M phosphate buffer (pH 7.4) for 60 minutes.
(3) Wash tissues in 0.15 M phosphate buffer (pH 7.4) for 60 minutes with three changes.
(4) Oxidize in 0.05 M sodium periodate in 0.15 M phosphate buffer at pH 4.2 for 15–60 minutes.
(5) Wash in 0.15 M phosphate buffer at pH 4.2 for 45 minutes, with three changes.
(6) React with a saturated solution of thiosemicarbazide in 0.28 M acetic acid for 1–3 hours (time varies with different tissues).
(7) Wash in 0.15 M phosphate buffer at pH 4.2 for 45 minutes, with three changes.
(8) Wash in 0.15 M phosphate buffer at pH 7.4, with three changes.
(9) Post-fix in 1% osmium tetroxide in pH 7.4 buffer for 60 minutes.
(10) Dehydrate, embed in Epon 812/Araldite.

Sections may also be contrasted with uranyl acetate and lead citrate if preferred.

Results

PAS-positive substances are electron dense.

Methods for glycogen

Glycogen, in colloidal solution, is found in the cytoplasm of certain cells. In adult life it may be demonstrated principally in the cells of the liver, but in fetal life it has a very wide distribution. After fixation it is seen as fine granules or an amorphous mass, dependent on the type of fixation employed.

It is a polysaccharide, which is derived from, and within 1 hour of death breaks down into sugar. Consequently, tissues must be fixed while fresh or frozen until fixation is possible. It is readily soluble in water before fixation, and tissues must not be rinsed or washed in water or saline solution prior to fixation.

Methods of demonstration

Methods of demonstration fall into the following four groups:

(1) iodine staining,
(2) carmine staining,
(3) oxidation–Schiff methods,
(4) silver impregnation.

Since the methods used may demonstrate other cell constituents, it is necessary to employ enzyme control to obtain specific demonstration of glycogen. This will therefore be discussed before the methods of demonstration are described.

Enzymic control for specific demonstration of glycogen

Glycogen is destroyed by the enzyme diastase (or amylase), which may be obtained from saliva or malt. Malt diastase is available commercially and is more reliable than saliva, but the latter is suitable for routine purposes and is readily available. If diastase is allowed to act on a section containing glycogen the glycogen present will be removed, and subsequent staining of this section and of a second untreated section will reveal those places where material has been removed by diastase. Diastase removes a variety of material other than glycogen (e.g. ribonucleic acid), but since this material is not PAS positive, or shown by Best's carmine, it is not a great disadvantage.

If sections are to be treated with celloidin it is essential that treatment with diastase be undertaken first. A celloidin film prevents the complete removal of glycogen by diastase for quite long periods, whereas treatment for 20–30 minutes at 37 °C before applying celloidin will remove all the glycogen present.

An enzyme-treated slide and known positive control should always be stained in parallel with the test slide; comparison between these slides will show specifically the presence of glycogen.

■ **Technique for digestion (stages 1–3) and celloidinization (stages 4–7)**

Method

(1) Bring sections to water.
(2) Digest with diastase (human saliva, or 1:1000 malt diastase in distilled water) for 30 minutes at 37 °C.
(3) Wash in water for 5–10 minutes.
(4) Wash with 90% alcohol, then absolute alcohol for $\frac{1}{2}$ minute.
(5) Transfer to a stoppered container of 1% celloidin in equal parts alcohol and ether for 2 minutes.
(6) Drain off the excess of celloidin, and transfer to 80% alcohol for 5 minutes to harden.
(7) Wash in running tap-water for 1–2 minutes.
(8) Stain by any desired technique.

Note: Test sections, and known positive controls which are not to be digested, are brought through xylol and alcohol directly to stage 4 above.

■ **Iodine technique**

Methods employing iodine are not as specific as Best's carmine or PAS, nor are they permanent; they are, however, simple and rapid in operation.

Method

(1) Bring sections to water.
(2) Place slide on rack, flood with Lugol's iodine and leave for 2–3 minutes.
(3) Drain, and flood with 1–2% iodine in absolute alcohol.
(4) Blot with filter paper.
(5) Place one to two drops of origanum oil on the section and lower a coverslip on to the oil, avoiding air bubbles.
(6) Seal the edges of the coverslip with paraffin wax or similar compound. After a few moments the origanum oil will clear and differentiate the section.

Results

Glycogen   Dark brown
Tissue   Yellow

■ **Best's carmine technique (1906)**

This gives a fairly permanent preparation, and is specific when controlled by enzyme digestion.

Reagents

(1) Alum haematoxylin

(2) Staining solution

> Best's stock solution (*see below*)   12 ml
> Concentrated ammonia (sp.gr. 0.880)18 ml
> Methyl alcohol   18 ml
> Filter before use.

The amounts given immediately above are sufficient for one Coplin jar, but smaller amounts may be used, and poured on to the slide.
  Best's stock solution is made as follows:

Carmine   2 g
Potassium carbonate 1 g
Potassium chloride   5 g
Distilled water   60 ml

The reagents, in a 250 ml flask, should be gently boiled until the colour deepens (3–5 minutes); the deeper the colour at this stage the deeper the staining of the glycogen. Cool, and add 20 ml of fresh concentrated ammonia (sp.gr. 0.880). This stock solution, in a tightly stoppered bottle, must be stored in a refrigerator (0–5 °C), but even then it will only keep for 6–8 weeks.

(3) Best's differentiating fluid*

> Absolute ethanol   20 ml
> Methanol   10 ml
> Distilled water   25 ml

Method

(1) Celloidinize, or digest sections (for technique *see above*).
(2) Place in alum haematoxylin (Ehrlich or Harris) for 10–15 minutes to stain nuclei.
(3) Rinse rapidly in 1% acid alcohol to clear the background.
(4) Wash in running water for 1 minute to remove acid (sections will be 'blued' by the ammonia in the carmine stain).
(5) Stain in a Coplin jar, or on a slide rack, with the staining solution for 10–15 minutes.
(6) Wash slide with Best's differentiating fluid until stain ceases to pour out, this usually

* Methanol alone may be used in place of this differentiating fluid for paraffin sections

takes only a few seconds: or wash rapidly with methyl alcohol if working with paraffin sections.
(7) Flood with alcohol or acetone to remove celloidin film (alcohol/ether mixture may be used if the film is difficult to remove).
(8) Clear in xylene and mount in Canada balsam or synthetic resin.

Results

Glycogen   Red
Nuclei   Blue

Oxidation Schiff methods

This group of methods (*see* page 217) is popular for the demonstration of glycogen, having the advantage that solutions do not require special preparation and, used in conjunction with enzyme digestion, are specific.

Schiff reagent, following oxidation with periodic acid, chromic acid, or potassium permanganate, gives a first-class demonstration of glycogen.

Following digestion of the control, celloidinize the control, test section and the positive control and treat the three sections as detailed on page 220.

Silver impregnation

Several methods of silver impregnation have been reported. Mitchell and Wislocki (1944) and Pritchard (1949) describe an ammoniacal silver technique. Gomori (1946) describes a methenamine silver method, which also colours mucin and melanin.

Methods for mucin (mucopolysaccharides and mucoproteins)

The term mucin is used to describe an intracellular secretion formed in a variety of cells. It is not a single entity and cells from different parts of the body secrete slightly differing substances having similar macroscopic appearances. Their chemical and histochemical differentiation are dealt with on page 214. This section will deal with their common characteristics and general demonstration, but although not listed below, the PAS technique is commonly used for this purpose.

In general, mucins have the following properties:

(1) They stain intensely with basic dyes.
(2) They are metachromatic, and therefore stain red to reddish-blue with thionin or toluidine blue.
(3) They are precipitated by acetic acid (except gastric mucin).
(4) They are soluble in alkaline solutions.

Mucin may be demonstrated in frozen, paraffin or celloidin sections by any of the methods described below.

The traditional methods used are the metachromatic techniques, mucicarmine and mucihaematein; of these the most popular is Southgate's mucicarmine. The histochemical methods will demonstrate mucins histologically and give more information.

Metachromatic staining

Metachromatic staining is a simple method of demonstrating mucin. The following method gives good results, but the buffered toluidine blue method is slightly more permanent.

■ **Feyrter's enclosure technique (1936)**

This method was developed by Feyrter to demonstrate myelin sheaths in frozen sections but, for the rapid demonstration of mucin, either frozen or paraffin sections may be used.

Reagent

Freshly prepared 1% thionin or toluidine blue in 0.5% aqueous solution of tartaric acid is used. In practice, keep a stock bottle of 0.5% tartaric acid, and add a few crystals of stain to 5 ml of the acid when required.

Method

(1) Bring section to water (frozen section mounted on slide).
(2) Filter a few drops of stain on to the section, and lower a coverslip on to the stain and section, taking care not to trap air bubbles.
(3) With blotting paper remove excess stain from the edge of the coverslip until the section can be seen.
(4) Ring the coverslip with paraffin wax or Vaseline and leave for a few minutes before examining.

Results

Metachromatic substances   Clear red
Other tissue   Shades of blue

The red will remain for a few days.

■ **Southgate's mucicarmine method (1927)**

This modification of Mayer's original method (which did not contain aluminium hydroxide) gives more consistent results. It demonstrates epithelial mucin well.

Reagent

Carmine   1 g
Aluminium hydroxide   1 g
50% Alcohol   100 ml

These constituents are mixed by shaking and to them is added

Aluminium chloride (anhydrous)   0.5 g

Boil in water-bath for $2\frac{1}{2}$–3 minutes. Cool, make up to original volume with 50% alcohol, and filter. The stock solution is stable for several months.

Method

(1) Bring section to water.
(2) Stain nuclei with haematoxylin.
(3) Differentiate in acid–alcohol and blue in tap-water.
(4) Stain for 30 minutes in the staining solution given above.
(5) Rinse in distilled water, dehydrate, clear and mount in Canada balsam or synthetic resin.

Results

Mucin   Red
Nuclei   Blue

■ **Mayer's mucihaematein**

Mayer's mucihaematein stains connective tissue mucin well, but is not recommended for gastric mucin.

Reagent

Dissolve 1 g of haematoxylin in 100 ml of 70% alcohol; add 0.5 g aluminium chloride, and 5 ml of 1% aqueous sodium iodate to ripen the solution immediately. The volume is then made up to 500 ml and the solution is ready for use. It remains stable from 4–6 months.

Method

(1) Bring sections to water, and wash well with distilled water.
(2) Stain with mucihaematein for 5–10 minutes.
(3) Wash in three 5-minute changes of distilled water.
(4) Dehydrate, clear and mount in Canada balsam or synthetic resin.

Results

Epithelial mucins   Deep blue-violet
Connective tissue mucins and cartilage matrix   Lighter violet

■ **Alcian blue–chlorantine fast red stain (Lison, 1954)**

Steedman (1950) reported the selective staining of mucin by Alcian blue: Lison combined it with chlorantine fast red to give, in addition, selective connective tissue staining.

Reagents

(1) Alcian blue solution

Alcian blue 8G, 1% aqueous   50 ml
Acetic acid 1% aqueous   50 ml

Filter and add:

Thymol   10–20 mg

(2) Phosphomolybdic acid (1%).
(3) Chlorantine fast red 5 B (0.5% in distilled water).

Method

(1) Bring sections to water.
(2) Stain in Ehrlich's haematoxylin for 10–15 minutes.
(3) Wash in tap-water until blue (the sections are differentiated by the succeeding steps).
(4) Stain in Alcian blue solution for 10 minutes.
(5) Rinse in distilled water for a few seconds.
(6) Treat for 10 minutes in 1% phosphomolybdic acid.
(7) Rinse in distilled water.
(8) Stain for 10–15 minutes in chlorantine fast red.
(9) Rinse in distilled water.
(10) Dehydrate, clear and mount in resinous mountant.

Results

Mucin, granules of mast cells, ground substance of cartilage, and some types of connective tissue fibres	Bluish-green
Nuclei	Purplish-blue
Collagen fibres and osteoid	Cherry-red
Cytoplasm and muscle	Pale yellow

■ Alcian green, phloxine–tartrazine (Attwood, 1958)

This method was introduced to demonstrate the mucin and squames in amniotic fluid embolism.

Method

(1) Bring sections to water.
(2) Stain in 1% Alcian green in 2% acetic acid for 2 minutes.
(3) Rinse in water.
(4) Stain with haematoxylin for 1 minute.
(5) Rinse in water and blue.
(6) Stain in 0.5% phloxine in 0.5% calcium chloride in a jar for 15–30 minutes.
(7) Rinse in water.
(8) Rinse in Cellosolve.
(9) Differentiate in Cellosolve saturated with tartrazine controlling microscopically.
(10) Wash in Cellosolve.
(11) Clear in xylene and mount in synthetic resin.

Results

Mucin	Green
Epithelial squames and fibrin	Red
RBCs	Yellow

Colloidal iron methods

Hale's colloidal iron technique (page 235) may be used to demonstrate epithelial and connective tissue mucins. It is preferred by some workers because it stains more deeply than Alcian blue.

Fluorescence methods

■ Acridine orange

Hicks and Matthaei (1958) discovered that a section previously stained by iron haematoxylin would, if subsequently stained with acridine orange, demonstrate mucins with some degree of specificity.

The preparations tend to fade on repeated examination.

Method

(1) Bring sections to water.
(2) Treat with 5% iron alum for 10 minutes.
(3) Wash in water.
(4) Stain in 0.1% aqueous acridine orange for 2–3 minutes.
(5) Wash in water.
(6) Mount in glycerin/phosphate buffer at pH 6 (9:1).

Results

Mucin and fungi fluoresce orange/red using BG12 exciter and OG4 barrier filters.

■ Atebrine

Vassar and Culling (1959a) used 1% aqueous atebrine in pH 3.95 sodium acetate–HCl buffer for 10 minutes.

Mucin fluoresces bright yellow, other tissue components pale green.

■ Fluorescence PAS (Culling and Vassar, 1961)

The fluorescent PAS reaction has the advantage of demonstrating minute quantities of reactive material. It demonstrates basement membranes, mucin and fungi exceptionally well.

The fluorescent Schiff reagent is given on page 188.

Method

(1) Bring sections to water.
(2) Treat with 1% aqueous periodic acid for 10 minutes.
(3) Wash briefly in distilled water.
(4) Place in fluorescent Schiff reagent for 20 minutes.
(5) Wash in 1% HCl in 70% alcohol and leave for 10 minutes. This removes the unreacted Schiff reagent.
(6) Transfer to fresh acid–alcohol for a further 10 minutes.

(7) Wash in a few changes of absolute alcohol to remove traces of acid.
(8) Clear in xylene and mount in synthetic resin.

Results

PAS-positive structures fluoresce bright golden yellow.
Other tissue components—green.
Examine using BG12 exciter and OG4 or OG5 barrier filters.

Methods for the demonstration of acid mucopolysaccharides and glycoproteins (COOH and OSO_3H groups)

As will be seen in the following pages, there is a multiplicity of methods available for the demonstration of acid groups. Many of these methods have been included to satisfy individual preferences, some because of their specificity and yet others because they are good histological methods (e.g. colloidal iron method).

As has been pointed out absolute specificity is difficult to achieve even with available chemical and enzymic controls. For general purposes the Alcian blue/PAS will demonstrate mucin and the degree to which it is composed of neutral (red) and acid (blue) components; similarly, the aldehyde fuchsin/Alcian blue, or high iron diamine/Alcian blue methods will stain acid mucins and demonstrate the degree to which they are carboxylated (blue) and/or sulphated (purple or black). The more specific techniques are the Alcian blue at pH 1.0 and/or 2.5, the diamine methods, Scotts CEC method, metachromasia with Azure A at controlled pH, together with methylation, saponification, enzymic digestion techniques and so on.

Metachromatic staining

The mechanism of staining is discussed on page 118. The question of alcohol stability is still in dispute and has not yet been resolved. The method described below avoids the use of alcohol, and it is of interest that colonic mucin (known to contain sulphate), which is metachromatic after clearing in xylene, loses most of its metachromasia if treated subsequently with alcohol.

The technique recommended for the demonstration of metachromasia is that of Vassar and Culling (1959b). This gives a permanent preparation.

Fixation

Formalin does not react with polysaccharides but it reacts with the proteins bound to polysaccharides; therefore a formalin fixative such as formal–calcium or formal–alcohol is recommended.

Reagent

Dissolve 0.25 g of toluidine blue in 100 ml of Michaelis's veronal acetate–hydrochloric acid buffer at pH 4.5.

Method

(1) Bring sections to water.
(2) Stain in buffered toluidine blue for 10 seconds.

(3) Rinse in distilled water.
(4) Blot section with fluffless filter paper, allow to dry and clear in xylene. If section does not completely clear, blot dry and immerse in fresh xylene.
(5) Mount in synthetic resin.

■ **Metachromasia with Azure A at controlled pH (Spicer, 1960; Gad, 1969)**

This technique is said to differentiate strongly acidic sulphomucins, which are metachromatic at pH 1.5 and 3.0, from weakly acidic mucosubstances which are metachromatic at pH 3.0 only. Sections are stained in 1:5000 Azure A in 0.1 M phosphate–citrate buffer or Walpole's buffer for 30 minutes, dehydrated through acetone and mounted in xylene cellulose caproate (Lillie, 1964). A full range of buffered stains from pH 0.5 to 5.0 may be prepared and used in a similar manner.

Alcian blue methods

Alcian blue is a water soluble copper phthalocyanin; its exact staining mechanism is not known although it is thought to stain by salt linkage to acidic groups. It must be used in acid solution, and has been shown to have a greater affinity for sulphate groups when used at a pH less than 2.0. Spicer has shown that it has a greater affinity for acid than for sulphated mucopolysaccharides. Although there is fairly general support for the above mechanism, Palladini and Lauro (1968) feel that the specificity of the dye is due to its inability to stain in the presence of a specific protein. In their opinion, this protein is soluble in various salt solutions and in 1 M sulphuric acid, but is insoluble in 3% acetic acid: it is also removable by peptic digestion. It is of interest to note that Quintarelli, Scott and Dellovo (1964) obtained increased staining with Alcian blue after pepsin treatment which they assumed was due to the fact that the removal of the protein had made the reactive tissue radicals accessible to the dye.

Each batch of Alcian blue 8 GX should be tested when it is received by staining known control sections (large and small intestine). The sections should be examined for depth of staining of mucins, and for non-specific background staining: in our experience there is considerable variation between different batches, some being so poor that they were useless.

Alcian blue was combined with chlorantine fast red by Lison (1954) to give a selective connective tissue stain. This is described on page 228, as a method for mucin, but should not be used as a histochemical method.

Lev and Spicer (1964) used Alcian blue at pH 1.0 and 2.5 to distinguish between acid and sulphated mucopolysaccharides or glycoproteins. At pH 1.0, carboxyl (COOH) groups are not ionized and do not stain, whereas sulphate (OSO_3H) groups are demonstrated. At pH 2.5 COOH groups stain well, while sulphated mucins may stain poorly (Spicer, Horn and Leppi, 1967).

■ **Standard Alcian blue method (pH 2.5) for acid groups (COOH and OSO_3H)**

Method

(1) Bring sections to water.
(2) Stain in freshly filtered 1% Alcian blue 8 GX in 3% acetic acid (pH 2.5) for 30 minutes.
(3) Wash in water.
(4) Dehydrate, clear and mount in synthetic resin.

Results

Acid polysaccharides (nuclei may stain faint blue)   Deep blue

■ **Alcian blue (pH 1.0) for sulphate groups**

Method

(1) Bring sections to water.
(2) Stain in 1% Alcian blue 8 GX in 0.1 N hydrochloric acid for 30 minutes. Rinse briefly in 0.1 N HCl.
(3) Blot dry with fine filter paper to prevent the staining which sometimes occurs after dilution with water (which will change the pH) in washing.
(4) Dehydrate in alcohol, clear in xylene and mount in resinous mountant.

Results

Sulphated mucosubstances stain blue.

■ **Alcian blue/PAS technique**

Steps (1)–(3) of standard Alcian blue method at pH 2.5 above, followed by steps (2)–(7) of the PAS technique (page 220), dehydration, clearing and mounting. This technique is sometimes useful for the differentiation of neutral and acid mucopolysaccharides.

■ **Aldehyde fuchsin/Alcian blue (Spicer and Mayer, 1960)**

Steps (2) and (3) of aldehyde fuchsin technique (page 238) are carried out before the standard Alcian blue technique at pH 2.5.

Results

Acid MPS   Blue
Sulphated MPS   Purple
Mixed acid and sulphated   Violet-purple

■ **Alcian blue–Alcian yellow method**

This method may be used to differentiate between sulphated (blue) and acid (yellow) mucopolysaccharides and glycoproteins. We have not found this method to be useful, it is included for the sake of completeness.

Method

(1) Bring paraffin sections fixed in Helly or formaldehyde to water.
(2) Stain for 30 minutes to 1 hour with 0.5% Alcian blue 8 GX in 0.1 N HCl.
(3) Wash for 10 seconds in buffer pH 0.5 (or 0.1 N HCl).
(4) Wash well in water.
(5) Stain 30 minutes to 1 hour with Alcian yellow GX 0.5% buffered at pH 2.5 (or in 3% acetic acid).
(6) Wash in water.

(7) Counterstain 30 seconds in 1% neutral red (optional).
(8) Wash in water, dehydrate, clear in xylene, mount in Canada balsam.

Results

Sulphate groups are coloured blue, carboxyl groups yellow; sites containing both carboxyl and sulphate groups are coloured blue-green.

■ **Alcian blue—ruthenium red method (Yamada, 1969)**

This method, also included for completeness, was used to differentiate between sulphated (blue) and acid (red) mucopolysaccharides and glycoproteins.

Method

(1) Bring sections to water, and rinse twice in 0.1 N hydrochloric acid at pH 1.0.
(2) Stain for 30 minutes in 0.5% Alcian blue 8 GX in 0.1 N hydrochloric acid at pH 1.0.
(3) Rinse in 0.1 N HCl, and then twice in 3% acetic acid at pH 2.5.
(4) Stain in 0.5% ruthenium red in 3% acetic acid (pH 2.5) for 5–20 minutes. Staining should be stopped when there is replacement of Alcian blue by ruthenium red.
(5) Rinse twice with 3% acetic acid and then twice with water.
(6) Dehydrate, clear and mount.

Results

Sulphate groups   Blue
Carboxyl groups   Red

Many mucins stain purple presumably indicating the presence of both acid (COOH) and sulphate (OSO_3H) groups.

■ **Alcian blue–safranin (Spicer, Horn and Leppi, 1967)**

This method has become popular in some laboratories as an alternative to the aldehyde fuchsin technique. It is used for the demonstration of human mast cells and can be recommended for this purpose.

Method

(1) Bring sections to water.
(2) Stain in 0.5% Alcian blue 8 GX in 3% acetic acid for 30 minutes.
(3) Wash in water for 5 minutes.
(4) Stain in 0.25% safranin in 0.125 N hydrochloric acid for 30 seconds.
(5) Dehydrate rapidly, clear and mount in synthetic resin.

Results

Strongly acidic (sulphated) mucins, mast cells   Red
Acid mucins (carboxylated)   Blue

Hale's colloidal iron technique (1946)

Hale's technique is based upon the affinity of acid groups for colloidal iron at a low pH. The iron forms a chelate with the acid groups and may then be demonstrated by the Prussian blue reaction.

While this method is excellent for the demonstration of acid mucins it is inferior to Alcian blue as a specific method for histochemical investigation.

Reagents

Dialysed iron solution

(1) Commercial

Dialysed iron (British Drug Houses or Merck)	1 volume
2 M Acetic acid	1 volume

(2) After Rinehart and Abu'l Haj (1951).

Dissolve gradually 75 g ferric chloride in 250 ml distilled water, adding 100 ml glycerol, followed by the gradual addition of 55 ml of 28% ammonia with constant stirring. This mixture is dialysed against regularly changed distilled water for 3 days.

Acid–ferrocyanide solution

Equal parts of 2% potassium ferrocyanide and 2% hydrochloric acid. Make fresh for use.

Technique

(1) Bring sections to water.
(2) Flood with dialysed iron solution (either solution works well) for 10 minutes.
(3) Wash well with distilled water.
(4) Flood with acid–ferrocyanide solution for 10 minutes.
(5) Wash well in water.
(6) Counterstain lightly with 0.1% neutral red or safranin.
(7) Rinse in water, and dehydrate rapidly.
(8) Clear in xylene and mount in synthetic resin.

Results

Acid mucopolysaccharides	Bright blue
Other tissue constituents	Shades of red

Spicer's diamine methods for acid mucosubstances

Spicer (1961, 1965) made yet another major contribution to histochemistry when he published his high iron, low iron and mixed diamine methods. The methods are based upon the formation of salt complexes between the cationic staining entity and the acid groups, in tissue. These diamines will also react with periodate engendered aldehyde groups to give yellow to brown Schiff bases.

The most useful of the methods at this time is the high iron diamine. This appears to be specific for ester sulphate (Gad and Sylven, 1969; Reid, Livingstone and Dunn, 1972), and although there is some slight coloration of nuclei and background tissue, a positive result is quite unmistakable. Some confusion arose when this method was first published since, due to an error, 'the concentration of ferric chloride given was 10% instead of 40%,' (Sheahan and colleagues, 1970). It is unfortunate that this incorrect formula has been republished in the literature, since it gives a very indifferent result.

The other diamine methods are described below with their expected results. It will be seen that their area of usefulness is in distinguishing between epithelial sialomucins and sulphomucins. Spicer has shown that some sialomucins are reactive, and others non-reactive, with the low iron diamine–Alcian blue pH 2.5 technique. The mixed diamine method distinguishes between periodate–reactive and periodate–unreactive acid mucosubstances (Leppi and Spicer, 1967).

■ High iron diamine method

Reagent–diamine solution

N,N-dimethyl-m-phenylenediamine dihydrochloride	120 mg
N,N-dimethyl-p-phenylenediamine hydrochloride	20 mg

Dissolve the diamines in 50 ml of distilled water then add 1.4 ml of 40% ferric chloride. The pH of the prepared solution should be 1.5–1.6. This solution must be freshly prepared and used immediately.

Method

(1) Bring sections to water.
(2) Stain in diamine solution in Coplin jar for 24 hours.
(3) Rinse rapidly in water.
(4) Dehydrate rapidly, clear and mount in resinous mountant.

Results

Sulphomucins   Grey-purple-black

Non-sulphated acid mucins are unstained unless an Alcian blue at pH 2.5 step is interposed after step 3, when they will be blue (high iron diamine–Alcian blue method).

■ Low iron diamine–Alcian blue method

Reagent–diamine solution

N,N-dimethyl-m-phenylenediamine dihydrochloride	30 mg
N,N-dimethyl-p-phenylenediamine hydrochloride	5 mg

Dissolve diamines in 50 ml of distilled water, and add 0.5 ml of 40% ferric chloride. This solution must be freshly prepared and used immediately.

Method

(1) Bring sections to water.
(2) Stain in diamine solution in a Coplin jar for 24 hours.

(3) Rinse quickly (in and out) in water.
(4) Stain in Alcian blue 8 GX (1% in 3% acetic acid) for 30 minutes.
(5) Rinse quickly (in and out) in water.
(6) Dehydrate, clear and mount in resinous mountant.

Results

Sulphated and many acid non-sulphated mucins stain black; few acid non-sulphated mucins stain blue. If demonstration of neutral polysaccharides is desired, oxidize an additional section in 1% periodic acid and then wash in water for 5 minutes before step 2, when they will be stained purple-grey.

■ Mixed diamine method

This method is extremely good for acidic mucosubstances.

Reagent–mixed diamine solution

N,N-dimethyl-m-phenylenediamine dihydrochloride   30 mg
N,N-dimethyl-p-phenylenediamine hydrochloride   5 mg

Dissolve diamines in 50 ml of distilled water, then adjust pH to between 3.4 and 4.0 with 0.2 M Na_2HPO_4 (0.15–0.65 ml). This solution must be freshly prepared.

Method

(1) Bring duplicate sections to water.
(2) Hydrolyse both sections in preheated N HCl at 60 °C for 10 minutes (Feulgen hydrolysis to remove interfering staining of nuclei).
(3) Wash in running water for 5 minutes.
(4) Oxidize one section in 1% aqueous periodic acid for 10 minutes, then rinse in running water for 5 minutes.
(5) Stain both sections in mixed diamine solution for 20–48 hours (usually 24 hours).
(6) Rinse and dehydrate in two changes of 95% alcohol.
(7) Treat with two changes of absolute alcohol, clear in xylene–alcohol and xylene.
(8) Mount in a resinous mountant.

Results

Periodate unreactive acidic mucosubstances   Purple
Periodate reactive neutral and acidic mucosubstances   Grey, grey-brown

Both types of acidic mucosubstances are purple in unoxidized sections.

■ Mixed diamine–sodium chloride method

The procedure for this method is identical to that of the mixed diamine method (*above*) except that 3–7 ml of 1 M sodium chloride replaces an equal volume of water in the mixed diamine solution.

Results

The inclusion of sodium chloride in the mixed diamine solution decreases the reactivity of many sialomucins but increases that of some sulphated mucins, especially in the cornea, ovarian follicles and some connective tissue.

Other methods

■ Saunders acridine orange–CTAC method (Pearse, 1968)

Saunders used CTAC–acridine orange staining followed by elution with different concentrations of sodium chloride to differentiate between hyaluronic acid, chondroitin sulphates and heparin.

Recommended fixation and processing of tissue

(1) Fix small pieces of tissue in Newcomer's fluid (page 42) for 12–24 hours.
(2) Transfer to equal parts of Newcomer's fluid and n-butanol for 30 minutes.
(3) Treat all three slides with ribonuclease (page 192) for 2 hours at 45 °C.
(4) Place in equal parts of n-butanol and wax for 30 minutes.
(5) Impregnate in three changes of wax for 30 minutes each.
(6) Embed tissue and cut 3–5 μm sections.

Method

(1) Treat three slides (A, B and C) with 1% cetyltrimethyl–ammonium chloride (CTAC) for 10 minutes.
(2) Wash in running water for 10 minutes.
(3) Treat all three slides with ribonuclease (page 192) for 2 hours at 45 °C.
(4) Treat slide A with CTAC (10 minutes); wash; 0.1% aqueous acridine orange (pH 7.2) for 3 minutes; running water 10 minutes, air dry and mount in fluorescent-free mountant.
(5) Treat slide B with 0.1% acridine orange in 0.01 M acetic acid (pH 3.2) for 3 minutes; rinse in running water and then differentiate in 0.3 M NaCl in 0.01 M acetic acid; wash in running water; air dry and mount in non-fluorescent mountant.
(6) Treat slide C as slide B but substitute 0.6 M NaCl for 0.3 M NaCl.

Results

Slide A   Red fluorescence due to hyaluronic acid
Slide B   Red fluorescence due to chondroitin sulphates and heparin
Slide C   Red fluorescence due to heparin

■ Gomori's Aldehyde fuchsin stain (Halmi's modification, 1952)

The combination of basic fuchsin and aldehyde in the presence of a strong mineral acid was described by Gomori in 1950, who noted its preferential staining for certain tissue constituents, for example, elastic tissue, mast cell granules, mucin and so on. Abu'l Haj and Rinehart (1953) noting these were polysaccharide in nature, concluded that the dye reacts with sulphated mucopolysaccharides. Although there is some dispute as to its absolute specificity, it is reasonable to assume that sites which are Alcian blue and aldehyde fuchsin positive, which become aldehyde fuchsin negative following methylation, and remain negative after saponification are sulphated mucopolysaccharides.

Reagents

Dissolve 0.5 g basic fuchsin in 100 ml of 60% alcohol, then add 1 ml paraldehyde (fresh) and 1.5 ml concentrated hydrochloric acid. Allow to 'ripen' for 24 hours before use.

Method

(1) Bring sections to 70% alcohol.
(2) Stain in fresh aldehyde fuchsin for 5–10 minutes. Older solutions may require a longer staining period, and give a less selective result.
(3) Rinse in 70% alcohol.
(4) Counterstain in 0.25% light green in 70% alcohol for 10 seconds (optional).
(5) Rinse rapidly in 70% alcohol.
(6) Dehydrate, clear and mount in synthetic resin mountant.

Results

Aldehyde fuchsin positive structures   Purple

■ Scott's critical electrolyte concentration technique

Scott and his colleagues (Quintarelli, Scott and Dellovo, 1964; Scott and Dorling, 1965) showed that carboxylated acid carbohydrates (e.g. hyaluronic acid, sialomucins) will not stain with Alcian blue in concentrations of magnesium chloride at or above 0.4 M, whereas sulphated mucins will stain at concentrations of 0.8 M and above. Carboxylated carbohydrates alone do not stain in concentration of MgCl above 0.1 M (Pearse, 1968).

Reagent

Dissolve 0.1% Alcian blue 8 GX in 0.05 M sodium acetate buffer at pH 5.7, add magnesium chloride to give molar concentrations of 0.1, 0.2, 0.4, 0.6, 0.8 and 1.0.

Method

(1) Bring sections to water.
(2) Stain serial sections in Alcian blue in each of the $MgCl_2$ concentrations for 30 minutes.
(3) Wash in running water.
(4) Dehydrate, clear and mount in resinous mountant.

Results

See above.

Use of radioactive isotopes (³⁵sulphur) for the specific localization of sulphated mucosubstances

The incorporation of ³⁵sulphur is the only truly specific method of localizing sulphate esters in tissues or tissue cultures. This may be done *in vivo* by injection of radioactive sulphate into laboratory animals, or *in vitro* by inclusion of the isotope in media for tissue cultures, minces and so on.

■ *In vivo* method

Leppi and Spicer (1967) injected rhesus monkeys with 2 mCi of carrier-free ³⁵sulphur (Na₂³⁵SO₄) intraperitoneally, the animals being sacrificed 6 hours later. Tissues were taken, fixed in formal–calcium for 24 hours, and radioautographs prepared using Kodak AR-10 stripping film and Alcian blue/PAS staining (*see* page 520 for technique).

■ *In vitro* method

Filipe (1971) recommended that tissues to be investigated be minced with a razor blade, placed on a stainless steel mesh support in a Petri dish, and tissue culture medium 199 containing 1 µCi/ml carrier-free ³⁵sulphur added until a thin layer was drawn over the surface of the tissue by capillary action. The specimens were then incubated in an oven at 37 °C in an atmosphere of 95% oxygen and 5% carbon dioxide for periods of 1, 2, 3 and 4 hours and overnight (3 hours' incubation was found to be the optimal time). Tissues were fixed in formal–calcium and embedded in paraffin. Autoradiographs were prepared as described above and on page 520.

Methods for sialic acids

Although several methods have been described for the purpose of specifically identifying sialic acids there are few that have been substantiated. Their identification is mainly dependent upon staining with Alcian blue and PAS both before and after sialidase (and mild acid hydrolysis) treatments, and possibly methylation, which removes most of the sialic acid from tissue sections (Quintarelli, Scott and Dellovo, 1964; Schmitz-Moorman, 1969). The only method that can be used to demonstrate the presence of sialic acids with certainty and also to determine whether or not it is labile to neuraminidase is the thiobarbituric acid assay technique of Warren (1959). Unfortunately, this is not a histochemical method.

The histochemical identification of sialic acid relies upon its removal by neuraminidase or KOH/neuraminidase (Culling and Reid, 1980). It is pointed out by Culling and colleagues (1981) that there is a variety of neuraminidases each with its own action pattern and that most do not remove sialic acids with C_4 or C_1 esters (Drzenick, 1973). Removal of these esters with alcoholic KOH usually, but not always, renders the sialic acid then labile to neuraminidase (Reid *et al.*, 1976).

The KOH/PAS effect was developed into a series of techniques by Culling and colleagues for the identification and differentiation of side chain acylated and non-acylated sialic acids. Veh and colleagues (1982) developed methods for the selective histochemical demonstration of sialic acids with unsubstituted, or only C_7 substituted, side chains based on mild periodic acid oxidation. Phenylhydrazine blockade was adapted by Spicer for differentiation of sialic acids and neutral and acidic mucopolysaccharides.

■ **BIAL reaction for sialic acids (Ravetto, 1964; Pearse, 1968)**

Reagent

Orcinol (5-methylresorcinol)	200 mg
Concentrated hydrochloric acid	80 ml
0.1 M Copper sulphate ($CuSO_4$)	0.25 ml

Dissolve the orcinol in the hydrochloric acid, add the copper sulphate solution and make up to 100 ml with distilled water. Allow to stand for 4 hours before using.

Method

(1) Spray cryostat or frozen dried formalin vapour fixed sections with above reagent.
(2) Place sections, face down, on a glass frame in a preheated container, which has on the bottom a thin layer of concentrated HCl, at 70 °C for 5–10 minutes.
(3) Dry sections in air.
(4) Clear in xylene and mount in resinous mountant.

Results

High concentrations of sialic acids   Red to red-brown (fades rapidly)

■ **KOH/PAS method (Culling, Reid and Dunn, 1971)**

This method has been shown to give greatly increased staining (compared with the PAS method) in human and rat ileocaecal valve, large intestine and rectum, and a moderate increase in the same areas in guinea pig and rabbit, Brunner's glands becoming strongly PAS positive from a faint reaction.

Method

(1) Bring serial sections to 70% alcohol.
(2) Saponify one section (*see* page 247).
(3) Stain both sections by routine PAS method.
(4) Counterstain lightly with haematoxylin.
(5) Dehydrate, clear and mount in synthetic resin.

Results

Compare section under comparison microscope for increased staining in saponified section.

■ **PB/KOH/PAS method (Reid, Culling and Dunn, 1975)**

This method is used to demonstrate the KOH/PAS reaction in isolation.

Method

(1) Bring sections to water.
(2) Oxidize in 1% periodic acid at room temperature for 1 hour.

(3) Wash in water for 10 minutes.
(4) Treat with 0.1% sodium borohydride in 1% disodium hydrogen phosphate for 30 minutes.
(5) Wash in water.
(6) Treat with 0.5% potassium hydroxide in 70% alcohol for 30 minutes.
(7) Wash in 70% alcohol.
(8) Wash in water.
(9) Stain by PAS technique.
(10) Dehydrate, clear and mount in synthetic resin.

Results

Mucin showing any red colour is interpreted as being KOH/PAS positive provided a parallel section treated by the PB/PAS technique is unstained (*see below*).

Notes

(1) A light haematoxylin counterstain is recommended.
(2) If a particular section treated by the PB/PAS technique, which is used as a negative control, shows any red colour then the long method of borohydride reduction should be used.

■ PB/PAS method

This technique is used to ensure that a normal PAS reactivity has been abolished.

Method

(1) Bring sections to water.
(2) Treat as above omitting steps (6)–(8).
(3) Dehydrate, clear and mount in synthetic resin.

Results

Any staining will indicate that the periodic–borohydride treatment is incomplete. This may be due to either insufficient time of oxidation with periodic acid or incomplete reduction by sodium borohydride.

■ PATS/KOH/PAS method (Culling, Reid and Dunn, 1976)

This technique allows the visualization of the normal PAS reactive material together with the KOH/PAS reactive sites. It uses a thionine–Schiff reaction to colour the normal PAS reactive material blue and a basic fuchsin–Schiff reaction to colour the KOH/PAS reactive material red.

■ Thionin–Schiff reagent (modified)

Dissolve 0.5 g thionin in 250 ml distilled water. Boil for 5 minutes, cool and make up to original volume. Add 75 ml N/1 HCl and 5 g sodium metabisulphite.

Stopper and leave for 24 hours at room temperature then 48 hours at 4 °C.
Filter.

Note: Charcoal should not be used.

Method

(1) Bring sections to water.
(2) Oxidize in 1% periodic acid for 30 minutes.
(3) Wash in water.
(4) Treat with thionin–Schiff reagent for 15 minutes.
(5) Wash in water.
(6) Proceed as in steps (6)–(10) of the PB/KOH/PAS method.

Results

PAS positive material will be blue and KOH/PAS positive material will be red.
Mixtures will be purple.

■ mPAS method (Veh *et al.*, 1982)

Method

(1) Bring sections to water.
(2) Wash in 0.1 M acetate buffer, pH 5.5 at 2 °C for 5 minutes.
(3) Oxidize in 0.001 M sodium iodate in 0.1 M acetate buffer, pH 5.5, at 2 °C for 10 minutes.
(4) Wash in 1% aqueous glycerol for 5 minutes.
(5) Wash in distilled water for 5 minutes.
(6) Treat with Schiff reagent for 30 minutes at room temperature.
(7) Wash in three changes of 0.5% potassium metabisulphite, 5 minutes in each
(8) Wash in running tap-water for 10 minutes.
(9) Wash in distilled water for 5 minutes.
(10) Dehydrate, clear and mount.

Results

Sialic acids with unsubstituted or C_7 only substituted side chains	Positive
Sialic acids with C_9 or $C_{7,9}$ substituted side chains	Negative

■ mPA/PD/AB method (Veh *et al.*, 1982)

Method

(1) Bring sections to water.
(2) Wash in 0.1 M acetate buffer, pH 5.5 at room temperature for 5 minutes.
(3) Oxidize in 0.005 M sodium iodate in 0.1 M acetate buffer, pH 5.5 at room temperature for 10 minutes.
(4) Wash in 1% aqueous glycerol.
(5) Wash in distilled water for 5 minutes.

(6) Schiff base formation with 0.2% aqueous N,N-dimethyl-m-phenylenediamine, pH 5.0 at room temperature for 1 hour.
(7) Wash in distilled water for 5 minutes.
(8) Stain in 1% Alcian blue in 3% acetic acid (pH 2.5) at room temperature for 30 minutes.
(9) Wash in two changes of distilled water, 5 minutes each.
(10) Dehydrate, clear and mount.

Results

Sialic acids with unsubstituted or C_7 only substituted
   side chains   Negative
Sialic acids with C_9 or $C_{7,9}$ substituted side chains   Positive

Note

Alkaline hydrolysis (0.5% KOH in 70% ethanol, 25 °C—5 mintes) before step 2 should give negative results with C9 or C7, 9 substituted side chains.

■ Periodic acid–phenylhydrazine–Schiff method (PAPS) (Spicer, 1961)

Sialomucins differ in their reactivity to the periodic acid–phenylhydrazine–Schiff technique. This is useful in the identification of some mucosubstances since phenylhydrazine blocks the Schiff staining of periodate-induced aldehydes from neutral mucosubstances; or when the neutral and acid moieties in the same mucin are sufficiently distant from each other that the reaction of the phenylhydrazine with anionic groups does not prevent its condensation with periodate-induced aldehydes. Conversely, when the neutral and acid moieties are close the aldehydes will be coloured.

Method

(1) Bring sections to water.
(2) Oxidize in fresh 1% periodic acid for 10 minutes.
(3) Wash in running water for 5 minutes.
(4) Block aldehydes (*see below*) in 0.5% aqueous phenylhydrazine hydrochloride for 30 minutes.
(5) Wash in water.
(6) Treat with Schiff reagent for 10–15 minutes.
(7) Wash in running water for 5 minutes.
(8) Counterstain with haematoxylin if desired.
(9) Dehydrate, clear and mount in synthetic resin.

Results

Phenylhydrazine blocks the staining of neutral polysaccharides and glycoproteins; some sialo-acid and sialo-sulphated glycoproteins are stained red.

Blocking techniques

A blocking technique is one that, although failing to give a colour reaction with a certain tissue element, will combine with that tissue element in such a manner as to prevent it from giving a colour reaction with other reagents. It may be used for the detection of those groups which react in this way.

Some of these techniques have been incorporated in techniques described previously but are included here for continuity.

Blocking of aldehyde groups

By blocking aldehyde groups in a periodic-acid-treated section, it can be shown that a positive Schiff reaction may be given by substances other than aldehydes, such as peroxide, ketone or ethylene oxide. Several blocking techniques have been devised, but those most commonly used are described below.

■ **Aldehyde blocking technique (Lillie and Glenner, 1957)**

After exposure of the sections to periodic acid, and washing, they are treated in the following solution for 30 minutes at room temperature.

Aniline	10 ml
Acetic acid	90 ml

The sections are then washed in distilled water and the PAS technique continued at stage 4.

Results

Only non-aldehyde PAS positive material (reducing lipid, and so on) will be stained red.

■ **Borohydride/aldehyde block (Lillie and Pizzolato, 1972)**

This method of blocking aldehyde groups with sodium borohydride is simple, quick and effective; alternatively, use steps (2), (3) and (4) of the method on page 248 in place of step (4) below, that is, uronic acid reduction.

Method

(1) Bring sections to water.
(2) Treat with freshly prepared 1% periodic acid.
(3) Wash in running water for 10 minutes.
(4) Treat with 0.1% sodium borohydride in 1% Na_2HPO_4.
(5) Treat slide with Schiff reagent.
(6) Treat by appropriate method, or dehydrate, clear and mount.

Results

Sections (at step 5) are Schiff negative.

■ **Spicer's phenylhydrazine blocking of aldehydes (Spicer, 1961)**

Sections are treated with a 0.5% aqueous solution of phenylhydrazine hydrochloride for 30 minutes.

Blocking technique for 1:2 glycol group (acetylation)

A PAS positive substance which, after treatment with acetic anhydride, gives a negative PAS reaction, indicates that the original reaction was due to a 1:2 glycol grouping (carbohydrate). Since acetylation is reversible by treatment with potassium hydroxide (saponification), the following technique of McManus and Cason (1950) is recommended.

■ *Method*

(1) Bring three sections to water.
(2) Treat two sections (A and B) in the following solution for 1–24 hours at room temperature.

Acetic anhydride   13 ml
Pyridine   20 ml

Note: One hour will usually suffice in this reagent, but longer periods may be required before a histochemical evaluation can be made.

(3) Wash sections A and B in water.
(4) Treat section B with 0.1 N potassium hydroxide for 45 minutes at room temperature (deacetylation).
(5) Wash section B in water.
(6) Treat all three sections by the PAS technique.

Results

A positive result in a given structure in sections B and C only indicates that the reaction was due to a 1:2 glycol grouping, and not to preformed aldehydes in the element.

Methylation

This procedure has been classified by Spicer (1960) as 'mild methylation' when performed at 37 °C for 4 hours, whereas the term 'active methylation' is used when it is performed at 60 °C for 4 hours. Spicer, Horn and Leppi (1967) state that 'mild methylation' eliminates basophilia of most COOH groups. Basophilia of all acid mucopolysaccharides is occluded after 4 hours at 60 °C. Schmitz-Moorman (1969) and Quintarelli, Scott and Dellovo (1964) suggest that sialic acid is mostly removed by active methylation (60 °C) and its staining cannot be restored by saponification. Active methylation (at 60 °C) is thought to methylate carboxyl groups (COOH) to methyl esters which can be restored to COOH by saponification.

Vilter (1968) supported by Sorvari and Stoward (1970) have suggested that the abolition of basophilia by methylation is due to the lactonization of carboxyl groups, rather than their esterification. Methylation has also been shown to desulphate the sulphated mucopolysaccharides and glycoproteins; staining of sulphate groups cannot be restored by saponification.

■ *Method*

(1) Bring sections to alcohol.
(2) Place in preheated 1% hydrochloric acid in methyl alcohol, for 4 hours at 60 °C (at 37 °C for mild methylation—*see above*).
(3) Rinse in alcohol.
(4) Stain by appropriate technique (parallel sections may be saponified (*see below*) then stained and compared).

Results

See above.

■ **Thionyl chloride methylation (Stoward, 1967; Sorvari and Stoward, 1970)**

For the reasons given below (*see* Results) this method is not useful in the routine laboratory. Culling (1974) used it as a research procedure together with the borohydride method of blocking carboxyl (COOH) groups.

Method

(1) Bring sections to methyl alcohol.
(2) Treat in 2% thionyl chloride in methyl alcohol for 4 hours at room temperature.
(3) Rinse twice in methyl alcohol and rinse in water.
(4) Stain by appropriate procedure.

Results

Basophilia due to COOH groups and RNA is said to disappear in 30 minutes and that due to sulphated mucopolysaccharides in 4 hours. It is, however, possible that in sulphomucins containing both COOH and sulphate groups that only the sulphate groups are esterified. A few sulphated mucins are desulphated completely (Pearse, 1968).

Saponification of methyl and acetyl esters

This procedure is used to restore reactions blocked by acetylation or methylation or to render acetylated hydroxyl groups PAS reactive.

Unless sections are firmly attached to slides they will become detached during this procedure. It is recommended that 0.1% chrome alum in 1% gelatin be used as an adhesive.

■ *Method*

(1) Bring sections to 70% alcohol.
(2) Treat with 0.5% potassium hydroxide (KOH) in 70% alcohol for 30 minutes at room temperature.
(3) Rinse carefully in 70% alcohol.
(4) Wash in slowly running tap-water for 10 minutes.

■ *Reduction of uronic acid esters (Reid, Culling and Day, 1970)*

Frush and Isbell (1956) described a method for the reduction of lactones and uronic acid esters to the corresponding primary alcohols; Reid and colleagues adapted this method for use in histochemistry.

This modification is based upon the esterification (by methylation) of the carboxyl groups (COOH), with the resultant uronic acid methyl esters or the lactones of Vilter (1968) and Sorvari and Stoward (1970) being reduced to primary alcohols with buffered sodium borohydride.

It had been intended to use this method together with the methanolic thionyl chloride (Stoward, 1967; Sorvari and Stoward, 1970) method, of esterification of COOH groups without desulphation, as a specific technique for sulphate esters. Unfortunately, it was found that partial desulphation took place.

Buffered borohydride reagent

Solution A

Boric acid (H_3BO_3)   2.45 g
Distilled water   100 ml

Dissolve boric acid in distilled water. This solution may be prepared and kept in a refrigerator until needed.

Solution B

Sodium borohydride ($NaBH_4$)   1.89 g
Distilled water   167 ml

Immediately before use dissolve the borohydride in distilled water. This should be done in a fume hood.

Method

(1) Methylate (thionyl chloride method) sections as described on page 247 or by preferred method.
(2) Place slides in glass (or stainless steel) holder in a container that will hold approximately 300 ml, but narrow enough that slides will be covered by 100 ml of ice-cold boric acid solution (solution A) that is first poured in. This container should be placed in crushed ice in a fume hood.
(3) Over a 30-minute period, add solution B to solution A. Leave sections in buffered borohydride in ice-bath for 1 hour.
(4) Wash sections in running water for 10–15 minutes.
(5) Stain sections by Alcian blue pH 2.5 or other appropriate method.
(6) Dehydrate, clear and mount in resinous mountant.

Result

Only sulphate esters (surviving methylation) are stained blue. A control section should be saponified after step (4) to ensure that reduction of esters has taken place, strongly positive alcianophilia (with Alcian blue at pH 2.5) after this step will indicate the absence or incompleteness of methylation or reduction.

Hydrolysis methods

■ **Smith oxidation hydrolysis (Reid, Culling and Day, 1970)**

This procedure (Goldstein and colleagues, 1965) was adapted to abolish existing PAS staining in tissue sections when investigating the KOH/PAS phenomenon. The method is based upon the oxidation of 1:2 glycols (vicinal diols) with periodic acid to dialdehydes, which are then reduced to primary alcohols with buffered borohydride (Lillie and Pizzolato, 1972). Subsequent hydrolysis with hydrochloric acid should cleave residues which have been oxidized with periodate, thus fragmenting the polymer into small diffusable molecules. The degree of fragmentation will depend upon the position of the oxidized residues.

Method

(1) Bring sections to water.
(2) Treat in freshly prepared 1% periodic acid for 10 minutes.
(3) Wash in running water.
(4) Treat with 0.1% sodium borohydride in 1% Na_2HPO_4 for 5 minutes.
(5) Immerse sections in 0.1 N hydrochloric acid for 6 hours at room temperature.
(6) Wash in running water.
(7) Perform PAS reaction.

Result

Sections will be PAS negative after reduction; following hydrolysis, however, certain structures may develop PAS positivity due to the oxidation of 1:2 glycols which were previously blocked.

(1) A control section should be stained with Schiff reagent after step (4) to ensure that aldehydes have been blocked (converted to primary alcohols).
(2) Following step (6), treatment of sections of human or rat large intestine with alcoholic KOH will result in areas of PAS positivity.

■ **Acid hydrolysis to remove sialic acid**

Since sialic acid is invariably a terminal group, it may be removed by mild acid hydrolysis (Quintarelli *et al.*, 1961). As is noted previously methylation is also said to remove most of the sialic acid from sections.

Method

(1) Bring sections to water.
(2) Treat sections in preheated 0.02 N sodium acetate–HCl buffer pH 2.5 (*see* page 129) at 75 °C for 2 hours (or in 0.1 N H_2SO_4 at 80 °C for 1 hour).
(3) Rinse in distilled water.
(4) Stain sections by Alcian blue/PAS technique.
(5) Dehydrate, clear and mount in resinous mountant.

Result

Removal of sialic acid is shown by loss of Alcian blue staining.

Enzyme digestion techniques

Hyaluronidase digestion

The histochemical identification of hyaluronic acid, chondroitin sulphates A and C (chondroitin-4-sulphate and chondroitin-6-sulphate) and chondroitin sulphate B (dermatan sulphate) is mainly dependent upon digestion with hyaluronidase allied with the staining and blocking methods described above. *Table 12.2* illustrates their mechanism of action, although it should be remembered that the results obtained will only be accurate if the enzymes are both pure and active, traces of protease activity can give misleading information. For the preparation of *Flavobacterium heparinum* extracts *see* Zugibe (1962, 1970).

Table 12.2 Activity of the various hyaluronidases (after Zugibe, 1962)

Enzyme	Acid mucopolysaccharide hydrolysed
Streptococcal hyaluronidase	Hyaluronic acid
Testicular hyaluronidase	Hyaluronic acid
	Chondroitin sulphate A
	Chondroitin sulphate C
Flavobacterium heparinum extract	Hyaluronic acid
(adapted to chondroitin sulphate A)	Chondroitin sulphates A, B and C
Flavobacterium heparinum extract	Hyaluronic acid
(adapted to heparitin sulphate)	Chondroitin sulphate A
	Chondroitin sulphate C
	Heparitin sulphate, heparin

Enzyme techniques

Serial sections should be used for this type of investigation and the test and control slides examined with a comparison microscope.

Methods   It should be remembered that a control section should always be incubated in buffer alone for the same time and at the same temperature as the test sections. A positive control section (umbilical cord, and so on) should also be treated with the test sections to ensure that the enzyme is active.

Testicular hyaluronidase technique

Method

(1) Bring sections to water.
(2) Treat slides for 2–6 hours in prewarmed (37 °C) hyaluronidase solution (50 mg/100 ml of acetic–acetate buffer pH 6.0, page 131) at 37 °C; place control slides in buffer alone for same time period.
(3) Rinse slides in buffer alone.
(4) Rinse in water.
(5) Stain with Alcian blue at pH 1.0 and/or 2.5.

Result

Loss of staining (by comparison with buffer control) is due to removal of hyaluronic acid and/or chondroitin sulphates A and/or B.

■ **Streptococcal hyaluronidase technique (Zugibe, 1962)**

Positive and negative control sections should be carried through with the test sections as described above.

Method

(1) Bring formal-fixed cryostat or paraffin sections to water.
(2) Rinse sections in acetic–acetate buffer at pH 5.0 (*see* page 131).
(3) Incubate sections in acetic–acetate buffer (pH 5.0) containing streptococcal hyaluronidase (1500 TRU/100 ml), 0.1 M NaCl and 0.05% gelatin, for 24 hours at 37 °C.
(4) Rinse in water.
(5) Stain with Alcian blue at pH 2.5.

Results

Loss of staining (by comparison with buffer control) is due to removal of hyaluronic acid.

Sialidase (neuraminidase) digestion

It has now been shown that some sialic acids are stable to sialidase treatment. Methods for enhancing their digestibility (described below) have all been found to be efficient in a given situation; however, it seems there are still some sialic acids (extracted from tissues after treatment) that are completely stable; these cannot be identified histochemically. Sialidase alone, and sialidase following potassium hydroxide treatment (as in (1) below) is recommended.

■ **Methods of enhancing digestibility of sialic acids before treatment with sialidase (Gad, 1969)**

(1) Pretreatment with 1% potassium hydroxide in 70% ethanol for 5 minutes (Spicer and Duvenci, 1964).
(2) Trypsin 1/1000 in M/100 phosphate buffer at pH 8.0 for 5 minutes to 4 hours at 37 °C (Lev and Spicer, 1964).
(3) Crystalline pepsin 2 mg/ml of 0.02 N sodium acctate–HCl buffer at pH 2.5 for 2 hours at 37 °C (Quintarelli, 1963).

■ **Sialidase technique (Quintarelli et al., 1961; Gad, 1969)**

Method

(1) Bring two (A and B) cryostat or paraffin sections of formal-fixed tissue to water, or air dry (Gad, 1969).
(2) Section A is incubated in sialidase (neuraminidase) 1 unit/ml in 0.05 M acetate buffer

at pH 5.5 (containing approximately 0.1% calcium chloride) (section B in buffer alone) for 24 hours at 37 °C (*see note below*).
(3) Rinse in water.
(4) Stain in Alcian blue pH 2.5 (*see* page 232).

Result

Loss of staining (by comparison with control **B**) is due to removal of sialic acids.

Note

Neuraminidase is now supplied in 1 ml vials containing *1 unit*. One unit is the amount of enzyme required to liberate one *micromole* of *N*-acetyl neuraminic acid from human α_1-acid glycoprotein/minute at 37 °C and pH 5.5.

The old system (100 units/ml) referred to the activity against *micrograms* of *N*-acetyl neuraminic acid.

Lectin histochemistry

Lectins are proteins or glycoproteins of plant or animal origin which bind to sugars. Lectins have a nominal polysaccharide specificity but in the histochemistry sense they may give quite different staining patterns on tissue sections since more complex polysaccharides are involved (Ponder, 1983). Cell membrane carbohydrates are important in characterizing cell types and in studying changes associated with cellular differentiation and neoplastic changes.

Some commonly used lectins are listed in *Table 12.3* along with their major sugar specificities. More comprehensive details are given by Goldstein and Hayes (1978) and Debray *et al.* (1981).

Table 12.3 Lectins

Source	Abbreviation	Major sugar specificity
Glycine max—soyabean	SBA	α-D-Gal NAc
Ricinus communis—castor bean	RCA 1	β-D-Galactose
Ulex europaeus—gorse	UEA	α-L-Fucose
Triticum vulgaris—wheat germ	WGA	β-D-Glc NAc(1 → 4), sialic acid
Arachis hypogaea—peanut	PNA	β-D-Gal-(1 → 3)-D-Gal NAc
Dolichos biflorus—horse gram	DBA	α-D-Gal NAc
Concanavalin—jack bean	Con A	α-D-Mannose
Bandeiraea simplicifolia	BSA	α-D-Galactose
Limulus polyphema—horse-shoe crab	LPA	Sialic acid

Gal NAc, *N*-acetylgalactosamine.
Glc NAc, *N*-acetylglucosamine.

Lectin binding is visualized by using lectins conjugated to fluorescein isothiocyanate or horse-radish peroxidase. They can be obtained commercially as conjugates and are simple to use. It is important to determine the correct concentration of lectin for any specific application to ensure minimum background staining. Control sections should be treated with lectin conjugate which has been absorbed by its specific monosaccharide at a concentration of 0.1 M.

Frozen sections are recommended but paraffin sections are often adequate.

■ **General method for peroxidase conjugated lectin labelling**

(1) Wash in phosphate buffered saline pH 7.5 containing 0.5% bovine serum albumin.
(2) Remove excess moisture.
(3) Add lectin conjugate and incubate for 1 hour at room temperature in a moist chamber.
(4) Wash with several changes of phosphate buffered saline.
(5) Demonstrate peroxidase activity. For most purposes the standard diamino-benzidine method may be used.
(6) Counterstain in haemalum and blue.
(7) Wash, dehydrate, clear and mount in synthetic resin.

References

ABU'L HAJ, S. K. and RINEHART, J. F. (1952–1953). Aldehyde–fuchsin staining of sulfated mucopolysaccharides and related sulfated substances. (Proc. Histochem. Soc.) *J. Natl Cancer Inst.*, **13**, 232

ALLISON, R. T. (1973). The effects of fixation on the subsequent demonstration of mucopolysaccharides. *Med. Lab. Technol.*, **30**, 27–31

ATTWOOD, H. D. (1958). The histological diagnosis of amniotic fluid embolism. *J. Pathol. Bacteriol.*, **76**, 211–215

BEST, F. (1906). Über Karminfarbung des Glykogens und der Kerne. *Z. Wiss. Mikr.*, **23**, 319–322

BRADEN, A. W. H. (1955). The reaction of isolated mucopolysaccharides to several histochemical tests. *Stain Technol.*, **30**, 19

COOK, H. C. (1959). A comparative evaluation of the histological demonstration of mucin. *J. Med. Lab. Technol.*, **16**, 1–6

COOK, H. C. (1974). *Histological Demonstration Techniques*. Butterworths, London

CULLING, C. F. A. (1974). *Handbook of Histopathological and Histochemical Techniques*. 3rd Ed. Butterworths, London

CULLING, C. F. A. and REID, P. E. (1980). Specific techniques for the identification of O-acylated sialic acids in colonic mucins. *J. Microscopy*, **119** (3), 415–425

CULLING, C. F. A., REID, P. E. and DUNN, W. L. (1971). The effect of saponification on certain histochemical reactions of the epithelial mucins of the gastrointestinal tract. *J. Histochem. Cytochem.*, **19**, 654–662

CULLING, C. F. A., REID, P. E. and DUNN, W. L. (1976). A new histochemical method for the identification and visualisation of both side chain acylated and non-acylated sialic acids. *J. Histochem. Cytochem.*, **24**, 1225–1230

CULLING, C. F. A., REID, P. E., DUNN, W. L. and FREEMAN, H. J. (1981). The relevance of the histochemistry of colonic mucins based upon their PAS reactivity. *Histochem. J.*, **13**, 889–903

CULLING, C. F. A. and VASSAR, P. S. (1961). Deoxyribose nucleic acid: A fluorescent histochemical technique. *Arch. Pathol.*, **71**, 76–80

DEBRAY, H., DECONT, D., STRECKER, G., SPIK, G. and MONTREUIL, J. (1981). Specificity of twelve lectins towards oligosaccharides and glycopeptides related to N-glycosylproteins. *Eur. J. Biochem.*, **117**, 41–55

DRZENICK, R. (1973). Substrate specificity of neuraminidases. *Histochem. J.*, **5**, 271–290

ENGFELDT, B. and HJERTQUIST, S. O. (1967). The effect of various fixatives on the preservation of acid glycosaminoglycans in tissues. *Acta Pathol. Microbiol. Scan.*, **71**, 219–232

FEYRTER, F. (1936). Über ein sehr einfaches Verfahren der Markscheidenfärbung, zugleich eine neue Art der Färberei. *Virchows Arch. Pathol. Anat.*, **296**, 645–654

FILIPE, M. I. (1971). Sulphur uptake in the mucosa adjacent to carcinoma of the large intestine. *Histochem. J.*, **3**, 27–35

FRUSH, H. L. and ISBELL, H. S. (1956). *J. Am. Chem. Soc.*, **78**, 2844

GAD, A. (1969). A histochemical study of human alimentary tract mucosubstances in health and disease. I. Normal and tumours. *Br. J. Cancer*, **23**, 52–63

GAD, A. and SYLVEN, B. (1969). On the nature of the high iron diamine method for sulphomucins. *J. Histochem. Cytochem.*, **17**, 156–160

GOLDSTEIN, I. J., HAY, G. W., LEWIS, B. W. and SMITH, F. (1965). *Methods in Carbohydrate Chemistry*. Ed. Whistler, R. L. Vol. 5. Academic Press, New York and London, p. 361

GOLDSTEIN, I. J. and HAYES, C. E. (1978). The lectins: carbohydrate-binding proteins of plants and animals. *Adv. Carbohydr. Chem. Biochem.*, **35**, 127–340

GOMORI, G. (1946). A new histochemical test for glycogen and mucin. *Am. J. Clin. Pathol.*, **10**, 177–179

GOMORI, G. (1950). Aldehyde fuchsin: a new stain for elastic tissue. *Am. J. Clin. Pathol.*, **20**, 665–666

GROCOTT, R. G. (1955). A stain for fungi in tissue sections and smears using Gomori's methenamine–silver nitrate technique. *Am. J. Clin. Pathol.*, **25**, 975–979.

HALE, C. W. (1946). Histochemical demonstration of acid polysaccharides in normal tissue. *Nature (Lond.)*, **157**, 802

HALMI, N. S. (1952). Differentiation of the two types of basophils in the adenohypophysis of the rat and mouse. *Stain Technol.*, **27**, 61–64

HICKS, J. D. and MATTHAEI, E. J. (1958). A selective fluorescence stain for mucin. *J. Pathol. Bacteriol.*, **75**, 473–476

HOOGHWINKEL, G. J. and SMITS, G. (1957). The specificity of the periodic-acid Schiff technique studied by a quantitative test tube method. *J. Histochem. Cytochem.*, **5**, 120–126

HOTCHKISS, R. D. (1948). A microchemical reaction resulting in the staining of polysaccharide structures in fixed tissue. *Arch. Biochem.*, **16**, 131–141

JEANLOZ, R. W. (1960). The nomenclature of mucopolysaccharides. *Arth. Rheumatol.*, **3**, 233–237.

LEPPI, T. J. and SPICER, S. S. (1966). The histochemistry of mucins in certain primate salivary glands. *Am. J. Anat.*, **118**, 833–851

LEPPI, T. J. and SPICER, S. S. (1967). Correlated histochemical staining and $^{35}SO_4$ labelling of salivary gland mucosubstances. *J. Histochem. Cytochem.*, **15**, 745–751

LEV, R. and SPICER, S. S. (1964). Specific staining of sulphate groups with Alcian blue at low pH. *J. Histochem. Cytochem.*, **12**, 309

LILLIE, R. D. (1947). *Bull. Invest. Ass. Med. Mis.*, **27**, 23

LILLIE, R. D. (1964). Histochemical acylation of hydroxyl and amino groups. Effect on the periodic acid Schiff reaction, anionic and cationic dye and Van Gieson collagen stains. *J. Histochem. Cytochem.*, **12**, 821–841

LILLIE, R. D. and GLENNER, G. G. (1957). Histochemical aldehyde blockade by aniline in glacial acetic acid. *J. Histochem. Cytochem.*, **5**, 161–169

LILLIE, R. D. and PIZZOLATO, P. (1972). Histochemical use of borohydrides as aldehyde blocking reagents. *Stain Technol.*, **47**, 13–16

LISON, L. (1954). Alcian blue 8G with chlorantine fast red 5B. A technique for selective staining of mucopolysaccharides. *Stain Technol.*, **29**, 131–138

McMANUS, J. F. A. (1946). Histological demonstration of mucin after periodic acid. *Nature (Lond.)*, **158**, 202

McMANUS, J. F. A. and CASON, J. E. (1950). Carbohydrate histochemistry studied by acetylation techniques: periodic acid methods. *J. Exp. Med.*, **91**, 651–654

MEYER, K. (1953). Some conjugated glycoproteins. *Proceedings of the Ninth Annual Conference on Protein Metabolism*. Ed. Cole, W. H. Rutgers University Press, New Brunswick, NJ

MITCHELL, A. J. and WISLOCKI, G. B. (1944). Selective staining of glycogen by ammoniacal silver nitrate; new method. *Anat. Rec.*, **90**, 261–266

MONTREUIL, J. and BISERTE, G. (1959). Sialic acid and specificity of the periodic acid Schiff's fuchsin reaction as applied to paper electrophoresis. Special example of orosomucoid. *Bull. Soc. Chim. Biol.*, **41**, 959–973

MONTREUIL, J., DEFRETIN, R., CLAY, A. and CAENEN, A. (1959). Sialic acid and specificity of the Hotchkiss–McManus histological reaction. *C. R. Soc. Biol.*, **153**, 1354–1357

PALLADINI, G. and LAURO, G. (1968). Observations sur la significativité de la coloration aux alcians pour les mucopolysaccharides. *Histochemie*, **16**, 15–22

PEARSE, A. G. E. (1968). *Histochemistry, Theoretical and Applied.* 3rd Ed. Vol. 1. Churchill, London

PONDER, B. A. J. (1983). Lectin histochemistry. In *Immunocytochemistry: Practical Applications in Pathology and Biology.* Eds Polak, J. M. and Van Noorden, S. Wright, Bristol

PRITCHARD, J. J. (1949). A new histochemical method for glycogen. *J. Anat.*, **83**, 30–31

QUINTARELLI, G. (1963). Masking action of basic proteins on sialic acid carboxyls in epithelial mucins. *Experientia*, **19**, 230–231

QUINTARELLI, G., SCOTT, J. E. and DELLOVO, M. C. (1964). The chemical and histochemical properties of Alcian blue. III. Chemical blocking and unblocking. *Histochemie*, **4**, 99–112

QUINTARELLI, G., TSUIKI, S., HASHIMOTO, Y. and PIGMAN, W. (1961). Studies of sialic acid-containing mucins in bovine submaxillary and rat sublingual glands. *J. Histochem. Cytochem.*, **9**, 176–183

RAVETTO, C. (1964). Histochemical identification of sialic (neuraminic) acids. *J. Histochem. Cytochem.*, **12**, 306.

REID, P. E., CULLING, C. F. A. and DAY, M. E. (1970). New methods for the histochemical investigation of the mucins of the gastrointestinal tract. *Proc. Can. Fed. Biol. Soc.*, **13**, 11

REID, P. E., CULLING, C. F. A. and DUNN, W. L. (1975). A histochemical method of differentiating lower gastrointestinal tract mucin from other mucins in primary or metastatic tumours. *J. Clin. Pathol.*, **28**, 656–658

REID, P. E., CULLING, C. F. A., DUNN, W. L. and CLAY, M. G. (1976). The use of a trans-esterification technique to distinguish between certain neuraminidase resistant epithelial mucins. *Histochemistry*, **46**, 203–207

REID, P. E., LIVINGSTONE, D. J. and DUNN, W. L. (1972). Staining of polymeric carbohydrate half sulphate esters with high iron diamine after cellulose acetate electrophoresis. *Stain Technol.*, **47**, 101–102

RINEHART, J. E. and ABU'L HAJ, S. K. (1951). An improved method for histologic demonstration of acid mucopolysaccharides in tissues. *AMA Arch. Pathol.*, **52**, 189–194

SCHMITZ-MOORMAN, P. (1969). Zur Histochemie der Neuraminsäure. *Histochemie*, **20**, 78–86

SCOTT, J. E. and DORLING, J. (1965). Difference of staining of acid glycosaminoglycans (mucopolysaccharides) by Alcian blue in salt solutions. *Histochemie*, **5**, 221–233

SCOTT, J. E. and HARBINSON, T. J. (1968). Periodate oxidation of acid polysaccharides. Inhibition by the electrostatic field of the substrate. *Histochemie*, **14**, 215–220

SHEAHAN, D. J., JERVIS, H. R., TAKEUCHI, A. and SPRINZ, H. (1970). The effect of staphylococcal enterotoxin on the epithelial mucosubstance of the small intestine of rhesus monkeys. *Am. J. Pathol.*, **60**, 1–18

SOCHOR, F. M. (1965). Effects of various fixatives on dissolution and staining characteristics of acid mucopolysaccharides in human aorta. *Am. J. Clin. Pathol.*, **44**, 636–638

SORVARI, T. E. and STOWARD, P. J. (1970). Some investigations of the mechanisms of the so-called 'methylation' reactions used in mucosubstance histochemistry. I. 'Methylation' with methyl iodide diazomethane and various organic solvents containing either hydrogen chloride or thionyl chloride. *Histochemie*, **24**, 106–113

SOUTHGATE, H. W. (1927). Note on preparing mucicarmine. *J. Pathol. Bacteriol.*, **30**, 729.

SPICER, S. S. (1960). A correlative study of the histochemical properties of rodent acid mucopolysaccharides. *J. Histochem. Cytochem.*, **8**, 18–35

SPICER, S. S. (1961). The use of cationic reagents in the histochemical differentiation of mucopolysaccharides. *Am. J. Clin. Pathol.*, **36**, 393–497

SPICER, S. S. (1965). Diamine methods for differentiating mucopolysaccharides histochemically. *J. Histochem. Cytochem.*, **13**, 211–234

SPICER, S. S. and DUVENCI, J. (1964). Histochemical characteristics of mucopolysaccharides in salivary and exorbital lacrimal glands. *Anat. Rec.*, **149**, 333–358

SPICER, S. S., HORN, R. G. and LEPPI, T. J. (1967). *The Connective Tissue*. Ed. Wagner, B. W. International Academic Monograph, No. 7. Williams and Wilkins, Baltimore

SPICER, S. S., LEPPI, T. J. and STOWARD, P. J. (1965). Suggestions for a histochemical terminology of carbohydrate-rich tissue components. *J. Histochem. Cytochem.*, **13**, 599–603

SPICER, S. S. and MAYER, D. B. (1960). Histochemical differentiation of acid mucopolysaccharides by means of combined aldehyde fuchsin–alcian blue staining. *Tech. Bull. Regist. Med. Technol.*, **30**, 53–60

STASTNA, J. and TRAVNIC, P. (1971). Electron microscopic detection of PAS-positive substances with thiosemicarbazide. *Histochemie*, **27**, 63–68.

STEEDMAN, H. F. (1950). Alcian blue 8GS. A new stain for mucin. *Quart. J. Micr. Sci.*, **91**, 477–479

STOWARD, P. J. (1967). The histochemical properties of some periodate-reactive mucosubstances of the pregnant Syrian hamster before and after methylation with methanolic thionyl chloride. *J. R. Micr. Soc.*, **87**, 77–103

VALLANCE-OWEN, J. (1948). Histological demonstration of glycogen in necropsy material. *J. Pathol. Bacteriol.*, **60**, 325–327

VASSAR, P. S. and CULLING, C. F. A. (1959a). Fluorescent stains with special reference to amyloid and connective tissues. *Arch. Pathol.*, **68**, 487–498

VASSAR, P. S. and CULLING, C. F. A. (1959b). Fibrosis of the breast. *Arch. Pathol.*, **67**, 128–133

VEH, R. W., MEESSEN, D., KUNTZ, H. D. and MAY, B. (1982). In *Colonic Carcinogenesis*. Eds Malt, R. A. and Williamson, R. C. N. Falk Symposium 31 (1981). MTP Press Ltd, pp. 355–365

VILTER, V. (1968). Contribution à l'étude du mécanisme de la 'méthylation-saponification' dans l'histochemie des mucines acides. *Ann. Histochem.*, **13**, 205–220

WARREN, L. (1959). The thiobarbituric acid assay of sialic acids. *J. Biol. Chem.*, **234**, 1971–1975

YAMADA, K. (1969). Combined histochemical staining of 1,2-glycol and sulphate groupings of mucopolysaccharides in paraffin sections. *Histochemie*, **20**, 271–276

ZUGIBE, F. T. (1962). The demonstration of individual acid-mucopolysaccharides in human aortas, coronary arteries and cerebral arteries. I. The Methods. *J. Histochem. Cytochem.*, **10**, 441–447

ZUGIBE, F. T. (1970). *Diagnostic Histochemistry*. Mosby, St Louis

13

Lipids

As early as 1823 it was established that common animal and vegetable fats were a combination of glycerol with fatty acids, but little further research occurred during the next 100 years.

The rather loose and indefinite terminology that has been applied to fats and fat-like substances is a reflection of the lack of systematic nomenclature in the early days. The use of the words lipoid, lipin, lipide and lipid has varied from author to author, the same name occasionally being used to mean all fats and fat-like substances, or fat-like substances alone (waxes, and so on).

Definitions

The term 'lipid' will be used to describe all naturally occurring fats and fat-like substances.

Lipids are usually defined as those naturally occurring substances which are insoluble in water but soluble in the so-called 'fat solvents' (chloroform, benzene, petroleum, ether, acetone and so on), which are related either actually or potentially to fatty acid esters, and which are capable of being utilized by the animal organism. For practical purposes this definition may be adopted but it cannot be accepted too rigidly since a typical lipid 'lecithin' is slightly soluble in water and insoluble in acetone; another lipid 'lysolecithin' is freely soluble in warm water and insoluble in ether, and sphingomyelin and the cerebrosides when purified are insoluble in a range of fat solvents (*see Table 13.1*).

Whereas certain pure lipids are insoluble in a particular fat solvent, the same lipids when contaminated with other lipids are rendered soluble in that solvent. An excellent solvent in general for crude lipids is a mixture of chloroform and methanol.

Fat and oil are terms used to describe the physical state of a lipid, a *fat* being a lipid which is solid at room temperature, an *oil* being liquid. A substance classified as a fat in a temperate climate may be an oil in the tropics.

General chemistry of lipids

The true fats (or oils) are the most abundant of the lipids. Chemically, they are neutral esters of fatty acids and glycerol. In nature, they are generally three fatty acid molecules (saturated or unsaturated) combined with one molecule of glycerol, with the splitting out of three molecules of water (*Figure 13.1*).

Table 13.1 Keilig extractions

	Hydrocarbons	Fatty acids	Glycolipids	Phospholipids	Sphingomyelin	Simple lipids	Cholesterol	Cholesterol esters
Cold acetone						+	+	+
Hot acetone			+					
Hot ether				+				
Hot chloroform methanol	+	+	+	+	+	+	+	+

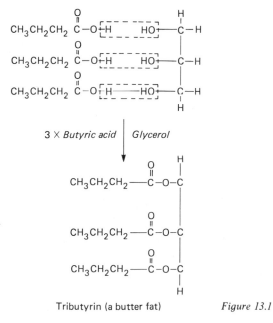

3 × Butyric acid   Glycerol

Tributyrin (a butter fat)   *Figure 13.1*

Most of the triglycerides which occur in nature are mixed triglycerides; that is, they contain two or three different fatty acids. Since most natural lipids contain glycerol their chemical and physical characteristics are determined by the nature of their fatty acid components. Some of the fatty acids are *saturated* with hydrogen, some are partially *unsaturated*. All have one property in common, in addition to the terminal carboxyl group (COOH), they contain an even number of carbon atoms if derived from naturally occurring fat. The latter is probably because of the mode of synthesis of fatty acids from 2-carbon fragments.

Physical properties

Triglycerides have a specific gravity of less than one (approximately 0.86) and are therefore lighter than water. The fact that they are solid *fat* or liquid *oil* will depend upon the room temperature and their melting point (MP). The MP will be dependent upon two factors:

(1) the chain length of the component fatty acids; and
(2) their degree of unsaturation.

In general, saturated fatty acids containing more than eight carbon atoms are solid (with four to eight they are liquid) and their MPs increase with the length of the chain. They confer these properties on the lipids containing them. The introduction of one carbon–carbon double bond into the fatty acid molecule will markedly lower the MP, so much so that even a fatty acid with 18 carbon atoms becomes an oil at room temperature (e.g. oleic acid).

The commonly occurring fatty acids are as follows. *Saturated*—stearic (18 carbons) and palmitic (16 carbons); *unsaturated*—oleic acid $CH_3(CH_2)_7$ $CH=CH(CH_2)_7COOH$.

Arichidonic acid, said to be found in animal fat and adrenal phosphatides, is a *polyunsaturated fatty acid* having 20 carbon atoms with four carbon–carbon double bonds.

Compound lipids

As will be seen below, compound lipids are those containing other components in addition to alcohols and fatty acids. They may contain sphingosine in place of glycerol (e.g. sphingomyelin and glycolipids).

Classification

Lipids may be classified according to their chemical structure and divided into three main groups, each of which may be further subdivided.

Group I—simple lipids

Simple lipids are neutral esters of fatty acids (palmitic, stearic or linoleic) with alcohols. They may be divided into the following.

(1) *Neutral lipids* comprising fats and oils in which the alcohol is glycerol.
(2) *Waxes*, which contain alcohols higher than glycerol (e.g. cholesterol esters).

Group II—compound lipids

These are lipids in which products other than fatty acids and alcohol are present. They comprise:

(1) Phospholipids.
    They contain a phosphoric acid molecule and may be divided into the glycerophospholipids and the sphingophospholipids.
    (a) Lecithin—glycerol, saturated and unsaturated fatty acid residues, phosphoric acid and choline.
    (b) Cephalin—similar to lecithin, the choline being replaced by ethanolamine.
    (c) Acetal phosphatides (plasmals)—similar to lecithin and cephalin but containing

acetals of fatty aldehydes in place of fatty acids, combined with cholamine glycerophosphate.

(d) Sphingomyelin—sphingosine (instead of glycerol), phosphoric acid, choline and fatty acid.

(2) Glycolipids.

They contain a sugar molecule and are either sphingosine based or glycerol based. The latter are not important in animals.

(a) Cerebrosides—sphingosine, hexose and fatty acid.

(b) Gangliosides—sphingosine, neuraminic acid, hexose and fatty acid.

(c) Sulphatides—cerebroside sulphate.

Group III—derived lipids

These are derivatives of Groups I and II, obtained by hydrolysis, and can be subdivided as follows.

(1) Fatty acids derived from natural products.

(a) Saturated fatty acids—such as palmitic or stearic acid which contain no double bond in the molecule.

(b) Unsaturated fatty acids—such as oleic acid, which contain double bonds in the molecule.

(2) Alcohols of higher molecular weight which are obtained by hydrolysis of waxes. Some authors include glycerol although it is water soluble.

(a) Sterols—containing the steroid nucleus, the commonest being cholesterol.

(b) Straight chain alcohols—these are not of importance histologically.

Hydrocarbons

These are non-saponifiable lipids containing only carbon and hydrogen.

Carotenoids (lipochrome, chromolipid)

These are coloured unsaturated hydrocarbons. These lipid pigments do not fall strictly into any of the above groups, but are included in this classification for the sake of completeness. Those of importance histologically are dealt with in Chapter 14 on Pigments (page 286).

Fixation of lipids

Whilst the most accurate procedures for the demonstration of lipids would utilize fresh cryostat sections, in practice fixation is commonly employed. Simple lipids are not affected by fixation in neutral buffered formalin. The compound lipids are best preserved by formal–calcium treatment but the plasmal reaction should be carried out on unfixed cryostat sections.

Identification of lipids

The histological identification of lipids is usually based on the following:

(1) solubility;
(2) examination by polarized light;

(3) reduction of osmium tetroxide;
(4) demonstration by fat-soluble dyes;
(5) other staining and histochemical methods.

Of these methods, only (1), (4) and (5) may be used with any certainty of identification, and for routine purposes (4) and (5) are the most commonly employed.

Solubility

Keilig (1944), using a continuous extraction apparatus, demonstrated that lipids may be differentiated by their solubility in various 'fat solvents'. Using a Soxhlet extraction apparatus and blocks of fresh human brain not more than 3 mm in thickness, tissues were extracted for 24 hours, with at least three changes of solvent (*Table 13.1*). The continuous extraction with equal parts of hot chloroform and methyl alcohol may be used to demonstrate that a given substance is a lipid. Following extraction, blocks are hydrated through descending strengths of alcohol to water, and frozen sections cut and stained by Sudan black B.

It is not anticipated that this method would often be employed in the routine laboratory, although occasionally it might assist in the identification of a tissue element in conjunction with other techniques.

Baker's hot pyridine method (1946) is still one of the few methods routinely employed. Zugibe (1970), using cryostat sections of unfixed tissue, notes that glycolipids and phospholipids are the only members of the major groups that are insoluble in cold acetone, and only phospholipids in hot acetone, which is a useful method to supplement the existing ones.

■ Baker's pyridine extraction test for phospholipids

Method

(1) Fix frozen sections of fresh, unfixed tissue for 20 hours in a dilute Bouin's fluid (saturated aqueous picric acid 50 ml, formalin 10 ml, glacial acetic acid 5 ml and distilled water 35 ml).
(2) Wash in 70% alcohol for 30 minutes.
(3) Wash in 50% alcohol for 30 minutes.
(4) Wash in running water for 1 hour.
(5) Dehydrate in two changes of pyridine at room temperature for 1 hour each.
(6) Extract in fresh, pure pyridine for 24 hours at 60 °C.
(7) Wash in running water for 2 hours.
(8) Transfer to stage 2 of the acid–haematein method.

Results

Phospholipids: lecithin, kephalin and sphingomyelin and cerebrosides   Colourless

Mucin, fibrinogen and other non-lipid elements are stained.

Examination by polarized light

Most lipids are highly refractile, and some are birefringent (anisotropic). By examining sections with polarized light it can be determined whether material is isotropic or anisotropic. In the past this method was considered to be of assistance in the identification of lipids, but in view of the variability of results (dependent on the state of the lipid at the time of examination) it is now accepted that the information gained by such examination is ambiguous.

Three types of refractility may be found (Lison, 1936).

Isotropic (monorefringent)

This occurs in neutral fats, fatty acids, cholesterol esters and lipids in any state which prevents the formation of liquid crystals.

Anisotropic (birefringent)

An appearance which may be found in any lipid in a crystalline state.

Maltese cross (birefringent)

A type of birefringence found in cholesterol esters of lipids (not neutral fats or fatty acids). If at first absent, this Maltese cross birefringence may sometimes be produced by heating and then cooling before examination.

Reduction of osmium tetroxide (osmic acid)

The reduction of osmium tetroxide from colourless OsO_4 to OsO_2, which is black, is of limited value histochemically for the identification of lipids, although it may be usefully employed for their demonstration (e.g. by Marchi's method). It does not react with all lipids, but does react with many non-lipid substances (e.g. tannic acid and eleidin).

Table 13.2 Lipid techniques

	Hydrocarbons	Fatty acids	Glycolipids	Phospholipids	Sphingomyelin	Simple lipids	Cholesterol	Cholesterol esters
Fat soluble dyes	+[1]	+	+	+	+	+	+[1]	+[1]
McManus Sudan black			+	+	+			
PFAS	+		+	+	+			
OTAN				+	+			
NaOH–OTAN					+			
Fischler		+						
Schultz							+	+
PAS			+	+	+			
Bismuth trichloride							+	

[1] When melted.
Notes: (1) Acetal phosphatides   Plasmal reaction positive
       (2) Sulphatides   Brown metachromasia with toluidine blue.

It remains, however, a useful method of demonstrating lipids in paraffin sections since the osmicated lipids are insoluble in the processing reagents.

Primary blackening with osmium tetroxide is said to be due to unsaturated fatty acids (oleic acid), but the secondary staining of fat (blackening which takes place only after alcohol treatment of certain lipids) has not been fully explained, although it is said to be due to the presence of saturated fatty acids (palmitic and stearic).

The use of osmium tetroxide histochemically should be limited to frozen sections of formal–calcium fixed tissue, when a positive reaction after 6 hours is regarded as specific for reducing lipids, provided that the only structures considered are those known to contain lipid.

Demonstration with fat-soluble dyes

The staining of neutral fat with a fat-soluble dye is still the most common routine method employed in histological laboratories. It is based on the fact that the dyes used are more soluble in fat than in the solvent employed (elective solubility).

The first of these dyes to be used was Sudan III (Daddi, 1896), and it is probably still the most commonly used fat stain today, in spite of the introduction of new and better dyes. The first solvent employed was 70% alcohol, for it was thought that this dilution of alcohol was not a lipid solvent; it has since been shown that small amounts of lipid may be dissolved out by this method. Herxheimer's method employs equal parts of acetone and 70% alcohol which gives a greater concentration of stain but again dissolves small amounts of lipid.

Of the more recent methods, that of Lillie and Ashburn using oil red O in isopropyl alcohol or Gomori (1952) using oil red O in tri-ethyl phosphate gives a more intense stain with minimal removal of lipid particles. Chiffelle and Putt's Sudan IV or Fettrot in propylene glycol, which does not remove even minute lipid particles, gives the best results and is recommended for both routine and research work.

Colloidal suspensions of Sudan dyes in gelatin give first-class results, and there is no danger of dissolving any lipids, but they have the disadvantage of being messy and time-consuming to prepare and are consequently not likely to become adopted as routine stains.

Bromination reduces the solubility of unsaturated lipids (Lillie, 1954). This has been developed by Bayliss and Adams (1972) and Bayliss High (1981) using Sudan black B for the demonstration of simple lipids and phospholipids. The question concerning the action of Sudan black B in staining both hydrophobic and hydrophilic lipids has been explained by Lansink (1968) who showed that it consists of two fractions, the first colouring hydrophobic lipids by elective solubility, the second acting as a basic dye and staining phospholipids.

Notes on technique

(1) Frozen sections of formalin-fixed material are used but cryostat sections, post-fixed in formalin, are often more convenient.

(2) To avoid precipitation on the sections due to evaporation of the solvent, these stains should always be employed in *closed vessels* (screw-capped wide-mouthed jars, or Petri dishes).

(3) Loose frozen sections stain more rapidly than sections attached to slides; 50% haematoxylin for 10 minutes should, therefore, be used to stain nuclei; 1%

hydrochloric acid in water should be used to differentiate fat sections as acid–alcohol will remove lipids.

(4) Carmalum may be used as a counterstain if Sudan black is the fat stain.

(5) The general rule is that the staining step is preceded by treatment with the solvent and the section is rinsed and differentiated in the solvent after staining. Tap-water is preferred for blueing the nuclei.

(6) Sections stained for the demonstration of lipids should never be blotted, or pressed with a needle to remove air bubbles under the coverslip, because such pressure will displace droplets of lipid. If air bubbles are present, wash off the coverslip in warm water and remount. The most common fault in mounting frozen sections is allowing them to get too dry before applying mountant. Sections should be just moist, with the excess water wiped from the slide.

Methods

Only details of the pre-staining, staining and post-staining steps are given. In each method sections should be washed prior to treatment and counterstained with haematoxylin before mounting in an aqueous medium.

■ (1) Chiffelle and Putt (1951)

Staining solution

Prepare a saturated solution of the dye by dissolving 1 g of Sudan IV, Sudan black or Fettrot in 100 ml of propylene glycol and heating to 100 °C for a few minutes. Filter while hot through Whatman No. 2 filter paper. Cool and refilter through a coarse sintered glass filter, or through glass wool using a vacuum pump.

Staining time	5–10 minutes
Pre-treatment	100% propylene glycol
Post-treatment	85% propylene glycol then 50% propylene glycol

■ (2) Lillie and Ashburn (1943)

Staining solution

A saturated solution of oil red O (0.25–0.5%) in isopropyl alcohol is kept in stock. For use dilute 6 ml of stock solution with 4 ml of distilled water, allow to stand for 5–10 minutes, then filter. This solution does not keep for more than 1–2 hours.

Staining time	10–15 minutes
Pre- and post-treatment	60% isopropyl alcohol

■ (3) Rinehart and Abu'l Haj (1951)

Staining solution

Sudan III, IV or black B saturated in absolute ethanol diluted 6 to 4 with distilled water for use.

Staining time	5 minutes
Pre- and post-treatment	50% ethanol

■ **(4) Herxheimer (1903); Lison and Dagnelie (1935)**

Staining solution

Sudan III, IV or black B saturated in equal parts acetone and 70% ethanol.

Staining time	5–10 minutes
Pre- and post-treatment	70% ethanol

■ **(5) Casselman (1959)**

Staining solution

Add 1 g oil red O to 100 ml of 60% aqueous tri-ethyl phosphate. Heat the mixture 56 °C for 2–3 hours. Filter the hot mixture and cool. Filter before using.

Staining time	10–15 minutes
Pre- and post-treatment	60% tri-ethyl phosphate

■ **(6) Govan (1944)**

Staining solution

Gelatin dye suspension

Add, drop by drop, a saturated solution of Sudan III or IV in acetone to 1% gelatin in distilled water containing 1% acetic acid. The stain solution is added, with constant stirring, until the gelatin becomes a bright red, milky fluid. The acetone is evaporated from the suspension in the 37 °C incubator for 2–3 hours. Filter through coarse filter paper.

Staining time	30 minutes
Pre- and post-treatment	1% gelatin for 2–3 minutes

■ **(7) Bayliss and Adams (1972)**

Staining solution

Saturated Sudan black B in 70% ethanol filtered before use.

Staining time	15 minutes
Pre-treatment	2.5% aqueous bromine 30 minutes
	Wash in water
	0.5% sodium metabisulphite 1 minute
	Wash in water
	Rinse in 70% alcohol
Post-treatment	70% alcohol

Other staining or histochemical methods

■ **Cain's Nile blue sulphate method**

The Nile blue method, which is usually described as a technique for differentiating neutral fat and fatty acids, is based on the fact that Nile blue sulphate normally contains a red oxazone (Nile red). The Nile blue is said to combine with fatty acids, and the oxazone (Nile red) to be more soluble in neutral fat than in the staining solution.

It is generally agreed that this method is not specific for fatty acids, but may be used to demonstrate acidic lipids if employed at a temperature above their melting points. Palmitic acid melts at 63 °C, stearic acid at 70 °C and oleic acid at 14 °C; the temperature suggested for this method by Cain (1947) is 60 °C, although 70 °C may be necessary to demonstrate stearic acid. While oleic acid (if liquid) will stain with concentrated solution, other fatty acids (if liquid) stain better with dilute solutions (*see* Note *below*).

Reagent

The staining solution—1% aqueous Nile blue sulphate—should be tested for the presence of oxazone (Nile red), by shaking a little of it with a small amount of xylene. The xylene, after 20–30 seconds, should be a definite red. A poor oxazone content may be improved by boiling 1% Nile blue sulphate in 5% sulphuric acid in a reflux condenser for 1–2 hours.

Method

(1) Fix tissue in Baker's formal–calcium fixative.
(2) Cut three frozen sections of 8–10 μm thickness.
(3) Stain one section (a) in saturated Sudan black B in 70% alcohol (or in isopropyl alcohol) as a control.
(4) Stain the other two sections (b) and (c) in Nile blue solution at 60–70 °C for 5–10 minutes.
(5) Wash all sections in warm water (60 °C).
(6) Differentiate in 1% acetic acid at 60 °C for 30 seconds.
(7) Re-stain section (c) in 0.02% Nile blue at 60 °C for 10–15 minutes.
(8) Wash in water.
(9) Mount in glycerin jelly.

Results

Neutral lipids	Red
Lecithin (and possibly kephalin and sphingomyelin) oleic acid	Blue
Nuclei	Blue
Cytoplasm and other tissue elements	Pale blue

Note

By comparison with the Sudan-black-stained section, differentiation of lipids and acidic lipids is possible (*see also* extraction methods on page 260). Compare sections (b) and (c) and if they are similar, discard (b). It is most likely that if a substance is equally well stained in (b) and (c) it is oleic acid. If sections (b) and (c) are dissimilar the deeper stained elements in section (c) are probably palmitic or stearic acid compounds.

■ Lillie's sulphuric Nile blue technique for fatty acids

This method is based upon the use of Nile blue sulphate at a very low pH (about 0.9). At such a pH carboxylic and phosphoric acid radicals should not be ionized, they should therefore be unable to bind the dye; the fatty acids, however, do bind the dye (Lillie, 1965).

Reagent

Acid Nile blue sulphate

Nile blue sulphate	0.05 g
Distilled water	99 ml
Conc. sulphuric acid	1 ml

Method

(1) Bring frozen, cryostat or paraffin sections to water.
(2) Stain in acid Nile blue sulphate for 20 minutes (for the reasons given above it is best to stain at 70 °C).
(3) Wash in running water for 10 minutes.
(4) Mount in Apathy's or glycerin jelly.

Results

Fatty acids	Dark blue
Neutral fats	Pink to red

Note

Dunnigan (1968) adds 10 ml of 1% sulphuric acid to 200 ml of 1% Nile blue sulphate, and boils it for 4 hours in a reflux condenser to generate more oxazone. He also extracts parallel sections with acetone at room temperature for 1 hour to remove hydrophobic lipids. He further notes that phospholipids give a more intense blue stain than free fatty acids.

■ Luxol fast blue methods for phospholipids

Luxol fast blue G has been recommended for phospholipids (Salthouse, 1965) as well as for myelin, collagen and elastin. Salthouse notes that the dye solvent employed is of prime importance since the tissue component–dye complex may be soluble. He showed that ethanol or isopropanol solutions of luxol fast blue G will stain phospholipids, but that metholic solutions stain collagen and elastin but not myelin or phospholipids.

■ Baker's acid haematein method for phospholipids (1946)

Baker's acid haematein method (used in conjunction with the pyridine extraction test) is superior to, and is given in place of, the Smith–Dietrich technique.

Reagents

(1) Formal–calcium fixative
(2) Dichromate calcium

Potassium dichromate	5 g
Calcium chloride	1 g
Distilled water	100 ml

(3) Acid haematein—to 0.05 g of haematoxylin in 49 ml of distilled water, add exactly 1 ml of 1% sodium iodate. Heat in a flask until boiling. Cool and add 1 ml of glacial acetic acid. This solution does not keep and can be used only on the day it is prepared.

(4) Borax ferricyanide differentiator

Potassium ferricyanide	0.25 g
Borax (sodium tetraborate 10 H_2O)	0.25 g
Distilled water	to 100 ml

This solution should be kept in the dark.

Method

(1) Fix small pieces of tissue in formal–calcium for 6–8 hours.
(2) Transfer to dichromate–calcium solution for 18 hours at room temperature.
(3) Transfer to dichromate–calcium solution for 24 hours at 60 °C.
(4) Wash well in distilled water and cut frozen sections at 8–10 μm.
(5) Mordant sections in dichromate–calcium solution for 1 hour at 60 °C.
(6) Wash in distilled water.
(7) Stain in acid haematein for 5 hours at 37 °C.
(8) Rinse in distilled water.
(9) Differentiate in borax ferricyanide for 18 hours at 37 °C.
(10) Wash in water.
(11) Mount in glycerin jelly, or for routine work, dehydrate, clear and mount in resinous mountant.

Results

Phospholipids: lecithin, kephalin and sphingomyelin (myelin sheaths) and nucleoprotein	Dark blue to black
Cerebrosides (in brain)	Pale blue to blue-black
Mucin, fibrinogen	Dark blue

■ Controlled chromatin procedure for phospholipids (Elftman, 1954)

This is a simplified form of Baker's acid haematein method. Elftman controlled the pH of the dichromate fixative and shortened the time of exposure of the tissue; he also omitted the iodate and added dichromate to the haematoxylin solution to prevent background staining of the tissue thus obviating the use of the borax–ferricyanide differentiation. The embedded tissues tend to be brittle and thicker sections may need to be used; *alternatively*, thin (2–3 μm) cryostat sections of fresh tissue may be mounted directly on to slides, and fixed and stained by this method. It is thought that the haematoxylin binds to the lipid chromous hydroxides.

Reagents

Buffered dichromate fixative

2.5% potassium dichromate adjusted to pH 3.5 with 0.2 M acetate buffer.

Buffered haematoxylin solution

0.2 M Acetate buffer pH 3.0
Potassium ferricyanide   0.25 g
Haematoxylin   50 mg

Method

(1) Fix fresh tissue (or cryostat sections of fresh tissue) in buffered dichromate at 56 °C for 18 hours.
(2) Wash tissues in running water (or syphon washer) for 4–6 hours (cryostat sections proceed directly to step 5).
(3) Dehydrate, clear and embed in paraffin wax.
(4) Section, and bring sections to water.
(5) Stain in buffered haematoxylin solution (preheated to 56 °C) at 56 °C for 2 hours.
(6) Rinse in distilled water, dehydrate, clear and mount in synthetic resin.

Results

Phospholipids dark blue. Staining a parallel section in oil red O will indicate that the structure stained is lipid in nature, or Baker's pyridine extraction test may be used.

■ **Osmium tetroxide—α-naphthylamine (OTAN) reaction for phospholipids (Adams, 1959)**

This method is useful for differentiating hydrophilic lipids (sphingomyelins, cerebrosides, gangliosides and so on) from hydrophobic triglyceride esters, cholesterol esters and fatty acids. It is based on the reaction of osmium tetroxide with the non-polar ethylene bonds of phospholipids and the subsequent chelation with α-naphthylamine to give an orange-red colour.

Reagents

Osmium tetroxide solution

1% osmium tetroxide   1 part
1% potassium chlorate ($KClO_3$)   3 parts

Saturated α-naphthylamine solution

Heat distilled water to 40 °C, and add α-naphthylamine to make a saturated solution, and filter. Since carcinogenic β-naphthylamine may be a contaminant it should be handled with care. The solution is used at 37 °C.

Method

(1) Cut frozen or cryostat sections of formal–calcium fixed tissue at 5–15 μm (depending upon the type of investigation or demonstration).
(2) Place free floating sections in osmium tetroxide solution for 18 hours. The container should be filled and stoppered tightly to prevent volatilization of osmium tetroxide.
(3) Wash sections in distilled water for 10 minutes and mount on slides.

(4) Treat with saturated α-naphthylamine solution at 37 °C for 15–20 minutes.
(5) Wash in distilled water for 5 minutes.
(6) Counterstain the sections with 2% Alcian blue in 5% acetic acid for 15–60 seconds (optional).
(7) Mount in an aqueous mountant such as glycerin jelly.

Results

Phospholipids   Orange-red
Cholesterol and triglyceride esters   Black

Note 1: Normal myelin will stain orange-red with degenerate myelin being black.
Note 2: Black staining hydrophobic lipids which may mask the orange-red phospholipid staining may be avoided by preliminary extraction of control sections with chilled acetones.

■ NaOH–OTAN technique for sphingomyelin (Adams, 1965)

If the OTAN method (above) is preceded by treatment with NaOH only alkali-resistant lipids are stained. The most important of these is sphingomyelin and this method may be used with some degree of specificity for its demonstration.

Method

As for the OTAN method above except that sections are pretreated in 2 N sodium hydroxide at 37 °C for 1 hour. They are then washed gently in water, rinsed in 1% acetic acid for 1 minute and again rinsed in water. Then transfer to osmium tetroxide solution (steps 2–7 above).

Result

The black staining of hydrophobic lipids can be avoided by acetone treatment (as above).

■ McManus's Sudan black B method for compound lipids in paraffin sections (1946)

A positive result with this method indicates that the substance demonstrated is a compound lipid. A negative result, however, has little significance since some compound lipids are not blackened. Myelin and mitochondria may be demonstrated using this technique. The method is based on the ability of calcium and formalin to render these lipids insoluble in acetone and the reagents used in paraffin processing. They may then be stained with Sudan black B whereas neither osmium tetroxide nor Sudan III gives a positive result.

Method

(1) Fix tissues for 2–4 weeks in Baker's formal–calcium fixative to which 1% cobalt nitrate or sulphate has been added. The precipitate which forms when the sulphate is used is covered with cotton wool, and the specimen laid upon the latter.
(2) Post-chrome for 24–48 hours in 3% potassium dichromate. Wash in running water overnight. (This stage is optional, but gives an improved result.)

(3) Process through paraffin keeping the length of time in alcohol, xylene and molten wax to a minimum. If fixation has been for less than 2 weeks. McManus recommends dehydration in three changes of acetone, each of 30 minutes; place directly into molten paraffin wax, change two or three times within 1 hour, and embed. Cut sections 4–6 μm in thickness and attach to slides.
(4) Bring sections to 70% alcohol.
(5) Stain for 30 minutes in saturated Sudan black B in 70% alcohol (sections of routine formal–saline fixed tissues should be stained for 30 minutes to 3 hours at 60 °C).
(6) Differentiate in 70% alcohol.
(7) Counterstain in carmalum (2% carmine in 5% ammonia alum) for 3 minutes.
(8) Wash in water, and mount in glycerin jelly.

Results

Compound lipids   Blue-black (*see above*)
Nuclei   Red

■ PAS methods for glycolipids

The hexose molecule of glycolipids may be demonstrated by the PAS technique but the reaction demonstrates other components. Adams and Bayliss (1963) introduced a series of blockades to increase the specificity of the reaction. The steps are as follows:

(1) Deamination in 10% aqueous chloramine T.
(2) Performic acid treatment to oxidize unsaturated bonds producing aldehydes which are then blocked with dinitrophenylhydrazine.
(3) A PAS reaction is then performed.
(4) A chloroform–methanol extracted section is used as a control.

Metachromatic methods for sulphatides

Cerebroside sulphate can be demonstrated by means of its brown metachromasia after cresyl fast violet (Hirsch and Peiffer, 1955), or toluidine blue (Bodian and Lake, 1963).

■ Cresyl fast violet–acetic acid method for sulphatides

(1) Stain frozen sections in 0.02% cresyl fast violet in 1% acetic acid for 5 minutes.
(2) Wash in water.
(3) Mount in glycerin jelly.

Results

Deposits of sulphatide in metachromatic leucodystrophy are stained metachromatically brown. Normal myelin and other tissues are stained orthochromatically lilac to violet.

Note

Sensitivity of this technique is improved by viewing the brown deposits by polarized light with a polarizer and analyser crossed. A specific lime green to yellow-green dichroism is seen.

■ **Fluorescence method for sulphatides (Hollander, 1963)**

(1) Stain frozen sections in 1 : 20 000 acriflavine in 0.1 M citrate–HCl buffer at pH 2.5 for
    6 minutes.
(2) Differentiate in 70% isopropanol for 1 minute.
(3) Dehydrate in increasing strengths of isopropanol.
(4) Clear in xylene and mount.

Results

Sulphatides gold-yellow on a greenish background with ultraviolet excitation.

Note

One minute's treatment with p-dimethyl aminobenzaldehyde solution (*see below*) after
step 2, followed by Mayer's haemalum, then step 3, allows examination by light
microscopy when sulphatides are reddish/yellow.

DMAB reagent

2% p-dimethyl aminobenzaldehyde in 20% HCl (5.5 N)   15 ml
Isopropyl alcohol   35 ml

■ **Fischler's method for fatty acids (1904)**

It is generally agreed that there is no specific histochemical method for the
demonstration of fatty acids. However, Fischler's method is known to demonstrate
fatty acids when present in large amounts.
   The method is based on the fact that fatty acids form calcium soaps if fixed in formal–
calcium. After mordanting with copper acetate, a lake is formed between the soaps and
the haematoxylin, which is very resistant to borax ferricyanide differentiator.

Reagents

(1) Weigert's lithium haematoxylin

   Solution A: 10% haematoxylin in absolute alcohol.
   Solution B: Saturated lithium carbonate   10 ml
               Distilled water   90 ml

   Mix equal parts of A and B just before use.

(2) Weigert's borax ferricyanide differentiator

   Borax   20 g
   Potassium ferricyanide   25 g
   Distilled water   to 1000 ml

Method

(1) Fix tissue in 10% formalin, which has been saturated with calcium salicylate
    (1.3–1.5%).

(2) Cut frozen sections 8–10 μm in thickness.
(3) Mordant sections in a saturated aqueous solution of copper acetate for 12–24 hours at 37 °C.
(4) Wash in distilled water.
(5) Stain in lithium haematoxylin for 20 minutes.
(6) Differentiate in borax ferricyanide (this may be diluted to give greater control) until red blood cells are very pale blue or colourless.
(7) Wash in distilled water. Counterstain, if desired, to show neutral lipid red.
(8) Mount in glycerin jelly.

The method may be controlled by extracting sections in alcohol–ether mixture for 24 hours before mordanting (stage 3); this will dissolve fatty acids, but not preformed calcium soaps.

Results

Fatty acids	Dark blue
Neutral lipid (if counterstained)	Red

■ Holczinger's method for fatty acids (1959)

Method

(1) Frozen sections of formal–calcium fixed material or post-fixed cryostat sections are dried on slides.
(2) Treat with N/1 HCl for 1 hour.
(3) Wash in distilled water and dry.
(4) Treat with 0.005% cupric acetate for 3 hours.
(5) Rinse in two changes of 0.1% ethylene diamine tetra-acetic acid (pH 7) for 10 seconds.
(6) Wash in distilled water.
(7) Treat with 0.1% rubeanic acid in 70% ethanol for 10 minutes.
(8) Rinse in 70% ethanol.
(9) Counterstain with carmalum.
(10) Wash and mount in glycerin jelly.

Results

Fatty acids   Dark green

Note

A control section should be extracted with acetone for 20 minutes at 4 °C.

■ Perchloric acid–naphthoquinone (PAN) method for cholesterol and cholesterol esters (Adams, 1961)

This method is based on the formation of cholesta-3,5-diene by the action of perchloric acid which subsequently reacts with naphthoquinone to give a dark blue-grey product. Although the mechanism of the latter is not known, its specificity has been shown to be high for cholesterol and related steroids. Tryptophan may give a pink colour as may some mucosubstances. It is recommended as a method of choice.

PAN reagent

0.1% 1,2-naphthoquinone-4 sulphonic acid in ethanol	4 ml
Perchloric acid (60%)	2 ml
Formalin (40% formaldehyde)	0.2 ml
Water	1.8 ml

Method

(1) Cut frozen or cryostat sections, leave in formal–calcium fixative for 1 week or more to allow oxidation of cholesterol to occur.
(2) Mount sections on slides and allow to dry.
(3) Cover sections with minimum amount of PAN reagent.
(4) Heat slides on hot plate at 60–70 °C for 5–10 minutes (until original red colour changes to blue).
(5) Place a drop of 60% perchloric acid on section and apply a coverslip (water or glycerin jelly cannot be used).

Results

Cholesterol and cholesterol esters   Dark blue

■ **Schultz method (Romieu's modification, 1927) for cholesterol and cholesterol esters**

Method

(1) Mount frozen sections (10–15 μm in thickness) on slides.
(2) Put one or two drops of concentrated sulphuric acid on the sections, leave for 5–15 seconds.
(3) Put three or four drops of acetic anhydride on the sections to develop the colour.
(4) Drain sections, and wash with a few drops of acetic anhydride.
(5) Mount in acetic anhydride, and examine immediately. (Stages 3, 4 and 5 should be performed rapidly.)

Result

Cholesterol and cholesterol esters   Red-violet, changing to green

■ **Bismuth trichloride method of differentiating between cholesterol and cholesterol esters (Grundland, Bulliard and Maillet, 1949)**

Reagent

Bismuth trichloride	0.2 g
Acetyl chloride	1.0 ml
Nitrobenzene (anhydrous)	to 100 ml

Method

(1) Fix the tissue (not more than 2–3 mm in thickness) in a saturated solution of digitonin in 70% alcohol for 36 hours.

(2) Press tissue gently between layers of filter paper to remove excess alcohol, and allow the remainder to evaporate in a 56 °C oven for 5–10 minutes.
(3) Infiltrate with paraffin wax, with 5% glycerol monostearate added, for 12–16 hours.
(4) Embed in paraffin wax.
(5) Cut sections 6–10 μm in thickness, and mount on slides.
(6) Without removing the wax, treat the sections with bismuth trichloride reagent for 15–45 minutes.
(7) Rinse rapidly in 10% acetyl chloride in nitrobenzene (anhydrous).
(8) Wash in 75% nitric acid (concentrated) in absolute alcohol.
(9) Rinse rapidly in absolute alcohol.
(10) Treat with 20% ammonium sulphide (yellow) for a few seconds.
(11) Wash in absolute alcohol.
(12) Clear in xylene, and mount in Canada balsam.

Results

Cholesterol   Dark brown
Cholesterol esters   Uncoloured

- **Pearse's peracetic or performic acid–Schiff method for phospholipids and cerebrosides (lipids containing unsaturated bonds) (1951)**

Fixation

Formal–saline or Zenker–formal should be employed.

Reagents

(1) Performic acid—to 40 ml of 98% formic acid, add 4 ml of 100 vol. (30%) hydrogen peroxide. Allow to stand for $1\frac{1}{2}$ hours before use. Fresh reagent must be made daily.
(2) Peracetic acid—peracetic acid (40%) is available commercially.
(3) Schiff reagent.

Method

(1) Bring paraffin or frozen sections to water. Remove mercury precipitate if present.
(2) Blot dry.
(3) Oxidize with performic or peracetic acid for 2–5 minutes.
(4) Immerse in Schiff reagent for 30 minutes.
(5) Wash in warm running water for 10 minutes.
(6) Mount in glycerin jelly.

Result

Lipids with unsaturated bonds (phospholipid or cerebroside)   Red

- **Bromine–silver method for unsaturated lipids (Norton, Korey and Brotz, 1962)**

This method is based on the bromination of unsaturated lipids, which is the combination of bromine at the site of double bonds. This is then reacted with silver to give a silver bromide and finally metallic silver. According to Adams (1965) this method has the advantage that it does not stain proteins; however, it also fails to react with double bonds of hydrophobic lipids (phospholipids and glycosphingosides) so that a negative result does not exclude them.

Method

(1) Cut frozen or cryostat sections of formal–calcium fixed tissue, mount on slides, dry in air.
(2) Treat with bromine–potassium bromide solution (1 ml of bromine in 390 ml of 2% potassium bromide) for 1 minute.
(3) Wash in water.
(4) Treat with 1% sodium bisulphite for 5 minutes.
(5) Rinse in several changes of distilled water.
(6) Treat with 1% silver nitrate in 1 N nitric acid for 18 hours.
(7) Rinse in several changes of distilled water.
(8) Reduce for 10 minutes in Kodak Dektol developer (diluted equal parts with water).
(9) Wash well and mount in an aqueous mountant such as glycerin jelly.

Results

Unsaturated lipids (*see above*)   Brown to black

■ Bromine/PAS method

Steps (2) and (3) above followed by the PAS method will obviate PAS staining of unsaturated lipids.

■ Plasmal reaction (Hayes, 1949)

Formal fixation should be avoided to reduce the possibility of pseudoplasmal reactions. The unsaturated ether bonds are hydrolysed by mercuric chloride, producing aldehyde which is demonstrated by Schiff reagent. A control section must be examined, for which the mercuric chloride step has been omitted. This will detect a pseudoplasmal reaction.

Method

(1) Frozen sections, or smears, are washed in distilled water.
(2) Transfer sections to 1% aqueous mercuric chloride for 5–10 minutes.
(3) Transfer to Schiff reagent for 5–15 minutes.
(4) Bring sections through three sulphite rinses (*see* page 220).
(5) Wash in water and mount in glycerin jelly, or float on slide, dehydrate, clear and mount in synthetic resin.

Results

Acetal lipids   Red-purple

Fluorescent methods for lipids

Fluorescent methods for lipids are much more sensitive than conventional methods, and therefore require some experience in interpretation. Popper (1944) described a method using phosphine 3R which, while not as sensitive as the 3:4 benzpyrene method, has some degree of permanency. The benzpyrene method is recommended for the demonstration of the finest lipid granules, but it must be remembered that the fluorescence fades rapidly.

■ **Phosphine 3R method (Popper, 1944)**

(1) Formalin fixation is preferred.
(2) Cut frozen or cryostat sections.
(3) Wash sections or smears in distilled water.
(4) Stain in 0.1% aqueous phosphine 3R for 3 minutes.
(5) Rinse quickly in water.
(6) Mount in 90% glycerin.

Results

All lipids, with the exception of fatty acids, soaps and cholesterol, give a silvery-white fluorescence. See benzpyrene method for recommended filter system.

■ **Benzpyrene method (Berg, 1951)**

Staining solution

Prepare a saturated aqueous solution of caffeine (about 1.5%) at room temperature and leave overnight. Filter, and add 0.002 g 3:4 benzpyrene to 100 ml of filtrate. Incubate at 37 °C for 2 days, filter and add an equal volume of distilled water.

Method

(1) Formalin fixation is preferred.
(2) Cut frozen or cryostat sections.
(3) Rinse sections or smears in distilled water.
(4) Filter staining solution on to smears or sections and leave for 20 minutes.
(5) Rinse in distilled water.
(6) Mount in distilled water and examine.

Results

Lipids, even the finest granules, give a brilliant blue-white fluorescence which fades rapidly.

Examine using a UG 1 or UG 2 (BG 12 if not available) exciter filter and a colourless ultraviolet barrier filter.

References

ADAMS, C. W. M. (1959). A histochemical method for the simultaneous demonstration of normal and degenerating myelin. *J. Pathol. Bacteriol.*, 77, 648–650

ADAMS, C. W. M. (1961). A perchloric acid–naphthoquinone method for the histochemical localisation of cholesterol. *Nature*, **192**, 331–332

ADAMS, C. W. M. (1965). In *Neurohistochemistry*. Elsevier, Amsterdam

ADAMS, C. W. M. and BAYLISS, O. B. (1963). Histochemical observations on the localisation and origin of sphingomyelin, cerebroside and cholesterol in the normal and atherosclerotic human artery. *J. Pathol. Bacteriol.*, **85**, 113–119

BAKER, J. R. (1946). The histochemical recognition of lipine. *Quart. J. Micr. Sci.*, **87**, 441–470

BAYLISS, O. B. and ADAMS, C. W. M. (1972). Bromine Sudan black: a general stain for lipids including free cholesterol. *Histochem. J.*, **4**, 505–515

BAYLISS HIGH, O. B. (1981). The histochemical versatility of Sudan black B. *Acta Histochem. (Jena) Suppl.*, **24**, 247–255

BERG, N. O. (1951). Histological study of masked lipids; stainability, distribution and functional variations. *Acta Pathol. Microbiol. Scand. Suppl.*, **90**, 1–192

BODIAN, M. and LAKE, B. D. (1962–63). The rectal approach to neuropathology. *Br. J. Surg.*, **50**, 702–714

CAIN, A. J. (1947). Use of Nile blue in the examination of lipoids. *Quart. J. Micr. Sci.*, **88**, 383–392

CASSELMAN, W. G. B. (1959). In *Histochemical Technique*. Methuen, London

CHIFFELLE, T. L. and PUTT, F. A. (1951). Propylene and ethylene glycol as solvents for Sudan IV and Sudan black B. *Stain Technol.*, **26**, 51–56

DADDI, L. (1896). Nouvelle méthode pour colorer la graisse dans les tissues. *Arch. Ital. Biol.*, **26**, 143–146

DUNNIGAN, M. C. (1968). The use of Nile blue sulphate in the histochemical identification of phospholipids. *Stain Technol.*, **43**, 249–256

ELFTMAN, H. (1954). Controlled chromation. *J. Histochem. Cytochem.*, **2**, 1–8

FISCHLER, F. (1904). Über die Unterscheidungen von Neutralfetten, Fettsäuren und Seisen in Gewebe. *Zentbl. Allg. Path. u. Pathol. Anat.*, **15**, 913–917

GOMORI, G. (1952). In *Microscopic Histochemistry*. Chicago University Press, Chicago

GOVAN, A. D. T. (1944). Fat staining by Sudan dyes suspended in watery media. *J. Pathol. Bacteriol.*, **56**, 262–264

GRUNDLAND, I., BULLIARD, H. and MAILLET, M. (1949). Détection histochimique du cholestérol par emploi du trichlorure de bismuth en solution dans nitrobenzène anhydre. *C. R. Soc. Biol. Paris*, **143**, 771–773

HAYES, E. R. (1949). A rigorous re-definition of the plasmal reaction. *Stain Technol.*, **24**, 19–23

HERXHEIMER, G. W. (1903). Zur Fettfärbung. *Zentbl. Allg. Path. u. Pathol. Anat.*, **14**, 841–842

HOLCZINGER, L. (1959). Histochemical demonstration of free fatty acids. *Acta Histochem. (Jena)*, **8**, 167–175

HOLLANDER, H. (1963). A staining method for cerebroside–sulphuric-esters in brain tissue. *J. Histochem. Cytochem.*, **11**, 118–119

KFILIG, I (1944). Über Spezifizitätsbreite und Grundlagen der Markscheidenfärbungen. *Virchows Arch. Pathol. Anat.*, **312**, 405–420

LANSINK, A. G. W. (1968). Thin layer chromatography and histochemistry of Sudan black B. *Histochemie*, **16**, 68–84

LILLIE, R. D. (1954). In *Histopathologic Technique and Practical Histochemistry*. 2nd Ed. Blakiston, New York

LILLIE, R. D. (1965). In *Histopathologic Technique and Practical Histochemistry*. 3rd Ed. Blakiston, New York

LILLIE, R. D. and ASHBURN, L. L. (1943). Supersaturated solutions of fat stains in dilute isopropanol for demonstration of acute fatty degenerations not shown by Herxheimer's technique. *Arch. Pathol.*, **36**, 432–435

LISON, L. (1936). In *Histochemie Animale*. Gauthier-Villard, Paris

LISON, L. and DAGNELIE, J. (1935). Méthodes nouvelles de coloration de la myéline. *Bull. Histol. Appl. Physiol. Pathol.*, **12**, 85–91

McMANUS, J. F. A. (1946). The demonstration of certain fatty substances in paraffin sections. *J. Pathol. Bacteriol.*, **58**, 93–95

NORTON, W. T., KOREY, S. R. and BROTZ, M. (1962). Histochemical demonstration of unsaturated lipids by a bromine–silver method. *J. Histochem. Cytochem.*, **10**, 83–88

PEARSE, A. G. E. (1951). A review of modern methods in histochemistry. *J. Clin. Pathol.*, **4**, 1–36

POPPER, H. (1944). Distribution of vitamin A in tissue as visualised by fluorescence microscopy. *Physiol. Rev.*, **24**, 205–224

RINEHART, J. F. and ABU'L HAJ, S. (1951). Histological demonstration of lipids in tissue after dehydration and embedding in a polyethylene glycol. *Arch. Pathol.*, **51**, 666–669

ROMIEU, M. (1927). Méthode de détection histochimique des lécithines. *C. R. Soc. Biol. Paris*, **96**, 1232–1234

SALTHOUSE, T. N. (1965). Selective staining of collagen and elastin by luxol fast blue G in methanol: A histochemical study. *J. Histochem. Cytochem.*, **13**, 133–140

VON HIRSCH, T. and PEIFFER, H. (1955). Über histologische Methoden in der Differentialdiagnose von Leukodystrophien und Lipoidosen. *Arch. Psychiat.*, **194**, 88–104

ZUGIBE, F. T. (1970). *Diagnostic Histochemistry*. C. V. Mosby, St Louis

14

Endogenous pigments

The pigments encountered in tissues in both normal and pathological conditions may be classified under the following headings:

(1) endogenous;
(2) exogenous;
(3) artefact.

The exogenous and artefact pigments are discussed in Chapter 15.

The endogenous pigments can be classified according to their derivation namely, haem, tyrosine and lipid pigments.

Haem pigments

Haem or haematogenous pigments are derived from haemoglobin.

Haemoglobin

Haemoglobin in red blood cells is stained by acid dyes such as eosin. It is well demonstrated in sections by one of the peroxidase techniques or by the patent blue method (page 324). We recommend the amido black method given below. Haemoglobin occurs pathologically (e.g. in renal casts) as droplets or granules of a yellow-brown colour. Distinction between the various types of haemoglobin (e.g. methaemoglobin) is only possible spectroscopically.

■ **Amido black method (Puchtler and Sweat, 1962)**

Reagent

Amido black. Saturate methanol/acetic acid mixture (9 parts/1 part) with amido black 10 B (naphthalene black 10 B).

Method

(1) Bring sections to water. (Zenker–formal fixation or mordanted sections are preferred.)
(2) Remove mercury deposit with iodine and hypo sequence.
(3) Treat with 5% aqueous tannic acid for 5 minutes.

(4) Wash well in distilled water.
(5) Treat with 1% aqueous phosphomolybdic acid for 10 minutes.
(6) Wash well in distilled water, drain and blot dry.
(7) Treat with amido black solution for 5 minutes.
(8) Rinse in methanol/acetic acid (9 parts/1 part).
(9) Rinse in water.
(10) Counterstain in neutral red.
(11) Wash, dehydrate, clear and mount in synthetic resin.

Results

Haemoglobin   Black

Haemosiderin

Haemosiderin is a breakdown product of haemoglobin and is thought to be composed of ferric iron and protein. It occurs in pathological conditions as yellow-brown granules.

The iron-containing pigments are soluble in acids, and insoluble in alkalis and fat solvents; they are demonstrated by Perls Prussian blue reaction. Tissues which are to be examined for iron-containing pigments must be fixed in non-metallic containers, and iron-free distilled water used for the reaction to avoid contamination. Acid fixatives may remove the iron or render it inactive (aposiderin).

Fixation

Although alcohol fixation was specified originally, buffered formal–saline gives equally good results, with improved preservation of tissue elements.

■ **Perls' Prussian blue reaction for ferric salts (Perls, 1867)**

Method

(1) Bring frozen, paraffin or celloidin sections to distilled water.
(2) Transfer to a fresh solution of equal parts of 2% aqueous potassium ferrocyanide and 2% hydrochloric acid, for 30 minutes. With a doubtful result, the reaction may be carried out at 60 °C, but this is not usually necessary.
(3) Wash thoroughly in several changes of distilled water.
(4) Counterstain lightly with 1% neutral red or safranin for 10–15 seconds.
(5) Wash in water, dehydrate, clear and mount in non-reducing synthetic resin.

Results

Ferric-iron-containing pigments (haemosiderin)   Blue
Nuclei   Red

■ **Tirmann–Schmelzer's Turnbull blue reaction for ferrous salts (Schmelzer, 1933)**

Method

(1) Bring sections to water.
(2) Treat with a dilute solution of yellow ammonium sulphide for 1–3 hours.

(3) Rinse in distilled water.
(4) Treat with a freshly prepared solution of equal parts of 20% potassium ferricyanide and 1% hydrochloric acid for 15 minutes.
(5) Wash thoroughly in several changes of distilled water.
(6) Counterstain nuclei lightly with 1% neutral red or safranin for 10–15 seconds.
(7) Wash in water, dehydrate, clear and mount.

Results

Ferrous salts and ferric salts converted by treatment
   with ammonium sulphide   Deep blue
Nuclei   Red

Note: If stage 2 is carried out ferric salts are converted to ferrous salts and are therefore demonstrated; to differentiate between the two, parallel sections are taken and stage 2 omitted in the treatment of one of them.

Haemozoin (malaria pigment)

This pigment is found in the parasites, and in brain capillaries, liver, spleen, bone marrow and lymph nodes in malaria. It is similar to formalin pigment in every respect except that it does not occur throughout the whole of the sections and is found intracellularly in phagocytes.

Haematoidin (bile pigment)

Haematoidin occurs as yellowish granules or masses. It is found in old haemorrhages, particularly in infarcts of the spleen or brain.

Of the methods of demonstration available, Gmelin's and Glenner's probably give the most consistent results, although Fouchet's reagent gives a much longer lasting reaction.

■ Fouchet's reaction for bile pigment (1917)

Fouchet's reagent

Dissolve 25 g of trichloroacetic acid in 100 ml of distilled water. Dissolve 1 g ferric chloride in 10 ml of distilled water and add to the trichloroacetic acid solution. Mix and store in a dark bottle.

Method

(1) Bring frozen or paraffin sections to water.
(2) Add three to four drops of Fouchet's reagent to sections, lower coverslip on to section and examine.

Result

Bile pigments are coloured green.

■ Glenner's method for bilirubin (1957)

This method is based on the oxidation of the pale yellow bilirubin pigment, by the potassium dichromate, to its oxidized form which is bright emerald green. The pH of the dichromate is critical since it must be low enough to ensure complete oxidation without being sufficiently acid to remove the pigment.

Reagent

3% Potassium dichromate	25 ml
N/10 hydrochloric acid	8 ml
N/10 potassium dihydrogen phosphate	17 ml

Mix and check to ensure that pH is 2.2.

Method

(1) Cut frozen or cryostat sections of fresh tissue, attach to slides.
(2) Treat with buffered dichromate in Coplin jar at room temperature for 15 minutes*.
(3) Wash in running water for 5 minutes.
(4) Fix in formal–calcium for 15 minutes.
(5) Wash in water and counterstain if desired.
(6) Mount in Apathy's or glycerin jelly.

Result

Bilirubin   Bright emerald green

■ Glenner's method for bilirubin, haemosiderin and lipofuscin (1957)

This method is a modification of the one above, with the Prussian blue and oil red O methods also being performed upon the section. It may prove useful in the identification of a yellow pigment.

Method

(1) Cut frozen or cryostat sections of fresh tissue and attach them to clean slides.
(2) Treat sections with 2% potassium dichromate for 5 minutes.
(3) Place sections in equal parts of 5% acetic acid and freshly prepared 2% potassium ferrocyanide for 20 minutes.
(4) Rinse in running water and treat with buffered dichromate solution (see above method) for 15 minutes.
(5) Rinse in water and rinse in 70% alcohol.
(6) Place in oil red O solution (see page 263) for 20 minutes.
(7) Rinse in 70% alcohol to remove excess stain.
(8) Wash in running water.
(9) Mount in Apathy's medium or glycerin jelly.

* An unoxidized control section (omitting step 2) should be carried through to ensure that any green colour present has been produced by oxidation.

Results

Bilirubin	Green
Haemosiderin	Blue
Lipofuscin	Red

It should be remembered that (a) neutral lipids will stain red, and (b) lipofuscin may stain faintly or not at all.

■ **Gmelin's reaction for bilirubin and haematoidin (Tiedemann and Gmelin, 1826)**

Method

(1) Bring frozen or paraffin sections to water.
(2) Wipe excess water from around sections and mount (in water) with coverslip avoiding air-bubbles.
(3) Place section on microscope stage, and focus with a 16 mm objective on the pigment to be identified.
(4) Using a pipette, place a few drops of 50% nitric acid at one end of the coverslip. Apply a small piece of filter paper to the other end of the coverslip to draw the nitric acid over the section.
(5) Watch the unidentified pigment under the microscope for a change of colour.
(6) Discard section as the reaction lasts only for a few seconds.

Results

Bilirubin and haematoidin change colour from yellow to green, then through blue to purple and red.

■ **Stein's technique for bilirubin (1935)**

Method

(1) Bring sections to water.
(2) Treat with a mixture of three parts Lugol's iodine and one part tincture of iodine for 6–12 hours.
(3) Decolorize with a 5% aqueous solution of sodium sulphite for 15–30 seconds.
(4) Counterstain nuclei in alum carmine for 1–3 hours (or in 1% neutral red for 5 minutes).
(5) Wash in distilled water.
(6) Dehydrate in acetone, clear in xylene and mount in Canada balsam.

Results

Bilirubin	Green
Nuclei	Red

Tyrosine pigments

Melanin

Melanin occurs normally as yellow-brown to black granules in hair, skin, eye and substantia nigra. It may be found pathologically in some skin diseases (in phagocytic cells), in benign naevi and in malignant melanomas and their metastases.

Melanin is formed from tyrosine by the enzyme action of tyrosinase producing dihydroxyphenylalanine which is further acted on to produce melanin. Tyrosine rich polypeptides are synthesized in the endoplasmic reticulum and are transferred into vesicles, the premelanosomes, where tyrosinase is incorporated. As melanin is synthesized it accumulates in granules, the melanosomes. It is thought that a single enzyme or enzyme complex is responsible for both stages in the synthesis and this enzyme is often referred to as DOPA-oxidase as well as tyrosinase.

The pigment may be demonstrated by reducing methods, enzyme methods, fluorescent methods or by its bleaching characteristics.

Reducing methods

Melanins have the ability to reduce solutions of ammoniacal silver nitrate to metallic silver, the methods most commonly used being modifications of the argentaffin reaction of Masson–Fontana (*see* page 475).

Melanins are also blackened by acid silver nitrate at pH 4 in less than 1 hour (Lillie, 1965).

Schmorl's ferric ferricyanide reaction is positive (*see* page 286).

These reactions are not specific for melanin, other pigments may react (*see Table 14.1*).

Enzyme methods

The DOPA-oxidase reaction (page 324) demonstrates the tyrosinase which converts tyrosine into DOPA and subsequently to melanin. The reaction therefore demonstrates cells capable of synthesizing melanin and is useful in the demonstration of amelanotic melanomas.

Table 14.1

	Solubility	Bleach (h)	Perls	Gmelin	Schmorl	Sudan black B	Long ZN	PAS	Diazo	Autofluorescence
Haemoglobin	Alcohol–water (slightly)									
Haemosiderin	Mineral acids		+							
Haematoidin	Chloroform (slightly)			+						
Haemozoin	Alcoholic picric acid									
Melanin	Strong NaOH	24/48				+				
Enterochromaffin	Alcohol					+			+	
Adrenal chromaffin						+		+	+	
Ceroid						+	+	+		+
Lipofuscin	Chloroform (slightly)	48+				+	+v	+v	+v	+
Dubin–Johnson pigment						+	±	+v	±	+v
Pseudomelanin		6/12				+		+	±	+

Notes: (1) Weak reaction = ±. Variable reaction but most often positive = +v.
(2) Iron may be bound to lipofuscin giving positive reactions with both Perls and Schmorl.

Fluorescence methods

The formaldehyde induced fluorescence method of Eranko (1955) has been used to demonstrate melanin precursors. Rost and Polak (1969) recommended fluorescence microscopy on formalin fixed material, using BG12 exciter filter and Zeiss 51/44 yellow barrier filter. Melanin precursors give yellow fluorescence.

Bleaching methods

Melanins are bleached by strong oxidizing agents. Hydrogen peroxide, potassium permanganate, ferric chloride and hydrochloric acid/potassium chlorate may be used. The time required for bleaching varies according to the site and the degree of pigmentation. Treatment with 0.25% potassium permanganate for $\frac{1}{2}$–4 hours followed by 1% oxalic acid is recommended. Culling (1974) prefers treatment with 20 volume hydrogen peroxide or Mayer's technique.

■ **Mayer's technique**

Method

(1) Place thin layer of potassium chlorate at the bottom of a Coplin jar and fill with 70% alcohol.
(2) Place hydrated section in the jar.
(3) Add 1 ml of concentrated hydrochloric acid to the bottom of the jar.

The nascent chlorine produced will bleach melanin within a few hours.

Other reactions

Melanins are insoluble in tissue processing agents, alcohol fat solvents, etc., as well as dilute acids and alkalis. Melanin is said to be soluble in strong alkali (Pearse, 1972).

Melanin is basophilic, staining with acidic solutions of methylene blue, thionin and azure dyes.

Ferrous ion uptake can be visualized by subsequent treatment with acidified potassium ferricyanide (Lillie, 1965). This reaction should not be confused with the Schmorl reaction which relies on *reduction* of ferric iron.

Enterochromaffin

The granules found in the enterochromaffin cells of the intestine are often listed among the tyrosine pigments. Although these cells are discussed in Chapter 27 it is appropriate to describe their reactions with the methods used for pigment identification. They are positive with Schmorl's method and are argentaffin with the Masson–Fontana alkaline silver techniques. Of the many other techniques available the alkaline diazo method is widely used (*see* page 481).

These cells are the type cells of carcinoid tumours. The tumour cells are usually, but not always, positive, the reaction depending on the functional state of the tumour. The reactions are dependent on the presence of 5-hydroxytryptamine which must be converted to the β-carboline derivative before the reactions can be demonstrated (Holcenberg and Benditt, 1961).

Adrenal chromaffin

The dark brown granular material found in the cells of the adrenal medulla after chrome fixation is derived from adrenaline and noradrenaline (*see* Chapter 27). This reaction is known as the chromaffin reaction.

To demonstrate the chromaffin reaction fresh material should be fixed in Regaud's fluid and frozen or paraffin sections prepared. Preliminary treatment with formalin should be avoided since the subsequent demonstration of the chromaffin will almost certainly be prevented. Acidic solutions of chrome salts should also be avoided.

Staining of the sections with Giemsa will show a characteristic yellowish-green colouring of the chromaffin cells.

Potassium iodate treatment of fresh tissue will produce a brown pigment with noradrenaline within a few minutes, whilst adrenaline requires up to 24 hours' treatment to produce a brown coloration (Pearse, 1972).

Chromaffin granules are argentaffin, Schmorl positive and appear grey red with PAS.

The tumour derived from these cells is the phaeochromocytoma.

Lipid pigments

Lipid pigments are derived from lipid or lipoprotein precursors by progressive oxidation. As oxidation proceeds the lipid gradually loses its fatty characteristics and darkens in colour. The lipid pigments are a heterogenous group which may be considered under the following titles.

Ceroid

Ceroid occurs usually as yellow globules of various sizes and although originally described in the liver can be found in a wide variety of situations. It is accepted as a lipid pigment at an early stage of oxidation. The fat type reactions are positive whilst the reducing reactions are negative.

Lipofuscin

Lipofuscin is often referred to as 'brown atrophy pigment' or 'wear and tear pigment' and is found as yellow-brown or brown granules in heart muscle, liver, adrenal, testis and in neurons. Since lipofuscins are the result of progressive oxidation the staining results are not consistent. Some of the earlier lipofuscins may still give positive fat type reactions whilst most are positive with the reducing reactions.

Dubin–Johnson pigment

The pigment described by Dubin and Johnson (1954) is considered to be a lipofuscin. It is found centrolobularly in otherwise normal livers in a type of chronic idiopathic icterus (Barone, Inferrera and Carrozza, 1969). It is positive with the reducing reactions and gives variable results with the fat type reactions.

Lipochromes

These are lipids which contain coloured hydrocarbons in solution. The hydrocarbons are of the carotenoid series and are present in the adrenal cortex and in corpora lutea. They are soluble in alcohol and in clearing agents used in tissue processing and for this reason are rarely found in paraffin sections.

Pseudomelanosis pigment

This pigment may be found in the lamina propria of colon, usually in macrophages. It is present in large quantities in pseudomelanosis coli, a condition of unknown aetiology, and may have to be distinguished from the pigment found in intestinal lipofuscinosis. It gives negative results with the fat-type stains (Pearse, 1972).

Methods for lipid pigments

The principal methods used to demonstrate lipid pigments are the Sudan black B, long Ziehl–Neelsen, Masson–Fontana and Schmorl methods. The PAS reaction and the detection of autofluorescence may be of value. Differential staining results are shown in *Table 14.1*.

■ **Schmorl's reaction for lipofuscin (Lillie, 1965)**

Method

(1) Bring sections to water.
(2) Treat with a freshly prepared solution of 30 ml of 1% ferric chloride, 4 ml of freshly prepared 1% potassium ferricyanide and 6 ml of distilled water for 10 minutes.
(3) Wash in running water.
(4) Counterstain nuclei with 1% neutral red or safranin for 15–30 seconds.
(5) Wash in water, dehydrate, clear and mount in resinous mountant.

Results

Lipofuscin, melanin and argentaffin	Dark blue
Chromaffin cells (after dichromate fixation)	Greenish blue
Nuclei	Red

Note

Sections may be differentiated after stage 3 with 1% potassium hydroxide in 50% alcohol. Differentiation is stopped by rinsing in 70% alcohol and water. Stages 4 and 5 are then proceeded with. Sudan black B may be used to demonstrate this pigment (*see* page 269).

■ **The long Ziehl–Neelsen method**

Reagent

Carbol–fuchsin

Basic fuchsin	1 g
Phenol	0.5 g
Absolute ethanol	10 ml
Distilled water	100 ml

Method

(1) Bring sections to water.
(2) Stain in carbol–fuchsin at 60 °C for 3 hours.
(3) Wash in water.
(4) Differentiate in 1% acid alcohol until background is pale pink or colourless.
(5) Wash in water.
(6) Counterstain lightly or, preferably, not at all.
(7) Wash, dehydrate, clear and mount in synthetic resin.

Result

Lipofuscin   Red

References

BARONE, P., INFERRERA, C. and CARROZZA, G. (1969). In *Pigments in Pathology*. Ed. Wolman, M. Academic Press, London, pp. 307–325

CULLING, C. F. A. (1974). *Histopathological and Histochemical Techniques*. 3rd Ed. Butterworths, London

DUBIN, I. N. and JOHNSON, F. B. (1954). Chronic idiopathic jaundice with unidentified pigment in liver cells: New clinico-pathologic entity with report of 12 cases. *Medicine*, **33**, 155–197

ERANKO, O. (1955). Distribution of adrenaline and noradrenaline in the adrenal medulla. *Nature*, **175**, 88.

FOUCHET, A. (1917). Méthode nouvelle de recherche et de dosage des pigments biliaires dans le serum sanguin. *C. R. Soc. Biol.*, **80**, 826–828

GLENNER, G. G. (1957). Simultaneous demonstration of bilirubin, haemosiderin and lipofuscin pigments in tissue sections. *Am. J. Clin. Pathol.*, **27**, 1–5

HOLCENBERG, J. and BENDITT, E. P. (1961). A new colour reaction for tryptamine derivatives. Histochemical application to enterochromaffin cells. *Lab. Invest.*, **10**, 144–158

LILLIE, R. D. (1965). In *Histopathologic Technic and Practical Histochemistry*. 3rd Ed. Blakiston, New York

PEARSE, A. G. E. (1972). *Histochemistry, Theoretical and Applied*. 3rd Ed. Vol. 2. Churchill-Livingstone, Edinburgh and London

PERLS, M. (1867). Nachweis von Eisenoxyd in gewisser Pigmentation. *Virchows Arch. Path. Anat. Physiol. Klin. Med.*, **39**, 42

PUCHTLER, H. and SWEAT, F. (1962). Amidoblack as a stain for hemoglobin. *Arch. Pathol.*, **73**, 245–249

ROST, F. W. D. and POLAK, J. M. (1969). Fluorescence microscopy and microspectrofluorimetry of malignant melanomas, naevi and normal melanocytes. *Virchows Arch. Abt. A Path. Anat.*, **347**, 321–326

SCHMELZER, W. (1933). Der mikrochemische Nachweis von Eisen in Gewebselementen mittels Rhodan-Wasserstoffsäure und die Konservierung der Reaktion in Paraffinöl. *Ztschr. Wissensch. Mikr.*, **50**, 99–102

STEIN, J. (1935). Reaction histochemique stable de détection de la bilirubine. *C. R. Soc. Biol.*, **120**, 1136–1138

TIEDEMAN, F. and GMELIN, L. (1826), *Die Verdauung nach Versuchen*. Vol. 1. K. Groos, Heidelberg and Leipzig

15

Deposits

The endogenous pigments of haem, tyrosine and lipid origins have been discussed in Chapter 14. This chapter will include artefact deposits, exogenous pigments and minerals, and some inorganic constituents which, being products of metabolism, could be correctly described as endogenous, for example, calcium and copper.

Artefact deposits

These deposits are the products of action of some reagent used in the processing of the tissue or section with tissue components, or by simple deposition.

Formalin pigment

Formalin pigment is acid formaldehyde haematin. It is formed in the tissues by the action of acid formaldehyde solutions on haemoglobin. It is therefore found in association with blood in tissues and is most commonly seen in spleen, liver, lung, bone marrow and in association with areas of haemorrhage and with blood vessels. It is dark brown in colour and is composed of small birefringent crystals. Its formation can be limited by fixing in non-acid formaldehyde, for example, buffered formalin. Formation of formalin pigment is not always prevented by the use of buffered formalin especially if fixation is prolonged.

Malarial and bilharzial pigments are similar to formalin pigment in all their reactions but may be differentiated from the latter by their intracellular distribution.

Formalin pigment may be removed by treating the section with alcoholic ammonia or alcoholic sodium or potassium hydroxide. These methods, however, have the tendency of removing the sections from the slide. The method of choice is that of Barrett (1944) using a saturated alcoholic solution of picric acid before the staining procedure. The time required for removal varies from 15 minutes to overnight.

Mercury pigment

Tissues fixed in solutions containing mercuric chloride contain a varying amount of a dark brown or grey deposit of granules or irregular masses. The deposit is found throughout the tissue. It is easily removed from the section by oxidation with iodine to mercuric iodide which can subsequently removed with sodium thiosulphate as follows:

(1) Remove paraffin wax with xylene.
(2) Rinse in absolute alcohol.
(3) Treat with 0.5% iodine in 80% alcohol for 3 minutes.
(4) Rinse in tap-water.
(5) Treat with 3% aqueous sodium thiosulphate until bleached (usually less than 3 minutes).
(6) Wash in running water for 2 minutes.

Chromate deposits

If tissues are not thoroughly washed in water after fixation in chromate-containing fixatives, the chrome salts will react with the dehydrating alcohol forming a yellow-brown to black precipitate within the tissue. This can be removed by treating the section for at least 30 minutes with 1% hydrochloric acid in 70% alcohol.

Stain deposits

Stain deposits may occur in tissue sections due to faulty technique. They may be amorphous or crystalline and are usually highly coloured. They are most likely to occur if concentrated solutions are allowed to evaporate on the sections. Care should be taken to ensure that surface layers of precipitated stain are removed from the staining-bath by filtration otherwise the precipitate will be deposited on the surface of the section as it is withdrawn from the staining-bath.

Paraffin wax

Paraffin wax is sometimes retained in the section, particularly in nuclei. It is easily recognized by its position, its refractile appearance and its birefringence. It can usually be removed by treatment in xylene at 60 °C.

Water

Water droplets in a section may occasionally simulate a light brown pigment.

Exogenous pigments, minerals and inorganic constituents

These are substances occurring as pigments which have gained entrance to the body or are products of metabolism. A variety of methods may be used to identify these substances:

Solubility studies
Staining and histochemical reactions
Polarizing microscopy
Micro-incineration
Electron microscope microprobe analysis

Carbon

Carbon occurs as black particles, or jagged masses, and is most commonly found in the lungs and associated glands. It may be found rarely in the liver, the spleen and the skin.

Carbon is distinguished from melanin, malaria pigment, formalin pigment and so on, by its insolubility in concentrated sulphuric acid (which dissolves all other pigments), and the inability of Mayer's chlorine method to bleach it (page 284).

Silica

Silica is found most commonly in the lungs and associated glands of stone-grinders (silicosis); in coal miners it occurs together with carbon (anthracosis). It occurs as greyish crystals, which are birefringent. Silica may be demonstrated by its resistance to micro-incineration, and the fact that it is birefringent.

Asbestos

Asbestos is a fibrous magnesium silicate. It is found in the lungs of asbestos workers causing a fibrous reaction which may lead eventually to the development of mesothelioma. The fibres are birefringent and resist micro-incineration. Soon after inhalation they become coated with an iron-containing protein and are known as asbestos bodies. These bodies have a characteristic beaded appearance and golden brown colour. Birefringence is lost because of the protein covering. The protein is destroyed by micro-incineration but the internal fibre remains unaffected. The bodies may be demonstrated by Perls' Prussian blue reaction. Asbestos bodies may be present in insufficient numbers to be identified in tissue sections. Freshly sliced lung may be smeared on slides and wet preparations examined unstained. Blocks of fresh or fixed lung tissue may be digested with 40% sodium hydroxide solution at 100 °C, centrifuged and wet preparations made from the deposit (Gold, 1967).

Silver

Silver may be found in skin, kidney or other parts of the body as a result of medical investigation or treatment, and as an occupational hazard among silver nitrate workers in the condition known as argyrea.

It occurs as a brown or black granular deposit, and is blackened by ammonium sulphide. It may be removed by borax ferricyanide differentiator (*see* page 271).

The granules can be demonstrated by the rhodanine method.

■ Rhodanine method for silver (Okamoto, Utamura and Akagi, 1939)

Frozen sections—reagent

0.2% *p*-Dimethylaminobenzylidene rhodanine in 10% alcohol	50 ml
Concentrated nitric acid	0.05 ml

Method

(1) Treat unmounted sections for 1–3 hours at 37 °C.
(2) Wash in 70% alcohol.
(3) Float onto slides and mount in glycerin jelly.

Paraffin sections—reagent

p-Dimethylaminobenzylidene rhodanine saturated in 90% alcohol	3.5 ml
N-nitric acid	3 ml
Distilled water	93.5 ml

Method

(1) Bring sections to water.
(2) Treat with reagent for 24 hours at 37 °C.
(3) Wash in distilled water.
(4) Mount in glycerin jelly.

Results

Silver deposits   Red-brown

Note

Diffusion of the reaction product occurs, therefore the short incubation of frozen sections is preferred. Examination should be carried out immediately.

Tattoo pigment

Under this heading is found a great variety of coloured pigments. They are, fortunately, usually confined to the skin which has been tattooed, but may be found in associated glands.

Iron-ore pigment

Iron-ore pigment may be encountered in the lungs in certain occupations (e.g. miners). The pigment may be black, blue, green, yellow or red, according to the composition. It is soluble in 5% oxalic or dilute acid (1 hour or more), and reacts in acid solutions with potassium ferricyanide or ferrocyanide, or both. It is, however, sometimes necessary to carry out the Prussian blue reaction at 60 °C, using stronger (even concentrated) hydrochloric acid to get a reaction.

Lead and copper

Lead and copper in tissues may be demonstrated with fresh alkaline haematoxylin. The colours described are for fresh unripened haematoxylin, and since the ripening may take place even in minutes, it is essential that the solution used is prepared immediately before use.

■ **Mallory and Parker's haematoxylin method for lead and copper (1939)**

Reagent

Dissolve 10 mg of haematoxylin in a few drops of 95% alcohol. Add 10 ml of a filtered 2% potassium dihydrogen phosphate.

Method

(1) Bring alcohol or formalin-fixed tissues to water.
(2) Stain in fresh haematoxylin solution for 2–3 hours at 50–60 °C.
(3) Wash in running water for 10 minutes.
(4) Dehydrate in 95% alcohol.
(5) Clear in terpineol and mount in terpineol balsam.

Results

Lead   Dark grey-blue
Copper   Blue

Copper is normally present in many tissues but in such small amounts that it cannot be demonstrated. In hepatolenticular degeneration (Wilson's disease) copper accumulates to such a degree that it can be demonstrated histochemically. This occurs in the liver, which is usually cirrhotic, and in the basal ganglia of the brain. It can be demonstrated by the method of Mallory and Parker but a more specific method is the rubeanic acid method of Howell (1959). Cobalt and nickel also produce rubeanates but these reactions can be blocked by using an acid solution containing sodium acetate (Uzman, 1956). Uzman also recommends releasing non-reactive protein-bound copper by exposing the sections to the fumes of concentrated hydrochloric acid.

■ Rubeanic acid method for copper

Reagents

Stock solution

Rubeanic acid (dithio-oxamide)   0.1 g
Ethanol   100 ml

Working solution

Stock rubeanic acid solution   2.5 ml
10% Aqueous sodium acetate   50 ml

Method

(1) Bring sections to water.
(2) Place in working solution overnight at 37 °C.
(3) Treat with 70% alcohol for 15 minutes.
(4) Place in absolute alcohol for 6 hours.
(5) Clear in xylene and mount in synthetic resin.

Results

Copper deposits   Greenish-black

■ Rhodizonate method for lead (Lillie, 1954)

Reagent

Sodium rhodizonate   0.2 g
Distilled water   99 ml
Glacial acetic acid   1 ml

Method

(1) Bring section to water.
(2) Treat with rhodizonate reagent for 1 hour.
(3) Wash in water.
(4) Counterstain in 0.1% light green in 1% acetic acid for 30 seconds.
(5) Rinse in water.

Results

Lead salts   Red
Tissue   Green

Note

See rhodizonate method for barium and strontium (*below*).

Bismuth

Bismuth in tissues is well demonstrated by the brucine-iodide method.

■ Wachstein and Zak's method for bismuth (1946)

Reagents

(1) Modified Castel's reagent—dissolve 0.25 g brucine sulphate in 100 ml of distilled
    water, add three drops of concentrated sulphuric acid and then 2 g of potassium
    iodide. This should be stored in a dark bottle and filtered before use.
(2) Castel's light green solution—add 0.1 ml of 1% aqueous light green to 10 ml of
    Castel's reagent.

Method

(1) Bring sections to water and blot dry.
(2) Treat with 100 vol. (30%) hydrogen peroxide for 1–15 seconds.
(3) Wash in running water for 1 minute.
(4) Treat with modified Castel's reagent for 1 hour.
(5) Transfer to 25% modified Castel's reagent in distilled water, and agitate gently to
    remove precipitate.
(6) Counterstain in Castel light green for 4 minutes.
(7) Mount in laevulose syrup (*see* page 148).

Results

Bismuth   Orange-red
Tissue   Shades of green

Calcium

The deposition of calcium is normally restricted to bone, although hyaline cartilage may show calcareous infiltration in old age. Calcium is not uncommonly found deposited in fibroids, tuberculous foci, mesenteric lymph glands and the thyroid gland: although calcium compounds are distributed throughout all the tissues and body fluids such compounds are in a state of solution and cannot be demonstrated histologically.

Fresh preparations

The solubility of calcium deposits in mineral acids may be used to demonstrate their presence in tissue, but it does not give their exact location. Treatment of smears or sections with concentrated hydrochloric acid may be used to determine whether the calcium present is carbonate or phosphate:

(1) The smear or section is mounted in water.
(2) Hydrochloric acid is run under the coverslip.
(3) Solution of the deposit *with* bubbles of CO_2 indicates the presence of calcium carbonate, whereas solution of the deposit *without* bubbles indicates calcium phosphate. Dilute sulphuric acid (15%) may also be used in this manner and the formation of gypsum crystals is specific for calcium. 2 M Acetic acid will dissolve calcium carbonate and calcium phosphate leaving calcium oxalate unaffected.

Sections

The methods for the demonstration of calcium in sections are based on the following:

(1) The conversion of the calcium salt into the salt of another metal which itself is opaque (e.g. von Kossa's technique) or, by further treatment, into a coloured compound.
(2) The ability of certain dyes to form lakes with calcium (such as purpurin or anthrapurpurin (alizarin), or even haematoxylin).

In spite of the new dyes and methods which have been evolved for the demonstration of calcium deposits in sections, the method usually employed is that of von Kossa, which was first described in 1901.

Lillie's oxalic acid technique is a more specific method for the presence of calcium, but does not show the location of the deposit. The use of the anthraquinone dyes (purpurin, anthrapurpurin) is usually confined to the demonstration of bones in embryos (page 535) on account of the technical difficulty of employing it and its low specificity.

The morin fluorescent technique for calcium may be confusing for an inexperienced observer in view of the autofluorescence of other material that may be present in some tissue sections (*see* page 583). Morin also reacts with aluminium and beryllium.

Calcium oxalate deposits, found in the kidney in oxalosis, give unreliable results with the von Kossa technique. They may be identified using the Pizzolato silver technique or by micro-incineration. Micro-incineration should be carried out at 450 °C when oxalate is converted to carbonate. When the preparation has cooled acid is introduced under a coverslip causing solution, with production of carbon dioxide bubbles.

■ von Kossa's technique (1901)

Method

(1) Bring two sections to water.
(2) Immerse one section in pH 4.5 citrate buffer for 20 minutes (*see* Note).
(3) Wash both slides well in distilled water.
(4) Flood slides with 5% silver nitrate.
(5) Expose to bright sunlight or ultraviolet light for 10–20 minutes or to a 60-watt electric bulb at a range of 4–5 inches for 30–60 minutes.
(6) Wash in several changes of distilled water.
(7) Treat with 5% sodium thiosulphate for 2–3 minutes.
(8) Counterstain with neutral red, safranin or Van Gieson's stain.
(9) Dehydrate, clear and mount in resinous mountant.

Result

Calcium deposits   Black

Note

This technique may be made more specific by removing the calcium from parallel sections with a 0.1 M citrate buffer at pH 4.5 for 20 minutes (Pearse, 1952). The buffer is prepared by mixing the following:

0.2 M Disodium hydrogen phosphate	9.09 ml
0.1 M Citric acid	10.91 ml

■ Lillie's oxalic acid technique (1954)

Method

(1) Mount the section in water.
(2) Draw 10% oxalic acid under the coverslip by placing a few drops of reagent at one end of the coverslip, and a piece of blotting paper at the other.

Results

The calcium deposits dissolve with the formation of characteristic envelope-shaped calcium oxalate crystals.

■ Silver peroxide method for calcium oxalate (Pizzolato, 1964; Pearse, 1972)

Reagent

2% Silver nitrate	1 part
30% Hydrogen peroxide (100 volumes)	1 part

Method

(1) Bring sections to water.
(2) Treat with 2 M acetic acid for 15 minutes.
(3) Treat with silver nitrate solution for 15 minutes at room temperature in bright daylight.
(4) Wash in distilled water.
(5) Counterstain as desired.
(6) Dehydrate, clear and mount in synthetic resin.

Results

Calcium oxalate deposits   Black
Calcium carbonate and phosphate   Negative (dissolved at step 2)

■ **Fluorescent technique for calcium and aluminium (Pearse, 1972)**

(1) Bring sections to 95% alcohol.
(2) Stain for 2–5 minutes in 0.2% Morin in 85% alcohol containing 0.5% acetic acid.
(3) Wash in 95% alcohol (differentiate if necessary in acid–alcohol).
(4) Rinse and mount in water; or, *preferably*, rinse rapidly in absolute alcohol, clear in xylene and mount in resin.
(5) Examine under fluorescent microscope.

Result

A greenish-white fluorescence indicates the presence of calcium or aluminium. By treating a control section in acid buffer (*see above*) they may be differentiated since aluminium is stable in acid solutions.

■ **Alizarin red S method (McGee-Russell, 1958)**

Reagent

Alizarin red S   1 g
Distilled water   50 ml

Add 0.5% ammonia until pH 4.1–4.3 is reached, using a pH meter. The pH is critical. The solution should be a deep iodine colour and keeps well.

Method

(1) Bring sections to water.
(2) Stain in alizarin solution for 30 seconds to 5 minutes, controlling with the staining microscope.
(3) Shake off excess stain and blot carefully.
(4) Transfer immediately to acetone for 10–20 seconds.
(5) Rinse in equal parts acetone and xylene for 10–20 seconds.
(6) Clear in xylene and mount in resinous mountant.

Results

Calcium deposits	Orange-red
Background	Pale pink

Aluminium and beryllium

Several methods are available for the demonstration of aluminium and beryllium which are usually demonstrated along with calcium, by the same method. The differentiation of these metals is described by Pearse (1972). The solochrome azurine method is given.

■ Solochrome azurine method (Pearse, 1972)

Reagent

Dissolve 0.1 g solochrome azurine in 50 ml of 2% aqueous sodium hydroxide.

Method

(1) Bring sections to water.
(2) Stain in solochrome azurine for 30 minutes.
(3) Rinse in distilled water.
(4) Dehydrate, clear and mount in synthetic resin.

Results

Beryllium deposits	Blue-black

Notes

(1) Aluminium deposits are dissolved in the staining bath.
(2) Treatment with dilute acid will dissolve calcium deposits and will convert beryllium deposits to brownish-orange.
(3) Staining in 0.2% aqueous solochrome azurine will stain both beryllium and aluminium blue.

Barium

■ Rhodizonate method (Waterhouse, 1951; Pearse, 1972)

Reagent

Sodium rhodizonate	0.1 g
Distilled water	50 ml

Prepare immediately before use.

Method

(1) Bring section to water.
(2) Incubate in rhodizonate solution at 60 °C for 1–2 hours.

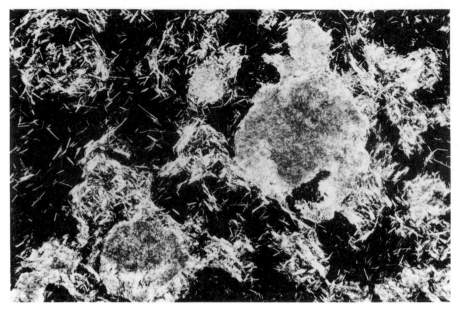

Figure 15.1 Wet preparation from gouty tophus showing birefringent sodium urate crystals. Polarizing microscopy. Original magnification × 40

(3) Wash in water.
(4) Dehydrate, clear and mount in synthetic resin.

Results

Barium deposits	Black
Strontium deposits	Black
Calcium deposits	Negative

Notes

(1) If section is treated for a few minutes in 20% hydrochloric acid, after step 3 barium deposits become red and strontium deposits are dissolved.
(2) Pretreatment with potassium chromate prevents the reaction with barium salts.
(3) Mercury and lead salts also react.

Urates

Urates occur in tissue (gouty tophi), or in synovial fluids from acute gouty joints, as acid sodium urate crystals. They may be demonstrated as argentaffin with methenamine silver (at 37 °C for 1–2 hours), or with the polarizing microscope (McCarthy and Hollander, 1961; Currey, 1968). Tissue should be fixed for the minimum time in formal–saline otherwise urate deposits will be removed. It is safer to fix in absolute alcohol. With either tissue or fluid the more specific method is examination with the polarizing microscope (*Figure 15.1*) (*see* page 591). In joint fluids, particularly, it is important to differentiate between sodium urate and calcium pyrophosphate dihydrate, which may occur in synovial fluid from acutely inflamed joints. This differentiation is relatively simple using polarizing microscopy.

References

BARRETT, A. M. (1944). On the removal of formaldehyde-produced precipitate from sections. *J. Pathol. Bacteriol.*, **56**, 135–136

CURREY, H. L. F. (1968). Examination of joint fluids for crystals. *Proc. R. Soc. Med.*, **61**, 969–971

GOLD, C. (1967). A simple method for detecting asbestos in tissue. *J. Clin. Pathol.*, **20**, 674

HOWELL, J. S. (1959). Histochemical demonstration of copper in copper fed rats and in hepatolenticular degeneration. *J. Pathol. Bacteriol.*, **77**, 473–484

LILLIE, R. D. (1954). *Histopathologic Technic and Practical Histochemistry*. Blakiston, New York

McCARTHY, D. J. and HOLLANDER, J. L. (1961). Identification of urate crystals in gouty synovial fluid. *Ann. Intern. Med.*, **54**, 452–460

McGEE-RUSSELL, S. M. (1958). Histochemical methods for calcium. *J. Histochem. Cytochem.*, **6**, 22–42

MALLORY, F. B. and PARKER, F. (1939). Fixing and staining methods for lead and copper in tissues. *Am. J. Pathol.*, **15**, 517–522

OKAMOTO, K., UTAMURA, M. and AKAGI, T. (1939). Biologische Untersuchungen des Silbers: Histochemische Silbernachweismethode. *Acta Scholae Med. Univ. Imp. Kioto*, **22**, 361–372

PEARSE, A. G. E. (1972). *Histochemistry, Theoretical and Applied*. 3rd Ed. Vol. 2. Churchill-Livingstone, Edinburgh and London

PIZZOLATO, P. (1964). Histochemical recognition of calcium oxalate. *J. Histochem. Cytochem.*, **12**, 333 336

UZMAN, L. L. (1956). Histochemical localization of copper with rubeanic acid. *Lab. Invest.*, **5**, 299–305

VON KOSSA, J. (1901). Nachweis von Kalk. *Beit. Pathol. Anat. Pathol.*, **29**, 163–202

WACHSTEIN, M. and ZAK, F. G. (1946). Bismuth pigmentation. Its histochemical differentiation. *Am. J. Pathol.*, **22**, 603–611

WATERHOUSE, D. F. (1951). Histochemical detection of barium and strontium. *Nature (Lond.)*, **167**, 358

16

Enzymes

The importance of enzymes has perhaps best been expressed by defining life as an orderly or disorderly function of enzymes, their state of function determining health or disease. Thus, enzymes control, regulate and maintain an orderly balance of physiological processes necessary for the preservation of life.

The number of enzymes recorded by Dixon and Webb in 1958 was over 800; of these only relatively few could be demonstrated histochemically. Dixon *et al.* (1979) now list over 2000 enzymes, of these over 100 can be demonstrated histochemically. It will be seen that this is a rapidly expanding field.

An enzyme is a catalyst of vital origin, that is, a substance that initiates or accelerates a chemical reaction. Although the enzyme takes part in the reaction its role is that of a 'bystander' who initiates a quarrel (or reaction) but takes no direct part in it and is not degraded by it. Enzymes are generally proteins with a very specific action, and they usually derive their name from this action; for example, the enzyme that hydrolyses sucrose to monosaccharides is a sucrase. The ending 'ase' indicates an enzyme, but some enzymes were named before this system was adopted and these usually end in 'in', such as trypsin, pepsin, ptyalin and so on. The substance (or kind of chemical bond) acted upon by an enzyme is known as its substrate and since enzymes are highly specific they tend to be limited to one type of substrate or group of related substances. The histochemical demonstration of enzymes, therefore, is dependent upon the effect they have upon a given substrate, either natural or artificial. In this way their visualization differs from that of other, inactive, tissue components, since enzymes must be active to be demonstrated histochemically. One cannot see the enzyme itself, only the effect it has had upon a substrate. This effect, to be seen, must result in the formation of an insoluble substance at the site of activity by the action of the enzyme on the specific substrate. This insoluble substance must be subsequently rendered coloured or opaque, if not already visible.

The recent introduction of immunocytochemical methods for the localization of enzymes, where the antigenic properties of the protein, rather than its activity, are utilized, shows great promise for the future. Some of the limitations due to fixation and sectioning can be overcome and increased specificity can be obtained. Pearse (1980) lists 22 enzymes which can be detected immunocytochemically, using standard techniques.

This chapter deals only with the histochemical demonstration of enzymes.

Preservation

Because of the nature of enzymes, their preservation is much more difficult than that of other tissue constituents. For a good demonstration it is important to preserve the maximum amount of enzyme activity, together with accurate localization by the prevention of diffusion.

Enzymes are sometimes classified as *lyo-enzymes* (e.g. glucuronidase) which are dissolved in the cytoplasm and thus are likely to diffuse; and *desmo-enzymes* (e.g. leucine amino-peptidase) which are attached to cytoplasmic constituents (mitochondria) and are much less likely to diffuse.

It will be obvious that tissue must be as fresh as possible and, although there are exceptions, autopsy tissue is generally unsuitable for the demonstration of enzymes. Although there have been papers published which record only a slight loss of alkaline phosphatase activity 5 hours after death, this should not be relied upon for an estimate of total enzyme activity. Tissue which cannot be treated immediately should be kept in a refrigerator. For most enzymes fresh preparations (cell cultures on coverslips), or frozen, cryostat or freeze-dried tissue sections are necessary. There are, however, some enzymes such as acid and alkaline phosphatases, esterase and so on, which will sufficiently resist fixation to allow their demonstration.

Fixatives, if used, should be refrigerator cold (4 °C) to preserve maximum enzyme activity. Following fixation they should be transferred to, and frozen for cutting in, 0.88 M sucrose (30%) in 1% gum acacia. Holt's ice-cold (0–4 °C) gum sucrose treatment improves cryostat section cutting, tissue morphology and enzyme localization: tissues should be left for 24 hours but may be left for longer periods (*Table 16.1*).

Methods of demonstration

These may be discussed under the four following headings.

(1) Simultaneous capture.
(2) Post-coupling (post-incubation coupling).
(3) Self-coloured substrate.
(4) Intramolecular rearrangement.

Two terms used in enzyme techniques are:

Primary reaction product (PRP), the product of the reaction of an enzyme on a substrate;
Final reaction product (FRP), the product of an insoluble uncoloured PRP which has been rendered coloured or opaque.

Simultaneous capture

This describes the procedure where a reagent, present in the incubation medium, combines with the PRP. An example of this technique is the diazo method for alkaline phosphatase. The diazonium salt, present in the incubation medium, combines with the PRP as soon as it is released from the substrate forming an insoluble coloured FRP.

Table 16.1 Effects of fixation upon enzyme activity

Enzyme	Fixative	Time	Temperature (°C)	Enzyme activity (%)	Reference
Alkaline phosphatase	Buffered formalin (pH 7.0)	60 minutes	4	80	Nachlas et al. (1956)
	10% formalin	2 hours	4	73	Seligman et al. (1951)
	Acetone	30 minutes	4	95	Nachlas et al. (1956)
	Ethanol	30 minutes	4	62	Nachlas et al. (1956)
Acid phosphatase	Buffered formalin	60 minutes	4	67	Nachlas et al. (1956)
	Formal–calcium	24 hours[1]	2	60	Holt (1959)
	Acetone	60 minutes	4	81	Nachlas et al. (1956)
	Ethanol	60 minutes	4	50	Nachlas et al. (1956)
β-Glucuronidase	Buffered formalin	15 minutes	4	38	Nachlas et al. (1956)
	Buffered formalin	60 minutes	4	16	Nachlas et al. (1956)
	Acetone	15 minutes	4	76	Nachlas et al. (1956)
	Acetone	30 minutes	4	73	Nachlas et al. (1956)
	Ethanol	15 minutes	4	33	Nachlas et al. (1956)
Esterase	Formal–calcium	24 hours[1]	2	50	Holt (1959)
	Acetone	30 minutes	4	68	Nachlas et al. (1956)
Leucine amino peptidase	Buffered formalin	60 minutes	4	85	Nachlas et al. (1956)
	Acetone	60 minutes	4	84	Nachlas et al. (1956)

[1] Post-fixation treatment in gum-sucrose at 2 °C.

Post-coupling reaction

This type of reaction is based on the production of an insoluble PRP which is then coupled with a coloured or opaque substance. The absence of diazonium salts in the substrate has two advantages:

(1) they have been thought by some workers to interfere with, or inactivate enzymes (Pearse, 1968); and
(2) long exposure of diazonium salts in an acid solution may result in non-specific staining (Nachlas, Young and Seligman, 1957).

The technique of Rutenberg and Seligman (1955) for acid phosphatase is an example of such a technique.

Self-coloured substrate

This type of reaction employs a water-soluble dye. This dye is then made insoluble, due to the removal of a hydrophilic group, by the enzyme. This gives a coloured precipitate at the site of enzyme activity. The fluorescent technique of Burstone's for alkaline phosphatase (*see* page 307) is an example of such a technique.

Intramolecular rearrangement

This type of reaction is based on the rearrangement of the molecular structure of a colourless substrate to give a coloured insoluble precipitate at sites of enzyme activity. Such a technique has been described by Nachlas, Crawford and Seligman (1957) for carboxylic acid esterase but the FRP is not sufficiently insoluble to give good localization.

The use of controls

Nowhere in the field of histochemistry are controls more important than in the demonstration of enzymes. Many substrates or their components break down on keeping which may lead to false negatives and on occasion to false positives. Therefore, control sections should always be carried through in parallel with the test sections. A positive control, if available, will demonstrate that the reagents are all working. A negative control is prepared by destroying the enzyme in the test section (of a positive control) by immersing in boiling water for 15 minutes, or by a specific chemical method for the enzyme to be demonstrated. A useful control is to incubate one of the test sections in the reaction mixture, without the substrate, for the same time that the test section proper is in the complete reaction mixture; both sections are then taken through the remainder of the technique together. A positive result in a given area in both sections indicates that this is not due to enzymic action. Appropriate control methods are given for each of the enzyme techniques.

Enzyme techniques

Alkaline phosphatase

Location of enzyme

Alkaline phosphatase is normally found in the bladder, suprarenal, kidney (convoluted tubules and Bowman's capsule), endothelial cells of liver and spleen, and in breast and ovary.

Calcium–cobalt methods

The Gomori method for the identification of this enzyme is based on the action of the enzyme (at pH 9) on a substrate containing organic phosphate, in the presence of calcium ions, to form calcium phosphate *in situ*. The calcium phosphate so formed may then be directly demonstrated by von Kossa's silver technique or by Gomori's method.

Controls

Among the disadvantages of this method is the danger of false positives, due to preformed calcium or other black pigment present in the section. For this reason two control sections should be carried through which are incubated in (a) distilled water, and (b) in substrate from which the glycerophosphate is omitted. Sites which are blackened in the uncontrolled section only and not in the two control sections are alkaline phosphatase.

■ Gomori's method (1952)

The technique depends on treatment, of the calcium phosphate formed, first with cobalt nitrate (when cobalt phosphate is formed) and then with ammonium sulphide to form cobalt sulphide, which is black.

Substrate solution

2% Sodium glycerophosphate	25 ml
2% Sodium barbitone	25 ml
Distilled water	50 ml
2% Calcium chloride	5 ml
2% Magnesium sulphate	2 ml
Chloroform	a few drops

This solution does not keep well and is best made up fresh for each batch of sections.

Method

(1) Fix *fresh* tissue in 80% alcohol for 24 hours, followed by normal paraffin wax processing, or better, fix in cold acetone at $-20\,°C$ for 24 hours, followed by two changes of acetone (at room temperature) of 2 hours; clear in xylene, two changes of 45 minutes; embed in paraffin wax as quickly as possible. The best results are usually obtained by the latter method.
(2) Cut thin paraffin sections.
(3) Bring sections to water.
(4) Leave in substrate for 1–3 hours at 37 °C.
(5) Rinse rapidly in distilled water.
(6) Treat with 2% cobalt nitrate for 2 minutes.
(7) Wash out the excess cobalt nitrate for 1 minute (this stage is critical).
(8) Treat with 1% yellow ammonium sulphide for 1 minute.
(9) Wash in water for 2–3 minutes.
(10) Counterstain in neutral red or safranin for 1 minute.
(11) Wash in tap-water.
(12) Dehydrate, clear and mount in resinous mountant.

Results

Structures possessing alkaline phosphatase activity,
and preformed calcium   Brown to black
Other structures   Red

Azo-coupling techniques

■ **Coupling with α-naphthyl phosphate (Menten, Junge and Green, 1944)**

The sections are incubated in a substrate containing a diazonium salt and sodium α-naphthyl phosphate. The enzyme liberates α-naphthol which couples with the diazonium salt to form an insoluble coloured precipitate (*Figure 16.1*).

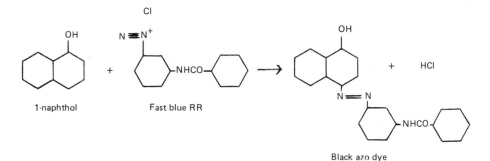

Figure 16.1 1-Naphthol (α-naphthol), released by the action of phosphatase on the phosphate ester, couples at the 4-carbon position with diazonium salts, Fast blue RR in this example, to produce highly coloured azo dyes. 2-Naphthol (β-naphthol) couples at the 1-carbon position

Controls

Treat control slides as above, omitting the α-naphthyl phosphate.

Substrate solution

Sodium α-naphthyl phosphate   10–20 mg
Michaelis's veronal–HCl buffer pH 9.2 (page 132)   20 ml
Fast blue RR or fast black B   20 mg

This substrate is prepared immediately before use.

Method

Frozen, cryostat or freeze-dried sections of fresh or cold formalin fixed tissue may be used. Paraffin sections of cold acetone fixed tissue also give good results.

(1) Bring paraffin sections to water.
(2) Filter enough substrate on to each slide to cover section adequately, and leave at room temperature for 30–60 minutes. Paraffin sections may require longer periods up to 4 hours, and should be put into a covered dish on wet blotting paper to control evaporation.

(3) Wash in running water for 2–3 minutes.
(4) Counterstain lightly with haematoxylin, and blue.
(5) Wash in running tap-water for 15 minutes.
(6) Mount in glycerin jelly or Apathy's medium.

Results

Sites of enzyme activity	Black if fast blue RR or fast black B is used
Nuclei	Pale blue

■ Coupling with substituted naphthol phosphate (Burstone, 1962)

The use of the phosphate ester of an arylide of 2-hydroxy-3-naphthoic acid, Naphthol AS (Naphtol Anilid Säure), as an alternative to 1-naphthyl phosphate or 2-naphthyl phosphate, led to the development of more complex arylides. The localization obtained with Naphthol AS phosphate revealed diffusion artefact but the more complex substituted Naphthol AS phosphates gave a more definite localization. Stained preparations are permanent, indicating the stable nature of the FRP obtained on coupling with a number of stable diazotates. The FRP has low solubility and high substantivity (affinity for protein). The substituted naphthols have very low solubility in water, so are first dissolved in an organic solvent, dimethylformamide being the most popular, before the addition of aqueous buffer solutions. The formula of one of these complex naphthols (Naphthol AS–BI phosphate) is compared with the formulas of sodium α-naphthyl phosphate and Naphthol AS phosphate in *Figure 16.2*.

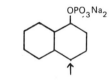

Sodium α-naphthyl phosphate

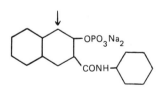

Naphthol AS phosphate

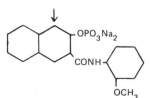

Naphthol AS-BI phosphate

Figure 16.2 Examples of substrates for phosphatases when using diazonium salts as couplers. The arrows show the coupling positions, *para* in the case of 1-naphthols, *ortho* in the case of 2-naphthols

■ Naphthol AS–BI phosphate method

Cold formal–calcium or cold acetone fixed paraffin sections may be used. Burstone (1961a) recommends fixation of cryostat sections in acetone for several minutes prior to incubation.

Stock substrate solution

Dissolve 50 mg of Naphthol AS–BI phosphate in 20 ml of *N,N*-dimethylformamide. Add 20 ml of distilled water and adjust to pH 8 with molar sodium carbonate. Add 600 ml of water then make up to 1 litre with 0.2 M tris buffer (pH 8.3). The solution is opalescent and is stable for several months at room temperature (Pearse, 1968).

Incubating substrate solution

Stock Naphthol AS–BI phosphate solution   40 ml
Fast red TR (or other suitable stable diazotate)   40 mg

Shake well and filter. The solution should be made up immediately before use.

Mountant

Polyvinyl pyrrolidone   50 g
Water   50 ml

Stand overnight then add 2 ml of glycerol and a crystal of thymol. Stir.

Method

(1) Bring sections to water.
(2) Incubate in working substrate solution for 5–15 minutes.
(3) Wash in water.
(4) Counterstain in 2% methyl green if desired.
(5) Mount in PVP mountant.

Results

Sites of alkaline phosphatase activity   Red
Nuclei (if counterstained)   Green

Note

The colour of the FRP depends on which diazotate is used.

Fluorescent method for alkaline phosphatase

This method, described by Burstone (1960) as one of several new techniques for this enzyme, is one of the first applications of fluorescence to enzyme histochemistry. The enzyme releases a fluorescent naphthol compound from the substrate in a non-coupling reaction (*see* page 303).

This approach has great significance since either the use of a substrate that gives a fluorescent reaction product, or the post-coupling of the reaction product with a fluorchrome would allow, because of the increased sensitivity of fluorescence, visualization of very low levels of activity.

■ Burstone's method

Substrate solution

Approximately 5 mg 5,6,7,8-β-tetralol carboxylic acid-β-naphthylamide phosphate and 0.5 ml *N,N*-dimethylformamide (DMF) substrate are placed in a 50 ml flask.

Twenty-five ml of distilled water is added, followed by 25 ml tris buffer pH 8.7 (24.2 g tris (hydroxymethyl) aminomethane, 16.5 ml N/1 HCl and distilled water to make 1 litre). Two drops of 10% magnesium chloride are then added, the solution is shaken several times and then filtered. The solution should be clear or slightly opalescent.

Method

(1) Bring frozen dried, cryostat cut or acetone-fixed paraffin embedded sections to distilled water.
(2) Incubate in substrate in a Coplin jar at 60 °C for 15 minutes, then remove Coplin jar to bench for remainder of incubation at room temperature. Incubation period may vary from 1–3 hours.
(3) Wash slides in two changes of 50% alcohol, then in running tap-water.
(4) Mount in 90% glycerin.

Examine using BG12 or UG1 or 2 exciter filter and colourless ultraviolet barrier filter.

Results

Sites of enzyme activity   Brilliant bluish-white fluorescence

5-Nucleotidase

Nucleotidase is an alkaline phosphatase having an optimum pH of about 7.8 in human tissue. Since by the following technique alkaline phosphatase is also demonstrated, an extra control section must be stained by the method for alkaline phosphatase at pH 7.5 (page 304) an an estimation of the 5-nucleotidase activity made by allowing for the amount of colour due to the alkaline phosphatase present.

Controls

Replacement of adenosine-5-phosphate with sodium-β-glycerophosphate in substrate, or 0.1 M sodium fluoride.

■ Pearse and Reis's method (1952)

Substrate solution

Barbiturate buffer (pH 7.5)*   30 ml

* This buffer is made as follows:

0.1 M sodium diethyl barbiturate	15 ml
N/10 hydrochloric acid	10 ml
Distilled water	5 ml

12% Calcium nitrate (Ca(NO$_3$)$_2$)	6 ml
2% Magnesium chloride (MgCl$_3$)	6 ml
0.04 M Adenylic acid (adenosine-5-phosphate)	6 ml

Method

(1) Cut thin sections of tissue fixed as for alkaline phosphatase.
(2) Incubate sections in the substrate at 37 °C for 3–18 hours (*see* note on control, *see above*).
(3) Wash all the sections with 2% calcium nitrate solution (pH 8) and then in distilled water.
(4) Expose to daylight for 1 hour in 1% silver nitrate.
(5) Rinse in distilled water.
(6) Transfer to 5% sodium thiosulphate for 10 minutes.
(7) Wash in running tap-water, dehydrate, clear and mount in resinous mountant.

Result

5-nucleotidase activity   Black

Unless the reaction is strongly positive it tends to be diffuse.

■ **Lead method (Wachstein and Meisel, 1952; Chayen and colleagues, 1969)**

This is the better of the two methods for the demonstration of 5-nucleotidase in all tissues.

Control

Same as for the calcium method above.

Substrate solution

Adenosine-5′-monophosphate	31 mg
0.1 M Acetate buffer pH 6.5	40 ml
0.1 M Lead nitrate	1 ml
0.1 M Magnesium sulphate	5 ml

This must be freshly prepared.

Method

(1) Incubate frozen or cryostat sections of fresh unfixed tissue in substrate at 37 °C for $\frac{1}{2}$–1 hour.
(2) Wash in running tap-water.
(3) Rinse in distilled water.
(4) Immerse in 0.5% ammonium sulphide for 1 minute.
(5) Rinse in distilled water.
(6) Float sections on to slides and mount in aqueous mountant.

Result

Site of enzyme activity　　Brown (precipitate of lead sulphide)

Adenosine triphosphatases

It is recognized that there are three types of adenosine triphosphatase:

(1) calcium activated myosin ATPase;
(2) magnesium activated mitochondrial ATPase;
(3) magnesium dependent, sodium and potassium activated, membrane associated ATPase (Na/K-ATPase).

This has led to a great deal of confusion in the literature. In relation to the Wachstein and Meisel (1957) lead method, Moses and colleagues (1966) showed that 3.6 mM lead nitrate inhibits ATPase in both unfixed sections (80% inhibition) and fixed sections (50% of remaining activity), and they showed that fixation itself inhibited 88% activity.

Rosenthal and colleagues (1966) showed that lead (in the concentration used in the method) hydrolysed ATP at pH 7.2 at 37 °C. Moses and colleagues (1966) also showed that increasing or decreasing the concentrations of either the lead or ATP resulted in a complete alteration in the reaction product. This method has therefore been the subject of considerable discussion in the literature since 1966.

There is today considerable doubt as to whether ATPase is actually demonstrated. In fact, Tormey (1966) obtained results which seemed to indicate the impossibility of the histochemical localization of Na/K-ATPase. Nevertheless, positive results for ATPase are obtained, at predictable sites, with the techniques described below. This suggests that the activity being demonstrated, if it is not in fact ATPase, may be used as a marker for the enzyme.

The special modification of the ATPase technique for the typing of muscle fibres is given in Chapter 23.

■ Calcium activated ATPase method (Niles and colleagues, 1964)

The method involved is essentially the same calcium trapping procedure discussed above for alkaline phosphatase but with adenosine triphosphate as the substrate.

Control

Substitute sodium-β-glycerophosphate for ATP in substrate, or use 2.5×10^{-3} M/p-chloromercuribenzoate as inactivator.

Substrate solution

0.1 M (2.06%) Sodium barbiturate	10 ml
0.18 M Calcium chloride solution	5 ml
Adenosine triphosphate	76 mg
2,4-Dinitrophenol	30 mg
Distilled water	35 ml

This solution must be freshly prepared.

Method

(1) Cut frozen or cryostat sections of unfixed tissue and incubate in substrate at 37 °C for 10–30 minutes.
(2) Wash sections in three changes of 1% calcium chloride.
(3) Transfer to three changes of 1% cobalt nitrate solution for 2 minutes each.
(4) Wash well in distilled water.
(5) Treat sections with 1% ammonium sulphide for 1 minute.
(6) Wash sections in distilled water, float on to slides and mount in aqueous mountant.

■ **Lead method for Mg-activated ATPase (Wachstein and Meisel, 1957; Chayen and colleagues, 1969)**

The calcium-trapping method (*above*) cannot be used in this technique since the magnesium (used as an activator) would compete for the enzyme released phosphate. The resultant magnesium phosphate being relatively soluble would then be lost. For this reason, in spite of the fact that lead may inhibit ATPase (*above*) Wachstein and Meisel use the lead-trapping procedure.

Control

As for Ca-activated ATPase.

Substrate solution

Adenosine triphosphate (ATP)	25 mg
Distilled water	22 ml
2% Lead nitrate	3 ml
0.25% Magnesium sulphate	5 ml

Dissolve the ATP in distilled water, and add the other reagents; 40 mg of 2,4-dinitrophenol may be added to the substrate to activate mitochondrial ATPase (Lehninger, 1960).

Method

(1) Cut frozen or cryostat sections of fresh tissue (formalin-fixed tissue may be used but is not as good).
(2) Incubate sections (free floating or mounted) in substrate at 37 °C for 2 hours.
(3) Wash in running water, then rinse in distilled water.
(4) Treat sections with 1% ammonium sulphide for 1 minute.
(5) Wash in distilled water.
(6) Mount in an aqueous mountant.

Results

Sites of enzyme activity   Brown-black precipitate

Acid phosphatase

The Gomori acid phosphatase method is based on the action (at pH 5.0) of the enzyme on a substrate containing organic phosphate in the presence of lead ions to form lead phosphate. This in turn is treated with ammonium sulphide to form lead sulphide *in situ*. The post-coupling technique will be found to give more reliable results, and is therefore recommended for fresh, fixed, frozen or cryostat sections.

Control

Add 0.01 M sodium fluoride to control substrate.

Location of enzyme

The enzyme is found in bone, the prostate and in certain tumours.

■ **Gomori's method (1941)**

Substrate solution

M/1 Acetate buffer, pH 5	3 parts
5% Lead nitrate	1 part
Distilled water	6 parts
2% Sodium glycerophosphate	3 parts

Shake well and stand for a few hours. Filter and dilute 1 : 3 with distilled water before use.

Method

(1) Fix *fresh* tissue in chilled acetone and leave in refrigerator for 24 hours. Dehydrate in two changes of acetone (at room temperature) each of 2 hours, clear in xylene (two changes each of 45 minutes). Embed in paraffin wax as quickly as possible.

(2) Cut thin sections, float on warm water (not above 35 °C if possible).

(3) Bring sections to water (including controls, page 304).

(4) Incubate in substrate at 37 °C for 1–24 hours (a moderately good result is usually obtained in 1 hour).

(5) Rinse rapidly in distilled water.

(6) Treat with 2% acetic acid for 1 minute.

(7) Rinse in distilled water.

(8) Treat with 1% ammonium sulphide for 1 minute.

(9) Wash in water for 2–3 minutes.

(10) Counterstain with neutral red or safranin for 1 minute.

(11) Wash in tap-water.

(12) Dehydrate, clear and mount in resinous mountant.

Results

Structures possessing acid phosphatase activity	Brown to black
Other structures	Red

Non-specific lead impregnation occasionally occurs. Such areas would be black in all three sections (*see* Control Sections, page 303). Structures which are black *only* in the test section show acid phosphatase activity.

■ **Post-coupling method for acid phosphatase (Rutenberg and Seligman, 1955)**

Substrate solution

Sodium 6-benzoyl-2-naphthyl phosphate	25 mg
Distilled water	80 ml
Walpole's acetate buffer pH 5.0	20 ml
Sodium chloride	2 g

Diazonium salt solution

Fast blue B or garnet GBC	50 mg
Distilled water	50 ml

This solution is made alkaline with sodium bicarbonate.

Method

Fresh or cold formalin fixed frozen or cryostat cut sections are used. Fresh tissues are placed sequentially in 0.85, 1 and 2% sodium chloride solutions for 2–3 minutes in each.

(1) Place sections into substrate at room temperature for 10–60 minutes (fresh tissue) and 1–2 hours (fixed tissue).
(2) Wash fresh sections in three changes of cold saline, and fixed tissues in three changes of water.
(3) Place in freshly prepared cold diazonium salt solution and agitate for 3–5 minutes.
(4) Wash in cold saline or water (fixed tissue), three changes of 5 minutes each.
(5) Mount in glycerin jelly.

Result

Sites of enzyme activity	Blue or red

Glucose-6-phosphatase

This enzyme, which is found chiefly in the liver, is absent in Von Gierke's disease.
    The method is based on the action of the enzyme on a substrate containing glucose-6-phosphate and lead nitrate to form lead phosphate, which is then converted to lead sulphide. Since this enzyme is easily destroyed, particularly by formalin, the reactions should be carried out on unfixed tissue.

Control

Substitute sodium β-glycerophosphate (25 mg/20 ml distilled water) for glucose-6-phosphate in substrate.

■ **Wachstein and Meisel's method (1956)**

Substitute solution

Potassium glucose-6-phosphate (0.125% solution)	20 ml
0.2 M Tris buffer pH 6.7	20 ml

2% Lead nitrate	3 ml
Distilled water	7 ml

Method

(1) Incubate cryostat or frozen sections of *fresh tissue* in the substrate at 32 °C for 5–15 minutes.
(2) Wash sections in distilled water.
(3) Treat sections with dilute ammonium sulphide for 1 minute.
(4) Wash in water.
(5) Post-fix in 10% formalin for 2 minutes.
(6) Mount in glycerin jelly.

Result

Sites of enzyme activity   Brownish-black deposit

Phosphamidase (phosphoamidase)

This enzyme acts upon phosphoamide bonds. The substrate used is *p*-chloroanilido-phosphonic acid, the released phosphate is trapped by lead, which is visualized as lead sulphide.

Control

Two controls should be used:

(1) omission of solution B from substrate to show reaction due to lead absorption; and
(2) the addition of 21 mg of sodium fluoride to 50 ml of substrate. This does not inhibit true phosphamidase activity.

■ Lead nitrate method (Gomori, 1948; Chayen and colleagues, 1969)

Substrate solution

Solution A

0.05 M Acetate buffer pH 5.4	50 ml
3.3% (0.1 M) Lead nitrate	1.9 ml
Sodium chloride	0.11 g
Polyvinyl alcohol	5 g

Add lead nitrate and sodium chloride to the buffer. Then dissolve the PVA by heating and stirring continuously; cool to 37 °C.

Solution B

p-Chloroanilidophosphonic acid	0.15 g
1 M Sodium hydroxide	0.5 ml

This must be prepared immediately before use. Add to solution A.

Method

(1) Place mounted cryostat sections of unfixed tissue in substrate at 37 °C for up to 20 minutes.
(2) Wash well in running water and rinse in distilled water.
(3) Treat with 1% ammonium sulphide for 1 minute.
(4) Wash in distilled water and mount in an aqueous mountant.

Result

Sites of enzyme activity   Brown-black precipitate

Esterase

The esterases are found in the liver, pancreas, stomach, kidney, pituitary and nerve cells. They may be demonstrated by the azo-coupling technique, or by the bromo-indoxyl acetate method. These enzymes are partially resistant to cold acetone fixation and paraffin embedding, but for maximum enzyme activity cryostat sections of unfixed tissue should be used.

Esterases may be classified according to their behaviour in the presence of organophosphates or organomercurials. The organophosphates most commonly used are di-isopropyl fluorophosphate (DFP) or diethyl *p*-nitrophenyl phosphate (E600). *p*-Chloromercuribenzoate (PCMB) may be used as the organomercurial inhibitor. DFP and E600 inhibit B-esterases, PCMB inhibits A-esterase and the alkaloid physostigmine (Eserine) inhibits the cholinesterases.

These reactions are summarized in *Table 16.2*.

Table 16.2 Esterase inhibitors

	A-esterase	B-esterase	C-esterase	Cholinesterase
E600		+		+
PCMB	+			
Eserine				+

+ = Inhibition.
(Concentrations: E600, 10^{-5} M; PCMB, 10^{-3} M; Eserine, 10^{-5} M.)

The esterases are useful differentiators of white cell types. Chloroacetate esterase withstands paraffin processing and is a useful marker of the granulocyte series. Non-specific esterase helps differentiate monocytes (i.e. histiocytes or macrophages), whilst α-naphthol acid esterase can be used as a T-lymphocyte marker. These methods are given in Chapter 22.

■ **Azo-coupling technique (after Burstone, 1962)**

This method depends upon the liberation of naphthol from the naphthol acetate. The naphthol then couples with fast blue RR to form an insoluble azo-dye. Control by the use of inhibitors (*see above*).

Substrate solution

Naphthol AS–LC acetate	3 mg
Acetone	0.3 ml
Distilled water	15 ml
0.1 M Phosphate buffer pH 7.2	15 ml
Fast blue RR (or fast garnet GBC)	15 mg

Dissolve the naphthol acetate in the acetone, then add in the order given. When the fast blue RR is added, stir to dissolve, filter and use immediately.

Method

(1) Cut frozen or cryostat sections of unfixed tissue (acetone fixed, paraffin sections may be used).
(2) Place free-floating or mounted sections in substrate at room temperature for 10–30 minutes, until sufficient red or blue colour develops. Leave for 2 hours to report a negative reaction (Lillie, 1965).
(3) Wash well in water and mount in aqueous mountant.

Result

Sites of esterase activity   Red (or blue)

■ **Hexazotized pararosanilin method (Barka and Anderson, 1963)**

Reagents

A. Phosphate buffer M/15 pH 7.6

0.3 M Monobasic sodium phosphate (NaH_2PO_4)	13 ml
0.3 M Dibasic sodium phosphate (Na_2HPO_4)	87 ml
Distilled water	200 ml

B. Pararosanilin

Pararosanilin hydrochloride	2 g
2 N HCl	50 ml

Heat gently, cool and filter.

C. 4% Sodium nitrate

D. α-Naphthyl acetate

α-Naphthyl acetate	10 mg
Acetone	1 ml

Filter before use.

Working solution

A. 8.9 ml
B. 0.3 ml ⎫ mix for 1 minute before adding
C. 0.3 ml ⎭
D. 0.5 ml

Method

(1) Cut frozen or cryostat sections of unfixed tissue (acetone fixed, paraffin sections may be used), mount on slides and dry.
(2) Incubate sections for $1\frac{1}{2}$–2 hours at room temperature.
(3) Wash in water.
(4) Counterstain in chloroform washed methyl green if desired.
(5) Wash, dehydrate, clear and mount.

Results

Sites of esterase activity   Red/brown

■ Indoxyl acetate method for esterases (after Holt and Withers, 1952)

This method will demonstrate non-specific esterase, lipase and cholinesterase and may be controlled by use of inhibitors (*see above*). It is based upon the liberation of the indoxyl group which is then oxidized by the ferri-ferro-cyanide oxidant to indigo.

Control

See above.

Reagents

Oxidant

Potassium ferricyanide	210 mg
Potassium ferrocyanide	155 mg
Distilled water	to 100 ml

Substrate solution

Tris buffer (0.2 M) at pH 8.3	2 ml
Oxidant	1 ml
1 M Calcium chloride	0.1 ml
2 M Sodium chloride	5 ml
Distilled water	2 ml

Dissolve 1.3 mg of 5-bromoindoxyl acetate in 1 ml of absolute ethanol in a small beaker, then add the above solution (separately mixed) agitating to mix.

Method

(1) Place frozen or cryostat sections of unfixed tissue in substrate at 37 °C, leave for 30–120 minutes (usually 30 minutes).
(2) Wash in distilled water.
(3) Float sections on to slides and mount in aqueous mountant.

Result

Sites of esterase activity   Blue

Lipase

The Tween compounds are esters of long-chain fatty acids and either Sorbitan or Mannitan. The Tween numbers indicate the type of fatty acid—20 (lauric), 40 (palmitic), 60 (stearic) and 80 (oleic). An appropriate Tween compound is used as the substrate, usually 60 or 80.

The method is based upon the fact that the enzyme splits off the fatty acid which is trapped *in situ* as an insoluble calcium soap. These are converted into lead soaps, which are then blackened by ammonium sulphide.

Control

Leave Tween compound out of the substrate.

■ **Gomori's method (1952)**

Substrate solution

2% Tween 60 or 80 in water	5 ml
0.2 M Tris buffer pH 7.2	20 ml
4% Calcium chloride (anhyd.)	5 ml
Distilled water	20 ml

Method

(1) Cryostat sections on slides, of unfixed tissue (taken directly to step 4), will show the maximum activity. Gomori's original technique may be used as follows. Fix *fresh* tissue in chilled acetone and leave in refrigerator for 24 hours. Dehydrate in two changes of acetone (at room temperature) each of 2 hours, clear in xylene (two changes each of 45 minutes); embed in paraffin wax as quickly as possible.
(2) Cut thin sections; float on warm water (not above 35 °C if possible).
(3) Bring sections to water.
(4) Incubate in substrate at 37 °C for 6–24 hours.
(5) Rinse in distilled water.
(6) Treat with 2% lead nitrate for 10–15 minutes.
(7) Treat with 1% ammonium sulphide for 1 minute.
(8) Stain nuclei lightly with haematoxylin.
(9) Mount in glycerin jelly.

Results

Sites of lipase activity	Brown
Nuclei	Blue

Cholinesterases

These may be classified as acetyl-cholinesterase (true cholinesterase) and cholinesterase (pseudo-). Although they may be demonstrated by the methods above, they are more specifically visualized by the following method.

■ **Acetylthiocholine method (after Karnovsky and Roots, 1964)**

The basis for the method is that the thiocholine ester is hydrolysed by the enzyme, and the liberated thiocholine is believed to reduce ferricyanide to ferrocyanide which combines with the copper ions to form the insoluble copper ferrocyanide (Hatchett's Brown).

Controls

(1) ISO-OMPA (tetraisopropylpyrophosphoramide; Burstone, 1962) in a concentration of 3×10^{-6} M should inhibit (pseudo-) cholinesterase. It is added to a portion of the substrate lacking acetylthiocholine, sections are incubated for 30 minutes at 37 °C, then the acetylthiocholine is added and the sections incubated for a further 30 minutes. A positive reaction after this treatment should be considered due to acetylcholinesterase.
(2) 3×10^{-5} M Eserine sulphate should inhibit both these enzymes, without affecting the A and B type esterases (*see above*). The eserine is added to the normal substrate mixture.

Substrate solution

Acetylthiocholine iodide	5 mg
0.1 M Acetate buffer pH 5.5	6.5 ml

Dissolve the acetylthiocholine in the buffer then add the following in order, with stirring between each addition.

0.1 M Sodium citrate	0.5 ml
30 mM Copper sulphate	1 ml
Distilled water	1 ml
5 mM Potassium ferricyanide	1 ml

If eserine sulphate is used as an inhibitor it is added instead of the distilled water.
The stock solutions keep in the refrigerator for several weeks. The prepared substrate, which is clear and greenish in colour, is only stable for a few hours.

Method

(1) Tissue is fixed overnight in cold formal–calcium, and then transferred to sucrose–gum solution (*see* page 301). The best results are obtained if tissues are left in the latter for 7–30 days, but reasonable results are possible after 24 hours. Blocks are washed in distilled water and frozen or cryostat sections are cut. The sections may be free-floating or affixed to slides or coverslips.
(2) Incubate sections in substrate at room temperature for 2–6 hours (brain sections take about 3 hours).
(3) Wash in water, float on to slides (if necessary) and mount in an aqueous mountant.

Result

Enzyme activity	Fine brown precipitate

Leucine aminopeptidase

This enzyme is found in highest concentration in kidneys or small intestine. It is also present in muscle, skin, CNS, spleen and lymph nodes.

■ Simultaneous coupling method (Burstone and Folk, 1956)

The aminopeptidase is demonstrated by its action on L-leucyl-β-naphthylamide, it releases β-naphthylamide which couples with the fast garnet GBC to produce an insoluble red precipitate at the sites of reaction.

Control

Omit L-leucyl-β-naphthylamide from substrate.

Substrate solution

1% L-Leucyl-β-naphthylamide	1 ml
Distilled water	40 ml
pH 7.1 tris buffer	10 ml
Garnet GBC (fast garnet GBC)	30 mg

This solution should be freshly prepared and filtered before use.

Method

(1) Bring frozen, cryostat or freeze-dried sections of *fresh* tissue to distilled water.
(2) Place sections into substrate at room temperature for 15 minutes to 3 hours.
(3) Wash well in water.
(4) Mount in glycerin jelly or Apathy's medium.

Result

Sites of enzyme activity   Red

■ Chelation method (Nachlas, Crawford and Seligman, 1957)

In this method copper is chelated to the azo-dye formed in the simultaneous coupling method. This allows sections to be dehydrated, cleared and mounted in a synthetic resin for better definition and more permanent preparation.

Stock substrate solution

(A) 0.8% L-Leucyl-β-naphthylamide
(B) 0.8% L-Leucyl-4-methoxy-β-naphthylamide

Either of these solutions may be used. They can be prepared and stored in the refrigerator for 2–3 months.

Substrate solution

Stock solution (A) or (B)	1 ml
0.1 M Acetate buffer pH 6.5	10 ml

0.85% Sodium chloride	8 ml
Potassium cyanide (2×10^{-2} M)	1 ml
Fast blue B salt	10 mg

Method

(1) Bring frozen, cryostat or freeze-dried sections of *fresh* tissue to distilled water.
(2) Incubate sections in substrate for 15 minutes to 4 hours at 37 °C (until sections are red).
(3) Rinse in 0.85% saline.
(4) Place in 0.1 M cupric sulphate.
(5) Rinse in 0.85% saline.
(6) Mount in glycerin jelly, or dehydrate, clear and mount in synthetic resin.

Results

Sites of enzyme activity   Red with (A); purple with (B)

β-Glucuronidase

This enzyme occurs in most tissues, with higher concentrations being reported in liver, kidney, spleen, lung, adrenal, thyroid and uterus. Within cells its location seems to be mainly in the mitochondrial or lysosomal fractions. The histochemical demonstrations of this enzyme is used to distinguish carcinomas (by its presence) from sarcomas in which it is minimal or absent.

■ Post-coupling method (Chayen and colleagues, 1969)

The simultaneous coupling technique is not recommended because of the possible inhibitor effect of the diazonium compounds, and because with post-coupling the substrate can be used at the optimal pH of the enzyme (4.5) at which the coupler is not efficient.

The method is based upon the liberation of the Naphthol AS–BI which is deposited at the site of enzyme activity, and subsequently coupled with the fast dark blue R to visualize it.

Controls

Potassium hydrogen saccharate, 0.05 g, is added to 22 ml of substrate. This gives complete inhibition of β-glucuronidase activity.

Stock substrate solution

Naphthol AS–BI glucuronide	11.4 mg
0.05 M Sodium bicarbonate (0.42%)	1 ml
0.2 M Acetate buffer (pH 4.5)	49 ml

Dissolve the Naphthol AS–BI glucuronide in the bicarbonate and add the buffer. This will keep indefinitely in the refrigerator.

PVA solution

Calcium chloride ($CaCl_2 . 6 H_2O$)   0.5 g
0.1 M Acetate buffer (pH 4.5)   100 ml
Polyvinyl alcohol   10 g

Dissolve the calcium chloride in the buffer. Add the PVA and heat (but not boil) with frequent mixing to dissolve. Cool before use.

Substrate solution

PVA solution   20 ml
Stock substrate   2 ml

Coupling solution

Fast dark blue R   8 mg
Ice-cold, 0.01 M phosphate buffer (pH 7.4)   20 ml

Dissolve fast blue in buffer at 4 °C, filter while still cold (4 °C) and use immediately.

Activator medium

Calcium chloride, 0.5%, in 0.1 M acetate buffer (pH 4.5). Sections may be immersed in this medium for 2 minutes prior to transfer to substrate.

Method

(1) Cut cryostat or frozen sections of unfixed tissue and attach to slides or coverslips.
(2) Immerse in substrate at 37 °C for 30–180 minutes. This time may be reduced by pretreatment with activator.
(3) Wash in activator medium.
(4) Immerse sections in ice-cold coupling solution for 5 minutes.
(5) Rinse in distilled water.
(6) Mount in glycerin jelly.

Results

Enzyme activity   Dark blue granules

Phosphorylases

Phosphorylase occurs in tissue in two forms, an enzymatically active form, *phosphorylase a* (α-glucan phosphorylase), and an enzymatically inactive form *phosphorylase b*. The 'inactive' (b) enzyme can be converted to the 'active' (a) by the enzymatic addition of two phosphate groups to each molecule of (b). This conversion is utilized in the technique below to give *total potential phosphorylase activity*, in addition to the *manifest existing activity*. Phosphorylases appear to play a major role in controlling glycogen metabolism in animal cells; the highest concentrations being found in the liver, and in voluntary and heart muscle. Myophosphorylase is absent in McArdle's disease. The demonstration of phosphorylase activity can be used to type skeletal muscle fibres.

■ Takeuchi's method (Takeuchi and Kuriaki, 1955; Chayen *et al.*, 1969)

The substrate contains glycogen, and glucose-1-phosphate, the phosphorylase (if present) will increase the size of the glycogen by accretion of glucose units from the glucose-1-phosphate. AMP is added as an activator. The extended molecules of glycogen, which should become attached to the section, are demonstrated by their reaction with the iodine. The iodine is thought to stain linear amylase blue, and branched polysaccharide red-brown; the latter is interpreted by some workers as demonstrating the presence of the *branching enzyme.*

Control

Leave glucose-1-phosphate out of substrate. Pretreatment of sections with diastase ensures that glycogen demonstrated has been formed during the reaction.

Substrate for manifest activity

Glucose-1-phosphate	50 mg
Sodium fluoride	15 mg
AMP (adenosine-5-phosphate)	10 mg
EDTA	10 mg
Glycogen	5 mg
Insulin	0.5 mg
Distilled water	15 ml
0.5 M Acetate buffer (pH 5.8)	10 ml

Substrate for total potential activity

As above, *plus* 10 mg of ATP and 10 mg of magnesium sulphate but *minus* the EDTA.

Glycerin–iodine solution

Equal parts of glycerin and Lugol's iodine.

Method

(1) Cut cryostat sections of unfixed tissue. Leave section at room temperature for 10 minutes to enhance binding of glycogen.
(2) Incubate in substrate for 20 minutes at 37 °C.
(3) Wash briefly in distilled water.
(4) Immerse in Gram's iodine, diluted 1:2 with distilled water for 30 seconds.
(5) Wash in water.
(6) Mount in glycerin–iodine solution.

Results

Blue or red-brown deposits of synthesized polysaccharide indicate sites of enzyme activity.

Haemoglobin peroxidase

Haemoglobin peroxidase is a relatively stable enzyme, resistant to short fixation in formalin. The peroxidase of the granular leucocyte and their precursors is almost as stable but not so resistant to the action of formalin.

■ **Lison–Dunn method (Dunn, 1946)**

Reagent

Leuco patent blue V

To 100 ml of a 1% aqueous solution of patent blue V, add 10 g of powdered zinc and 2 ml of glacial acetic acid. Boil this mixture until it is a pale straw colour (approximately 10 minutes). Cool, filter and store in a stoppered bottle. The stock solution is stable.

Just before use, add 2 ml of glacial acetic acid and 1 ml of 3% (10 vol.) hydrogen peroxide to 10 ml of the stock leuco patent blue.

Method

(1) Fix tissues in buffered formalin for not more than 48 hours.
(2) Embed in paraffin wax and cut sections 5–7 μm thick.
(3) Bring sections to water.
(4) Stain for 5 minutes in leuco patent blue reagent.
(5) Rinse in water.
(6) Counterstain nuclei in safranin for 1 minute.
(7) Rinse in water.
(8) Dehydrate, clear and mount in resinous mountant.

Results

Haemoglobin   Dark blue
Oxidase granules   Dark blue
Nuclei   Red

Dopa-oxidase (tyrosinase)

Dopa-oxidase is thought to be responsible for the conversion of tyrosine into melanin. The initials DOPA stand for dihydroxyphenylalanine, and this was originally thought to be the precursor of melanin, and it is for this reason the enzyme concerned in this conversion was called Dopa-oxidase.

Controls

Pre-incubate sections in 10^{-3} potassium cyanide (3.25 mg/50 ml), also add 10^{-3} of potassium cyanide to control substrate (step 3).

■ **Dopa-oxidase reaction (Becker, Praver and Thatcher, 1935)**

Method

(1) Fix pieces of tissue 5 mm thick in 10% formalin for 1 hour at room temperature.

(2) Wash in running water for 3–4 minutes.
(3) Place in 0.1% DOPA in 0.1 M phosphate buffer (pH 7.4) at 37 °C and leave for 1 hour.
(4) Change into fresh DOPA reagent, and leave for 12 hours at 37 °C.
(5) Wash in running water.
(6) Fix in Bouin's fluid for 24 hours.
(7) Dehydrate, clear in xylene and embed in paraffin wax.
(8) Cut thin sections, attach to slides.
(9) Bring sections to water, counterstain with haematoxylin and eosin (or tartrazine in Cellosolve).
(10) Dehydrate, clear and mount in resinous mountant.

Results

Dopa-oxidase (tyrosinase)   Dark brown granules
Other structures   Depending on the counterstain

Cytochrome oxidase

The demonstration of this enzyme is based on the fact that cytochrome oxidase will act as a catalyst for the oxidation reaction between α-naphthol and a dimethyl-*p*-phenylaminediamine hydrochloride to form indophenol blue ('Nadi' reaction).

Controls

Add 10^{-3} M of potassium cyanide (3.25 mg/50 ml) to control Nadi reagent.

■ Gräff's G–Nadi reaction

Reagents

(1) α-Naphthol solution. α-Naphthol, 0.1 g, is dissolved in 1 ml of alcohol, and then made up to 100 ml with distilled water.
(2) Oxidase reagent. Dissolve dimethyl-*p*-phenylaminediamine hydrochloride, 0.12 g, in 100 ml of distilled water. This solution should be colourless, or just tinted, otherwise it should be discarded. If this reaction is performed infrequently it is better to prepare small amounts fresh for each batch of sections. It should be stored in a dark brown bottle.
(3) Nadi reagent. Mix 20 ml each of α-naphthol solution and oxidase reagent, and to the mixture add 8 ml of 0.1 M phosphate buffer pH 7.5.

Method

(1) Cut frozen sections of fresh, unfixed tissue.
(2) Incubate in Nadi reagent at 37 °C for 1 hour.
(3) Transfer sections to normal saline solution.
(4) Counterstain nuclei (optional).
(5) Float on to slides, drain and mount in 20% potassium acetate solution.
(6) Ring coverslip with paraffin wax, and examine. These preparations are not permanent.

Results

Cytochrome oxidase   Blue-violet

Burstone proposed several methods for the demonstration of cytochrome oxidase using different amines and different couplers. The most popular amine was *p*-amino-diphenylamine (N-phenyl-*p*-phenylene diamine) which may be used with several different couplers. Metal chelation is sometimes employed. One method is given below.

■ **Amine–amine method (Burstone, 1961b)**

Substrate solution

p-Aminodiphenylamine	10 mg
p-Methoxy-*p'*-aminodiphenylamine (Variamine blue B base)	10 mg
Ethanol	0.5 ml
Distilled water	35 ml
0.2 M Tris–HCl buffer (pH 7.4)	15 ml

Dissolve the amines in the ethanol (reagent grade), then add the distilled water and buffer. Filter before use. If tissues are known to have low enzyme activity add 10–20 mg cytochrome C and dissolve.

Method

(1) Incubate fresh frozen mounted and air-dried sections in substrate solution for $\frac{1}{4}$–2 hours.
(2) Wash briefly.
(3) Counterstain in 1% methyl green for 2 minutes.
(4) Wash briefly.
(5) Mount in aqueous mountant.

Result

Sites of cytochrome oxidase activity   Brownish red

Dehydrogenases and diaphorases

These enzymes oxidize their substrates by removing hydrogen from the substrate and transferring it to an appropriate acceptor. Many of the dehydrogenases transfer the hydrogen to either of the two co-enzymes nicotinamide-adenine-dinucleotide (NAD) or nicotinamide-adenine-dinucleotide phosphate (NADP). The reduced co-enzymes are themselves oxidized by the enzymes NADH-diaphorase or NADPH-diaphorase.

The demonstration of NADH-diaphorase or NADPH-diaphorase activity therefore indicates the presence of an NAD- or NADP-linked dehydrogenase. A particular dehydrogenase can be demonstrated using the specific substrate with either NAD or NADP as co-enzyme.

The diaphorase transfers the hydrogen to a tetrazolium salt. The tetrazolium salt can accept two atoms of hydrogen producing an insoluble coloured formazan.

$$C_6H_5-N-N$$
$$C-C_6H_5 + 2\ H \longrightarrow$$
$$C_6H_5-N^+=N$$
$$Cl^-$$

$$C_6H_5-NH-N$$
$$C-C_6H_5 + HCl$$
$$CC_6H_5-N=N$$

Many new tetrazolium compounds based on triphenyl tetrazolium chloride (TTC) have been introduced for use in dehydrogenase histochemistry. They are either monotetrazolium salts (e.g. INT and MTT) or ditetrazolium salts (e.g. Nitro-BT and TNBT), the chemical names being abbreviated. Tetrazolium salts must be capable of being easily reduced, intercepting hydrogen atoms which would otherwise pass along the electron transport chain resulting in the formation of a highly coloured, insoluble formazan. The distribution of the formazan will reflect the distribution of the diaphorase, not necessarily that of the specific dehydrogenase.

Phenazine methosulphate (PMS) can, however, be used to transfer the hydrogen directly from the reduced co-enzyme (NADH or NADPH) to the tetrazolium salt, by-passing the diaphorase, and thus showing the distribution of the specific dehydrogenase.

Succinate dehydrogenase and α-glycerophosphate dehydrogenase (EC1.1.99.5) are examples of dehydrogenases transferring hydrogen to a different co-enzyme (co-enzyme Q_{10}). For the demonstration of these enzymes, menadione is often included in the incubation medium. This compound will accept hydrogen from the enzymes and transfer it to the tetrazolium salt thus compensating for low levels of endogenous Q_{10}.

■ Standard method for dehydrogenases and diaphorases (after Pearse, 1972)

Stock 0.2 M tris buffer (pH 7.4)

2.42% Tris (hydroxymethyl) aminomethane	20.7 ml
0.2 M Hydrochloric acid	79.3 ml

Table 16.2 Stock substrate solutions (pH 7.0)

	Amount	Distilled water	NHCl
Bound enzymes			
Disodium succinate	6.75 g	8 ml	0.05 ml
Sodium D-3-hydroxybutyrate	1.27 g	8 ml	0.15 ml
Sodium L-glutamate monohydrate	1.87 g	8 ml	0.05 ml
Disodium glycerol-3-phosphate[1]	3.15 g	8 ml	0.7 ml
Soluble enzymes			
Sodium-L-malate	1.87 g	8 ml	[3]
Trisodium-DL-isocitrate	2.76 g	8 ml	0.9 ml
Sodium-DL-lactate	1.25 ml	—	—
Disodium glycerol-3-phosphate[2]	3.15 g	8 ml	0.7 ml
Disodium glucose-6-phosphate	3.04 g	8 ml	0.6 ml
Barium-6-phosphogluconic acid	4.3 g	8 ml	0.6 ml
Ethanol	0.58 ml	8 ml	[4]

After neutralization the volume is made up to 10 ml. These solutions are stable at $-20\ ^\circ$C for several months.
[1] Add 5 mg menadione to 1 ml stock solution, incubate for 1 hour at 37 $^\circ$C and filter before use.
[2] For the soluble enzyme the stock solution should be made up in 0.06 M phosphate buffer instead of 0.2 M tris buffer.
[3] Neutralization with 0.9 ml 40% sodium hydroxide.
[4] Neutralization with 1 drop stock tris buffer pH 10.4.

Stock incubating solution

Nitro-BT (4 mg/ml)	2.5 ml
Tris buffer pH 7.4	2.5 ml
50 mM Magnesium chloride	1.0 ml
Distilled water	3.0 ml

pH should be adjusted to pH 7.0–7.2 with 0.2 M tris (hydroxymethyl) aminomethane. Store at −20 °C.

Stock respiratory chain inhibitor

Sodium cyanide 0.1 M (prepare freshly).

Table 16.3 Incubating media

	Stock incubating solution (ml)	Stock substrate solution (ml)	Distilled water (ml)	NaCN (ml)	Co-enzyme (2 mg)	PVP (optional) (mg)
Bound enzymes						
NADH	0.9	—	0.1	—	NADH	—
NADPH	0.9	—	0.1	—	NADPH	—
Succinate	0.9	0.1	—	—	—	—
Hydroxybutyrate	0.9	0.1	—	—	NAD	—
Glutamate	0.9	0.1	—	—	NAD or NADP	—
α-Glycerophosphate	0.9	0.1	—	—	—	—
Soluble enzymes						
Malate	0.9	0.1	—	—	NAD	—
Isocitrate	0.9	0.1	—	0.1	NAD or NADP	—
Lactate	0.9	0.1	—	—	NAD	75
α-Glycerophosphate	0.9	0.1	—	—	NAD	75
Glucose-6-phosphate	0.9	0.1	—	0.1	NADP	75
Phosphogluconate	0.9	0.1	—	0.1	NADP	75
Alcohol	0.9	0.1	—	—	NAD	—

Add co-enzyme just before use and adjust to pH 7.0–7.1 if necessary.
Note: If PMS is to be used with any of the above media 1 mg should be added (per ml) and incubation carried out in the dark.

Method

(1) Mount cryostat sections on coverslips.
(2) Cover sections with incubating medium (0.2 ml) and incubate at 37 °C for 10–60 minutes.
(3) Pour off incubating medium and immerse in 15% formal–saline for 15 minutes.
(4) Wash in distilled water for 2 minutes.
(5) Counterstain in carmalum.
(6) Rinse in distilled water.
(7) Dehydrate, clear in xylene and mount in synthetic resin.

Result

Sites of enzyme activity   Purple formazan deposit

Note

If MTT is the tetrazolium salt used, the sections should be mounted in glycerin jelly.

References

BARKA, T. and ANDERSON, P. J. (1963). *Histochemistry*. Harper & Row, New York

BECKER, S. W., PRAVER, L. L. and THATCHER, H. (1935). An improved (paraffin section) method for the DOPA reaction. *Arch. Derm. Syph.*, **31**, 190–195

BURSTONE, M. S. (1960). Postcoupling, noncoupling and fluorescence techniques for the demonstration of alkaline phosphatase. *J. Nat. Cancer Inst.*, **24**, 1199–1207

BURSTONE, M. S. (1961a). Histochemical demonstration of phosphatases in frozen sections with naphthol AS-phosphates. *J. Histochem. Cytochem.*, **9**, 146–153

BURSTONE, M. S. (1961b). Modifications of histochemical techniques for the demonstration of cytochrome oxidase. *J. Histochem. Cytochem.*, **9**, 59–65

BURSTONE, M. S. (1962). *Enzyme Histochemistry*. Academic Press, New York

BURSTONE, M. S. and FOLK, J. E. (1956). Histochemical demonstration of aminopeptidase. *J. Histochem. Cytochem.*, **4**, 217–226

CHAYEN, J., BITENSKY, L., BUTCHER, R. and POULTER, L. (1969). *A Guide to Practical Histochemistry*. Oliver and Boyd, Edinburgh

DIXON, M. and WEBB, E. C. (1958). *Enzymes*. Longman, London

DIXON, M., WEBB, E. C., THORNE, C. J. R. and TIPTON, K. F. (1979). *Enzymes*. 3rd Ed. Longman, London

DUNN, R. C. (1946). A haemoglobin stain for histologic use based on the cyanol-haemoglobin stain. *Arch. Pathol.*, **41**, 676–677

GOMORI, G. (1941). Distribution of acid phosphatase in the tissues under normal and under pathologic conditions. *Arch. Pathol.*, **32**, 189–199

GOMORI, G. (1948). Histochemical demonstration of sites of phosphoamidase activity. *Proc. Soc. Exp. Biol. Med.*, **69**, 407–409

GOMORI, G. (1952). Histochemistry of esterases. *Int. Rev. Cytol.*, **1**, 323–335

HOLT, S. J. (1959). Factors governing the validity of staining methods for enzymes and their bearing upon the Gomori acid phosphatase technique. *Exp. Cell. Res. Suppl.*, **7**, 1–27

HOLT, S. J. and WITHERS, R. F. J. (1952). Cytochemical localisation of esterases using indoxyl derivatives. *Nature*, **170**, 1012–1014

KARNOVSKY, M. J. and ROOTS, L. (1964). A 'direct-colouring' thiocholine method for cholinesterases. *J. Histochem. Cytochem.*, **12**, 219–221

LEHNINGER, A. L. (1960). The enzymic and morphologic organisation of the mitochondria. *Pediatrics*, **26**, 466–475

MENTEN, M. L., JUNGE, J. and GREEN, M. H. (1944). A coupling histochemical azo dye test for alkaline phosphatase in kidney. *J. Biol. Chem.*, **153**, 471–477

MOSES, H. L., ROSENTHAL, A. S., BEAVER, D. L. and SCHUFFMAN, S. S. (1966). Lead ion and phosphatase histochemistry. II. Effect of adenosine triphosphate hydrolysis by lead ion on the histochemical localisation of adenosine triphosphatase activity. *J. Histochem. Cytochem.*, **14**, 702–710

NACHLAS, M. M., CRAWFORD, D. T. and SELIGMAN, A. M. (1957). The histochemical demonstration of leucine aminopeptidase. *J. Histochem. Cytochem.*, **5**, 264–278

NACHLAS, M. M., PRINN, W. and SELIGMAN, A. M. (1956). Quantitative assessment of lyo- and desmoenzymes in tissue sections with and without fixation. *J. Biophys. Biochem. Cytol.*, **2**, 487–502

NACHLAS, M. M., YOUNG, A. C. and SELIGMAN, A. M. (1957). Problems of enzymatic localisation by chemical reactions applied to tissue sections. *J. Histochem. Cytochem.*, **5**, 565–583

NILES, N. R., CHAYEN, J., CUNNINGHAM, G. J. and BITENSKY, L. (1964). The histochemical demonstration of adenosine triphosphatase activity in myocardium. *J. Histochem. Cytochem.*, **12**, 740–743

PEARSE, A. G. E. (1968). *Histochemistry, Theoretical and Applied*. 3rd Ed. Vol. 1. Churchill-Livingstone, London

PEARSE, A. G. E. (1972). *Histochemistry, Theoretical and Applied*. 3rd Ed. Vol. 2. Churchill-Livingstone, Edinburgh and London

PEARSE, A. G. E. (1980). *Histochemistry, Theoretical and Applied.* 4th Ed. Vol. 1. Preparative and optical technology. Churchill-Livingstone, Edinburgh

PEARSE, A. G. E. and REIS, J. L. (1952). The histochemical demonstration of a specific phosphatase (5-nucleotidase). *Biochem. J.,* **50,** 534–536

ROSENTHAL, A. S., MOSES, H. L., BEAVER, D. L. and SCHUFFMAN, S. S. (1966). Lead ion and phosphatase histochemistry. I. Nonenzymatic hydrolysis of nucleoside phosphates by lead ion. *J. Histochem. Cytochem.,* **14,** 698–701

RUTENBERG, A. M. and SELIGMAN, A. M. (1955). The histochemical demonstration of acid phosphatase by a post-incubation coupling technique. *J. Histochem. Cytochem.,* **3,** 455–470

SELIGMAN, A. M., CHAUNCEY, H. H. and NACHLAS, M. M. (1951). Effect of formalin fixation on the activity of five enzymes of rat liver. *Stain Technol.,* **26,** 19–23

TAKEUCHI, T. and KURIAKI, H. (1955). Histochemical detection of phosphorylase in animal tissues. *J. Histochem. Cytochem.,* **3,** 153–160

TORMEY, J. McD. (1966). Significance of the histochemical demonstration of ATPase in epithelia noted for active transport. *Nature (Lond.),* **210,** 820–822

WACHSTEIN, M. and MEISEL, E. (1952). Histochemical demonstration of 5-nucleotidase activity in cell nuclei. *Science,* **115,** 652–653

WACHSTEIN, M. and MEISEL, E. (1956). On the histochemical demonstration of glucose-6-phosphatase. *J. Histochem. Cytochem.,* **4,** 592

WACHSTEIN, M. and MEISEL, E. (1957). Histochemistry of hepatic phosphatases at a physiologic pH with special reference to the demonstration of bile canaliculi. *Am. J. Clin. Pathol.,* **27,** 13–23

17

Micro-organisms

Bacteria

Bacteria in sections are usually stained by slight modifications of those stains employed for smears, such modifications usually being designed to demonstrate the tissue constituents; for example, Gram–Weigert.

Gram-positive bacteria

Gram-positive bacteria may be stained by the simple acetone–Gram technique which will suffice for routine purposes, or by the Gram–Weigert method in which the Gram's stain is superimposed on a haematoxylin and eosin stain.

■ Gram's method (modified)

Reagent

Lugol's iodine

Iodine	1 g
Potassium iodide	2 g
Distilled water	to 100 ml

Dissolve the potassium iodide in 4–5 ml of water; dissolve the iodine in this. Dilute to 100 ml to make Lugol's iodine, or to 300 ml to make Gram's iodine.

Method

(1) Bring sections to water.
(2) Stain with 0.5% aqueous methyl violet 6 B for 1–3 minutes.
(3) Rinse with water.
(4) Pour on Lugol's iodine for 1–3 minutes (or Gram's iodine for 2 minutes).
(5) Differentiate rapidly with acetone (1–2 seconds) and wash immediately in running water.
(6) Counterstain with 1% neutral red or safranin for 1 minute.
(7) Wash in water.
(8) Dehydrate, clear and mount.

Results

Gram-positive organisms	Blue-black
Other tissue structures	Shades of red

■ **Gram–Weigert method**

Reagent

Aniline crystal violet

Crystal violet (*see note below*)	5 g
Absolute alcohol	10 ml
Aniline	2 ml
Distilled water	88 ml

This solution keeps well.

Note: An explanation of the relationship of methyl, crystal and gentian violet to each other is thought worthwhile. These violet dyes consist of a *para*-rosanilin structure with a varying number of methyl groups attached, the number of which decide the actual shade of violet ranging from reddish to bluish violet. Methyl violet may be obtained as 2 R, R, B, 2 B, 6 B, and in that range the number indicates the depth of colour, and the letter the shade, therefore 6 B is a bluer shade than B, or 2 B. Gentian violet is a misture of ill-defined rosanilins and is in no way standardized. Crystal violet is a hexamethyl *para*-rosanilin, and is sometimes known as methyl violet 10 B. It is a definite bluish violet in colour, with a specific formula.

For these reasons, methyl violet of a specified shade or crystal violet should always be used to obtain standardized results.

Method

(1) Bring sections to water.
(2) Stain nuclei lightly with alum haematoxylin.
(3) Blue in tap-water.
(4) Stain in 2.5% aqueous phloxine or eosin for 10 minutes at 56 °C.
(5) Wash in water.
(6) Stain in aniline crystal violet for $\frac{1}{2}$–1 hour.
(7) Rinse in water.
(8) Treat with Lugol's iodine (*see above*) for 1 minute.
(9) Blot with fine filter paper.
(10) Differentiate with equal parts of xylene and aniline until only bacteria and fibrin are blue-black (it is almost impossible to overdifferentiate).
(11) Rinse in xylene to remove aniline, and mount in synthetic resin.

Results

Gram-positive organisms	Blue-black
Nuclei	Blue
Other tissue constituents	Shades of red

Gram-negative bacteria

Gram-negative bacteria may usually be demonstrated by staining sections with Leishman or Giemsa stain in addition to 'control' sections stained by Gram's stain. Organisms present in the Leishman slide which are not Gram-positive are assumed to be Gram-negative. In practice this method works well.

There are a number of other methods described for the differentiation of Gram-positive and Gram-negative bacteria, but of these only the following has given consistent results.

■ Ollett's modification of Twort's stain

This method (Ollett, 1951) is simple and gives reasonable contrast between Gram-positive bacteria, Gram-negative bacteria and tissues. The light green in Twort's stain is replaced by fast green FCF to avoid fading.

Reagent

Modified Twort's stain

0.2% Alcoholic neutral red	90 ml
0.2% Alcoholic fast green FCF	10 ml

For use, dilute one volume of the above stock solution with three volumes of distilled water.

The pH of this stain, like that of Twort's stain, is 4.9; it may depend on the dye samples used, but uniformity can be secured by diluting the stock solution in M/5 acetate buffer instead of distilled water.

The proportions of the dyes given are only approximate, and the optimum formula will depend on the dye content of the samples used. The stock alcoholic solution should be of reddish-magenta tint; too much green will weaken the red bacterial staining; the total dye concentration is less critical.

Method

(1) Fix material in 5% formal–saline, pass through the alcohols and embed in paraffin.
(2) Cut sections 3 μm in thickness.
(3) Bring sections to distilled water.
(4) Stain in aniline crystal violet for 3–5 minutes.
(5) Pour off stain and wash quickly in distilled water.
(6) Treat with Gram's iodine for 3 minutes.
(7) Pour off the iodine, wash quickly in distilled water and blot dry.
(8) Decolorize with 2% acetic acid in absolute alcohol until no more colour comes away—the section should be a dirty straw colour at this stage.
(9) Wash quickly in distilled water.
(10) Counterstain in the modified Twort's neutral red–fast green stain, diluted 1 part with 3 parts of distilled water, or pH 4.9 buffer, for 5 minutes.
(11) Wash quickly in distilled water.
(12) Differentiate with 2% acetic acid alcohol until no more red stain (neutral red) comes away (15–30 seconds).
(13) Clear in xylene and mount in synthetic resin.

Results

Nuclei	Red
Cytoplasm	Light green
Red blood corpuscles	Green
Gram-positive bacteria	Dark blue
Gram-negative bacteria	Pink

■ Brown and Brenn method (1931)

Reagents

Crystal violet stain

1% Crystal violet in distilled water	4 parts
5% Sodium bicarbonate in distilled water	1 part

   Mix together immediately before use.

Basic fuchsin stain

0.25% Basic fuchsin in distilled water. Dilute with an equal part of distilled water for use.

Differentiator

Picric acid	0.1 g
Acetone	100 ml

Method

(1) Bring sections to water.
(2) Stain with crystal violet solution for 1 minute.
(3) Wash in water.
(4) Flood slide with Gram's iodine and leave for 1 minute.
(5) Rinse in water and blot with filter paper to complete dryness.
(6) Decolorize with a mixture of equal parts acetone and ether dropped on the slide until no more blue colour runs off.
(7) Stain with basic fuchsin for 1 minute.
(8) Wash in water and blot gently but do not dry completely.
(9) Dip in acetone.
(10) Differentiate immediately with the picric acid differentiator until the sections are yellowish pink.
(11) Rinse quickly in acetone followed by equal parts acetone/xylene.
(12) Clear in xylene and mount.

Results

Gram-positive bacteria	Blue
Gram-negative bacteria and nuclei	Red
Other tissue elements	Yellow

Legionella pneumophilla

This coccobacillus is found in the lungs in legionnaire's disease. It is difficult to detect being weakly Gram-negative. Modifications of the Dieterle silver impregnation technique (1927), Van Orden and Greer (1977), have given unsatisfactory results in our hands with tissue sections although the results were satisfactory with smears. The Levaditi block impregnation method gave satisfactory results.

Immunocytochemical techniques seem to show most promise.

Actinomyces

Actinomyces, sometimes referred to as the 'ray fungus', has a characteristic appearance, both to the naked eye and microscopically. The yellow pus present in actinomycosis contains numerous small granules (so-called 'sulphur granules'), which on section are seen to consist of a matted mass of branching mycelia; the mass may be surrounded by radiating club-shaped bodies. The filaments are sometimes segmented and give the appearance of cocci or short bacilli.

Staining reactions

The mycelium is Gram-positive, PAS-negative and non-acid-fast; the clubs are Gram-negative, PAS-positive and acid-fast (using Ziehl–Neelsen's stain).

Gridley's method (page 342) may be used to demonstrate these organisms, as may the Giemsa or Leishman stains.

Acid-fast bacilli

In spite of the multiplicity of methods now available, the author prefers the traditional Ziehl–Neelsen technique for the demonstration of *Mycobacterium tuberculosis* as a conventional method. If the equipment is available the fluorescent technique (*see* page 337) should be used. A satisfactory alternative is the use of night blue or Victoria blue R in place of basic fuchsin, with a safranin or tartrazine in Cellosolve counterstain; this gives blue bacilli.

Fixation

Formal–saline gives excellent results, although any of the routine fixatives may be used with the possible exception of Carnoy's fluid, which would tend to remove lipid material from the bacilli, and render them non-acid-fast.

Processing

Although the use of water-soluble wax has been recommended to avoid clearing reagents, for routine purposes this is unnecessary.

■ Ziehl–Neelsen method

Reagent

Carbol–fuchsin

Basic fuchsin	1 g
Absolute alcohol	10 ml
5% Phenol (aqueous)	100 ml

Dissolve the basic fuchsin in the alcohol, then add the 5% phenol.

Method

(1) Bring section to water.
(2) Stain in hot carbol–fuchsin, *either* in a Coplin jar in a 56 °C oven for 30 minutes, *or* by covering section with a small square of filter paper (to avoid precipitate on sections), flooding the slide with stain, heating until the stain steams and leaving for 10 minutes.
(3) Wash in water to remove excess stain.
(4) Differentiate in 3% hydrochloric acid in 70% alcohol until tissue is a very pale pink colour when washed in water (approximately 5–10 minutes).
(5) Wash in water.
(6) Counterstain lightly in 0.1% methylene blue for 10–15 seconds (if too heavy a counterstain is used, bacilli may be difficult to find).
(7) Wash in water.
(8) Dehydrate, clear and mount in synthetic resin.

Results

Acid-fast bacilli	Red
Nuclei	Blue
Other tissue constituents	Pale blue

Note: In a well-stained section tubercle bacilli should be clearly visible when using a ×40 objective.

■ Modified Ziehl–Neelsen technique for *Mycobacterium leprae*

Since this organism is not so acid-fast as *M. tuberculosis*, either a 1% acid alcohol should be used to differentiate in the above technique, or the Wade–Fite method should be employed. *M. tuberculosis* will also stain.

■ Wade–Fite method for *M. leprae* in paraffin sections (modified from Wade, 1957)

According to the originators of this method, the bacilli are protected from extraction of their lipids during the deparaffinization, but Azulay and Andrade (1954) suggest that this new technique is not exclusively one of protection of the acid-fastness of *M. leprae* in the lesions, but that it also has the property of restoring acid-fastness which has been lost in the processing.

Method

(1) Deparaffinize sections with a mixture of equal parts of liquid petrolatum and rectified turpentine.
(2) Blot with filter paper until of semi-dry appearance.
(3) Wash in water for 5 minutes.
(4) Stain in carbol–fuchsin for 25–30 minutes at room temperature.
(5) Wash in water, and blot with filter paper.
(6) Decolorize with 10% sulphuric acid.
(7) Wash in water.
(8) Stain with alum haematoxylin for 5–10 minutes.
(9) Wash in water for 10 minutes.
(10) Blot with filter paper in an incubator at 56 °C to dry.
(11) Clear in xylene and mount in Canada balsam or synthetic resin.

Results

| *M. leprae* | Red |
| Nuclei | Blue |

■ Fluorescent demonstration of acid-fast bacilli in sections and smears

Fluorescence microscopy for the detection of acid-fast bacilli has been used widely for years. It has probably not become universally used due to the lack of, or inadequacy of, fluorescence equipment. However, with the equipment now available the fluorescence method is reliable, sensitive and permits very rapid screening of sections and smears. By using the method in duplicate with Ziehl–Neelsen technique, organisms have on several occasions been found reasonably quickly, which could only be found on repeated examinations by the conventional method. Wellman and Teng (1962) found that positive cases are three times as likely to be overlooked by the ZN method as they are by the fluorescence method.

Fixation

This does not appear to be critical. Formalin or Zenker fixatives give good results.

Reagent

Staining solution

Auramine O	1.5 g
Rhodamine B	0.75 g
Glycerol	75 ml
Phenol cryst. (liquified at 50 °C)	10 ml
Distilled water	50 ml

Method (*Kuper and May, 1960*)

(1) Bring sections or smears to water (use thin, scratch-free slides).
(2) Stain with filtered auramine–rhodamine at 60 °C for 10 minutes.
(3) Wash in tap-water for 2 minutes.

(4) Differentiate in 0.5% aqueous HCl in 70% alcohol for 2 minutes. Use 0.5% aqueous HCl for *M. leprae.*
(5) Wash in tap-water for 2 minutes.
(6) Differentiate in 0.5% potassium permanganate for 2 minutes. This step quenches background fluorescence.
(7) Wash in tap-water for 2 minutes, blot dry.
(8) Dehydrate, clear and mount in Fluormount.

Examine using a high dry objective, with a UG1 or 2 exciter filter, and a colourless ultraviolet barrier filter.

Spirochaetes

In fluids

In fresh fluid material, such as exudates, spirochaetes are best demonstrated by darkground illumination or phase contrast. Smears may be stained with dilute Giemsa (1 drop to 1 ml of distilled water) if heat is applied, and five to ten changes of stain made over a period of 10–15 minutes. The addition of one or two drops of 0.1% sodium carbonate to 100 ml of the staining solution sometimes increases the intensity of staining.

The traditional and better method of demonstrating spirochaetes in smears is that of Fontana, modified by Hage.

■ **Hage–Fontana method (Fontana, 1925–26)**

Reagents

(1) Fixative (Ruge's fluid)

Acetic acid	1 ml
Formalin	20 ml
Distilled water	to 100 ml

(2) Mordant

Phenol	1 g
Tannic acid	5 g
Distilled water	to 100 ml

Method

(1) Make film and allow to dry in the air.
(2) Pour on fixative and leave for 1 minute.
(3) Wash in running water for 10 seconds.
(4) Pour on mordant, heat gently until it steams and leave for 30 seconds.
(5) Wash in running water for 20 seconds.
(6) Rinse in distilled water.
(7) Flood slide with 0.5% silver nitrate; add one drop of concentrated ammonia; heat until steam rises and leave for 20 seconds.
(8) Rinse in distilled water.
(9) Blot dry and examine.

Results

Spirochaetes   Black
Cells and general background   Shades of yellow

In tissue

Spirochaetes in blocks of tissue are best demonstrated by Levaditi's method (*Figure 17.1*).

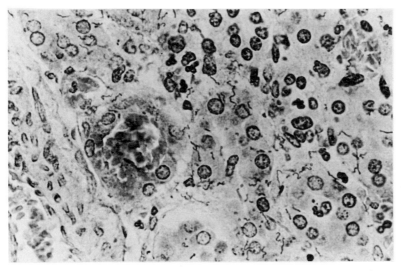

Figure 17.1 Treponema pallidum demonstrated by Levatiti's block silver impregnation method. Original magnification × 160

■ Levaditi's method (1905)

Reagent

Reducing fluid

Pyrogallic acid   4 g
Formalin   5 ml
Distilled water   to 100 ml

Method

(1) Fix small thin pieces (1 mm in thickness) of tissue in 10% formal–saline for 24 hours.
(2) Wash for 1 hour in water, and then place in 96% alcohol for 24 hours.
(3) Transfer to 1.5% silver nitrate in a dark bottle for 3 days at 37 °C.
(4) Wash in distilled water for 30 minutes.
(5) Place in reducing fluid for 48 hours at room temperature in the dark.
(6) Wash well in water, dehydrate, clear and embed. Cut thin sections and mount in the usual way.
(7) Remove paraffin from sections and mount in Canada balsam or synthetic resin.

Results

Spirochaetes   Black
Tissue   Shades of yellow

In paraffin sections

■ **Warthin–Faulkner method (Faulkner and Lillie, 1945)**

The Warthin–Faulkner method gives reasonably reliable results on sections of paraffin-embedded tissue. Formal–saline should be used for fixation.

Reagent

Stock gelatin (for use with developer solution)

Gelatin   5 g
Walpole's sodium acetate–acetic acid buffer (pH 3.6)   to 100 ml

Add 1 ml of 1:10 000 merthiolate to prevent the growth of moulds.

Method

(1) Bring paraffin sections to water.
(2) Wash in 1:25 dilution of stock pH 3.6 acetate–acetic acid buffer (page 130) for 5 minutes.
(3) Impregnate with 1% silver nitrate in dilute pH 3.6 buffer (as in (2)) for 45 minutes at 60 °C.
(4) While sections are in silver nitrate prepare the following developer solution. Mix 15 ml of the stock gelatin solution and 3 ml of 2% silver nitrate in pH 3.6 acetate–acetic acid buffer, both previously heated to 60 °C. Add 1 ml of fresh 3% hydroquinone in pH 3.6 acetate–acetic acid buffer. Mix and use immediately.
(5) Place slides on staining rack and flood with freshly prepared developer. When sections become brown to greyish-yellow, and the developer turns brownish-black, rinse with warm water (55–60 °C), and then with distilled water.
(6) Dehydrate, clear and mount in Canada balsam or synthetic resin.

Results

Spirochaetes   Black
Tissue elements Shades of yellow

Note: Overdevelopment will give precipitation and thickened black spirochaetes, and should be overcome by carrying through two or three sections with varying times of developments.

■ **Modified Dieterle method for spirochaetes (Van Orden and Greer, 1977)**

Reagents

Gum mastic

Add 100 g gum mastic to 1000 ml absolute ethanol. Stand for 2 or 3 days till dissolved. Filter and store in the refrigerator in a well-stoppered bottle.

Developer

Hydroquinone	15 g
Sodium sulphite	2.5 g
Distilled water	600 ml
Acetone	100 ml
Formalin (40%)	100 ml
Pyridine	100 ml
10% Alcohol gum mastic	100 ml

Mix in order, swirling gently as each solution is added. The developer is ready for use after 6 hours and may be used until the colour becomes dark brown.

Method

(1) Bring sections to water.
(2) Treat with preheated 5% alcoholic uranyl nitrate at 56 °C for 1 hour.
(3) Dip in distilled water.
(4) Dip in 95% ethanol.
(5) Treat with 10% alcoholic gum mastic for 3 minutes.
(6) Dip in 95% alcohol.
(7) Treat with distilled water for 1 minute, then allow slides to drain for 15–20 minutes until almost dry.
(8) Place in preheated 1% aqueous silver nitrate at 56 °C for 4 hours in the dark.
(9) Dip twice in distilled water.
(10) Dip in developer until the sections are pale yellow to light tan.
(11) Dip twice in distilled water.
(12) Dip twice in 95% alcohol.
(13) Dip twice in acetone.
(14) Clear in xylene and mount in synthetic resin.

Results

Spirochaetes and some bacteria are impregnated brown to black on a yellow to light tan background.

Fungi

Most fungi in sections may be demonstrated, at least in part, by Gram's method, the branching mycelium (hyphae) being Gram-positive and the spores (conidia) Gram-negative. Gridley's method is the best for their selective demonstration. Since practically all fungi are PAS-positive, these techniques may be used for their general demonstration. The standard technique gives good results, the fluorescent method of Culling and Vassar (1961) gives bright yellow fungi on a dark background, especially if tissue sections are prestained in Weigert's haematoxylin for 2 minutes before treating with periodic acid. Gomori's silver methenamine technique gives excellent results for photography (see page 221) (Figure 17.2).

Cryptococcus neoformans can be demonstrated by virtue of its mucoid capsule. Metachromatic toluidine blue or thionin methods, Alcian blue or Southgate's mucicarmine may be used.

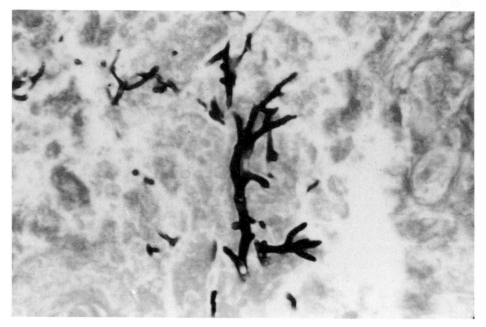

Figure 17.2 Methenamine silver technique demonstrating fungal hyphae. Original magnification × 100

Histoplasma capsulatum, which is PAS-positive, may be differentiated from morphologically similar organisms by its positive birefringence (*Figure 17.3a* and *b*).

Skin scrapings may be smeared on to slides, fixed in alcohol and stained by the above techniques.

■ Gridley's method (1953)

Method

(1) Bring sections to water.
(2) Oxidize in 4% chromic acid for 1 hour.
(3) Wash in running water for 5 minutes.
(4) Transfer to Schiff reagent (page 186) for 15–20 minutes.
(5) Take through two sulphite rinses (as in Feulgen technique, page 186).
(6) Wash in running water for 15 minutes.
(7) Stain for 15–20 minutes in Gomori's aldehyde fuchsin (*see* page 177).
(8) Rinse in 95% alcohol, and wash in running water for 5–10 minutes.
(9) Counterstain in 0.25% metanil yellow in 0.25% acetic acid for 2–5 minutes.
(10) Wash in water.
(11) Dehydrate, clear and mount in synthetic resin.

Results

Hyphae   Deep blue
Conidia   Rose to purple

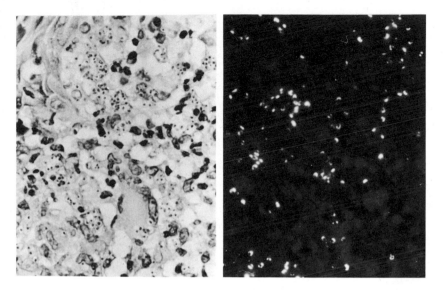

Figure 17.3 (a) *Histoplasma capsulatum* showing positive PAS reaction. Original magnification × 160. (b) *Histoplasma capsulatum* showing positive birefringence in an adjacent field. Original magnification × 160

Elastin and mucin	Deep blue
Yeast capsules	Deep purple
General background	Yellow

■ Fluorescent PAS (Culling and Vassar, 1961)

The fluorescent PAS reaction has the advantage of demonstrating minute quantities of reactive material. It demonstrates basement membranes, mucin and fungi exceptionally well; it has a high degree of specificity and may be controlled in the same manner as the conventional method (*see* page 188). Because of the degree of specificity and the brilliance of the fluorescence, some experience of the method is required in interpreting results, as compared with the conventional technique.

Method

(1) Bring sections to water.
(2) Treat with 1% aqueous periodic acid for 10 minutes.

Steps 3–8 and method of examination are as for the fluorescent Feulgen technique (*see above*).

Results

PAS-positive structures	Fluoresce bright golden yellow
Other tissue components	Green

Rickettsiae and inclusion bodies

Rickettsiae and inclusion bodies may be stained by Giemsa, using a pH 7.2 buffer as a diluent, or alternatively by Macchiavello's method (1937). Most of the inclusion bodies may be demonstrated with Lendrum's phloxine–tartrazine method which is given on page 457. This will not stain Negri bodies, which may be stained with Giemsa, Macchiavello or Mann's methyl blue–eosin. DNA inclusions may be demonstrated by the Feulgen techniques.

■ **Macchiavello's method (modified)**

Method

(1) Bring paraffin sections to water.
(2) Stain in 0.25% aqueous basic fuchsin for 30 minutes.
(3) Differentiate rapidly (about 3 seconds) in 0.5% citric acid.
(4) Wash in tap-water.
(5) Counterstain for 15–30 seconds in 1% methylene blue.
(6) Wash in water.
(7) Dehydrate, clear and mount in Canada balsam or synthetic resin.

Results

Rickettsiae, inclusion bodies   Red
Tissue elements   Blue

■ **Mann's methyl blue–eosin method**

Staining solution

1% Aqueous methyl blue	35 ml
1% Aqueous eosin	45 ml
Distilled water	100 ml

This solution keeps well.

Method

(1) Tissues are fixed in Zenker or formal–saline.
(2) Bring paraffin sections to water.
(3) Stain for 8–24 hours (dependent on the age of the stain) in a Coplin jar.
(4) Wash in water.
(5) Differentiate in absolute alcohol to which two to three drops of N/1 sodium hydroxide/100 ml have been added.
(6) Wash rapidly in several changes of absolute alcohol.
(7) Clear in xylene and mount in neutral mounting medium or synthetic resin.

Results

Negri bodies, red blood cells, oxyphil cytoplasm and granules   Red
Nuclei and other tissue elements   Blue

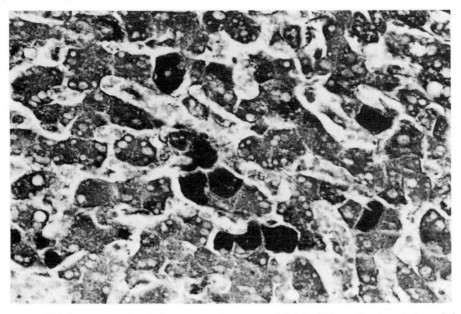

Figure 17.4 Australia antigen in hepatocytes demonstrated by the Shikata–Orcein technique. Original magnification ×160

■ Shikata's orcein method (1974)

This method is used to demonstrate Australia antigen in the liver of hepatitis B affected cases (*Figure 17.4*). The surface antigen stains with orcein, as does elastic. Aldehyde fuchsin can also be used but gives a less intense reaction. Some batches of orcein are not suitable, staining elastic fibres only, consequently all batches should be tested on positive control sections. The most specific demonstration techniques are immunocytochemical techniques using the specific antibody.

Reagents

Acidified potassium permanganate

Potassium permanganate	1.5 g
Concentrated sulphuric acid	1.5 ml
Distilled water	100 ml

Orcein stain

Orcein	1 g
70% Alcohol	100 ml
Concentrated hydrochloric acid	1 ml

Method

(1) Bring sections to water.
(2) Oxidize in permanganate.

(3) Bleach in 1.5% oxalic acid.
(4) Wash in water.
(5) Stain in orcein at room temperature for 4 hours.
(6) Differentiate in 1% acid alcohol.
(7) Dehydrate, clear and mount in synthetic resin.

Results

Hepatitis B surface antigen and elastic   Brown
Background   Pale brown

Protozoa

Pathogenic protozoa are best demonstrated in smears of body fluids. A review of practical methods is given by Drury and Wallington (1980).

Protozoa may be encountered in tissue sections. Most common fixatives are compatible with their demonstration, though when closely associated with red blood cells Zenker–formal may be preferred. Haematoxylin and eosin, and Giemsa often give satisfactory results. Heidenhain's iron haematoxylin or PAS can be used to demonstrate amoebae, and Grocott or PAS techniques are recommended for the demonstration of *Pneumocystis carinii*.

References

AZULAY, R. D. and ANDRADE, L. M. C. (1954). Demonstration of *Mycobacterium leprae* in sections in 532 cases of leprosy; comparative study between Ziehl–Klingmuller and Wade–Fite techniques. *Int. J. Leprosy*, **22**, 195–199

BROWN, J. H. and BRENN, L. (1931). Method for differential staining of Gram-positive and Gram-negative bacteria in tissue sections. *Bull. Johns Hopkins Hosp.*, **48**, 69–73

CULLING, C. F. A. and VASSAR, P. S. (1961). Desoxyribose nucleic acid: a fluorescent histochemical technique. *Arch. Pathol.*, **71**, 76–80

DIETERLE, R. R. (1927). Method for demonstration of *Spirochaeta pallida* in single microscope sections. *Arch. Neurol. Psychiat.*, **18**, 73–80

DRURY, R. A. B. and WALLINGTON, E. A. (1980). In *Carleton's Histological Technique*. 5th Ed. Oxford University Press, Oxford

FAULKNER, R. R. and LILLIE, R. D. (1945). A buffer modification of the Warthin–Starry silver method for spirochaetes in single paraffin sections. *Stain Technol.*, **20**, 81–82

FONTANA, A. (1925–26). Über die Silberdarstellung des *Treponema pallidum* und anderer Mikroorganismen in Ausstrichen. *Derm. Z.*, **46**, 291–293

GRIDLEY, M. F. (1953). A stain for fungi in tissue sections. *Am. J. Clin. Pathol.*, **23**, 303–307

KUPER, S. W. A. and MAY, J. R. (1960). Detection of acid-fast organisms in tissue sections by fluorescence microscopy. *J. Pathol. Bacteriol.*, **79**, 59–68

LEVADITI, C. (1905). Sur la coloration du *Spirochaete pallida* Schaudin dans les coupes. *C. R. Soc. Biol.*, **59**, II, 326

MACCHIAVELLO, A. (1937). Rickettsia. *Reveta Chil. Hig. Med. Prev.*, **1**, 5–25

OLLETT, W. S. (1951). Further observations on the Gram–Twort stain. *J. Pathol. Bacteriol.*, **63**, 166

SHIKATA, T., UZAWA, T., YOSHIWARA, N., AKATSUKA, T. and YAMAZAKI, S. (1974). Staining methods for Australia antigen in paraffin section—detection of cytoplasmic inclusion bodies. *Jap. J. Exp. Med.*, **44**, 25–36

VAN ORDEN, A. E. and GREER, P. W. (1977). Modification of the Dieterle spirochaete stain. *J. Histotechnol.*, **1**, 51–53

WADE, H. W. (1957). A modification of the Fite formaldehyde (Fite 1) method for staining acid-fast bacilli in paraffin sections. *Stain Technol.*, **32**, 287–292

WELLMAN, K. F. and TENG, K. P. (1962). Demonstration of acid-fast bacilli in tissue sections by fluorescence microscopy: a study with clinical and histopathological associations. *Can. Med. Ass. J.*, **87**, 837–841

Part V

Immunocytochemistry

18

Immunofluorescence

Creech and Jones (1940) showed that various proteins, including antibodies, could be labelled with a fluorescent dye (phenylisocyanate) without material effect on their biological or immunological properties. The complex gave a blue fluorescence which was difficult to distinguish from the blue autofluorescence of tissue. Coons, Creech and Jones (1941) described the preparation of fluorescein isocyanate (FIC) which imparted an apple-green fluorescence to the labelled antibody and was easily distinguished from tissue autofluorescence. FIC was soon replaced by fluorescein isothiocyanate (FITC) (Riggs et al., 1958), which gave a more intense fluorescence. Several other fluorochomes have proved reliable for protein labelling:

(1) sulphonyl chloride of 1-dimethylaminonaphthalene-5-sulphonic acid (DANS);
(2) Lissamine rhodamine B (RB200);
(3) tetramethylrhodamine isothiocyanate (TMRITC).

Conjugates

Antibodies can be produced by a series of injections of antigen, into a suitable animal. After an appropriate period of time the animal is bled and the serum is separated. The gamma globulin fraction is precipitated with saturated ammonium sulphate and recovered by centrifugation. The globulin is dissolved in distilled water and dialysed extensively against sodium chloride solution to remove residual ammonium ions which interfere with the conjugation procedure. Immunoglobulin G (IgG) and immunoglobulin M (IgM) fractions can be obtained by DEAE-cellulose or Sephadex fractionation. The protein concentration is brought to 25 mg/ml by ultrafiltration.

Numerous methods exist for the conjugation of FITC and immunoglobulin. The concentration of protein, proportion of FITC to protein, FITC solvent, buffer, pH, time and temperature, all vary according to the author. These are reviewed by Pearse (1980). The conjugation method of The and Feltkamp (1970) is as follows:

(1) FITC is dissolved in 0.15 M sodium phosphate ($Na_2HPO_4.2H_2O$) at pH 9.0 at a strength of 1 mg/ml, immediately before use.
(2) 10 ml of FITC solution is added to the protein solution for each gram of protein, while stirring at room temperature.
(3) Adjust to pH 9.5, while stirring, by adding 0.1 M trisodium orthophosphate ($Na_3PO_4.12H_2O$).

(4) Stirring is continued for 60 minutes at room temperature, while maintaining pH 9.5.
(5) Purification procedures are then carried out (*see below*).

Purification of conjugates

Unreacted fluorescent material (UFM) was originally removed by dialysis against saline over a period of several days, but this method is not as effective as the charcoal or Sephadex methods.

Extraction is carried out with powdered activated charcoal, which has been washed well with saline and dried at 100 °C. The charcoal, moistened with saline to avoid undue loss of protein, is added in the proportion of 2.5 mg/mg of protein in the sera. The mixture is shaken for 1 hour and the charcoal is then removed by centrifugation. The only disadvantage of this technique is the loss of protein (20–30%) which may be important when conjugating small amounts of a weak antiserum.

The method of choice is gel filtration with a cross-linked dextran, Sephadex (Pharmacia Fine Chemicals AB, Box 175, S-75104, Uppsala 1, Sweden). This depends on the diffusion of small molecules into the pores of the gel, the larger molecules being excluded because of their size. Separation takes place in a column, with the large protein molecules travelling more rapidly than the small molecules, which diffuse into the gel. Pore size G 25 or G 50 are the commonly used grades for this purpose. The manufacturers describe the method of preparation and use in detail. For volumes of conjugate up to 20 ml a column 20 cm in length and 3 cm in diameter, which has been washed with buffered saline, is adequate. The conjugate, having been centrifuged, is allowed to soak into the column, and a suitable head of buffered saline applied. As the solution passes down the column, two bands separate, the faster one being the conjugate. The loss of protein by this method is very small. Dilution of the conjugate may be overcome by reprecipitation of the globulins.

Using the conjugation procedure of The and Feltkamp (1970) the average FITC/protein ratio is about 2.5.

The conjugate can be further fractionated by gradient elution on a DEAE–Sephadex A 50 column. The optical densities at 280 and 495 nm of the fractions are determined and FITC/protein ratios calculated.

Fractions with the optimal FITC/protein ratio are dialysed against phosphate buffered saline and concentrated by ultrafiltration to 10 mg/ml. One ml aliquots are freeze-dried and vacuum sealed for storage.

Absorption by tissue powders

The removal of conjugated non-specific serum proteins may be carried out by absorption with tissue powders, if possible with the same type as the tissue to be examined, provided that it does not contain any appreciable amount of the specific antigen. The precipitation of the globulin fraction will also remove these to a great degree, but more elaborate fractionation of sera by chromatography on modified cellulose (Goldstein, Slizys and Chase, 1961) reduces them to almost undetectable levels.

The tissue powders, usually liver or bone marrow (to inhibit non-specific staining of granulocytes) are prepared as follows.

Wash the organ free of blood with physiological saline, chop into small pieces with scissors or scalpel and rewash with saline. Grind up the material in a low-speed homogenizer (or pestle and mortar) with acetone, and filter through coarse filter paper. Wash several times with acetone until completely dehydrated, and dry at 37 °C. Grind to powder in a mortar, sieve through wire mesh to remove coarse material and store at room temperature. For absorption purposes approximately 100 mg of tissue powder is used for each ml of original serum. The mixture is shaken at room temperature for 1 hour, and centrifuged at about 10 000 g (preferably in a refrigerated centrifuge) for about 15 minutes. The high speed is essential to give maximum return of conjugate. The supernatant fluid is now ready for use. The conjugate should be divided in small aliquots and stored in a deep-freeze, otherwise there will be a protein–dye breakdown which will necessitate re-absorption before use.

Commercial conjugates

A wide range of reliable conjugates are available commercially. They usually do not require further purification before use.

Techniques

The fluorescent antibody technique is used for the detection and localization of animal and human tissue antigens or antibodies and has wide use in identifying bacterial, parasitic and viral antigens.

Direct staining

The fluorescent antibody is used to directly locate an antigen (*Figure 18.1a*). The conjugated antibody is applied to the section or smear, left for the appropriate time (*see below*) and washed off with buffered saline. After further washing to remove unreacted antibody the preparation is mounted in buffered glycerol saline.

Sandwich technique

Antibody in tissues or smears is reacted with unlabelled antigen. After washing, fluorescent labelled antibody is applied (*Figure 18.1b*). This will react with the antigen and so will demonstrate the site of the original antibody.

Indirect or multiple layer technique

This is an extension of the sandwich technique. A tissue antigen is reacted with an unlabelled antibody (or succession of antibodies) followed by a final FITC labelled antibody (*Figure 18.1c*). This widely used technique provides the most economical method of identifying a wide range of tissue antigens or serum antibodies. For example, when testing human serum for the presence of immunoglobulins against tissue antigens, the various antigen–antibody complexes formed in substrate sections can be identified by one single rabbit–antihuman immunoglobulin–FITC conjugate.

It is assumed that there are several antigenic determinants on each molecule of antibody; using additional layers will therefore increase the final number of fluorescent molecules on the tissue so producing a more intense fluorescence (*Figure 18.2*).

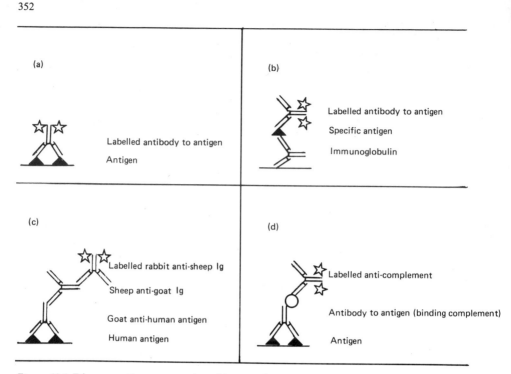

Figure 18.1 Diagrammatic representation of immunofluorescent techniques. (a) Direct, (b) sandwich, (c) indirect (multiple layer), and (d) complement techniques. *See Figure 8.2* for further discussion

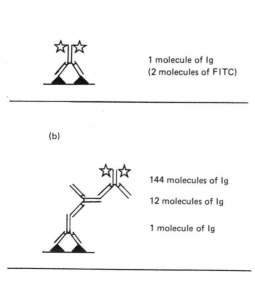

(a)

1 molecule of Ig
(2 molecules of FITC)

(b)

144 molecules of Ig

12 molecules of Ig

1 molecule of Ig

Figure 18.2 Diagrammatic illustration of the increased fluorescence intensity of the indirect method of immunofluorescence (b) compared with the direct method (a). Ideally there are two fluorescent molecules (FITC) per molecule of immunoglobulin. In the indirect technique 12 molecules of secondary antibody have the potential to combine with one primary antibody molecule (Cammisuli and Wofsy, 1976), thereby increasing the two fluorescent molecules in the direct technique to a theoretical total of 24 (2×12) in the indirect technique (or $12^2 \times 2$ with a third layer). This potential increase may be reduced by steric hindrance in situations of high antigen density (prozone phenomenon)

Complement techniques

When an antigen–antibody reaction involving complement takes place the complement may be demonstrated using FITC-labelled anti-complement (*Figure 18.1d*).

Preparation of material

Cryostat sections

These are by far the most commonly employed histological preparations. Unfixed tissue is quick frozen or quenched and sections cut in the cryostat. They may be used fresh (after air-drying) or fixed in cold 95% alcohol either before or after air-drying. Tissues which tend to detach during staining may need to be air-dried before fixing. The type of fixative used will depend on the antigen/antibody involved in the reaction, but cold 95% alcohol has been employed successfully in a number of investigations.

Smears

Tissue and bacterial smears, touch preparations and tissue culture monolayers on coverslips have all been used with great success for fluorescent antibody staining techniques.

Smear preparations of tissue are best made by brushing the cut surface of the tissue with a camel hair brush which has been dipped into 7.5% PVP (polyvinylpyrolidone). Several strokes are then made on to a clean slide. One advantage of this technique is that the experimental and control smears can easily be made on the same slide.

Wax sections

Sections of polyester wax embedded, freeze-dried or freeze substituted material have been used. Conventional paraffin sections have been used but are generally unsuitable unless some special procedures are adopted. Huang, Minassian and Morse (1976) and Curran and Gregory (1978) used the enzymatic action of trypsin to 'unmask' proteins, including immunoglobulins for reaction with FITC-conjugated antibodies. They treated the sections with 0.1% trypsin in 0.1% calcium chloride at pH 7.8 for times varying between 5 minutes and 4 hours, before carrying out the immunofluorescence staining technique.

Sainte-Marie (1962) approached the problem by preventing the loss of immunological activity during fixation and processing. Fixation and dehydration were carried out at 4 °C in 95% and absolute alcohol, respectively. Xylene at 4 °C was used as a clearing agent, and tissues were impregnated in paraffin wax at 56 °C. The author claimed more precise localization and increased sensitivity when compared with cryostat sections.

▪ Staining technique

Reagents

Phosphate buffered saline (pH 7.1)

Sodium chloride	8.5 g
Disodium hydrogen phosphate (anhyd.) (Na_2HPO_4)	1.07 g

| Sodium dihydrogen phosphate ($NaH_2PO_4 . 2 H_2O$) | 0.39 g |
| Distilled water | to 1 litre |

Buffered glycerin mountant

| Glycerin | 9 ml |
| Phosphate buffered saline | 1 ml |

Method

(1) Sections or smears may be rinsed with buffered saline. This facilitates spreading of the conjugate.
(2) Slides or coverslips are placed in a moist chamber, for example, Petri dish, with moist filter paper in the bottom. The preparation is covered with a drop (or two) of the conjugate which is applied with a platinum loop or Pasteur pipette. The chamber is kept at room temperature. The reaction time may vary (with the strength of antisera or type of antigen) from 10 minutes to 2 hours; from 15–30 minutes is usually adequate.
(3) The preparations are rinsed in several changes (not less than three) of buffered saline over a period of 10–15 minutes. This step is critical and should be carried out for a longer, rather than a shorter time. A magnetic stirrer to agitate the buffer during washing is recommended. The slides to be washed are suspended in an open-type slide holder in a beaker, over a magnetic stirrer; three changes are usually adequate.
(4) Excess buffered saline is wiped off and the specimens mounted in buffered glycerin. After examination they may be rinsed in distilled water and stored dry in the dark.

Or

(5) Rinse briefly in distilled water and blot dry.
(6) Place in xylol until section is clear; it may be necessary occasionally to blot again before complete clearing is achieved.
(7) Mount in non-fluorescing mountant.

Results

Antigen–antibody reaction sites give an apple-green fluorescence (with FITC or DANS) or orange fluorescence with rhodamine B.

Background fluorescence will be blue (unless counterstained with rhodamine B) except for autofluorescent sites. An unstained slide should be used to check autofluorescence.

A UG1 exciter filter with a GG9 barrier filter may be adequate but the use of special filters for selective FITC observations are recommended. The exciter filter is a band pass filter, BP 450–490, and the barrier filter is also a band pass filter, BP 520–560 or BP 525/20. If incident illumination is used a 510 nm beam splitter is incorporated.

Counterstains

Counterstains may be used in FITC-immunofluorescence techniques either to eliminate the background fluorescence or to increase cell and tissue detail or to accomplish both functions. Immunofluorescence counterstains were investigated by

Schenk and Churukian (1974). Flazo orange, Congo red, Evans blue, brilliant cresyl blue and eriochrome black eliminate background fluorescence. Methyl green produces red fluorescent nuclei without eliminating the background. These authors recommend the Lissamine–rhodamine conjugated bovine serum albumin counterstain of Smith, Marshall and Eveland (1959) when there is FITC staining of nuclei, and methyl green as the counterstain when there is FITC staining of cytoplasmic constituents. Pearse (1980) recommends the PAS technique which gives a dull red background without nuclear staining.

Tests of specificity

Tests of specificity are modelled on those used in established immunological techniques. Those most commonly employed are as follows.

Blocking

Staining should be inhibited by pretreatment of the specimen with unconjugated antisera (at room temperature for 30 minutes) before staining. The unconjugated sera should bind all the reactive sites on the antigen, and block a reaction with the conjugated antibody. This is referred to as a *blocking test*. It will sometimes be found that only a reduction in intensity of staining can be obtained by this test.

The blocking test should also be performed with a non-specific (control) serum to prove that the blocking is due to the presence of the specific antibody.

Absorption

Staining should be inhibited if the conjugate has been previously absorbed (usually twice) with the specific antigen (specific absorption), the conjugate being centrifuged after absorption to remove reacted material (if possible).

The staining should not be inhibited by absorption with a different antigen (non-specific absorption) using the same technique.

Absorption of the antisera with an antigen is simple when the antigen is pure, but it must be remembered that when an antigen is impure there is no guarantee that positive staining of the antibody may not be due to a non-specific antigen (impurity) blocking a non-specific antibody.

Control conjugate

Occasionally it may be necessary to prove that staining is due to an induced antibody, and not a naturally occurring one. This is tested for by conjugation of a normal control serum from the same species of animal. There should be no staining of the antigen with this serum (*Table 18.1*).

Applications

Fluorescent antibody techniques are used for the identification of antigen–antibody complexes in tissue, principally in the study of glomerulonephritis and the identification of pemphigus and pemphigoid in skin biopsies. The identification of tissue antigens is more reliably carried out by immunoenzyme techniques (*see* Chapter 9).

Table 18.1

Treatment (as detailed above)	Results if sera are specific
(1) Conjugated antisera alone	Staining $(+++)$
(2) Unconjugated antisera, followed by conjugated antisera (blocking test)	No staining $(-)$
(3) Unconjugated control sera, followed by conjugated antisera (control blocking test)	Staining $(+++)$
(4) No treatment. Slide mounted unstained to control autofluorescence	No staining $(-)$

The most important application of fluorescent antibody techniques is in the field of autoimmune disease. A wide range of substrate sections may be used to demonstrate the presence of autoantibodies in human serum.

Routine screening for circulating autoantibodies

Screening for antibodies to thyroid colloid, thyroid microsomes, gastric parietal cells, mitochondria, smooth muscle and nuclei can be carried out on one slide.

A cryostat section of fresh surgical thyroid is mounted on a microscope slide and fixed for 3 minutes in methanol at 60 °C. This section allows the demonstration of the antibodies to thyroid colloid. A further section of thyroid is mounted adjacent to the fixed section followed by sections of fresh surgical gastric fundus and kidney cortex, these are air-dried but not fixed. The unfixed thyroid is used to demonstrate thyroid microsomal antibody, the stomach, for parietal cell antibody and smooth muscle antibody. The kidney section is an excellent substrate for mitochondrial antibody while all three fresh sections are substrates for antibodies to nuclei. Serum may be used undiluted but many authors recommend using serum diluted 1:10. It is advisable to use an FITC-conjugated polyvalent immunoglobulin antiserum at the predetermined optimum dilution.

Additional blocks of frozen tissues should be kept for the more specialized investigations, some of which are detailed below.

Thyroid

Fresh surgical thyroid gland should be used as substrate. It should be thyrotoxic and have tall follicular cells and small acini containing dense colloid. It is important to test the substrate sections using direct immunofluorescence with FITC–antihuman immunoglobulin since immune complexes are often deposited on the acinar basement membranes and between the follicular cells. Such sections are not suitable. The water soluble thyroglobulin is retained *in situ* by methanol fixation. In an indirect immunofluorescence technique, antibodies to thyroglobulin will produce a floccular or crazed pattern of fluorescence. Homogeneous staining is attributed to an antibody against a non-iodine containing protein (the second colloid antigen) which is of no diagnostic significance.

Unfixed sections are necessary to demonstrate the thyroid microsomal antibody which produces fluorescence in the follicular cell cytoplasm.

Thyroid antibodies are found in a small percentage of normal subjects and in association with a number of other autoimmune states. Higher titres are found in Grave's disease and in Hashimoto's thyroiditis.

The antibodies are organ-specific but not species-specific.

The haemagglutination reactions for antibodies to thyroglobulin and thyroid microsomes are replacing the immunofluorescence tests in some laboratories.

Methods for the demonstration of cell-surface antibodies and TSH–receptor antibodies are described by Fagraeus and Jonsson (1970) and Rees Smith (1977), respectively.

Stomach

Circulating antibodies to gastric parietal cells are found in patients with gastric atrophy, atrophic gastritis and pernicious anaemia. The fundal mucosa is the area involved in these conditions (Type A gastritis). These antibodies are also present to some degree in a number of other autoimmune conditions, notably autoimmune thyroid disease.

Intrinsic factor antibodies may also be present but their presence is demonstrated by radioimmunoassay. Cryostat sections of human Group O fundal mucosa, obtained at operation, should be used for immunofluorescence.

In antral gastritis (Type B gastritis) antibodies to gastrin cells are found in about 8% of cases, parietal cell antibody being absent. Fresh cryostat sections of Group O human antrum, devoid of parietal cells, are used as substrates. The specificity of the reaction can be demonstrated using a double immunofluorescence technique (Vandelli et al., 1979), the gastrin antibody reaction being identified with FITC–anti-IgG, while the gastrin cell is identified with rabbit antigastrin and rhodamine–antirabbit IgG.

Pancreatic islet cells

Cryostat sections of fresh pancreas from blood group O surgical cases are the preferred substrate.

Since the exocrine pancreas secretes blood group antigens, test sera which contain high titres of ABH isoagglutinin may produce immunofluorescence in the exocrine cells.

An antibody which produces immunofluorescence in all the islet cells may be found in insulin dependent diabetes (Type I). The reaction is not confined to the B-cells and absorption of positive serum with insulin, glucagon or somatostatin does not abolish the immunofluorescence (Bottazzo and Doniach, 1978). The antibodies are thought to react with the intracellular membranes and not with the hormones. These antibodies are found in non-diabetics with polyendocrine autoimmune disease and in healthy relatives of Type I diabetics.

Using an indirect immunofluorescence technique complement-fixing islet cell antibodies may be demonstrated which show selective staining of some islet cells. These antibodies are more closely related to the expression of disease.

Striated muscle

Antibody to acetylcholine receptor (AChR) in muscle endplates is present in the serum of 85–90% of patients with generalized myasthenia gravis and a third of all patients have antibody reacting with muscle striations (Leibowitz and Hughes, 1983) and with some cells in the thymus.

The AChR antibodies can be demonstrated by an indirect immunofluorescence technique using cryostat sections of striated muscle as substrate. Suitable human muscle is not always available so rat diaphragm is often used. The receptors can be identified using FITC–α-bungarotoxin. Bender *et al.* (1975) claim that the binding of α-bungarotoxin is blocked by the previous application of a serum containing AChR antibody. Sondag-Tschroots *et al.* (1979) found no clear inhibition of α-bungarotoxin binding by previous application of serum containing AChR antibodies. They used a double staining technique where the AChR antibody was located by FITC–antihuman IgG. This was followed by α-bungarotoxin, rabbit–antibungarotoxin and finally TRITC–antirabbit IgG. The location of the green and red fluorescence was the same.

It is known that the binding sites on the acetylcholine receptors for the antibody and the toxin are different and that the binding of the antibody is not blocked by previous binding of the toxin.

In our experience the results of attempted blockade of α-bungarotoxin binding by AChR antibody have been equivocal. This is perhaps not surprising in the light of the paucity of α-bungarotoxin site blocking antibodies in myaesthenic patients' sera (Vincent and Newsom-Davies, 1982).

The antibody which produces a striated fluorescence pattern with all striated muscle (including cardiac muscle) is said to play no part in the pathogenesis of the disease.

The patient's serum should be diluted 1:40 for the striated muscle immunofluorescence technique.

Skin

Circulating autoantibodies to skin components are present in several skin diseases.

Immunoglobulins may be demonstrated in skin biopsies by direct immunofluorescence techniques. Frozen sections are used with FITC labelled antihuman IgA, IgG, IgM, complement and fibrinogen (*see also* Chapter 22).

Circulating antibodies are detected with an indirect immunofluorescence technique using sections of guinea pig lip or oesophagus, monkey oesophagus or human skin. Chu, Bhogal and Black (1983) report fewer false negative results using monkey oesophagus as substrate. Polyvalent FITC antihuman Ig should be used for screening.

Pemphigus vulgaris

In skin biopsies there is an intercellular deposition of immunoglobulin in the epithelium. It is usually IgG, but IgA and IgM may be present. Complement may also be present (*Figure 22.4a*).

Circulating immunoglobulin level frequently reflects the severity of the disease, falling with treatment and rising with relapse. It is usually IgG.

Low titre antibodies giving similar staining patterns are present in a variety of other conditions: complement may be fixed and demonstrated by the indirect complement immunofluorescence technique.

Bullous pemphigoid

Skin biopsies may show a linear basement membrane deposition of immunoglobulin. IgG is most common and complement may be present (*Figure 22.4b*).

Circulating antibody, detected by an indirect immunofluorescence technique is usually IgG. Complement may also be demonstrated. There is no correlation between titre and severity of the disease.

Dermatitis herpetiformis

Skin biopsies may show a granular deposition of IgA in the tips of the dermal papillae, but occasionally the deposition may be of the linear basement membrane pattern. Complement is frequently found.

Indirect immunofluorescence for circulating antibodies is usually negative but circulating IgA giving a basement membrane zone pattern may be present.

Antibodies to reticulin (IgG) may also be found.

Liver

Circulating autoantibodies are found in cases of chronic active hepatitis (CAH) and primary biliary cirrhosis (PBC) and in other liver diseases.

Smooth muscle antibody

Seventy to 90% of patients with autoimmune CAH have smooth muscle IgG antibodies (Lidman, 1976). They act against many muscles and non-muscle tissues. In CAH associated with hepatitis-B virus, IgM antibodies to smooth muscle are found (Farrow *et al.*, 1970). Broad specificity smooth muscle antibodies (CAH) are absorbed by actin, while those acting against smooth muscle only (other diseases) are not absorbed by actin. Bottazzo *et al.* (1976) classified smooth muscle antibodies according to their reaction with kidney smooth muscle, namely tubule (SMA-T), glomeruli (SMA-G) and vessels (SMA-V). SMA-T is associated with autoimmune CAH. The association with primary biliary cirrhosis is not so great. The reader is referred to the review by Toh (1979).

Mitochondrial antibody

Circulating mitochondrial antibodies are strongly associated with PBC. They are non-species specific. The immunofluorescence is seen in cells containing numerous mitochondria, principally in the cells of the proximal tubule of the renal cortex, but also in distal tubule and ascending loop of Henlé in the renal medulla. The antibody is directed against a lipoprotein constituent of the mitochondrial inner membrane. Swana *et al.* (1977) described a human specific mitochondrial antibody which reacted with mitochondria-rich cells in many organs.

Microsomal antibody

The liver–kidney–microsomal antibody (LKM) gives immunofluorescence mainly with liver and kidney. The kidney microsomal reaction can be differentiated from the mitochondrial reaction by the former's reaction with proximal tubules only (Rizzetto, Bianchi and Doniach, 1974).

Liver-specific antibodies

Two liver-specific autoantigens have been isolated. They are F antigen (Silver and Lane, 1975) and liver-specific membrane lipoprotein (LSP) (Meyer Zum Büschenfelde and Miescher, 1972).

Technique

Substrate sections for demonstration of smooth muscle antibody can be obtained from human surgical stomach, prostate, cervix or uterus. Animal tissues may also be used. It is advisable to use polyvalent immunoglobulin–FITC conjugates for screening purposes in order to detect IgM as well as IgG antibodies.

Human or rat kidney sections are often used to detect mitochondrial antibodies but human tissue is preferred since the human specific mitochondrial antibody is not detected using rat tissues.

Unfixed cryostat sections should be used. Cultured fibroblasts were used by Kurki *et al.* (1977) to differentiate the subtypes of smooth muscle antibody. It should be remembered that the mitochondrial antibody will also react with gastric parietal cells in the standard screening protocol.

Nuclei

A group of autoimmune diseases are characterized by the presence of circulating antibodies to many nuclear antigens. These diseases include, for example, systemic lupus erythematosis (SLE), rheumatoid arthritis, Sjögren's syndrome, scleroderma, dermatomyositis and a clinical syndrome known as mixed connective tissue disease (MCTD).

Antibodies to different nuclear antigens produce different immunofluorescent staining patterns but it should be remembered that antibodies of multiple specificities may be present giving mixed staining patterns.

There are four well recognized patterns of nuclear immunofluorescence, namely homogeneous, peripheral (or rim), speckled and nucleolar; however, Burnham and Bank (1974), emphasizing strict attention to morphology, describe 15 separate patterns.

Antigen, immunofluorescence pattern and some associated diseases are shown in *Table 18.2*, which is derived largely from Tan (1979). Diseases other than those detailed in this table may give a reaction whilst only a percentage of those named will react.

Speckled (RNP) pattern is found in high titre in a high proportion of patients with MCTD and in lower titre in other collagen vascular diseases. The speckled (Sm) pattern is highly specific for SLE. The speckled (RANA) pattern is associated only with Sjögren's syndrome when it occurs in conjunction with rheumatoid arthritis. Antibodies to ssDNA may be present in drug induced lupus but dsDNA antibodies are not. The peripheral anti-dsDNA pattern is less frequent in patients with SLE than the homogeneous pattern but when the rim pattern is present it indicates a greater likelihood of active disease (Coffey, Zile and Luskin, 1981).

A leucocyte-specific nuclear antibody giving a homogeneous pattern of immunofluorescence may be found in SLE and in rheumatoid arthritis. Leucocyte preparations should not be used for general screening since speckled patterns will not be seen (Holborow and Johnson, 1969).

Many human and animal tissue sections and cell impression smears have been used for nuclear antibody studies. Unfixed cryostat sections of rat liver are a convenient substrate. Some authors recommend acetone fixation but this does not appear to be necessary.

FITC-conjugated polyvalent antihuman immunoglobulin should be used. A potent serum should be used to allow a dilution which ensures absence of non-specific staining.

Table 18.2 Antinuclear fluorescence patterns

Antibodies to:	Nuclear pattern	Disease association
DNA		
Native double stranded DNA (dsDNA)	Peripheral	SLE
Single stranded DNA (ssDNA)	Speckled	Rheumatic and some chronic infectious diseases
dsDNA/ssDNA		SLE and rheumatic diseases
Deoxyribonucleoprotein (DNP)		
Complex of DNA and histones	Homogeneous	Idiopathic and drug induced LE
Histones		
All histone fractions	Homogeneous	SLE
H2A and H2B sub-fractions	Homogeneous or patchy	Drug induced LE
Non-histone nuclear proteins		
Sm antigen (Smith)	Speckled	Idiopathic SLE
Ribonucleoprotein (RNP)	Speckled	MCTD
SS-A and SS-B antigens	Speckled	Sjögren's disease
Scl-I antigen	Speckled	Scleroderma
Rheumatoid arthritis nuclear antigen (RANA)	Speckled	Rheumatoid arthritis
Nucleolar antigens		
4-6S nucleolar RNA	Nucleolar	Raynaud's disease and scleroderma

Antinuclear techniques

■ **Detection of antibodies to histones (Tan, Robinson and Robitaille, 1976)**

(1) A section (A) is treated with 0.1 N IICl for 30 minutes. This results in the elution of all proteins.
(2) Another extracted section (B) is now reacted with purified histone (20 µg/ml) for 1 hour. This forms complexes with DNA. Histone fractions may also be used.
(3) Excess histone is removed by washing.
(4) Sections are used as specific substrates for detection of antibodies to histone since no non-histone protein antigens are present. Section A will be negative but reconstituted sections (B) will be positive in the presence of antibodies to histone.

■ **Detection of antibodies to dsDNA using haemoflagellates**

The haemoflagellate *Crithidia luciliae* contains an organelle called the kinetoplast. This is a giant mitochondrion in which the mitochondrial DNA is concentrated in a single large network. The DNA is entirely double stranded and is unassociated with histones. This organism is non-pathogenic to man and contains about six times more dsDNA than *Trypanosoma gambiense* which was originally used (Thivolet *et al.*, 1965).

Method (after Aarden, de Groot and Feltkamp, 1975)

Substrate

(1) *C. luciliae* is grown in Bacto tryptose medium (pH 7.4) at 24 °C.
(2) After low speed centrifugation (10 minutes at 3000 *g*), the organisms are washed and centrifuged three times with phosphate buffered saline at pH 7.4.
(3) A suspension is prepared containing 20×10^6 organisms/ml.

(4) 10 μl drops are applied to glass slides and dried with a fan.
(5) Fix in 96% ethanol for 10 minutes at room temperature.
(6) Slides may be used immediately or stored at $-20\,°C$.

Control

A slide is stained with ethidium bromide (1 mg/ml in PBS) for 1 minute and washed in PBS for 1 minute. The kinetoplast and nucleus can be examined with fluorescence microscopy using the FITC filters.

Immunofluorescence

(1) The substrate slides are washed in PBS and dried around the *C. luciliae* spot.
(2) Serum diluted 1:10 with PBS is applied to the *C. luciliae* spot, mixed and incubated in a moist chamber for 30 minutes at room temperature.
(3) Wash for 30 minutes in PBS.
(4) FITC-conjugated polyvalent antihuman Ig at the optimum dilution is added and the slides are again incubated in a moist chamber for 30 minutes at room temperature.
(5) Wash in PBS.
(6) Mount in 90% glycerin in PBS.

Results

With anti-dsDNA sera, the kinetoplast appears as a fluorescent ring or circle lying against the cytoplasmic membrane between the nuclear and flagellar ends of the organism.

Sometimes nuclear and kinetoplast fluorescence occur simultaneously. Flagellar base staining is not associated with anti-dsDNA (Sontheimer and Gilliam, 1978).

If undiluted serum is used the cytoplasm of the organism may show diffuse non-specific staining.

■ **Detection of antibodies to dsDNA using human metaphase chromosomes (Somerfield and Wilson, 1980)**

Peripheral blood leucocytes are cultured for 72 hours in the presence of phytohaemagglutinin. Colchicine, 20 μg/ml, is added to arrest the growth of lymphocytes in metaphase and left for 2 hours.

The cell suspension is fixed in 3:1 methanol/acetic acid.

The cells are spotted onto microscope slides and air-dried. They may be used immediately or stored at room temperature.

Controls and immunofluorescence are performed as above.

Results

Positive sera produce diffuse immunofluorescence with all chromosomes. Serum with high antibody titres produce brighter marginal immunofluorescence.

Steroid producing cells

A majority of patients with idiopathic Addison's disease have autoantibodies to steroid producing cells of the adrenal. In a minority of these patients the autoimmune reaction is directed against antigens which are not confined to the adrenal cortex but are found in one or more of the other steroid producing cells, for example, theca cells of corpus luteum and granulosa cells of Graafian follicles, Leydig cells of testis and syncitial cells of the placenta.

Sera of the majority of these patients react with all three layers of the adrenal cortex. Some sera of patients with gonadal failure *and* Addison's disease react only with specific zones of the cortex. The adrenal cortex synthesizes oestrogens, progesterone and androgens as well as cortisol, so it is not surprising that the adrenals and other steroid producing tissues have common antigens.

Unfixed cryostat sections for immunofluorescence studies are obtained from *suitable* surgical specimens of human adrenal, ovary and testis. Placenta should be included.

Ovaries from rabbits at various stages of the oestrous cycle contain a larger number of ova and luteal cells than human specimens and, with rabbit testis, should be included in a composite block.

The antibodies are IgG and are easily detected using an indirect immunofluorescence technique. Autoimmunity against steroid producing tissues is described by Irvine (1978). Staining patterns are well illustrated by Kamp, Platz and Nerup (1974).

Kidney

Circulating antibodies against glomerular basement membrane occur in Goodpasture's syndrome, a condition characterized by multiple pulmonary haemorrhages in association with glomerular nephritis. Activity is also observed against lung basement membrane (Pasternack, Linder and Kuhlbäck, 1965). The antibody is detected in patient's serum using unfixed cryostat sections of kidney as substrate, giving a uniform fluorescence in the glomerular basement membrane using antihuman IgG–FITC.

Glomerulonephritis is studied using unfixed cryostat sections of needle biopsies of kidney. The distribution and type of immune-complexes are demonstrated using direct immunofluorescence techniques. The FITC-conjugated antisera used are anti-IgA, anti-IgG, anti-IgM, anticomplement (C_3) and antifibrinogen.

Kidney biopsy procedures and the principal reactions are given in Chapter 22.

Miscellaneous

In addition to those mentioned above, circulating autoantibodies have been demonstrated by immunofluorescence in other tissues and cells (Nairn, 1976; Polak and van Noorden, 1983) (*Table 18.3*).

Table 18.3

Early Type I diabetes	Pituitary prolactin cells
Primary hypoparathyroidism	Chief cells of parathyroid
Primary gonadol insufficiency	Sperm and ovum
Endocrine exophthalmos	Ocular muscles
Diabetes insipidus	Arginine vasopressin cells of hypothalamus
Coeliac disease	Endocrine cells of duodenum
Small intestine enteropathy	Gut mucosal epithelium
Ulcerative colitis	Colon mucosa
Rheumatic and ischaemic heart disease	Heart muscle
Dermatitis herpetiformis	Reticulin
Guillain Barré syndrome and multiple sclerosis	Myelin

Autoantibodies have been demonstrated against tumours.

References

AARDEN, L. A., DE GROOT, E. R. and FELTKAMP, T. E. W. (1975). Immunology of DNA III. *Crithidia luciliae*, a simple substrate for the determination of anti-dsDNA with the immunofluorescence technique. *Ann. N.Y. Acad. Sci.*, **254**, 505–515

BENDER, A. N., ENGEL, W. K., RINGEL, S. P., DANIELS, M. P. and VOGEL, Z. (1975). Myasthenia gravis: a serum factor blocking acetylcholine receptors of the human neuromuscular junction. *Lancet*, **1**, 607–609

BOTTAZZO, G-F., FLORIN-CHRISTENSEN, A., FAIRFAX, A., SWANA, G., DONIACH, D. and GRÖSCHEL-STEWART, U. (1976). Classification of smooth muscle antibodies detected by immunofluorescence. *J. Clin. Pathol.*, **29**, 403–410

BOTTAZZO, G-F. and DONIACH, D. (1978). Islet cell antibodies (ICA) in diabetes mellitus: evidence of an autoantigen common to all cells in the islet of Langerhans. *Ric. Clin. Lab.*, **8**, 29–30

BURNHAM, T. K. and BANK, P. W. (1974). Antinuclear antibodies. I. Patterns of nuclear immunofluorescence. *J. Invest. Dermatol.*, **62**, 526–534

CAMMISULI, S. and WOFSY, L. (1976). Hapten sandwich labelling. III. Bifunctional reagents for immunospecific labelling of cell surface antigens. *J. Immunol.*, **117**, 5, pt 1, 1695–1704

CHU, A. C., BHOGAL, B. and BLACK, M. M. (1983). Immunochemistry in dermatology. In *Immunochemistry. Practical Applications in Pathology and Biology*. Eds Polak, J. M. and van Noorden, S. Wright PSG, Bristol, London, Boston, pp. 302–333

COFFEY, R. L., ZILE, M. R. and LUSKIN, A. T. (1981). Immunologic tests of value in diagnosis. 1. Acute phase reactants and autoantibodies. *Postgrad. Med.*, **70**, 163–178

COONS, A. H., CREECH, H. J. and JONES, R. N. (1941). Immunological properties of an antibody containing a fluorescent group. *Proc. Soc. Exp. Biol. (N.Y.)*, **37**, 200–202

CREECH, H. J. and JONES, R. N. (1940). The conjugation of horse serum albumin with 1,2-benzanthryl isocyanates. *J. Am. Chem. Soc.*, **62**, 1970–1975

CURRAN, R. C. and GREGORY, J. (1978). Demonstration of immunoglobulin in cryostat and paraffin sections of human tonsil by immunofluorescence and immunoperoxidase techniques. *J. Clin. Pathol.*, **31**, 974–983

EVANS, D. J. (1982). Immunocytochemistry in histopathology with particular reference to renal disease. In *Immunocytochemistry. Practical Applications in Pathology and Biology*. Eds Polak, J. M. and van Noorden, S. Wright PSG, Bristol, London, Boston, pp. 334–345

FAGRAEUS, A. and JONSSON, J. (1970). Distribution of organ antigens over the surface of thyroid cells as examined by immunofluorescence test. *Immunology*, **18**, 413–416

FARROW, L. J., HOLBOROW, E. J., JOHNSON, G. D., LAMB, S. G., STEWART, J. S., TAYLOR, P.E. and ZUCKERMAN, A. J. (1970). Autoantibodies and the hepatitis associated antigen in acute infective hepatitis. *Br. Med. J.*, **2**, 693–695

GOLDSTEIN, G., SLIZYS, I. S. and CHASE, M. W. (1961). Studies on fluorescent antibody staining. *J. Exp. Med.*, **114**, 89–110

HOLBOROW, E. J. and JOHNSON, G. D. (1969). The immunofluorescent test for serum antinuclear factor. *Ass. Clin. Pathol. Broadsheet*, **65**, 1–5

HUANG, S-N., MINASSIAN, H. and MORSE, J. D. (1976). Application of immunofluorescent staining on paraffin sections improved by trypsin digestion. *Lab. Invest.*, **35**, 383–390

IRVINE, W. J. (1978). Autoimmunity against steroid producing organs. In *The Menarini Series on Immunopathology*. Eds Miescher *et al.* Vol. 1. Schwabe, Basel, pp. 35–49

KAMP, P., PLATZ, P. and NERUP, J. (1974). 'Steroid-cell' antibody in endocrine diseases. *Acta Endocrinol.*, **76**, 729–740

KURKI, P., LINDER, E., VIRTANEN, I. and STENMAN, S. (1977). Human smooth muscle autoantibodies reacting with intermediate (100 Å) filaments. *Nature (Lond.)*, **268**, 240–241

LEIBOWITZ, S. and HUGHES, R. A. C. (1983). *Immunology of the Nervous System*. Edward Arnold, London

LIDMAN, K. (1976). Clinical diagnosis in patients with smooth muscle antibodies: a study of a one-year material. *Acta Med. Scand.*, **200**, 403–407

MEYER ZUM BÜSCHENFELDE, K. H. and MIESCHER, P. A. (1972). Liver specific antigens. Purification and characterisation. *Clin. Exp. Immunol.*, **10**, 89–102

NAIRN, R. C. (1976). *Fluorescent Protein Tracing*. 4th Ed. Churchill-Livingstone, Edinburgh, London, New York

PASTERNACK, A., LINDER, E. and KUHLBÄCK, B. (1965). Glomerulonephritis with initial pulmonary haemorrhage. *Acta Med. Scand.*, **177**, 601–605

PEARSE, A. G. E. (1980). *Histochemistry, Theoretical and Applied*. 4th Ed. Vol. 1. Preparative and optical technology. Churchill-Livingstone, Edinburgh, London and New York

POLAK, J. M. and VAN NOORDEN, S. (1983). *Immunocytochemistry. Practical Applications in Pathology and Biology*. Wright PSG, Bristol, London, Boston

REES SMITH, B. (1977). Membrane receptors for polypeptide hormones. *Adv. Clin. Chem.*, **19**, 91–124

RIGGS, J. L., SEIWALD, R. J., BURCKHALTER, J. H., DOWNS, C. M. and METCALF, T. G. (1958). Isothiocyanate compounds as fluorescent labelling agents for immune serum. *Am. J. Pathol.*, **34**, 1081–1097

RIZZETTO, M., BIANCHI, F. B. and DONIACH, D. (1974). Characterisation of the microsomal antigen related to a subclass of active chronic hepatitis. *Immunology*, **26**, 589–601

SAINTE-MARIE, G. (1962). A paraffin embedding technique for studies employing immunofluorescence. *J. Histochem. Cytochem.*, **10**, 250–256

SCHENK, E. A. and CHURUKIAN, C. J. (1974). Immunofluorescence counterstains. *J. Histochem. Cytochem.*, **22**, 962–966

SILVER, D. M. and LANE, D. P. (1975). Dominant nonrepressiveness in the induction of autoimmunity to liver-specific F antigen. *J. Exp. Med.*, **142**, 1455–1461

SMITH, C. W., MARSHALL, J. D. and EVELAND, W. C. (1959). Use of contrasting fluorescent dye as counterstain in fixed tissue preparations. *Proc. Soc. Exp. Biol. (N.Y.)*, **102**, 179–181

SOMERFIELD, S. D. and WILSON, J. D. (1980). The detection of double stranded DNA antibody using human metaphase chromosomes. *J. Clin. Lab. Immunol.*, **3**, 203–207

SONDAG-TSCHROOTS, I. R. J. M., SCHULZ-RAATELAND, R. C. M., VAN WALBEEK, H. K. and FELTKAMP, T. E. W. (1979). Antibodies to motor end-plates demonstrated with the immunofluorescence technique. *Clin. Exp. Immunol.*, **37**, 323–327

SONTHEIMER, R. D. and GILLIAM, J. N. (1978). An immunofluorescence assay for double-stranded DNA antibodies using the *Crithidia luciliae* kinetoplast as a double-stranded DNA substrate. *J. Lab. Clin. Med.*, **91**, 550–558

SWANA, G. T., SWANA, M. R., BOTTAZZO, G-F. and DONIACH, D. (1977). A human-specific mitochondrial antibody. Its importance in the identification of organ-specific reactions. *Clin. Exp. Immunol.*, **28**, 517–525

TAN, E. M. (1979). Autoimmunity to nuclear antigens. In *The Cell Nucleus*. Ed. Busch, H. Vol. 7. Academic Press, London, pp. 457–477

TAN, E. M., ROBINSON, J. and ROBITAILLE, P. (1976). Studies on antibodies to histones by immunofluorescence. *Scand. J. Immunol.*, **5**, 811–818

THE, T. H. and FELTKAMP, T. E. W. (1970). Conjugation of fluorescein isothiocyanate to antibodies. II. A reproducible method. *Immunology*, **18**, 875–881

THIVOLET, J., MONIER, J. C., LALAIN, F. and RICHARD, M. M. (1965). Recherche quantitative simultanée des anticorps antinucléaires totaux et anti acide désoxyribonucléique sur frottis de sang de souris parasitées par *Trypanosoma gambiense*. *Ann. Inst. Pasteur*, **109**, 817–829

TOH, B. H. (1979). Smooth muscle autoantibodies and autoantigens. *Clin. Exp. Immunol.*, **38**, 621–628

VANDELLI, C., BOTTAZZO, G-F., DONIACH, D. and FRANCESCHI, F. (1979). Autoantibodies to gastrin-producing cells in antral (Type B) chronic gastritis. *New Engl. J. Med.*, **300**, 1406–1410

VINCENT, A. and NEWSOM-DAVIS, J. (1982). Acetylcholine receptor antibody characteristics in myasthenia gravis. I. Patients with generalized myasthenia or disease restricted to ocular muscles. *Clin. Exp. Immunol.*, **49**, 257–265

19

Immunoenzyme technique

Immunofluorescence techniques, the first kind of immunocytochemical methods to be developed (Coons and Kaplan, 1950), suffer from many disadvantages. The primary disadvantage is that fresh tissue is required, fixed paraffin-embedded tissue being generally unsuitable. The sections have to be examined in an aqueous mountant and are therefore not permanent, a feature which is complicated by the fact that the specific fluorescence decays with time and exposure to light. Furthermore expensive fluorescence equipment and suitable accommodation are required, and photography presents problems. Electron microscopy is not applicable.

The introduction of antibody directed enzyme labels, as an alternative to fluorochromes, has overcome all these disadvantages and has led to an incredible and rapid expansion of immunocytochemistry as both a research and a diagnostic tool (Falini and Taylor, 1983).

Several enzymes have been used as labels, for example, peroxidase (Nakane and Pierce, 1966), alkaline phosphatase (Engvall and Perlman, 1971) and glucose oxidase (Masseyeff and Maiolini, 1975), and many variations in technical methods have evolved (*see below*). Advances in specificity have occurred primarily with the introduction of monoclonal antibodies (Kohler and Milstein, 1976).

Types of method (*see Figure 19.1*)

Direct

The label is bound to the primary antibody.

Indirect

The primary antibody is applied to the section. A second labelled antibody from another species raised to the immunoglobulin of the species producing the primary antibody is then applied. The primary antibody thus acts as an immunoglobulin antigen at the second stage. The advantage of this method is that one labelled secondary antibody can be used to detect a number of primary antibodies from one species without the necessity of labelling each primary antibody.

Unlabelled antibody

A bridging antibody is interposed between the primary antibody and the final antibody, the latter being raised against horseradish peroxidase in the same species as

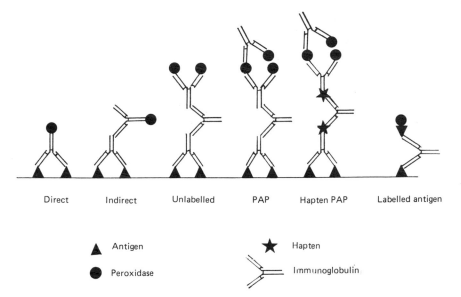

Direct   Indirect   Unlabelled   PAP   Hapten PAP   Labelled antigen

▲ Antigen   ★ Hapten

● Peroxidase   ⤙ Immunoglobulin

Figure 19.1 Diagrammatic representation of main types of immunocytochemical staining

the primary antibody. The last step is the application of horseradish peroxidase which binds immunologically to the final antibody, thus avoiding the necessity of any conjugation procedures. Single or double bridges may be used.

Peroxidase antiperoxidase

This modification of the antibody bridge method uses a preformed stable immune complex consisting of three peroxidase molecules and two antibody molecules as the third step (Sternberger *et al.*, 1970). This method is simpler to perform, allowing the use of much higher dilutions of primary antibody resulting in low background staining.

Labelled antigen

The primary antibody is applied to the section in high excess followed by labelled primary antigen (Mason and Sammons, 1979).

Hapten methods

A hapten is a small chemically well-defined molecule which will combine with hapten-specific antibodies, despite the fact that, by itself, it is unable to stimulate antibody formation. The advantage of hapten is that it can be linked covalently to antibodies without loss in their specific binding activity, thus allowing their tissue localization with the use of hapten-specific antibodies. For example, hapten, when combined with the primary antibody, can be localized with a labelled antibody to the hapten (Cammisuli and Wofsy, 1976). Jasani, Wynford-Thomas and Williams (1981) labelled both the primary antibody and the PAP complex with hapten (dinitrophenyl group, DNP) and used a monoclonal anti-DNP as the bridge. This hapten-bridging technique has been shown to produce intense labelling with low background staining.

Other methods

Avidin, a tetravalent glycoprotein from egg white, has a high affinity for biotin. Biotin can be linked to antibodies without causing any loss in their specific binding activity, and avidin may be used as a bridging agent to bring an enzyme label into close juxtaposition to the primary antibody (Guesdon, Ternynck and Avrameas, 1979; Hsu, Raine and Fanger, 1981).

Protein A from *Staphylococcus aureus* has the property of attaching to the Fc portion of immunoglobulins. Suitably labelled with an enzyme it may be used as a second layer agent (Roth, Bendayan and Orci, 1978).

Notes on technique

Endogenous peroxidase

Enzymatically active endogenous peroxidase in tissue sections is capable of reacting with hydrogen peroxide and oxidatively polymerizing diaminobenzidine. Since this would be confused with the immunoperoxidase reaction product it should be blocked at the start of the procedure. This can be accomplished by treating the section with 0.5% hydrogen peroxide in methanol for 30 minutes.

■ Enzyme digestion

Fixation and processing may mask antigens rendering them non-immunoreactive. Curran and Gregory (1977) and Mepham, Frater and Mitchell (1979) used proteolytic enzymes to unmask them. Masking is most pronounced in buffered formalin fixed material. Other fixatives such as Bouin, formaldehyde–mercury and formaldehyde–acetic acid are said not to mask antigens (Isaacson and Wright, 1983). Since these fixatives have disadvantages and because formalin is most widely used, trypsin digestion is often necessary to procure a satisfactory reaction, particularly for the detection of tissue immunoglobulins.

Great attention should be paid to the conditions of the reaction. Optimum time and temperature must be ascertained for each tissue since the conditions of fixation vary from tissue to tissue.

Reagent

0.1% Trypsin in tris buffer at pH 7.8. Warm the solution to 37 °C and check the pH.

Method

(1) Bring section to water.
(2) Block endogenous peroxidase.
(3) Place in pretreated trypsin reagent at 37 °C for the required time.
(4) Rinse well in cold distilled water.
(5) Rinse in phosphate buffered saline (PBS).
(6) Proceed with the reaction sequence.

Since sections tend to become detached from slides during trypsin digestion they must be firmly attached to the slide with adhesive. Slides can be treated with either 0.01% aqueous poly(L-lysine) or a water soluble wood glue emulsion.

Buffers

(1) 0.01 M Phosphate buffered saline pH 7.1 (PBS)

NaCl	8.5 g
Na$_2$HPO$_4$	1.07 g
NaH$_2$PO$_4$.2 H$_2$O	0.39 g
Distilled water	to 1000 ml

(2) 0.05 M Tris–HCl-buffered saline pH 7.6 (TBS)

Trizma base (Sigma)	6.05 g
Distilled water	100 ml

Adjust to pH 7.6 with 0.5 M HCl. For use dilute 1:10 with 0.9% sodium chloride.

Peroxidase development

Several developers have been used, the classical being diaminobenzidine (DAB). The probability that this reagent is carcinogenic has encouraged the introduction of alternative reagents.

■ **DAB (after Graham and Karnovsky, 1966)**

In order to avoid repeatedly weighing small quantities of DAB it is best to make a large batch of concentrated DAB solution, for example, ten times, dispense into vials and store frozen.

Reagent

Stock

DAB	2.5 g
0.2 M Tris buffer pH 7.6	500 ml

Dispense in 5 ml amounts and store frozen.

For use

0.2 M Tris buffer pH 7.6	45 ml
Stock DAB	5 ml
30% Hydrogen peroxide (100 vol.)	0.015 ml

Method

(1) Treat with the reagent for 5 minutes.
(2) Rinse in tris buffer.
(3) Wash in water.
(4) Counterstain lightly with haematoxylin.
(5) Dehydrate, clear and mount in synthetic resin.

■ **Phenylenediamine-pyrocatechol (PDP)**

The peroxidation of *p*-phenylenediamine is accelerated by pyrocatechol producing a dark brown reaction product. The mixture is available commercially as Hanker–Yates reagent (Hanker *et al.*, 1977), consisting of one part *p*-phenylenediamine and two parts pyrocatechol.

Reagent

Hanker–Yates reagent   75 mg
0.1 M Tris buffer pH 7.6   100 ml

For use add 0.1 ml 30% hydrogen peroxide (100 vol.).

Method

Treat with the reagent for 5–20 minutes at room temperature and continue as above.

■ Amino-ethylcarbazole (after Kaplow, 1975)

The reaction product using this reagent is red in colour and soluble in alcohol but sections may be mounted in synthetic resin after the sections have been thoroughly dried.

Reagent

0.4% 3-Amino-9-ethylcarbazole in dimethylformamide	0.5 ml
0.05 M Acetate buffer pH 5	9.5 ml
30% Hydrogen peroxide (100 vol.)	0.01 ml

Method

(1) Filter the reagent onto slides and incubate for 5 minutes at room temperature.
(2) Counterstain lightly in haematoxylin (do not differentiate).
(3) Wash in water.
(4) Mount in aqueous mountant or dry thoroughly and mount in synthetic resin.

Blocking of non-specific reactive sites

Non-immune serum from the same species as that producing the second layer antibody (e.g. normal swine serum), applied to the section at the beginning of the procedure, blocks protein binding sites by non-specific adsorption or by the binding of specific but unwanted serum antibodies (van Noorden and Polak, 1983).

  Since these reactions are of low affinity the serum is simply drained and not washed off, before the primary antibody is applied.

Antibodies

Before an antibody is brought into routine use its optimum working dilution should be ascertained by titration. In this way the dilution giving the strongest specific reaction with the least non-specific background staining is found.

  In sensitive methods such as the PAP method and the hapten-labelled antibody technique, it is often possible to use very low concentrations producing little non-specific staining and ensuring the economical use of reagents which are often very expensive. High dilutions also reduce the possibility of non-specific ionic binding and complement binding.

Controls

To ensure the reliability of an immunocytochemical technique several controls should be used.

(1) Treatment of test sections with negative control serum.
(2) Parallel staining of negative control sections with test serum.
(3) Absorption of primary antibody with excess antigen should abolish staining.
(4) Adsorption of the specific antibody to affinity column should abolish the staining reaction.
(5) Treatment of primary antibody with inappropriate antigen should produce no impairment of staining.
(6) Parallel staining of positive control sections.

General procedure

■ **Indirect method**

(1) Bring section to water.
(2) Block endogenous peroxidase.
(3) Rinse well in PBS or TBS.
(4) Treat with trypsin if desired.
(5) Treat with 3% normal swine serum.
(6) Drain off without washing.

Table 19.1

	Direct	Indirect	Unlabelled	PAP	Hapten–PAP	Labelled antigen
Hydrogen peroxide/methanol	●	●	●	●	●	●
Normal swine serum	●	●	●	●		
Normal rabbit serum					●	●
Primary rabbit antiserum		●	●	●		●
Primary rabbit antiserum/peroxidase labelled	●					
Primary rabbit antiserum/hapten labelled					●	
Swine anti-rabbit Ig			●	●		
Swine anti-rabbit Ig/peroxidase labelled		●				
Anti-hapten monoclonal antibody					●	
Rabbit anti-peroxidase			●			
PAP				●		
PAP/hapten labelled					●	
Peroxidase			●			
Antigen/peroxidase labelled						●
Development reaction	●	●	●	●	●	●

(7) Apply appropriate dilution of primary antiserum and incubate at room temperature for the predetermined time in a moist chamber.
(8) Wash off with PBS or TBS.
(9) Rinse in three changes of buffered saline, 2 minutes in each.
(10) Incubate in appropriate dilution of peroxidase-labelled secondary antiserum.
(11) Develop peroxidase.
(12) Counterstain as desired.
(13) Mount as appropriate.

The various techniques are detailed by Sternberger (1979). The outline steps of the various techniques are shown in *Table 19.1.*

Applications

While either immunofluorescence or immunoenzyme techniques may be used in similar situations the latter are becoming standard in the identification of tumour markers. Tumour marker demonstration is used to determine the site of occult primary tumours and in differential diagnosis. It is used in the functional classification of tumours and is important in determining prognosis and treatment.

These techniques are used in many areas, examples of tumour markers are given below:

Lymphocyte markers
Pituitary hormones
Endocrine polypeptides
Enzymes
Oncofetal antigens
Epithelial antigens
Immunoglobulins

References

CAMMISULI, S. and WOFSY, L. (1976). Hapten sandwich labelling. III. Bifunctional reagents for immunospecific labelling of cell surface antigens. *J. Immunol.*, **117**, 1695–1704

COONS, A. H. and KAPLAN, M. H. (1950). Localisation of antigens in tissue cells. II. Improvements in a method for the detection of antigen by means of fluorescent antibody. *J. Exp. Med.*, **91**, 1–30

CURRAN, R. C. and GREGORY, J. (1977). The unmasking of antigens in paraffin sections of tissue by trypsin. *Experientia*, **33**, 1400–1401

ENGVALL, E. and PERLMAN, P. (1971). Enzyme linked immunosorbent assay (ELISA). Quantitative assay of immunoglobulin G. *Immunocytochemistry*, **8**, 871–874

FALINI, B. and TAYLOR, C. R. (1983). New developments in immunoperoxidase techniques and their applications. *Arch. Pathol. Lab. Med.*, **107**, 105–117

GRAHAM, R. C. and KARNOVSKY, M. J. (1966). The early stages of absorption of injected horseradish peroxidase in the proximal tubules of the mouse kidney. Ultrastructural cytochemistry by a new technique. *J. Histochem. Cytochem.*, **14**, 291–302

GUESDON, J. L., TERNYNCK, T. and AVRAMEAS, S. (1979). The use of avidin–biotin interaction in immuno-enzymatic techniques. *J. Histochem. Cytochem.*, **27**, 1131–1139

HANKER, J. S., YATES, P. E., METZ, C. B. and RUSTIONI, A. (1977). A new specific, sensitive and non-carcinogenic reagent for the demonstration of horseradish peroxidase. *Histochem. J.*, **9**, 789–792

HSU, S. M., RAINE, L. and FANGER, H. (1981). A comparative study of the PAP method and avidin–biotin complex method for studying polypeptide hormones with radioimmunoassay antibodies. *Am. J. Clin. Pathol.*, **75**, 734–738

ISAACSON, P. and WRIGHT, D. H. (1983). Immunocytochemistry of lymphoreticular tumours. In *Immunocytochemistry. Practical Applications in Pathology and Biology.* Eds Polak, J. M. and van Noorden, S. Wright PSG, Bristol

JASANI, B., WYNFORD-THOMAS, D. and WILLIAMS, E. D. (1981). Use of monoclonal antibodies for immuno-localisation of tissue antigens. *J. Clin. Pathol.*, **34**, 1000–1002

KAPLOW, L. S. (1975). Substitute for benzidine in myeloperoxidase stains. *Am. J. Clin. Pathol.*, **63**, 451

KOHLER, G. and MILSTEIN, C. (1976). Derivation of specific antibody-producing tissue culture and tumor lines by cell fusion. *Eur. J. Immunol.*, **6**, 511–519

MASON, D. Y. and SAMMONS, R. E. (1979). The labelled antigen method of immuno-enzymatic staining. *J. Histochem. Cytochem.*, **27**, 832–840

MASSAYEFF, R. and MAIOLINI, R. (1975). A sandwich method of enzyme immunoassay. Application to rat and human α-fetoprotein. *J. Immunol. Methods*, **8**, 223–234

MEPHAM, B. L., FRATER, W. and MITCHELL, B. L. (1979). The use of proteolytic enzymes to improve immunological staining by the PAP technique. *Histochem. J.*, **11**, 345–357

NAKANE, P. K. and PIERCE, G. B. JR (1966). Enzyme labelled antibodies: preparation and application for the localisation of antigen. *J. Histochem. Cytochem.*, **14**, 929–931

ROTH, J., BENDAYAN, M. and ORCI, L. (1978). Ultrastructural localisation of intracellular antigen by the use of protein A–gold complex. *J. Histochem. Cytochem.*, **26**, 1074–1081

STERNBERGER, L. A. (1979). *Immunocytochemistry*. 2nd Ed. Wiley, New York

STERNBERGER, L. A., HARDY, P. H., CUCULIS, J. J. and MEYER, H. G. (1970). The unlabelled antibody–enzyme method of immunochemistry. Preparation and properties of soluble antigen–antibody complex (horseradish peroxidase–anti-horseradish peroxidase) and its use in the identification of spirochaetes. *J. Histochem. Cytochem.*, **18**, 315–333

VAN NOORDEN, S. and POLAK, J. M. (1983). Immunocytochemistry today. In *Immunocytochemistry. Practical Applications in Pathology and Biology*. Eds Polak, J. M. and van Noorden, S. Wright PSG, Bristol

Part VI

Tissues of special interest

20

The nervous system

Neurohistology has always been regarded as a series of very highly specialized methods which are difficult even for the practised routine technologist. Little specialized work of this nature enters the ordinary routine histology laboratory, and many of the techniques employed are lengthy and require the use of solutions with an involved preparation. These points are probably largely responsible for the apprehension with which many technologists approach neurohistology, either in their own laboratory or in preparation for their Institute of Medical Laboratory Sciences examinations. In spite of this, any competent technologist should be able to perform most of the techniques involved with a small amount of practice, and given an understanding of what he is demonstrating. It is for the latter reason that the beginning of this section has been devoted to the anatomy and composition of the nervous system, since the cells and fibres, and the nomenclature, are peculiar to it.

Anatomy

The central nervous system (CNS) is made up of the following six parts (*Figure 20.1*).

(1) The *cerebrum* is composed of right- and left-paired halves or hemispheres which are separated above, in front and behind to a depth of approximately $1\frac{1}{2}$ inches by the great longitudinal fissure; deep to this is the corpus callosum, composed of nerve fibres, which connects the two hemispheres. Each hemisphere is composed of a mass of white matter covered with a superficial layer of grey matter.

(2) The *cerebellum* is composed of two hemispheres, the surfaces of which are divided by a series of deep fissures known as sulci, which are close together. As with the cerebrum, there is a core of white matter with a superficial layer of grey matter.

(3) The *midbrain* and *pons* connect with the medulla and spinal cord; it is from here that the optic nerves emanate.

(4) The *medulla* connects the spinal cord to the midbrain and cerebellum.

(5) The *spinal cord* connects the nervous structures to the peripheral (skeletal) nerves. The cord is composed of a core of grey matter—which increases in proportion as the nerves leave it (*Figure 20.2*)—surrounded by white matter. The cervical enlargement (where the nerves of the upper body and arms branch off), and the lumbar enlargement (where the nerves of the lower limbs leave) give characteristic shapes on cross-section (*Figure 20.2*).

(6) The *meninges* surround and protect the central nervous system. They are composed of connective tissue proper and comprise three membranes: (a) the dura mater; (b)

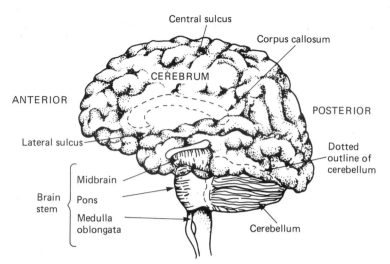

Figure 20.1 Diagram of the brain

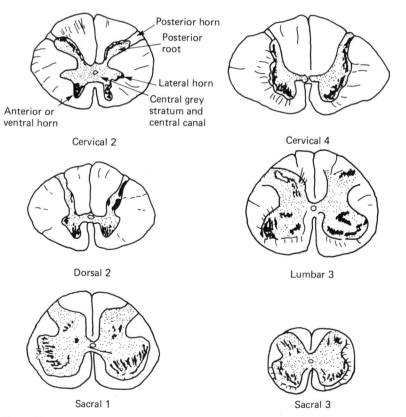

Figure 20.2 Drawings illustrating the characteristic shapes of the spinal cord at different levels, note the increase in grey matter (shaded) as compared with the white matter at the lower end of the cord

the arachnoid; and (c) the pia mater. These membranes are composed of collagen fibres, a small number of elastic fibres and endothelial cells.

Composition

The nervous system is composed of three types of tissue:

(1) *Nervous tissue proper:* nerve cells and their processes.
(2) *Neuroglia:* the special connective tissue of the nervous system.
(3) *Connective tissue proper:* the meninges (the dura mater, the arachnoid and pia mater).

Nervous tissue proper

Nervous tissue proper consists of neurons (nerve cells) and their processes. These processes (nerve fibres) may be very long and are known as axons (those conducting impulses from the cell) and dendrites (those conducting impulses to the cell). A nerve axon ends by branching into a series of smaller, finer fibres which make contact with the next neuron; where these meet the dendrites of another cell (without their actually touching) the result is known as a *synapse*. Although there is a natural tendency to think of nerve cells and nerve fibres as separate entities, because of the near impossibility of preparing sections to show the whole, one should remember that the nerve fibres are processes of the cell and that they are a single unit, although for convenience they will be dealt with separately.

Nerve cells

These may vary in size from 4 to 5 µm in diameter (the pigment cells of the cerebellum) up to 150 µm in diameter (motor cells of the anterior horn of the spinal cord). They are usually classified by the number of their processes: unipolar (rare), bipolar (retina and cochlea) and multi-polar (most common and found throughout most of the nervous system) (*Figure 20.3a*).

The nucleus is pale-staining, large and usually circular, containing a nucleolus.

Within the cytoplasm of nerve cells are found the following.

Neurofibrils

These are fine fibres which are arranged throughout the cytoplasm, extending into the processes.

Nissl substance

This material in fixed tissue is granular in nature and stains intensely with basic aniline dyes. The Nissl substance is usually evenly distributed throughout the cytoplasm except for the area immediately surrounding the origin of the axon; it may, however, spread into the dendrites. Damage to the nerve fibre usually results in the loss of Nissl substance (*Figure 20.3b*).

Mitochondria and Golgi apparatus

These may be well demonstrated in nerve cells.

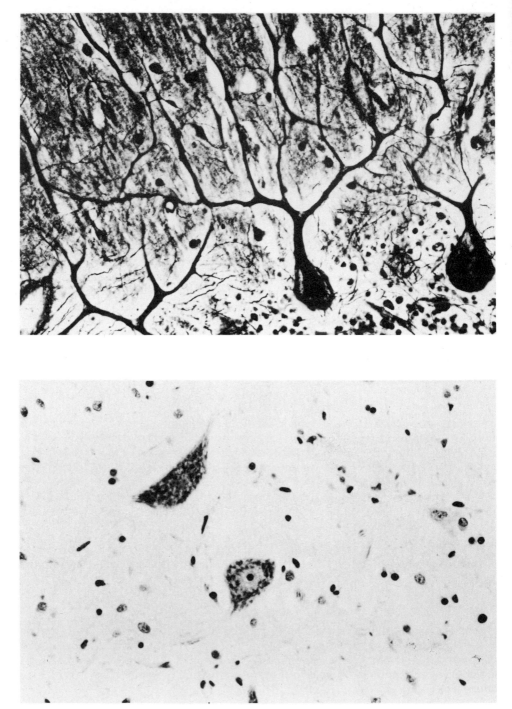

Figure 20.3 (a) Purkinje cells in cerebellum. Paraffin section. Glees and Marsland silver impregnation. Original magnification × 100. (b) Ganglion cells in spinal cord showing Nissl granules. Paraffin section Cresyl fast violet. Original magnification × 100.

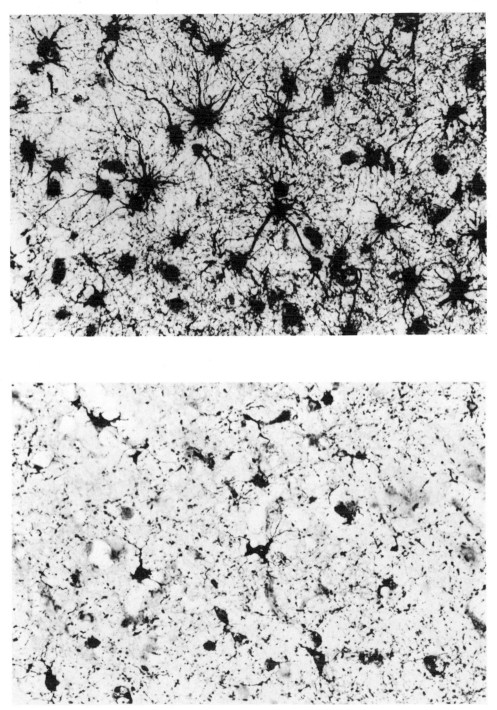

Figure 20.3 (cont.) (c) Astrocytes in cerebrum. Frozen section Cajal's gold sublimate technique. Original magnification ×100. (d) Oligodendroglia and microglia in cerebrum. Paraffin section. Modified Weil–Davenport. Original magnification ×100

Granules

Certain cells, such as those in the substantia nigra, contain melanin, and all ageing nerve cells may contain yellow lipofuscin granules.

Nerve fibres

These may consist of the following.

Naked axons (axis cylinders)

These are without any form of covering and are found in the grey matter in the brain and spinal cord.

Axons with a neurilemmal sheath

These are surrounded only by flattened cells of Schwann, the nuclei of which stain intensely (nucleated sheath of Schwann). They are usually found in the sympathetic nervous system.

Myelinated nerve fibres

These are axons surrounded by a lipid sheath (myelin sheath), which is in turn surrounded by a neurilemmal sheath.

In peripheral nerve fibres the myelin sheath is constricted at regular intervals, these constrictions being known as the nodes of Ranvier. Myelinated fibres are also found in the white matter of the brain and spinal cord.

Nerve endings

Nerve fibres end in a peripheral organ and may be either of the following.

Sensory or receptor

These transmit nerve impulses from the peripheral organ to the nervous system. They are dendrites of a nerve cell and may end in a simple branching structure or in a complex organ.

Motor or effector

These transmit nerve impulses from the nervous system to the peripheral organ. They are terminations of a nerve axon (myelinated in voluntary muscle and non-myelinated in cardiac and in striped muscle and glands). The nerve endings are either special motor end-plates (voluntary muscle), or simple branching of the axon terminating in thickened ends. (For details of the more complex organs a textbook of histology should be consulted.)

Neuroglia

The name neuroglia (meaning nerve glue) is given to the special type of connective tissue which is found in the nervous system. It is composed of neuroglia fibres and cells.

The astrocytes and their processes form a complicated meshwork which supports the neurons and insulates them from each other; the oligodendroglia are thought to be concerned in the formation and maintenance of myelin; and the microglia, which may become amoeboid and phagocytic, act as a defence mechanism for the nervous system.

The neuroglia cells are divided into two types.

Macroglia

Ectodermal in origin, macroglia may be protoplasmic astrocytes, fibrous astrocytes or oligodendroglia.

Microglia

These are mesodermal in origin.

Macroglia

These are the neuroglia proper, as classified below (*Figure 20.3c*).

Protoplasmic astrocytes

These cells have a large nucleus and a granular cytoplasm with long branching processes which are protoplasmic in nature. Some of the processes are attached to blood vessels by 'sucker feet'. The cells contain no fibres. They are found most abundantly in the grey matter.

Fibrous astrocytes

These cells (as the name implies) contain thick fibres which branch outside the cell. They are also found attached to capillaries by vascular feet, but the processes tend to be longer and finer than those of the protoplasmic astrocyte. They are most abundant in the white matter.

Oligodendroglia

These cells are small and stain intensely. They have no fibres or vascular feet, but the processes are fine and rarely branch (*Figure 20.3d*).

They are abundant in the white matter where they are found in rows along the myelinated fibres. In the grey matter they are found close to nerve cells or blood vessels.

Microglia

Microglia are small oval-shaped cells which contain a deeply staining nucleus. From each end of the cell a thick process arises which branches freely to give numerous small processes ending in terminal spines (*Figure 20.3d*).

Meninges (connective tissue proper)

The brain and spinal cord are covered by three membranes: the dura mater, the arachnoid and the pia mater.

Dura mater

The strong outermost coat, the dura mater is composed of white fibrous tissue (collagen) and a few elastic fibres.

Arachnoid

This is a very thin membrane of fine connective-tissue fibres clothed on both sides with endothelial cells. Between the arachnoid and the pia mater is the subarachnoid space which contains the cerebrospinal fluid. The space has innumerable fine trabeculae crossing it.

Pia mater

The pia mater consists of white fibrous tissue and elastic fibres, and is highly vascular.

The pia mater and the arachnoid are sometimes known collectively as the pia–arachnoid membrane because of their close attachment to each other.

Processing and section cutting of the central nervous system

Fixation

For some techniques special fixatives are given, but as a routine the best fixative is formal–saline. This will enable special fixatives and techniques to be used subsequently if desired. Whole brains should always be fixed by perfusion via the basilar artery after first washing through with isotonic saline solution to remove the blood. After injection of the fixative, the basilar artery is tied off with a long length of thread. The brain is then transferred to a bucket containing fixative and suspended by the thread from a glass or wooden rod laid over the top of the bucket so that the brain remains suspended in the fixing fluid without touching the bottom of the container.

Processing

Sections may be prepared from either paraffin or celloidin-embedded tissue, or frozen tissue, depending on the technique to be employed. While routine methods for celloiding embedding or freezing may be used, processing by paraffin embedding requires extra care.

Paraffin embedding

Vacuum bath embedding is not recommended for tissue of the central nervous system, since this method tends to render the sections brittle, and often causes them to float off the slides during staining or silver impregnation techniques. Such tissue should be impregnated thoroughly with paraffin wax giving at least four changes of wax during this period.

Section cutting

Sections are cut routinely at a thickness of 7 μm, but sections for myelin techniques should be at least 12 μm in thickness. Those sections in which complete neurons are to be demonstrated (dendrites and axons) should be even thicker (15–20 μm).

Methods of demonstration

As routine methods, haematoxylin and Van Gieson, and Mallory's PTA haematoxylin are employed as with other tissues.

Other methods, such as those for elastic tissue, reticulin, mucin and fat, are often employed for differential diagnosis.

The special methods employed for the demonstration of the various elements in nervous tissue are dealt with under the following headings.

Neurons (nerve cells and their processes)
Nissl substance
Normal and degenerate myelin
Neuroglial cells and fibres
Peripheral nerves
Rapid methods

Neurons (nerve cells and their processes)

The most popular technique in Great Britain for the demonstration of neurons is that of Bielschowsky, or one of its variants. Three such methods are given:

(1) the long standard method;
(2) Glees and Marsland's modification for paraffin sections; and
(3) Holmes' technique, a very reliable and simple technique, used either with or without Luxol fast blue.

All of these methods are reliable and give good results with human tissue and most animal tissue. Eager's method for degenerating axons is also given. As with all silver impregnation procedures, dishes and flasks should be thoroughly cleaned and rinsed several times in distilled water before use.

■ Bielschowsky's method (1909)

Reagent

Ammoniacal silver

To 5 ml of 20% silver nitrate add six drops of 40% sodium hydroxide. Add strong ammonia (0.880) drop by drop until the resultant precipitate is just dissolved. Add distilled water to a total volume of 25 ml and filter.

Technique

(1) Tissue should be fixed in formal–saline (once adequately fixed, the length of time in formal–saline is not important).
(2) Rinse tissue in water before cutting.
(3) Frozen sections are cut at 10 μm for neurofibrils, or 15–20 μm to show cells and processes.
(4) Wash sections in distilled water for 1 hour, giving several changes.
(5) Transfer to a dish of 4% silver nitrate; place in the dark for 24–48 hours (sections must be flat and without creases).
(6) Rinse rapidly in distilled water.
(7) Treat with fresh ammoniacal silver nitrate for 2–10 minutes until sections, which are a very light brown, darken in shade to a deep tobacco brown.
(8) Rinse rapidly in two changes of distilled water.
(9) Transfer to 10% formalin in tap-water for 5–10 minutes to reduce the silver.

(10) Wash in distilled water, two to three changes, for 5–10 minutes.
(11) Tone in 0.2% gold chloride for 10–15 minutes.
(12) Rinse in distilled water.
(13) Transfer to 5% sodium thiosulphate for 5 minutes.
(14) Wash in tap-water for 5 minutes.
(15) Float on to clean slides, dehydrate, clear and mount in Canada balsam or synthetic resin.

Results

Nerve cells (and neurofibrils), axons and dendrites   Brown to black

Note: Toning (stage 11) is optional and need not be employed: as it tends to clear the background and make the neurons appear more deeply impregnated it is generally included.

■ **Glees and Marsland's modification of Bielschowsky's method for paraffin sections (Marsland, Glees and Erikson, 1954)**

This method gives excellent results with paraffin sections of formal-fixed material and is sufficiently reliable to be used as a routine method.

Reagent

Ammoniacal silver

To 30 ml of 20% silver nitrate add 20 ml of absolute alcohol and mix; add strong ammonia (sp.gr. 0.880) drop by drop until the precipitate first formed is just dissolved, then add a further five drops of strong ammonia.

Method

(1) Treat sections with xylene for $\frac{1}{2}$–1 minute to remove wax.
(2) Flood with alcohol for 30 seconds.
(3) Flood slide with 1% celloidin for 20 seconds, or put into a glass-stoppered jar containing 1% celloidin for 20–30 seconds.
(4) Wipe off excess celloidin from back of slide, and flood with 70% alcohol to harden the remainder.
(5) Rinse in distilled water (two changes).
(6) Treat with 20% silver nitrate at 37 °C for 25–30 minutes.
(7) Rinse in distilled water.
(8) Flood twice, 10 seconds each time, with 10% formalin in tap-water.
(9) Impregnate with ammoniacal silver for 30 seconds.
(10) Drain off silver solution and flood slide with two changes of 10% formalin for 1 minute each.
(11) Rinse in distilled water.

Note: Sections may be toned in 0.2% gold chloride for 10 minutes, followed by a rinse in distilled water. Stages 12–15 should then be continued.

(12) Fix in 5% sodium thiosulphate for 5 minutes.

(13) Wash in tap-water.
(14) Blot and flood with absolute alcohol to remove celloidin film. The metallic precipitate which often occurs is usually confined to the celloidin film and is removed with it.
(15) Clear in xylene and mount in Canada balsam or synthetic resin.

Results

Neurons (nerve cells, axons and dendrites)   Black

■ Holmes' silver technique (1947)

This method gives good results when used in conjunction with Luxol fast blue to show the myelin sheaths.

Reagents

Impregnating solution

Dilute 100 ml of Holmes' boric acid–borax buffer pH 8.4 (page 133) to 494 ml with distilled water. Add 1 ml of 1% aqueous silver nitrate, then 5 ml of 1% aqueous solution of pure pyridine. Mix well. This solution should be freshly prepared.

Reducing solution

Hydroquinone	1 g
Sodium sulphite (cryst.)	10 g
Distilled water	to 100 ml

Method

(1) Bring formalin fixed paraffin sections to water.
(2) Place in 20% aqueous silver nitrate, in the dark, at room temperature for 1 hour.
(3) Wash in distilled water (three changes) for 10 minutes.
(4) Place in impregnating solution, cover container and leave overnight at 37 °C. There should not be less than 20 ml of solution for each slide.
(5) Remove slides from impregnating solution, shake off excess fluid and place in reducing solution for 2–3 minutes.
(6) Wash in running water for 3 minutes.
(7) Rinse in distilled water.
(8) Tone in 0.2% gold chloride for 3 minutes.
(9) Rinse in distilled water.
(10) Place in 2% oxalic acid for 3–10 minutes. The impregnation of the neurons is controlled at this stage, they become progressively pale red, deep red, then black. If Luxol fast blue is being used to counterstain myelin the impregnation should be stopped while axons are reddish-black.
(11) Rinse in distilled water.
(12) Place in 5% sodium thiosulphate for 5 minutes.
(13) Wash in tap-water.
(14) Dehydrate, clear and mount in synthetic resin.

Or

(14) Rinse in 95% alcohol.

(15)–(20) As steps (2)–(7) in Luxol fast blue–cresyl violet stain on page 392.

(21) Dehydrate, clear and mount in synthetic resin.

Results

Neurons	Red-black
Myelin (if stained)	Blue

■ Eager's method for the demonstration of degenerating axons (1970)

Several modifications of the Nauta–Gygax (1951) method for degenerating axons have been introduced. Most of these rely on the suppression of the staining of the normal fibres and enhancement of the staining of the degenerating fibres.

Fixation

Formal–saline.

Reagents

Ammoniacal silver

1.5% Silver nitrate	40 ml
95% Ethanol	24 ml
Ammonia	4 ml
2.5% Sodium hydroxide	3.6 ml

Reducer

Ethanol	90 ml
Distilled water	810 ml
1% Citric acid	27 ml
10% Formalin	27 ml

Method

(1) Frozen sections rinsed in water from 2% formalin.

(2) Treat with 2.5% uranyl nitrate for 5 minutes.

(3) Rinse in distilled water.

(4) Place in ammoniacal silver for 3–15 minutes until brown.

(5) Transfer directly to reducer for 2–5 minutes until there is no further change in colour.

(6) Rinse in distilled water.

(7) Fix in 5% sodium thiosulphate.

(8) Wash, dehydrate, clear and mount in synthetic resin.

Results

Degenerating fibres	Brown to black
Normal fibres	Pale yellow

Nissl substance

This granular material for which the standard method of demonstration has been thionin or toluidine blue followed by Gothard's differentiator, is, in fact, almost pure ribonucleic acid. It is well demonstrated by the Luxol fast blue–cresyl violet technique, or specifically by the acridine–orange or Unna–Pappenheim methods which stain it an intense red. After treatment with the enzyme ribonuclease (page 192), the substance cannot be demonstrated either with Unna–Pappenheim stain or the basic aniline dyes.

■ Thionin or toluidine blue methods

Fixation

Although alcohol fixation was originally specified, formal–saline fixation gives good results.

Reagent

Gothard's differentiator

Creosote	50 ml
Cajuput oil	40 ml
Xylene	50 ml
Absolute alcohol	150 ml

This original formula is really too powerful and it is advisable to dilute it with an equal amount of absolute alcohol before use.

Method

(1) Bring paraffin, celloidin or frozen sections to water.
(2) Stain for 30 minutes at 56 °C (or overnight at room temperature) in 1% toluidine blue in 1% borax, or in 0.1% thionin.
(3) Rinse in water.
(4) Treat with 90% alcohol for 10–30 seconds.
(5) Differentiate in Gothard's differentiator until the Nissl substance stands out against a clear background. This stage should be controlled with a microscope.
(6) Rinse in absolute alcohol.
(7) Clear in xylene and mount in resinous medium.

Results

Nissl substance	Deep blue to mauve
Nucleoli and chromatin	Blue
Other tissue elements	Colourless

■ Cresyl fast violet method

Fixation

Formal–saline or alcohol.

For paraffin sections

Method

(1) Bring sections to water.
(2) Stain in 1% aqueous cresyl fast violet for 20–30 minutes.
(3) Rinse in water.
(4) Dehydrate in ethanol and place in xylene.
(5) Differentiate in 95% alcohol containing a few drops of cajuput oil
(6) Rinse in 95% alcohol.
(7) Dehydrate, clear and mount in synthetic resin.

Results

Nissl substance   Deep violet
Background   Colourless

For celloidin sections

Differentiator (Cook, 1974)

95% Alcohol   100 ml
Chloroform   2 ml
Acetic acid   8 drops

Method

(1) Place celloidin sections in 70% ethanol overnight.
(2) Rinse in distilled water.
(3) Place sections in 0.1% cresyl fast violet and heat until a temperature of 60 °C is reached. Allow to cool for 1 hour.
(4) Wash in water.
(5) Partially dehydrate in 75 and 95% ethanol.
(6) Place in xylene and leave overnight.
(7) Rinse in absolute ethanol and 95% ethanol.
(8) Complete differentiation in special differentiator.
(9) Arrest differentiation in xylene.
(10) Mount in Canada balsam.

Results

Nissl substance   Violet
Background   Colourless

Normal myelin

The classical method of demonstrating normal myelin is the Weigert–Pal technique which is performed on paraffin or, preferably, celloidin sections. Loyez has been the routine method for its demonstration in paraffin sections and it is well demonstrated by the Luxol fast blue–cresyl violet technique. McManus's Sudan black method (page 269) demonstrates myelin well, but it is not specific. Normal myelin in frozen sections may be demonstrated by the fat-soluble stains (pages 262–264), by Baker's acid haematein method (page 266) and by the peracetic acid–Schiff technique (page 274). The method of choice for myelin in peripheral nerves is that of Page (1970) (*see* page 403).

■ **Weigert–Pal technique (Kultschitzky's modification) (1890)**

The Kultschitzky's modification of the Weigert–Pal method is based on the formation of chromium dioxide by the interaction of chrome salts with the phosphatides and cerebrosides which are constituents of normal myelin. It is this chromium dioxide which subsequently acts as a mordant and forms a lake with the haematoxylin.

Reagents

(1) Weigert's primary mordant

Potassium dichromate	5 g
Fluorchrome (chromium fluoride)	2.5 g
Distilled water	to 100 ml

Add the dichromate to the water, bring to the boil and add the fluorchrome. Stir the solution well; cool and filter.

(2) Gliabeize*

Fluorchrome (chromium fluoride)	2.5 g
Copper acetate	5 g
Distilled water	to 100 ml

Add the fluorchrome and copper acetate to the water and bring to the boil. While the solution is boiling, add 3 ml of acetic acid. Cool, filter and keep in a well-stoppered bottle.

(3) Kultschitzky's haematoxylin

10% Haematoxylin in absolute alcohol (ripened)	10 ml
Glacial acetic acid	2 ml
Distilled water	90 ml

This solution should be freshly prepared.

(4) Pal's solution

Oxalic acid	1 g
Sodium sulphite	1 g
Distilled water	to 100 ml

Method

(1) Fix tissue in formal–saline.
(2) Transfer to Weigert's primary mordant for 5–10 days.
(3) Wash in running water overnight.
(4) Dehydrate and embed in celloidin.

* The use of gliabeize is not essential, stage (6) being optional, but since it gives improved staining in many cases, it is advisable to use it as a routine.

(5) Cut sections 12–20 μm in thickness (cross-section of the spinal cord need not be thicker than 12 μm).
(6) Treat with gliabeize for 30 minutes (this stage is optional, but is preferred, *see footnote** on previous page).
(7) Wash in water.
(8) Stain in Kultschitzky's haematoxylin for 12–24 hours.
(9) Rinse in distilled water.
(10) Treat with 0.25% potassium permanganate for $\frac{1}{2}$–1 minute.
(11) Rinse rapidly in distilled water.
(12) Treat with Pal's solution for 1–2 minutes.
(13) Wash sections in several changes of tap-water for 10–20 minutes.
(14) Dehydrate, clear and mount in Canada balsam or synthetic resin.

Note: Stages (10)–(12) are the stages of differentiation. From stage (12) the section is returned via stage (11) to stage (10) and the sequence repeated until only the myelin sheaths are blue on a nearly colourless background. Sections may be left in Pal's solution, or in fresh distilled water, but never for longer than 1 minute in the 0.25% potassium permanganate.

Results

Myelin sheaths and red blood cells	Deep blue-black
Other tissue elements	Colourless to creamy yellow

■ **Luxol fast blue–cresyl violet for myelin (modified Kluver and Barrera, 1953)**

This method is excellent for staining myelin fibres with good cellular definition.

Reagents

Luxol fast blue solution

Luxol fast blue	1 g
95% Alcohol	1000 ml
10% Acetic acid	5 ml

Alternative Luxol fast blue solution (Salthouse, 1964)

Isopropanol	100 ml
Luxol fast blue	0.1 g

Cresyl violet solution

Cresyl violet	0.1 g
Distilled water	100 ml

Lithium carbonate solution

0.05% Aqueous solution lithium carbonate

This can be diluted to slow down differentiation.

Cresyl violet differentiator

95% Alcohol	90 ml
Chloroform	10 ml
Glacial acetic acid	3 drops

Method

(1) Bring sections to 95% alcohol.
(2) Stain in Luxol fast blue overnight at 37 °C.
(3) Wash in 95% alcohol, then in distilled water.
(4) Commence differentiation by immersing sections in lithium carbonate solution for not more than 20 seconds.
(5) Differentiate in 70% alcohol until grey and white matter are clearly distinguished (30 seconds–1 minute).
(6) Rinse in distilled water and examine under microscope. If differentiation is not complete repeat steps (4)–(6) with reduced times (lithium carbonate, 2–3 seconds).
(7) Wash well in distilled water.
(8) Stain in cresyl violet for 10 minutes at room temperature.
(9) Wash in distilled water.
(10) Wash in 70% alcohol.
(11) Differentiate in cresyl violet differentiator for 1–2 seconds.
(12) Rinse in 95% alcohol to remove differentiator.
(13) Rinse in absolute alcohol and clear in xylene.
(14) Check differentiation under microscope to *ensure* only nuclei (and Nissl substance) are stained, repeat (11), (12), (13) and (14) if necessary.
(15) Mount in synthetic resin.

Results

Myelin	Blue
Nuclei	Purple

■ **Luxol fast blue–PAS**

Sections are taken through the Luxol fast blue technique (*above*) from stages (1)–(7), following which the standard PAS technique is performed.

■ **Luxol fast blue–phosphotungstic acid haematoxylin**

Sections are brought to water, left in 0.25% potassium permanganate for 5 minutes, rinsed in distilled water, decolorized in 5% oxalic acid for 3–5 minutes and washed in running water for 5 minutes. Then stages (1)–(7) of the Luxol fast blue technique (*above*) are carried out, followed by stages (11)–(13) of the phosphotungstic acid haematoxylin technique (page 399).

■ **Loyez's technique for myelin in paraffin-embedded material (modified) (Loyez, 1910; La Manna, 1937)**

This technique, which for many years has been a standard method for paraffin sections, may be applied with equal success on frozen or celloidin sections.

Reagents

(1) La Manna's fluid

Potassium dichromate	9.5 g
Zinc chloride	4.5 g
Distilled water	to 100 ml

(2) Lithium carbonate haematoxylin

10% Haematoxylin in absolute alcohol (ripened solution)	10 ml
Saturated aqueous solution of lithium carbonate	2 ml
Distilled water	to 90 ml

   Lithium carbonate haematoxylin should be freshly prepared from stock solution.

(3) Loyez's differentiator

Borax	2 g
Potassium ferricyanide	2.5 g
Distilled water	to 200 ml

Method

(1) Fix tissue in formal–saline. By post-mordanting in La Manna's fluid for 24 hours at 56 °C (to render the myelin insoluble in the fat solvents) before paraffin processing a much better result may be obtained.
(2) Cut paraffin, celloidin or frozen sections to a thickness of 15–20 μm.
(3) Bring to distilled water.
(4) Treat paraffin or frozen section (on slides) with alcohol, then coat with celloidin.
(5) Mordant in 4% iron alum for 12–24 hours.
(6) Rinse in distilled water.
(7) Stain in haematoxylin for 2–4 hours at 56 °C, or 6–8 hours at 37 °C.
(8) Wash well in tap-water.
(9) Partially differentiate in 4% iron alum until myelin sheaths stand out bluish-black on a pale grey background.
(10) Wash in tap-water for 10 minutes.
(11) Complete differentiation in Loyez's differentiator (borax ferricyanide) for 2 minutes. This renders the myelin an intense deep blue against a creamy background.
(12) Wash well in tap-water.
(13) Dehydrate, clear and mount in Canada balsam or synthetic resin.

Degenerate myelin

The demonstration of degenerate myelin depends on the period of time that has elapsed since the original damage responsible for the degeneration; this period may be divided approximately into the following three stages.

Up to 10 days

Myelin tract will stain more heavily with normal myelin techniques.

10–60 days

Positive demonstration with osmium tetroxide techniques.

Over 60 days

Degenerate myelin will have been removed by phagocytic cells, and evidence of degeneration will be given by unstained areas using the normal myelin techniques (negative demonstration method).

Positive demonstration of degenerate myelin is carried out by the classical method of Marchi, by the Swank–Davenport method or by one of the fat-soluble stains (pages 262–264) which may be used in conjunction with a normal myelin method, such as the Luxol fast blue–oil red O technique.

■ **Marchi's technique (Marchi and Algeri, 1895)**

Marchi's technique is based on the fact that after normal myelin has been oxidized by chrome salts it will not react with osmium tetroxide. Degenerate myelin contains oleic acid which is not oxidized by chrome salts, it will therefore reduce osmium tetroxide, and is blackened.

Reagent

Marchi's fluid

3% Potassium dichromate	40 ml
1% Osmium tetroxide	20 ml

Fixation

Tissue should be fixed in formalin and post-chromed for 4–8 days in 3% potassium dichromate; it is said that Marchi's fluid may be used directly as a fixative. Prolonged fixation in formalin (after 8–10 days) may reduce the intensity of the reaction and should be avoided if possible.

Method

(1) Fix small pieces of tissue (not more than 2 mm in thickness) in formalin, and treat with potassium dichromate as described above.
(2) Transfer to Marchi's fluid for 8–12 days for spinal-cord sections, or 12–15 days for brain tissue. Tissues should be supported on glass wool to avoid the precipitate which forms, and to aid penetration. The fluid should be changed every 4–5 days.
(3) Wash in running water for 24 hours.
(4) Dehydrate rapidly and embed in celloidin, or clear and embed in paraffin wax.
(5) Cut sections 20–30 μm in thickness and mount them in Canada balsam or synthetic resin.

Results

Degenerate myelin (10–60 days after injury)	Black
Neutral fat (e.g. adipose tissue)	Black

■ **Swank–Davenport method (1935)**

The Swank–Davenport method gives better demonstration of degenerate myelin than the classical Marchi technique.

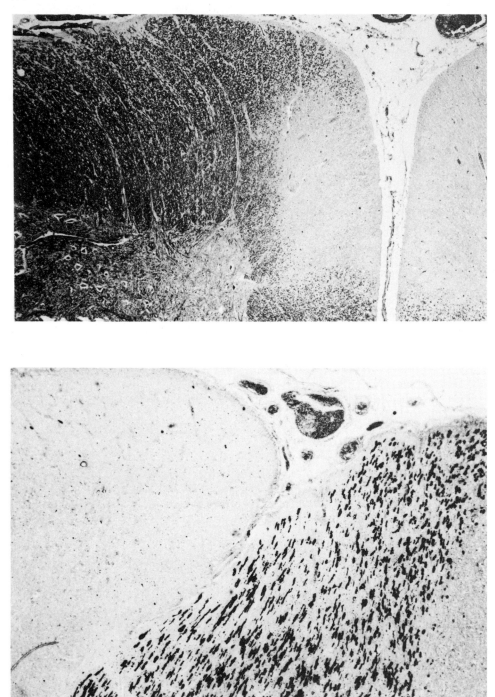

Figure 20.4 (a) Negative demonstration of late myelin degeneration in spinal cord. Luxol fast blue. Original magnification × 10. (b) Positive demonstration of early myelin degeneration in spinal cord. Marchi. Original magnification × 10

Method

(1) Fix tissue in 4% formal–saline.
(2) Transfer without washing to the following solution for 7–10 days.

1% Potassium chlorate	60 ml
1% Osmium tetroxide	20 ml
Commercial formalin	12 ml
Glacial acetic acid	1 ml

Approximately 15 volumes of fluid to one of tissue should be used, the solution shaken and the tissues turned over daily to improve penetration.

(3) Wash in running tap-water overnight.
(4) Embed in celloidin.
(5) Cut sections 20–30 µm in thickness, and mount in neutral mountant.

Results

Degenerate myelin	Black
Neutral fats	Black

■ Luxol fast blue–oil red O technique

This technique quite often gives a very pretty result, but the myelin staining is not as deep as when counterstained with cresyl violet.

Method

(1) Cut frozen sections of formalin-fixed tissue at 15–20 µm and wash in tap-water.
(2) Rinse briefly in 50% and then 70% alcohol.
(3) Place in Luxol fast blue solution (*see* page 392), and leave at room temperature for 3 hours.
(4) Rinse briefly in 70% and then 50% alcohol.
(5) Place in distilled water for 30 seconds.
(6) Commence differentiation by immersing sections in lithium carbonate solution for not more than 20 seconds.
(7) Differentiate in 70% alcohol until grey and white matter are clearly distinguished (30 seconds–1 minute).
(8) Rinse in distilled water and examine under microscope. If differentiation is not complete repeat steps (6)–(8) with reduced times (lithium carbonate 2–3 seconds).
(9) Wash well in distilled water.
(10) Stain by Lillie and Ashburn's oil red O method (page 263) from stages (3)–(10).

Results

Normal myelin	Blue-green
Degenerate myelin	Red

Neuroglia fibres and astrocytes

The demonstration of all the various elements of neuroglia can rarely be achieved by one technique.

The methods described below are the most reliable of a great variety of techniques and their modifications, and are recommended.

Neuroglia fibres and astrocytes

Anderson's Victoria blue technique
Mallory's PTA haematoxylin
Cajal's gold sublimate technique
Scharenberg's triple impregnation

Oligodendroglia and microglia

Penfield's silver carbonate technique
Weil–Davenport's technique

■ **Anderson's Victoria blue method (1929)**

Anderson's method gives good results with both paraffin and frozen sections; the latter are preferable.

Reagent

Neuroglia mordant

Distilled water	to 100 ml
Sodium sulphite	5 g
Oxalic acid	2.5 g
Potassium iodide	5 g
Iodine	2.5 g

Dissolve in the above order, then add 5 ml of acetic acid and keep in a well-stoppered bottle. If the solution turns brown, add one or two crystals of sodium sulphite.

Method

(1) Frozen or paraffin sections of formalin-fixed tissue are cut to a thickness of 15–20 μm.
(2) Frozen sections are washed in, or paraffin sections brought to, distilled water for 3–4 minutes.
(3) Transfer to equal parts of neuroglia mordant and 5% ferric chloride for 10–15 minutes.
(4) Wash in water, and transfer to 0.25% potassium permanganate for 5 minutes.
(5) Transfer directly to Pal's solution (page 391) until sections are white (sections may remain in this solution for up to 24 hours).
(6) Rinse in distilled water.
(7) Float frozen sections on to clean albuminized slides, and drain off excess water. Blot with fine filter paper.
(8) Boil a quantity of 1.5% Victoria blue in a test tube and pour immediately on to sections. Allow the stain to remain for 1–5 minutes.
(9) Drain slide and flood directly with Lugol's iodine for 1 minute.

(10) Blot section with fine filter paper and flood with xylene; if the section is not clear, repeat the blotting and xylene flooding process.
(11) Differentiate section with a mixture of equal parts of aniline oil and xylene. This must be controlled with a microscope until neuroglia fibres and astrocytes show up as blue on a pale blue or colourless background. All nuclei are stained by this method.
(12) Wash with xylene to remove aniline oil.
(13) Mount in Canada balsam or synthetic resin.

Results

Neuroglia fibres and astrocytes	Blue
Cell nuclei	Blue

Both fibrous and protoplasmic astrocytes are demonstrated by this technique.

■ Mallory's phosphotungstic acid haematoxylin (modified)

Method

(1) Mordant in saturated aqueous mercuric chloride for 30 minutes.
(2) Wash in water.
(3) Place in Anderson's neuroglia mordant for 10 minutes.
(4) Transfer to Lugol's iodine and leave for 15 minutes.
(5) Wash in two changes of 95% ethanol till colourless.
(6) Wash in distilled water.
(7) Place in 0.25% potassium permanganate for 15 minutes.
(8) Wash in distilled water.
(9) Treat with 5% oxalic acid until bleached.
(10) Wash well in distilled water.
(11) Stain in phosphotungstic acid haematoxylin for 18–24 hours at room temperature.
(12) Without washing transfer directly to 95% ethanol and leave for 2 minutes.
(13) Dehydrate, clear and mount.

Results

Nuclei, neuroglial fibres and fibrin   Deep blue

■ Cajal's gold sublimate method for astrocytes (1913)

This technique is the classical method for the demonstration of astrocytes, both protoplasmic and fibrous.

Reagents

(1) Formal–ammonium bromide (FAB)

Formalin	15 ml
Ammonium bromide	2 g
Distilled water	85 ml

(2) Gold sublimate solution

Mercuric chloride	0.4 g
1% Gold chloride (brown)	10 ml
Distilled water	60 ml

Dissolve the mercuric chloride in the distilled water with the aid of gentle heat; cool and then add the gold chloride. This solution should be prepared immediately before use.

Method

(1) Fix pieces of tissue 3–5 mm in thickness in FAB for 3–8 days.
(2) Cut frozen sections to a thickness of 15–20 µm.
(3) Store sections in FAB until ready for staining.
(4) Rinse well in distilled water (two to three changes).
(5) Treat in gold sublimate solution, in a flat covered dish in the dark at 22 °C for 4–8 hours or longer until sections are deep purple in colour. Sections must lie flat without creasing or overlapping.
(6) Rinse rapidly in distilled water.
(7) Fix in 5% sodium thiosulphate.
(8) Wash in distilled water.
(9) Float on to clean slides.
(10) Dehydrate, clear and mount in Canada balsam or synthetic resin.

Result

Astrocytes (protoplasmic and fibrous)   Red-black

Note: Frozen sections of formal–saline-fixed tissue may be impregnated, but they should be treated overnight in FAB (*above*) or for 1 hour in 5% hydrobromic acid (supplied commercially as a 50% solution) at 37 °C; then continue from stage (4) above.

■ **Scharenberg's triple impregnation method (1954) (modified) for glial cells and fibres**

Scharenberg's method is a very trustworthy one and usually gives excellent results on both normal and pathological material, particularly gliomatous tissue. Occasionally, with refractory material, superior results may be obtained by omitting stage (7) (*see below*) and using a double rather than a triple impregnation.

As with the majority of silver methods, sections may be mounted either toned in gold chloride or untoned, but in either case tissues should always be fixed in sodium thiosulphate.

Reagents

(1) Stock silver carbonate solution

10% Silver nitrate AR	100 ml
5% Sodium carbonate AR (anhydrous)	300 ml

Add strong ammonia, drop by drop, until the creamy yellow precipitate is just dissolved; scrupulous care must be taken not to add an excess of ammonia. Dilute to a total volume of 700 ml. The solution may be used for up to 3 months if kept in a dark bottle.

(2) Ammoniacal silver solution

Add strong ammonia to a 2% solution of silver nitrate until the precipitate, formed instantaneously, is just dissolved. Again, there must be no excess ammonia. The solution keeps indefinitely if stored in the dark.

Method

(1) Fix tissue in 10% formal–saline. (In the original technique it was stated that tissue must be fixed in formal–ammonium–bromide, page 399, but the technique given here gives equal if not better results.)

(2) Cut frozen sections to a thickness of 15–20 μm and receive in distilled water.

(3) Wash sections overnight in 1% ammonia water.

(4) Transfer direct to 5% hydrobromic acid for 2–3 hours at 37 °C. Rinse in two changes of 1:5000 ammonia and then in distilled water.

(5) Sensitize sections for 15 minutes at 60 °C in 50 ml of 2% silver nitrate, to which 20 drops of pyridine have been added.

(6) Without rinsing, transfer to 50 ml of silver carbonate solution for 15 minutes at 60 °C, to which 20 drops of pyridine have been added.

(7) Transfer direct to 2% ammoniacal silver nitrate at room temperature for 5 minutes.

(8) Reduce in 1% formaldehyde for 2–3 minutes.

(9) Wash in distilled water.

(10) Tone in 0.2% gold chloride for 10–15 minutes.

(11) Wash in distilled water.

(12) Fix in 5% sodium thiosulphate for 5 minutes.

(13) Wash in distilled water and mount on an albuminized slide.

(14) Carefully blot and dehydrate in absolute alcohol.

(15) Clear in xylene and mount in Canada balsam or synthetic resin.

Note: Although this technique does not demonstrate oligodendroglia or microglia, the stock silver carbonate solution may be used with Penfield's technique (*below*). For oligodendroglia it is used undiluted, and for microglia diluted 1:4 with distilled water.

Results

Protoplasmic and fibrous astrocytes and neuroglia fibres   Jet black

■ Penfield's modification of Hortega's technique for oligodendroglia and microglia (1928)

Oligodendroglia are best demonstrated by Penfield's technique (with increased strength of silver solution), or, when this fails, by the Weil–Davenport method which occasionally gives a good result.

Reagents

Silver carbonate solution

10% Silver nitrate	5 ml
5% Sodium carbonate	20 ml

Mix and add strong ammonia (sp.gr. 0.880) drop by drop until the precipitate, which is first formed, is dissolved. Make up the total volume to 75 ml with distilled water. For *oligodendroglia specifically*, better results may be obtained by using 10 ml of 20% silver nitrate when preparing this silver carbonate solution.

Method

(1) Cut frozen sections of formalin-fixed tissue to a thickness of 10–15 µm.
(2) Remove traces of formalin by washing sections overnight in 1% ammonia in distilled water.
(3) Transfer directly to 5% hydrobromic acid* in distilled water for 1 hour at 37 °C.
(4) Wash in three changes of distilled water.
(5) Transfer to 5% sodium carbonate for 1 hour (up to 6 hours).
(6) Transfer to silver carbonate solution for 3–5 minutes, until sections turn light brown in colour.
(7) Transfer to 1% formalin and agitate sections by blowing on the surface of the fluid for 2–3 minutes.
(8) Wash in distilled water.
(9) Tone in 0.2% gold chloride for 10–15 minutes.
(10) Rinse in distilled water.
(11) Fix in 5% sodium thiosulphate.
(12) Wash in water.
(13) Mount on clean slides, dehydrate, clear and mount in synthetic resin.

Result

Oligodendroglia and microglia   Black

■ Weil–Davenport's technique (1933)

Demonstration of microglia cells is best achieved by the Weil–Davenport method, but Penfield's silver carbonate technique gives less brilliant but more reliable results.

The Weil–Davenport method was devised for frozen sections, but sometimes gives good results with loose paraffin sections which have been de-waxed and treated as frozen sections.

Reagent

Silver solution

To 2–3 ml of strong ammonia (sp.gr. 0.880) in a flask, add 10% silver nitrate, drop by drop, until about 18 ml have been added and the solution is still slightly opalescent. This solution is reported to give the best results if it is prepared in a silvered flask (with a

---

* Hydrobromic acid is supplied commercially as a 50% solution.

deposit of silver on the inside) which should be kept for the purpose.

The reader is referred to Wallington (1965) concerning the explosive qualities of silver nitrate, and therefore we recommend that silvered flasks should NOT be used.

Method

(1) Cut frozen or paraffin sections to thickness of 12–15 μm.
(2) Bring sections (frozen or loose de-waxed paraffin) to three changes of distilled water.
(3) Transfer to silver solution for 15–20 seconds.
(4) Transfer to 15% formalin; gently agitate section until it is coffee-brown in colour.
(5) Rinse in three changes of distilled water.
(6) Tone in 0.2% gold chloride for 10–15 minutes.
(7) Rinse in distilled water.
(8) Fix in 5% sodium thiosulphate for 5 minutes.
(9) Wash in water.
(10) Float on to clean slides, dehydrate, clear and mount in Canada balsam or synthetic resin.

Result

Oligodendroglia and microglia   Black

Notes: Toning (stages (6)–(7)) is optional and sections may be mounted untoned. Shorter time at stage (3) and weaker formalin at stage (4) may be used to reduce the chance of over-impregnation.

Peripheral nerves

Nerve fibres and sheaths of the peripheral nervous system can often be demonstrated by the methods previously described. However, because of their different structure (small bundles and solitary nerves) it may be advantageous to use the following methods.

■ Osmium tetroxide for myelin sheaths

Fresh or formalin-fixed tissue of small dimension is placed in 1% osmium tetroxide for a few days and after thorough washing frozen or paraffin sections are prepared. Treatment with low grade alcohol may be prolonged but thereafter the times should be kept to the minimum. Chloroform is the antemedium of choice (Drury and Wallington, 1980). After removing the paraffin wax with xylene the sections are mounted directly in synthetic resin.

■ Solochrome cyanine for myelin sheaths (Page, 1970)

Paraffin sections of formalin-fixed tissue are suitable.

Reagent

Solochrome cyanine RS	0.2 g
Distilled water	96 ml

| 10% Iron alum | 4 ml |
| Concentrated sulphuric acid | 0.5 ml |

Method

(1) Bring sections to water.
(2) Stain for 10–20 minutes at room temperature.
(3) Wash in running water.
(4) Differentiate in 10% iron alum. Wash in water and examine microscopically.
(5) Counterstain if desired.
(6) Dehydrate, clear and mount in synthetic resin.

Results

Myelin sheaths   Bright blue

■ Schofield's method for peripheral nerve axons (1959)

Frozen sections are preferred for the demonstration of peripheral nerve axons because thicker sections can be obtained more easily. Of the many modifications of the Bielschowsky silver method which are available, that of Schofield gives minimum impregnation of the background. Toning is not recommended.

Fixation

Formal–saline.

Reagents

Ammoniacal silver

To 10 ml of 20% silver nitrate add strong ammonia, drop by drop, until the precipitate first formed is just dissolved.

Pyridine alcohol

50% Ethanol	50 ml
Marble chips	A few
Pyridine	15 drops

Formalin solutions

Formalin solutions should be made up in tap-water.

Method

(1) Place frozen sections in pyridine–alcohol for at least 1 hour at 37 °C.
(2) Rinse in distilled water.
(3) Place in 20% silver nitrate for 15–20 minutes at room temperature in the dark.
(4) Blot sections gently.
(5) Place sections into three baths of 10% formalin for 30 seconds in each bath.

(6) Place sections in 2% formalin for 30 seconds.
(7) Wash in two changes of distilled water.
(8) Treat with ammoniacal silver for 30–60 seconds and blot.
(9) Treat with 1% formalin until golden brown.
(10) Wash.
(11) Fix in 5% sodium thiosulphate.
(12) Wash, mount on slides and blot.
(13) Dehydrate, clear and mount in synthetic resin.

Results

Nerve fibres	Dark brown to black
Other tissues	Pale brown

Nerve endings

Nerve endings may be demonstrated by the metallic impregnation method of Ranvier (1880) or one of its many modifications. This gold impregnation technique used a lemon juice pretreatment followed by gold chloride and formic acid treatment. Of the silver impregnation methods derived from the Bielschowsky technique that which is recommended is the Schofield method (*see above*).

Intravital and supravital methylene blue staining will demonstrate motor end-plates well (page 453) but a more popular and simpler technique for use in the routine laboratory is the technique for cholinesterase (page 319).

Methods for rapid diagnosis

Toluidine blue staining, as used for frozen sections, can be used for the rapid diagnosis of brain smears following fixation in absolute ethanol. Excellent results are often obtained with haematoxylin and eosin or with May Grunwald–Giemsa. The following method gives a good differential picture.

■ **Morris's smear technique (1947) for the rapid histological diagnosis of tumours of the central nervous system**

This technique, which is rapid and gives a good nuclear and cytoplasmic picture, need not be restricted to brain tumours. It may be used for a variety of tissues, notably smears of fresh pituitary, when a useful differential picture is obtained.

Reagents

(1) Dichromate–eosin

Eosin (water soluble)	1 g
Potassium dichromate	1 g
Distilled water	to 100 ml

This stain keeps indefinitely.

(2) Acetone–alcohol

Absolute alcohol	30 ml
Acetone	25 ml

(3) Polychrome blue

Methylene blue	1 g
Potassium carbonate	1 g
Distilled water	to 300 ml

Place the constituents in a 500 ml flask and boil for 10–15 minutes. Add 3 ml of glacial acetic acid drop by drop, shaking vigorously until the precipitate is dissolved. Reduce the volume to 100 ml by boiling; then allow to cool. The stain remains stable for at least 1 year.

Method

(1) Fix smears by drying or, better, in absolute alcohol for 3–5 minutes.
(2) Rinse in distilled water.
(3) Stain for 5–10 seconds in dichromate–eosin.
(4) Wash in tap-water.
(5) Differentiate in acetone–alcohol.
(6) Wash in tap-water.
(7) Stain 10–30 seconds in polychrome blue.
(8) Wash in tap-water.
(9) Dehydrate in acetone–alcohol (*as above*).
(10) Clear first in chloroform, then in toluol.
(11) Mount in Canada balsam.

Results

| Nuclei | Blue |
| Other tissue elements | Shades of pink |

References

ANDERSON, J. (1929). *How to Stain the Nervous System*. Livingstone, Edinburgh

BIELSCHOWSKY, M. (1909). Eine Modifikation meines Silberimpregnationsverfahrens zur Darstellung der Neurofibrillen. *J. Psychol. Neurol. (Lpz.)*, **12**, 135–137

CAJAL, S. RAMON, Y. (1913). Sobre un nuevo proceder de impregnación de la neurología y sus resultados en los centricos nerviosos del hombre y animales. *Trav. Lab. Recher. Biol. Univ. Madrid*, **2**, 219

COOK, H. C. (1974). *Histological Demonstration Techniques*. Butterworths, London

DRURY, R. A. B. and WALLINGTON, E. A. (1980). *Carleton's Histological Technique*. 5th Ed. Oxford University Press, Oxford

EAGER, R. P. (1970). Selective staining of degenerating axons in the central nervous system by a simplified method: spinal cord projections to external cuneate and inferior olivary nuclei in the cat. *Brain Res.*, **22**, 137–141

HOLMES, W. (1947). In *Recent Advances in Clinical Pathology*. Ed. Dyke, S. C. Churchill, London

KLUVER, H. and BARRERA, E. (1953). A method for the combined staining of cells and fibres of the nervous system. *J. Neuropathol. Exp. Neurol.*, **12**, 400–403

KULTSCHITZKY, N. (1890). Über die Farbung der markhältigen Nervenfasern in den Schnitten des Zentralnervensystems mit Hamatoxylin und mit Karmin. *Anat. Anz.*, **5**, 519–524

LA MANNA, S. (1937). Zeitschrift für wissenschaftliche Mikroskopie und für mikroskopische Technik. Die Markscheidenfarbung. *Z. Wiss. Mikr.*, **54**, 257–287

LOYEZ, M. (1910). Coloration des fibres nerveuses par la méthode à l'hématoxylaine au fer après inclusion à la celloîdine. *C. R. Soc. Ciol.*, **69**, 511–513

MARCHI, V. and ALGERI, G. (1885). Rivista sperimentale di freniatria e medicina legale delle alienazioni mentali. Sulle degenerazioni discendenti consecutive a lisione della corteccia cerebrale. *Riv. Sper. Freniat.*, **11**, 492

MARSLAND, T. A., GLEES, P. and ERIKSON, L. B. (1954). Modification of Glees' silver impregnation for paraffin sections. *J. Neuropathol. Exp. Neurol.*, **13**, 587–591

MORRIS, H. L. (1947). Use of smear technique in rapid histological diagnosis of tumours of central nervous system; description of new staining method. *J. Neurosurg.*, **4**, 497–504

NAUTA, W. J. H. and GYGAX, P. A. (1951). Silver impregnation of degenerating axon terminals in the central nervous system. 1. Technic. 2. Chemical notes. *Stain Technol.*, **26**, 5–11

PAGE, K. M. (1970). Histological methods for peripheral nerves. Part 1. *J. Med. Lab. Technol.*, **27**, 1–17

PENFIELD, W. (1928). A method of staining oligodendroglia and microglia (combined method). *Am. J. Pathol.*, **4**, 153–157

RANVIER, L. (1880). On the terminations of nerves in the epidermis. *Quart. J. Micr. Sci.*, **20**, 456–458

SALTHOUSE, T. N. (1964). Luxol fast blue G as a myelin stain. *Stain Technol.*, **39**, 123

SCHARENBERG, K. (1954). Blastomatous oligodendroglia as satellites of nerve cells. A study with silver carbonate. *Am. J. Pathol.*, **30**, 957–967

SCHOFIELD, G. (1959). In *Leprosy in Theory and Practice*. Ed. Cochrane, R. G. Wright PSG, Bristol

SWANK, R. L. and DAVENPORT, H. A. (1935). Chlorate–osmic–formalin method for staining degenerate myelin. *Stain Technol.*, **10**, 87–90

WALLINGTON, E. A. (1965). Explosive properties of ammoniacal silver nitrate. *J. Med. Lab. Technol.*, **22**, 220–223

WEIL, A. and DAVENPORT, H. A. (1933). Staining of oligodendroglia and microglia in celloidin sections. *Arch. Neurol. Psychiat. Chicago*, **30**, 175–178

21

Hard tissue

For the purposes of this chapter, three types of hard tissue are recognized: soft tissue in which calcification has occurred, bone and teeth. Calcification of soft tissues occurs as a result of pathological or age changes.

Bone

Bone is a tissue. Bones are organs.

Cellular components of bone

Three types of bone cell are recognized, each having a specific function:

(1) *Osteoblasts* are concerned with the formation of bone.
(2) *Osteocytes* are concerned with the maintenance of bone as living tissue.
(3) *Osteoclasts* are concerned with the resorption of bone.

   These cells almost certainly derive from a common ancestor and may, during growth, transform from one type to another yet still retain their common potencies. The morphology of a particular cell will depend upon the function it is called upon to perform at that moment. Even in adult bone, transformations occur during the healing of fractures. Osteoblasts form a continuous layer on the surface of new bone. They are plump cuboidal cells of regular size. The nucleus is distal to the bone and the cytoplasm is deeply basophilic due to the high RNA content. When the cell is active, PAS-positive granules are present and it is rich in alkaline phosphatase. When quiescent, it becomes almost indistinguishable from surrounding fibroblasts.

   Ultrastructurally, osteoblasts are rich in granular endoplasmic reticulum and have a well-defined Golgi region (*Figure 21.1*).

   As bone formation continues, osteoblasts become embedded in the new bone matrix and become osteocytes. They are plump cells with many branching processes, although they may appear shrunken due to processing artefact. The cells are enclosed within spaces termed *lacunae*, and the processes within *canaliculi*. These form an inter-connected network within bone. The cell remains basophilic with moderate amounts of endoplasmic reticulum, mitochondria and some electron dense granules. A narrow, uncalcified zone containing collagen fibres separates the cell from bone.

   Osteoclasts are multinucleate giant cells with up to 15 or even 20 nuclei (*Figure 21.2*). They are found in a close relationship to bone surfaces, usually in characteristic

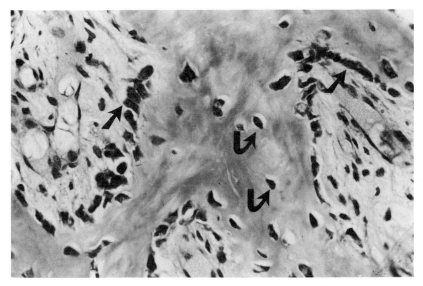

Figure 21.1 Decalcified section of bone showing both osteoblasts (straight arrows) and osteocytes (curved arrows). H and E. Original magnification × 100

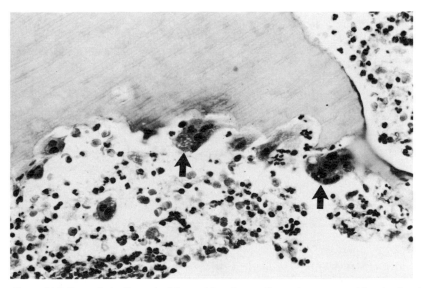

Figure 21.2 Osteoclasts. Several of the multinucleate cells can be seen resorbing dentine (arrows). The typical scallop shaped areas of resorption termed Howship's lacunae are clearly seen. H and E. Original magnification × 100

scallops of the resorbed front—*Howship's lacunae*. A brush border is present between the cell and bone and this has been shown to be a very active and undulating membrane. The bone itself shows a margin of rarefaction facing the osteoclast. Crystals of resorbed material can often be demonstrated within osteoclast cytoplasm.

Bone matrix

The organic matrix of bone is composed essentially of collagen fibres similar to those found in other connective tissues together with a ground substance containing chondroitin sulphate.

Calcification occurs as the deposition within the soft organic matrix of a virtually insoluble calcium salt, hydroxyapatite.

Calcification depends upon humoral conditions and a local trigger mechanism. Humoral conditions provide the constituent ions, calcium and phosphate, in the relative concentrations necessary for nucleation of the crystals. Collagen acts as the catalyst for nucleation of apatite crystals due to the macromolecular aggregation of the fibrils, and the ground substance has a regulatory effect. The whole complicated system involves a specific form of collagen, sulphated mucopolysaccharides, enzyme systems including glycolysis and the citric acid cycle, the energy sources ATP and UTP and a system for concentrating calcium and phosphate ions.

Calcification occurs as true crystal formation and not as simple precipitation. Calcium phosphate acquires hydroxyl ions to form a crystal lattice of hydroxyapatite. Other ions may be taken up by substitution of the calcium, including strontium, magnesium, etc., and is the mode of action by which fluoride is included in the crystal structure of tooth enamel. Hydroxyapatite crystals are small (20 nm) and needle shaped.

Small numbers of reticulin fibres are present in the organic matrix of bone, occupying, biochemically, a position intermediate between collagen and the mucopolysaccharides of ground substance.

Water has been estimated to make up 3.7% of adult bone by weight and about 8% by volume. Figures for organic matrix are 24% by weight and 38% by volume. The remainder forms the mineral phase.

The external surfaces of bones are covered by a connective tissue membrane termed the *periosteum*. In rapidly growing bone the periosteum consists of a dense outer layer of collagen and fibroblasts and a loose inner layer of osteoblasts. When bone is quiescent, the periosteum forms an anchorage for tendons.

The inner surface, lining the marrow spaces of bone, is termed *endosteum*. This membrane also lines the *Haversian canals* of compact bone and retains both osteogenic and haemopoietic potency. Like periosteum, endosteum is active in fracture repair.

Bone structure

Bone is laid down sequentially as lamellae, each normally 4–12 μm wide. Collagen fibrils in adjacent lamellae lie in different directions, giving strength and resistance to shearing forces in particular.

Two types of bone are normally recognized.

(1) *Cancellous, trabecullar* or *spongy* bone is found at the ends of long bones, within marrow spaces and at the centre of flat bones. Thin trabecullae of fairly uniform diameter interconnect to form a three-dimensional network. Each trabecullum consists of a few lamellae which appear to have been laid down in parallel and are, in fact, concentric. This formation gives bone its strength and weight bearing properties.

(2) *Compact* or *cortical* bone appears solid, is very hard and strong. It forms the shafts of long bones and the outer plates of flat bones such as skull. The lamellae form concentric structures through which runs a central canal containing connective

tissue and blood vessels. These are the *Haversian* systems into which are connected the canaliculi. Channels which contain blood vessels and connect adjacent Haversian systems are termed *Volkmann's canals*. The entire shaft of long bones is surrounded by the *circumferential* lamellae.

The term *woven bone* is often used in pathology to denote immature bone formed during a healing process. Random orientation of collagen fibres is a characteristic of this bone. Special stains may be used to demonstrate this feature, but it is most striking when sections are viewed in polarized light, producing the pattern from which the name is derived.

Bone growth

'Normal' bone growth (i.e. developmental growth) is referred to as *epiphyseal plate growth* and occurs during embryonic and post-fetal life. When bone is formed to replace cartilage, the process is called *endochondral ossification*; when no cartilage is present it is called *intramembranous ossification*.

During embryonic life most skeletal bones are formed in cartilage. At a specific stage, the surrounding *perichondrium* infiltrates the cartilage, replacing hypertrophied cartilage cells by mesenchymal cells to form primitive marrow with both osteogenic and haemopoietic potential.

On the outer surface, the perichondrium slowly acquires the characteristics of periosteum and provides foci from which ossification begins. Osteoblasts differentiate and invade the degenerating cartilage, depositing osteoid which becomes calcified. Growth centres of active cartilage remain at the ends of long bones. At a time characteristic for each species and each bone this *epiphyseal cartilage* is invaded by mesenchymal cells which eventually differentiate to form a dense network of trabecullar bone.

Once bones are fully developed, subsequent growth may only occur by the apposition of new bone, which increases the girth of long bones. In certain pathological conditions active and characteristic concomitant resorption and new bone formation occurs (Paget's disease). New bone growth also occurs following fractures, of course. This is characterized by direct osteogenesis and primitive cells appear in the medullary cavity. A mass of new bone is formed termed a *callus* (*Figure 21.3*).

Specimens

The treatment of small biopsies is relatively straightforward. Before sections can be cut it is usually, although not invariably, necessary and desirable to remove the calcium salts. To be of value, sections must reveal detail of both the bone and any adjacent soft tissue as well as the relationship between the two.

Larger specimens, such as resections or amputations, require special attention. It is good practice to take X-rays of these specimens as a routine. It is often easy to obtain radiographs of laboratory specimens that are of better quality than the clinical ones. It is desirable to dissect these specimens as soon as possible so that the unwanted attached soft tissue, that may hinder fixation, can be removed.

A band saw is a most useful tool for dividing large specimens but precautions should be taken to minimize the hazards of airborne dust. Freezing the specimen before cutting is *not* recommended, severe ice-crystal artefacts may result. Smaller specimens may be

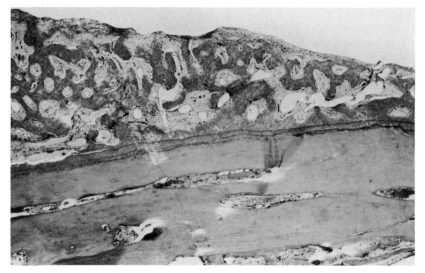

Figure 21.3 Callus formation on compact bone following a fracture. H and E. Original magnification × 10

divided using a geological cutting machine fitted with a diamond impregnated cutting disc. With practice, cross-sections of whole bones may be cut thin enough for processing. Bone dust should be carefully washed from the cut surfaces with saline or fixative solution.

Fixation

Formal–saline is the fixative of choice. It must be remembered that penetration of fixative into large specimens, particularly dense cortical bone, will be slow. The sooner the specimen can be divided into smaller portions, the more successful will be fixation. Black and white photographs of the specimen can be marked with a felt-tipped pen to indicate exactly from where the blocks are taken.

Decalcification

Calcium salts are removed from tissue either by the action of acids, by chelation or by electrolysis. Whichever method is chosen, the resultant tissue will remain tough and difficult to cut.

Acid decalcification

Treating tissue with acid results in tissue damage. The stronger or more concentrated the acid, the harsher the effects. A balance therefore has to be struck between the urgency of the specimen and the deleterious effects of acid. Nucleic acids are particularly intolerant to acid decalcification, so that haematoxylin staining may be much less effectual. Staining times need to be prolonged and it is beneficial to use a stronger haematoxylin such as Ehrlich's. Acid dyes, especially eosin, tend to stain more strongly, so that shorter times are required. Methyl green–pyronin staining of nucleic acids is severely affected.

Acids may be used as simple solutions, in a mixture with other reagents, especially fixatives, or in buffered solution. Both organic and inorganic acids have been used. For a description of the physicochemical factors involved the reader is referred to Brain (1966). For most routine laboratory procedures a choice of two or three decalcifying reagents is sufficient. The criteria of a good decalcifying agent remain the same as they were in the first edition of this book:

(1) complete removal of calcium;
(2) minimal damage to cells and tissue;
(3) non-impairment of subsequent staining;
(4) reasonable speed.

Several factors influence the speed of decalcification, in particular, heat, the strength of the acid and agitation. The first two are inversely proportional to the damage caused to tissue. Decalcification is usually carried out at room temperature and the concentration of acid in solution has been designed to strike a compromise between speed and damage. We recommend constant agitation to ensure removal of calcium saturated solution from around the tissue. There are several agitators available commercially.

Decalcifying fluids

There are numerous formulas for decalcifying fluids: those that follow are the ones we recommend.

Formic acid

Formic acid (90%)	100 ml
Distilled water	900 ml

Gooding and Stewart's fluid (1932)

Formic acid (90%)	100 ml
Formalin	50 ml
Distilled water	850 ml

Both of the above solutions are suitable for routine use, giving reasonable speed with a minimum of damage to tissue.

Nitric acid

Nitric acid	80 ml
Distilled water	900 ml

Carefully add the acid to the water.

A disadvantage of the use of nitric acid is the yellow colour which develops. This discolours the tissue and may interfere with subsequent staining. The addition of 0.1% urea obviates this colour formation, although further amounts may be required if left standing.

The formula is rapid and causes little damage to tissue if it is removed as soon as decalcification is complete. Most staining reactions can be performed following its use.

Commercial decalcifiers

Although the exact composition of these proprietary reagents is unknown, most are believed to contain a fairly high concentration of hydrochloric acid. They are rapid in action, but in our hands interfere badly with subsequent staining.

There has been some concern over the possible formation of a potent carcinogen, bischloromethyl ether (BCME), by the reaction of formaldehyde and hydrochloric acid. However, this reaction occurs between the vapour phases of these reagents and not the solutions. Gill (1982) explains in detail the relevance of this particular hazard and preliminary investigations by the Health and Safety Executive (personal communication) suggests that no hazard exists, even at concentrations far exceeding those normally used in histopathology.

Surface decalcification

Occasionally, an unexpected area of calcification may only become apparent whilst a paraffin-wax block is being trimmed. If only a small area is involved, it is possible to decalcify the surface layer by inverting the block in 5% hydrochloric acid for 1 hour or so. This is less drastic than returning the tissue to aqueous solutions. As only the top 30 μm or so is likely to be decalcified, care should be exercised to collect the first sections cut. Before cutting, the block should be rinsed in water to avoid contaminating knife or microtome with acid.

Once decalcification is complete, surface acid should be washed from the tissue with water. If there is any delay before processing the tissue should be returned to formal-saline. Although there are advocates of neutralizing the acid before processing, it is probable that it will all be washed out by the processing fluids.

Chelating agents

These are organic compounds which have the power of binding certain metals. EDTA (ethylene diamine tetra-acetic acid) is able to bind calcium, its use as a decalcifying agent being first described by Hilleman and Lee (1953). It is a slow process as calcium is removed layer by layer from the hydroxyapatite lattice.

Tissues decalcified by this method show a minimum of artefact, and may subsequently be stained by most techniques with first class results. These qualities make it the decalcifying agent of choice for electron microscopy.

EDTA solution

EDTA (disodium salt)   55 g
Formalin   100 ml
Distilled water   900 ml

EDTA is sometimes known as Sequestrene, or Versene.

Ion exchange resins

Ion exchange resins in decalcifying fluids are used to remove the calcium ions from the fluid, thus ensuring a more rapid rate of solubility of the calcium from the tissue and a reduction in the time of decalcification.

The resin, commonly an ammonium form of a sulphonated polystyrene resin, is layered on the bottom of the container to a depth of approximately 1 cm (it should not be less than 10% of the bulk of the decalcifying agent), and the specimen allowed to rest on it. The volume of the fluid by this technique need be only 20 to 30 times the bulk of the specimen.

The use of resins is limited to those decalcifying fluids not containing mineral acids: formic acid is recommended. After use, the resin may be regenerated by washing twice with dilute (N/10) hydrochloric acid, followed by three washes in distilled water. This procedure allows the resin to be used over a very long period without renewal.

Complete decalcification can only be determined by X-ray (*see below*).

Electrophoretic decalcification

This method depends, in theory, upon the solution of calcium ions in the electrolyte and their attraction to the cathode. The method has found very little favour, any advantages which it may have in speeding up the process most probably being due to the heat generated (Clayden, 1952).

The endpoint of decalcification

Because of the harmful effects of acid on tissue, they must be left in decalcifying fluids for the minimum time possible. Accurate determination of the endpoint of decalcification is therefore necessary. Experience will enable a value judgement to be made upon the approximate time required, depending on the tissue structure and size of the block. Small biopsies of cancellous bone should be examined after 24 hours, and other specimens daily after two to three 24-hour changes of fluid.

Experienced hands can tell by the 'feel' of the tissue if decalcification is virtually complete. Whilst probing the tissue with a needle is not recommended, judicious bending or trimming can be valuable—a fact often derided in textbooks. However, such methods are no substitute for accurate determination using either chemical tests or X-rays. Although not always easy, it is worth the effort of visiting the radiography department if suitable equipment is not available in the laboratory.

Radiography is the most efficient test for the endpoint, as well as being invaluable in detecting foreign bodies in specimens. Several specimens can be exposed on the same X-ray if care is taken over identification (*Figure 21.4*).

Chemical test

This method depends upon the identification of calcium in the decalcifying solution. It therefore follows that the endpoint can only be detected by sampling the fluid change following completion. This method cannot be used following EDTA decalcification.

Method

Five ml of decalcifying fluid is nearly neutralized with N/2 sodium hydroxide or strong ammonia. This may be adjudged using pH paper. Add 5 ml of saturated ammonium oxalate solution. Absence of turbidity after a delay of 5 minutes indicates that the fluid is free of calcium and decalcification is therefore complete.

A precipitate that forms after the addition of sodium hydroxide (calcium hydroxide) indicates that large amounts of calcium are still present in the fluid. A precipitate following the addition of ammonium oxalate suggests decalcification is nearly complete.

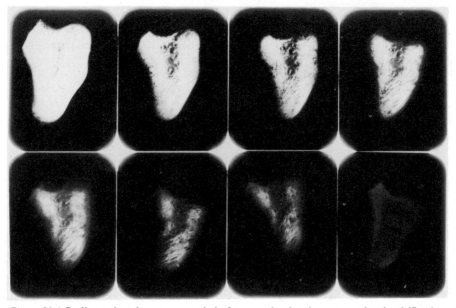

Figure 21.4 Radiographs taken over a period of two weeks showing progressive decalcification of a cross-section of cortical bone

Processing

Small blocks of cancellous bone, or tissue blocks containing small amounts of bone, may be processed routinely. Larger or dense blocks require special attention. The processing schedule should be prolonged with extended periods in molten wax. Three changes of wax, under vacuum, of 2 hours each is not unreasonable. A hard wax is an advantage.

The double embedding procedure using LVN and paraffin wax, detailed in Chapter 4, is unlikely to appeal as a routine process, but it can produce better results than paraffin wax alone.

Microtomy

A substantial microtome and knife contribute greatly to successful microtomy of bone. A base sledge microtome and wedge-shaped steel or tungsten carbide edged knife are recommended. The rake of the knife should be less than for conventional microtomy, even though this may result in some compression. The blocks should be well iced before cutting. Slightly thicker sections, 6–7 μm, are acceptable when cutting bone.

It often helps if tissue is embedded obliquely in the wax, as described in Chapter 5.

The floating out bath may need to be hotter than for soft tissues, as bone has a tendency to crinkle when cut. Sections should be picked up on chrome gelatin coated slides, to reduce the chance that they may lift from the slide during staining.

Staining

Acid treated tissue is less susceptible to haematoxylin staining, so that routine haematoxylin and eosin sections may be disappointing. Ehrlich's haematoxylin is a good nuclear stain in these conditions and has the added advantage that it stains mucopolysaccharides and thus demonstrates cement lines (or reversal lines) and cartilage well. Gill's haematoxylin (3 ×) is also a useful stain for decalcified bone. Eosin staining is enhanced by acid decalcification, so that some reduction in staining time is required.

General bone structure, as opposed to cellular detail, is well demonstrated by silver reticulin methods (page 173) and particularly by picro–thionin (page 427).

Undecalcified sections of bone

In certain metabolic bone diseases, there is an increase in the width of non-mineralized bone (osteoid) on the outer surfaces of trabecullar bone. In the diagnosis of osteomalacia, in particular, it is valuable to assess the ratio of mineralized to non-mineralized bone. Traditionally, it has been necessary to produce undecalcified bone sections for this purpose, so that calcium salts may be demonstrated in mineralized areas. However, there now exist at least three successful methods for demonstrating the osteoid seam. Iliac crest biopsies are the usual source of tissue for these investigations.

Adhesive tape method for undecalcified tissue (Duthie, 1954; Ball, 1957)

Formal-fixed, paraffin-embedded tissue is generally suitable, although double-embedding was originally specified. It is almost possible to diagnose osteomalacia by the ease with which sections are cut!

Although sections may be cut on a rotary microtome, a base sledge is recommended. Once the tissue has been carefully trimmed to expose the surface of the tissue, a strip of adhesive tape (such as Sellotape) is pressed firmly onto the surface of the block. The leading edge is raised above the edge of the knife as a section is slowly cut. The quality of the section can be immediately assessed.

Press the section bearing tape flat onto a chrome gelatin coated slide. Place a clean slide over the tape and firmly clamp the two together using a bulldog clip at each end. Place in an oven at 56 °C and leave overnight.

Remove the covering slide and place wet filter paper over the adhesive tape. Leave for 30 minutes. The backing tape may then be removed, leaving the adhesive covering the section. This is removed by immersing in warm xylene for 30–60 minutes. Wash in fresh xylene, then perform the von Kossa technique.

■ von Kossa technique for calcium salts (1901)

This method depends on treating the section with silver nitrate so that silver phosphate is formed by salt substitution with the calcium phosphates present in the mineral phase of bone. This is reduced to black metallic silver by the action of light (*Figure 21.5*).

Method

(1) Bring sections to water.
(2) Rinse in distilled water.
(3) Place in 5% silver nitrate in a glass Coplin jar (*see note below*).
(4) Wash well in distilled water.
(5) Treat with 5% sodium thiosulphate (hypo) for 5 minutes.
(6) Wash in running water for 3 minutes.

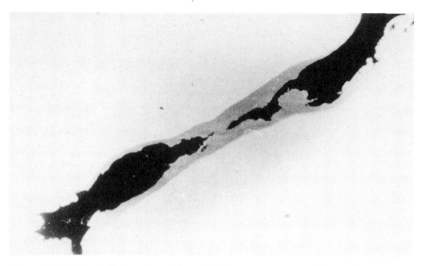

Figure 21.5 Undecalcified section of bone. Black areas represent calcium salts. There is excessive unmineralized osteoid present in this single bony trabeculum. Von Kossa technique. Original magnification × 63

(7) Counterstain in Van Gieson's stain for 3 minutes.
(8) Dehydrate rapidly, clear and mount in synthetic resin.

Results

Mineralized bone	Black
Osteoid seams	Red

Notes

The type of light to which the silver solution is exposed will determine the time of exposure. A bench light, illuminating the Coplin jar from the side at a distance of 2–3 inches will take approximately 1 hour. Ultraviolet light will require only 10 minutes. Strong sunlight will take somewhere in between. Reduction of the silver is easily detected macroscopically.

■ Block impregnation method for osteoid seams (Tripp and Mackay, 1972)

In this method, a modified von Kossa technique is performed on blocks of tissue prior to processing and microtomy. Once reduced silver has been deposited on mineralized sites, the tissue can be decalcified and sectioned (*Figure 21.6*).

Chemical reduction of the formed silver phosphate is necessary, and the method suffers from uneven impregnation. The following method is taken from Cook (1974).

Solution—reducer

Sodium hypophosphite	5 g
0.1 N Sodium hydroxide	0.2 ml
Distilled water	100 ml

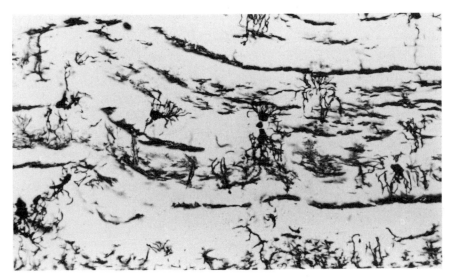

Figure 21.6 Cementocytes blackened by silver in a modified block impregnation method after Tripp and Mackay. Original magnification ×100

Method

(1) Fix thin blocks of bone in formal–saline.
(2) Wash in several changes of large volumes of distilled water. A mechanical agitator and three changes over 6 hours are recommended.
(3) Place in 2% aqueous silver nitrate in the dark for a period of 2–4 days.
(4) Wash in three changes of distilled water for 20 seconds each time.
(5) Wash in running tap-water for 4 hours.
(6) Treat with reducer over 2 days.
(7) Wash in running tap-water for 1 day.
(8) Treat with 5% sodium thiosulphate (hypo) for 1 day.
(9) Wash in running tap-water for 1 hour.
(10) Decalcify in 10% formic acid.
(11) Process into paraffin wax.
(12) Cut 7–8 μm sections and dry in oven.
(13) Take sections to water.
(14) Stain with Van Gieson's stain for 3 minutes.
(15) Dehydrate rapidly, clear and mount in synthetic resin.

Results

Mineralized bone	Black
Osteoid seams	Red

Resin embedded sections

Small blocks of undecalcified bone are processed into methyl methacrylate as described in Chapter 4. If using hydroxyethyl methacrylate the addition of 2% polystyrene improves the cutting qualities of the final block.

An exceptionally rigid microtome is required to cut sections of these blocks. The Jung K microtome is one such instrument, being a heavy duty base sledge type microtome, fitted with a motorized drive and employing specially designed tool-edged knives. Sections are cut at a slow speed with the block face and knife edge moistened with 70% alcohol. Individual sections are stored in 70% alcohol until required. Sections are usually stained before mounting, in the manner of frozen sections (Chapter 5).

Osteoid may be differentiated from mineralized bone by many techniques, using undecalcified sections, including haematoxylin and eosin and trichromes. The most useful techniques are solochrome cyanine staining and the modified trichrome method of Goldner (1938).

■ Solochrome cyanine staining for osteoid in resin sections

Solochrome cyanine, by some mechanism which is unknown, differentiates bone and osteoid into blue and red stained structures.

Solution (after Hyman and Poulding, 1961)

Solochrome cyanine R	1 g
Concentrated sulphuric acid	2.5 ml

Mix all the dye into a slurry.

0.5% Aqueous iron alum	500 ml

Filter.

Method

(1) Loose resin sections are washed in water.
(2) Stain in solochrome cyanine solution for 60 minutes.
(3) Differentiate in warm (30 °C) tap-water. A colour shift from red to blue will occur and should be controlled microscopically.
(4) Dehydrate, clear, mount on slides, then with synthetic resin.

Results

Mineralized bone	Blue
Osteoid	Red
Nuclei	Blue

Notes

Cook (1974) recommends 1% solochrome cyanine in 2% acetic acid, staining for 10 minutes only. This is a simpler, although less intense, stain.

Trichrome methods

Most of the trichrome stains will differentiate unmineralized osteoid from bone. MSB (Chapter 25) shows red-stained osteoid particularly well against blue bone, but the method of Goldner is preferred because of the clarity in cellular detail.

■ Goldner's method for osteoid (1938)

The method is a modification of Masson's trichrome.

Solutions

(1) Solution A

Ponceau de xylidine	0.75 g
Acid fuchsin	0.25 g
Acetic acid	1.0 ml
Distilled water	100 ml

Mix both dyes in the acetic acid before adding the distilled water.

Solution B

Azophloxin	0.5 g
Acetic acid	0.6 ml
Distilled water	100 ml

Add the dye to the acid before adding water.

Working solution

Solution A	10 ml
Solution B	2 ml
0.2% Acetic acid	88 ml

(2) Alkaline alcohol

80% Alcohol	90 ml
25% Ammonia	10 ml

Method

(1) Place free floating resin sections in alkaline alcohol solution for 1 hour.
(2) Wash in water for 15 minutes.
(3) Stain with celestine blue/haemalum sequence (page 161).
(4) Wash in water, then rinse in distilled water.
(5) Stain in Ponceau/fuchsin/azophloxin solution for 5 minutes.
(6) Rinse in 1% acetic acid for 15 seconds.
(7) Stain in 0.2% orange G in 1% phosphomolybdic acid for 20 minutes.
(8) Rinse in 1% acetic acid for 25 seconds.
(9) Stain in 0.2% light green in 0.2% acetic acid for 3 minutes.
(10) Rinse in 1% acetic acid.
(11) Rinse in water, dehydrate rapidly, clear and mount on slides.
(12) Mount in synthetic resin.

Results

Mineralized bone	Green
Osteoid	Red/orange
Nuclei	Blue

Rális and Ráliš (1975, 1976, 1978) have described a method of phosphotungstic acid staining and a 'tetrachrome' stain which they claim will differentiate five types of mineralized and non-mineralized bone in health and disease. These methods have not been particularly successful in our hands.

Fluorescent labelling of bone

The antibiotic tetracycline is brilliantly autofluorescent and quickly deposited in bone and teeth following administration. It not only forms an interesting artefact, but may be used to assess bone deposition if two doses are administered at known intervals. It is particularly useful in the study of bone healing.

Tetracycline deposited in developing teeth causes discoloration of dental tissues (*Figure 21.7*). The antibiotic is incorporated into both enamel and dentine, and because of the detailed knowledge of the chronological development of teeth, an experienced observer can estimate very accurately the age at which the drug was administered.

There is some argument over whether alcohol is the best fixative. Formal–saline certainly preserves tetracycline staining of teeth and undecalcified bone well in our experience. However, the resultant fluorescence is much brighter in ground sections than in decalcified paraffin-wax embedded material.

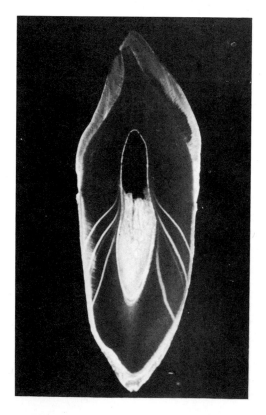

Figure 21.7 Discrete bands of tetracycline fluorescence in dentine following oral administration of the antibiotic several times during tooth development. Original magnification × 1.25

Microradiography

Microradiographs are high resolution X-ray films of undecalcified sections. Modern technology permits a very high degree of detail to be visualized. Whilst Haversian systems have for long been visible on microradiographs, it is now possible to produce pictures which show dentinal tubules, in longitudinal section, in 50 μm thick tooth sections (Davies, personal communication) (*Figures 21.8* and *21.9*).

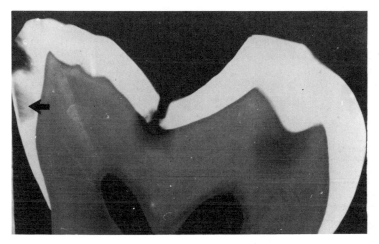

Figure 21.8 Microradiograph of a ground section of a human tooth showing three carious lesions at different stages. The lesion arrowed is represented by the densitometric trace in *Figure 21.9*. The strip at the extreme left of the illustration represents the aluminium wedge included for quantitative measurement. Original magnification × 3.2. (Reproduced by permission of the Editor, *Medical Laboratory Sciences*)

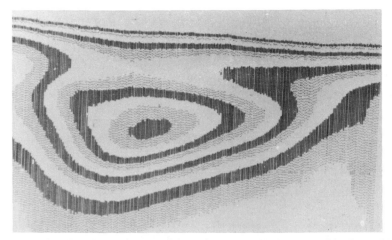

Figure 21.9 Densitometric trace of the carious enamel lesion arrowed in *Figure 21.8*. (Reproduced by permission of the Editor, *Medical Laboratory Sciences*)

Detailed densitometric measurements may be made by including a grey-step wedge of aluminium foil with known densities in the microradiograph.

Suitable microradiographs can be made by using clinical X-ray generators at low kV and fine grain high contrast film, by using soft X-ray generators designed primarily for X-ray crystallography or by using a purpose built instrument for producing soft radiographs from clinical specimens (e.g. Faxitron, Vinten Instruments Ltd, Jessamy Rd, Weybridge, England).

Teeth

The routine laboratory is rarely called upon to produce sections of teeth. However, it is not as difficult a procedure as is often presumed. Most of the technique applied to bone is equally applicable to teeth.

Structure and function

Teeth are identified numerically by the position they occupy in the jaws and by whether they are on the left or right. Thus the jaws may be divided into four quadrants and teeth are referred to by the position in the patient's mouth (not as the observer sees them). The quadrants are abbreviated by the symbols ∟ (upper left), ⌐ (upper right), Γ (lower left) and ⌐ (lower right) and numbered from the midline. Four types of teeth are recognized: incisors, canines, premolars and molars. Thus the symbol ⫇ denotes an upper left central incisor and ⁸⌐ a lower right molar (the 'wisdom' tooth).

Three distinct calcified tissues are recognized in teeth, but interest most often lies in the associated soft tissues of the pulp and supporting tissues.

Enamel

Enamel is the hardest body tissue and is composed of some 98% inorganic material. It is produced as a secretory product of specialized cells—*ameloblasts*—and subsequently becomes fully calcified. Ameloblasts, which are only seen in association with developing teeth, buried in the jaws, are epithelial in origin (*Figure 21.10*). They are recognized as columnar cells with a nucleus distal to the formative front. The cytoplasm is basophilic and granular, containing the organelles and enzymes usually associated with an actively secreting cell. Once enamel formation is completed, the ameloblasts become flatter and eventually fuse with the overlying cells of the outer enamel epithelium. They may have a role in tooth eruption.

The organic matrix of developing enamel is proteinaceous and appears to be a specialized form of collagen unique to enamel. Enamel crystals are very much longer than the calcified crystals of bone, although still composed essentially of hydroxyapatite. Small crystallites unite to form the larger crystals which are bound together by intercellular substance containing only small amounts of acid mucopolysaccharide. Although the general direction of the crystals is from the surface to the junction with dentine, the crystals may follow more tortuous routes, as in the occlusal plane of molar teeth, giving greater strength to withstand the forces of chewing and grinding.

Because of the exceptionally high inorganic content, special methods are required to preserve enamel in microscopic preparations.

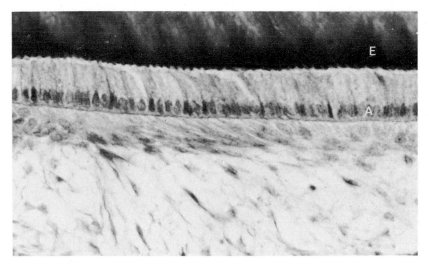

Figure 21.10 Section through developing tooth showing immature enamel (E) laid down by ambeloblasts (A)

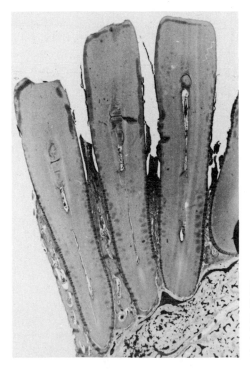

Figure 21.11 Decalcified section through lower incisor teeth. Note that the enamel has been lost from these teeth during decalcification, and that the plane of section shows only parts of the pulp chambers. The alveobar bone has been replaced by tumour in the bottom right of the photomicrograph. Original magnification ×1.0

Dentine

Dentine results from the activity of highly specialized cells, arising from the undifferentiated mesenchyme, termed *odontoblasts*. These cells lay down the ground substance of dentine in apposition to the enamel, retreating towards the pulp chamber as dentinogenesis proceeds. Odontoblasts remain vital even after the tooth has completed development, and may, with suitable stimulus, be reactivated to form new dentine. Conversely, they are susceptible to insult and may be killed. Each odontoblast has a cytoplasmic extension, the dentinal or odontoblast process which extends from the cell, through tubules in the dentine, terminating virtually at the amelo–dentinal junction.

Dentine contains a much higher proportion of organic matrix than enamel and remains following conventional decalcification and paraffin-wax processing. In haematoxylin and eosin-stained sections of dentine cut longitudinally, dentinal tubules may be faintly discerned. With specialized stains they are a striking feature. In cross-section, three distinct features are seen: tubules containing odontoblast processes, peritubular dentine and intertubular dentine. The MSB technique (page 471) is a useful method to differentiate these structures. A further structure that may be identified is 'interglobular' dentine which results from areas of incomplete calcification as foci of calcification coalesce. MSB is again useful.

Cementum

Cementum lines the external root of the tooth. It is remarkably similar to bone in morphology and composition. Cementoblasts may line the external surface and cementocytes lie within the matrix. Extra cementum may be laid down in response to infection, for example. Specialized connective tissue fibres—Sharpey's fibres—run from the supporting periosteum and enter the cementum thus 'anchoring' the tooth in its socket.

Fixation

Formal–saline is suitable for teeth, although penetration may be a problem. Access to the pulp chamber is limited to the apex, which becomes progressively narrower with age. It is sometimes recommended that the apex should be cut off to allow easier penetration. Unfortunately, the apex may be the area of greatest interest. Fixation should therefore be prolonged.

Decalcification

A variety of specialized formulas have been recommended for decalcifying teeth many of which seek to speed up the process. As the appearance of the associated soft tissues is likely to be at least as important as that of the hard tissue, the same arguments about the merits of these apply to teeth as they do to bone. Fifteen per cent formic acid is recommended.

The endpoint of decalcification must be determined by X-ray. One particular hazard may cause artefacts in decalcified tooth sections; that is recalcification. This is prone to occur particularly if the decalcifying solution remains unchanged. There is little opportunity for the calcium removed from the calcified structures to escape. It may reach sufficient concentration in the pulp to precipitate out, giving rise to artefactual, haematoxyphil, star-shaped crystal aggregates.

Processing

It is rarely worthwhile examining decalcified sections of teeth unless the plane of section includes the pulp. Because of the difficulties of successfully embedding whole teeth in paraffin wax, it is recommended that the sides of the tooth be shaved off prior to processing. The exact plane will depend upon the pathology.

Processing should be more leisurely than for soft tissues, and paraffin-wax infiltration thorough. The use of a specialized wax such as Ralwax (Raymond A. Lamb, 6 Sunbeam Rd, London, England) or Histoplast Special (Shandon Southern Products Ltd, Astmoor, Cheshire, England) is recommended. Best results are obtained by double embedding (Chapter 4) and if the relationship between hard and soft tissue is to be critically examined, LVN is the embedding medium of choice.

It is often advantageous to embed teeth so that they lie at an angle to the plane of section as described in Chapter 4.

Microtomy

A heavy microtome and sharp steel or tungsten carbide-edged knife are essential. It is rarely possible to cut sections of permanent teeth using disposable blades.

Blocks should be carefully trimmed until the pulp is exposed. Sections may be cut at 6–7 µm. Floating out may be a problem, particularly with multirooted teeth. The water-bath should be maintained just below the melting point of the wax.

Sections are mounted onto gelatin coated slides (Chapter 5), and left in a drying oven maintained at the melting point of the wax for 60 minutes. Unfortunately, tooth sections often have a depressing habit of lifting from the slide. Coated slides help prevent this, as does absolutely water free alcohol used in the final dehydration sequence in processing (Brain, personal communication).

Staining

Morphological stains recommended for bone are equally applicable to teeth. Thus Ehrlich's haematoxylin and eosin is preferred to Harris's or Meyer's. Silver reticulin methods show more detail of the hard tissues, but Schmorl's picro–thionin is the method of choice. Other methods may be used to demonstrate specific components such as nerves in the pulp and oxytalan fibres in the periodontium.

■ Picro–thionin method (Schmorl, 1934)

Method

(1) Take sections to water, wash well.
(2) Stain in half saturated aqueous thionin for 2–10 minutes.
(3) Wash well in running water.
(4) Stain in saturated aqueous picric acid for 30–60 seconds.
(5) Dehydrate *thoroughly*. This stage need not be rushed.
(6) Clear and mount in synthetic resin.

Results

Dentinal tubules, incremental lines in bone, lacunae and
    canaliculae   Dark brown
Cartilage, nuclei   Red/brown
Background   Yellow

Notes

(1) In recent years, it has become difficult to obtain samples of thionin satisfactory for this method. An ideal sample should stain adequately in 2 minutes. Poor samples of thionin can be improved by adding one to two drops of ammonia immediately before use.

(2) If hydration is less than complete at stage (5), the background will turn green. It is often advantageous to return to alcohol after taking to xylene and then to re-clear and mount.

(3) Modifications to this method have included the addition of phenol to the thionin solution (carbol–thionin) and the introduction of phosphotungstic or phosphomolybdic acid which gives a sky-blue background.

(4) Washing well following hydration helps minimize the deleterious effects of formal–saline fixation. Washing after thionin, removes excess dye which may be indiscriminately precipitated by the picric acid.

Ground sections

It is rarely necessary to produce ground sections of bone or teeth unless it is specifically desired to examine enamel. This material has never been successfully sectioned on any microtome to the authors' knowledge, despite claims to the contrary.

Apparatus with which undecalcified teeth may be cut and polished have been designed primarily for cutting, grinding and polishing geological specimens. In the authors' laboratories, teeth are embedded in a cold curing methacrylate and sections approximately 100 μm thick cut on a Microslice 2 (Cambridge Instruments, Rustat Rd, Cambridge, England). Cutting is effected by a diamond-edged disc, which may be of annular or peripheral configuration. Annular cutting discs are more accurate and less prone to distortion. However, they are less tolerant of stress—an important consideration in view of their cost. The cutting process must be cooled with a continuous drip feed of water or light oil. It should be a slow process, with the rate of feed being controlled by a system of weights. It is tempting, but counterproductive, to apply too much weight.

In the absence of precision equipment, it is possible to divide a tooth into two or three thick slices using a dental handpiece and diamond impregnated, or carborundum, wheel (Carborundum Co. Ltd, Trafford Park, Manchester, England). The slices may subsequently be ground to an acceptable thickness. There are occasional references in the literature to the possibility of dividing teeth longitudinally using a fine, diamond impregnated, fretsaw.

Thick sections of teeth may be ground and polished by simply rubbing on a glass plate using an abrasive slurry. Specimens perfectly satisfactory for simple morphological study may be prepared in this way. However, for more sophisticated examination, by critical polarization microscopy or microdensitometry, plano-parallel sections of known thickness are required. Suitable apparatus, for example, the Logitech polishing machine (Logitech Ltd, Alexandria, Scotland), will provide such sections if the manufacturers' instructions are carefully followed.

Sections need not be less than 15–20 μm for microscopy. If sections are allowed to dry, air in hard tissue spaces will dramatically increase the contrast. This may be advantageous on some occasions but on others will obscure detail. A hazard is that thin sections may curl irreversibly if allowed to dry out.

If the final preparation is not to be spoiled, meticulous attention must be given to

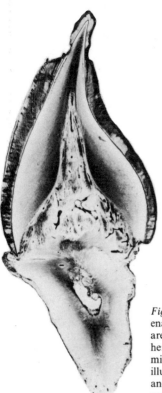

Figure 21.12 Ground section of a human tooth. Note that the enamel is still present covering the crown, although there are areas near the incisal edge which feature developmental, hereditary enamel hypoplasia. This tooth has suffered further misfortune during development, the aftermath of which is illustrated by the abnormal dentine in the centre of the section and the diminutive root. Unstained section. Original magnification × 1.25

removing scratches and small particles of abrasive which show a marked tendency to embed themselves into the section. Progressively finer abrasives should be used during polishing—we have found certain domestic scouring powders to be the most suitable final abrasive, followed by soapy water (*Figure 21.12*).

After washing, the sections should be dehydrated and mounted in synthetic resin. A thin coat of the mountant is applied to the slide, the section placed on top and that in turn covered by more mountant. The coverslip is then carefully placed over the section and laid down from one edge. The preparation must be allowed to dry completely while still flat. Sections may float to the surface of viscous media if placed on edge too soon.

Although suggestions for staining ground sections of teeth have been made, wide experience has shown that these procedures are largely unhelpful and frequently unsuccessful. Normal intact enamel resists most stains, although where it has been subject to carious attack it will take up common dyes.

Brain (1951, 1962) and Goland, Tagger and Engel (1965) have pioneered two techniques whereby enamel may survive decalcification. The first involves the use of carefully buffered decalcifying fluids and the second alternate treatment using special fixation—with procion dyes (ICI Ltd, Alderley Park, Macclesfield, Cheshire, England)—and conventional acid decalcification. The enamel which survives this treatment assumes the consistency of wet chalk and is therefore difficult to handle. Sections prepared by these methods permit study not only of the matrix, but also of the crystalline structure of enamel.

References

BALL, J. (1957). A simple method of defining osteoid in undecalcified sections. *J. Clin. Pathol.*, **10**, 281–282

BRAIN, E. B. (1951). Serial sections of decalcified human enamel and dentine. A modified method of *in situ* preparation in paraffin wax. *Dent. Radiog.*, **24**, 45–49

BRAIN, E. B. (1962). A new method for the preparation of decalcified sections of human enamel *in situ. Arch. Oral Biol.*, **7**, 757–760

BRAIN, E. B. (1966). *Preparation of Decalcified Sections.* Charles C. Thomas, Illinois

CLAYDEN, E. C. (1952). A discussion on the preparation of bone sections by the paraffin wax method with special reference to the control of decalcification. *J. Med. Lab. Technol.*, **10**, 103–123

COOK, H. C. (1974). *Manual of Histological Demonstration Techniques.* Butterworths, London

DUTHIE, R. B. (1954). A simple method for cutting sections from undecalcified bone for subsequent autoradiography and microscopy. *J. Pathol. Bacteriol.*, **68**, 296–297

GILL, G. (1982). Bis-chloro-methyl ether (BCME): a response. *Histo-Logic*, **12**, 176–177

GOLAND, P., TAGGER, E. S. and ENGEL, M. (1965). Enamel preservation during decalcification following fixation by some reactive halogen compounds. *J. Dent. Res.*, **44**, 342–349

GOLDNER, J. (1938). A modification of the Masson trichrome technique for routine laboratory purposes. *Am. J. Pathol.*, **14**, 237–243

GOODING, H. and STEWART, D. (1932). A comparative study of histological preparations of bone which have been treated with different combinations of fixatives and decalcifying fluids. *Lab. J.*, **7**, 55–65

HILLEMAN, H. H. and LEE, C. H. (1953). Organic chelating agents for decalcification of bones and teeth. *Stain Technol.*, **28**, 285–287

HYMAN, J. M. and POULDING, R. H. (1961). Solochrome cyanin–iron alum for rapid staining of frozen sections. *J. Med. Lab. Technol.*, **18**, 107

RÁLIŠ, Z. A. and RÁLIŠ, H. M. (1975). A simple method for demonstration of osteoid in paraffin sections. *J. Med. Lab. Technol.*, **32**, 203–213

RÁLIŠ, Z. A. and RÁLIŠ, H. M. (1976). Phosphotungstic acid–iron–haematoxylin staining method for osteoid, boundary bone and bone components in paraffin sections. *Microscopica Acta (Basle)*, **78**, 407–425

RÁLIŠ, H. M. and RÁLIŠ, Z. A. (1978). Poorly mineralised osteoid bone and its staining in paraffin sections. *Med. Lab. Sci.*, **35**, 293–303

SCHMORL, G. (1934). *Die Pathologisch-histologischen Untersuchungmethoden.* 16th Ed. Vogel, Berlin

TRIPP, E. J. and MACKAY, E. M. (1972). Silver staining of bone prior to decalcification for quantitative determination of osteoid in sections. *Stain Technol.*, **47**, 129–136

VON KOSSA, J. (1901). Über die in Organismus künstlich erzeugbaren Verkalukungen. *Beitr. Z. Path. Anat. u. Z. Allg. Path.*, **29**, 163–202

22

Miscellaneous biopsies

Kidney

The successful application of percutaneous needle biopsy technique, thin paraffin sections (2–3 μm), the 'Ralph' knife, resin sections (1–2 μm) and electron microscopy have greatly increased the role of histopathology in the diagnosis and classification of renal disease.

Many renal diseases arise as a result of immune reactions, either directly, as in the case of antibasement membrane antibody, or indirectly, when immune complexes may be deposited in the kidney. Immune complexes, of varying size and solubility, are regularly formed in response to insult and they are disposed of by the reticulo-endothelial system (RES). Large or insoluble complexes are readily disposed of by the liver and roving phagocytic cells. Small, soluble complexes may accumulate in the kidneys of some individuals as deposits on the glomerular basement membrane or in the mesangium. It is the appearance, site and reactivity of these deposits that help in the classification of many renal diseases. Thus, in immune complex disease, granular deposits may be found along the glomerular basement membrane, whilst with antibasement membrane antibody a linear reactivity is found. Where only a few lobules of a glomerulus are involved, the disease is said to be segmental or local; in diffuse disease the whole glomerular basement membrane or all lobules are affected. Focal disease refers to few affected glomeruli whereas in general disease most glomeruli are affected.

These changes are detected by immunocytochemical techniques, but conventional staining is also important in diagnosis, as may be electron microscopy in certain pathological states. The proper investigation of renal biopsies requires a combination of staining reactions (e.g. methenamine silver for foot processes on the basement membrane), immunocytochemistry (e.g. immunofluorescence for linear deposits in frozen sections) and electron microscopy (e.g. in minimal change disease). As each of these requires special treatment, it is desirable that the biopsy receives special attention.

Specimen

By the use of a modified Vim–Silverman needle (Colodny and Reckler, 1975) a core of tissue 10–12 mm in length and 1–2 mm in diameter may be obtained. Cortex must be present for the biopsy to be of value. It is most important that the specimen should not be allowed to dry. It should be transported to the laboratory on saline dampened gauze. If a delay of more than a few minutes is anticipated before receipt, the specimen should be immersed in a transport medium such as Michel's or Histocon (Histo-Lab Division of Bethlehem Instruments, PO Box 101, Hemel Hempstead, Herts., England).

■ Michel's transport medium

Anhydrous citric acid (0.025 M)	4.803 g
Ammonium sulphate (3.12 M)	412.3 g
N-ethylmaleimide (0.005 M)	0.625 g
Magnesium sulphate (0.005 M)	1.23 g

Make up to 1 litre. Keeps for 6 months when refrigerated.

Once received in the laboratory, the specimen should be divided into three using a sharp razor. A dissecting microscope helps identify glomeruli. A suitable way of dividing the biopsy is shown in *Figure 22.1*. The specimen for light microscopy should have priority, so that if only a few glomeruli are identified, that portion of tissue is fixed in 10% neutral formal–saline. It is possible to reprocess paraffin sections for electron microscopy and to use immunoenzyme methods on these sections for immunocytochemistry.

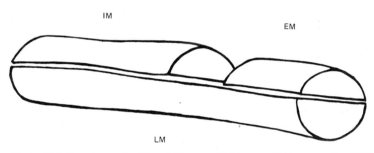

Figure 22.1 Popular method by which a needle biopsy of kidney may be divided to satisfy three investigative methods. LM = light microscopy, EM = electron microscopy, IM = immunocytochemistry

A choice must be made between paraffin-wax processing and resin embedding. Thin sections are necessary to study the morphology of the glomerular basement membrane; 2 μm sections are readily produced using disposable microtome blades, especially if a modified wax such as Ralwax 1 (Raymond A. Lamb, 6 Sunbeam Rd, London, England) or Histoplast Special (Shandon Southern Products Ltd, Chadwick Rd, Astmoor, Cheshire, England) is employed. It is advantageous, but not essential, to have a short processing schedule reserved for these and other small biopsies.

One portion of the biopsy should be snap frozen for immunofluorescence, this technique having a great sensitivity with weak immunoreactivity. Elias (1982) suggests that frozen sections may be post-fixed in 1% paraformaldehyde containing 20% dimethyl sulphoxide to give good morphology and staining.

This fixative is also reported to give a greater preservation of antigenicity (Johnson and Ham, 1980). It is an added advantage that tissue may be stored frozen at − 70 °C for at least a year without loss of reactivity.

Tissue for electron microscopy should be fixed in cold 3% neutral buffered glutaraldehyde, processed and stained as described in Chapter 34. It should be remembered that glutaraldehyde-fixed tissue is unsuitable for the PAS technique. If it should be necessary to reprocess paraffin-wax sections for electron microscopy, a Beem capsule containing unpolymerized epoxy resin is inverted over the section and allowed to polymerize. The capsule can then be carefully removed, the resin bringing the section off the glass with it. The block may then be sectioned on an ultramicrotome.

Microtomy

It is important to trim the blocks with great care. If the microtome chuck holder is not premanently set at one position, it is advised that the block is not removed from the holder until all sections have been cut. All sections that contain tissue should be kept, as there may be few glomeruli present in the specimen. Short ribbons should be cut, and up to four sections, cut at different levels, mounted on each slide; for example, sections 1, 8, 15 and 22 on the first slide, 2, 9, 16 and 23 on the second and so on.

Staining

A haematoxylin and eosin stained section is a prerequisite for morphological study, giving information on inflammatory infiltrates, cellularity, necrosis, etc.

Periodic acid–Schiff demonstrates basement membranes, immune complexes and the mesangium.

Methenamine–silver demonstrates glomerular basement membrane particularly well, including 'spiky' protrusions which are difficult to visualize by other methods. It is important not to over or under impregnate, as the basement membrane thickness is an important diagnostic criterion.

Other methods for amyloid, fibrin and hyaline deposits (trichrome stains) may be employed.

Immunofluorescence

Direct immunofluorescence (Chapter 18) is perfectly suitable for immune complexes. Routine screening should include antisera to IgA, IgG, IgM, the C_3 component of complement and fibrinogen.

If immunoenzyme methods are to be employed (Chapter 19) it may be necessary to use an indirect method if conjugated antisera are not available to all the antigens.

■ **Methenamine–silver method for basement membranes (Jones, 1957)** (*Figure 22.2*)

This method is a variation of the Gomori–Grocott method, periodic acid replacing chromic acid as the oxidizing agent.

Reagent

3% Hexamethylenetetramine (abbreviated to methenamine or hexamine)	100 ml
5% Silver nitrate	5 ml

A precipitate is formed when the silver nitrate is added to the methenamine solution; it dissolves on shaking. This solution should be freshly prepared.

Immediately before use add 3 ml of 5% sodium tetraborate (borax) to 50 ml of the above solution.

Table 22.1 Immunolocalization in the main glomerulonephropathies (from Elias, 1982)

Appearance	Major protein antigen	Disease
Continuous linear deposit on BM	IgG, C_3	Anti-GBM glomerulonephritis (Goodpastures' syndrome)
Irregular granular deposit in the subendothelial mesangium	C_3, variable IgG, IgM	Membrane proliferative glomerulonephritis
Granular subepithelial and/or subendothelial deposits	IgG, C_3	Acute glomerulonephritis
Fine subepithelial and intramembranous granular deposits	IgM, IgG, possibly C_3	Membranous glomerulonephritis
Mesangial deposits	IgA and IgG, variable C_3	Focal glomerulonephritis
Diffuse granular deposit on BM	IgG, IgM, IgA	Lupus glomerulonephritis Group II
Granular mesangial and subendothelial deposits	IgG, IgM, IgA, C_1, C_3	Lupus glomerulonephritis Group III
EM changes only	—	Minimal change disease

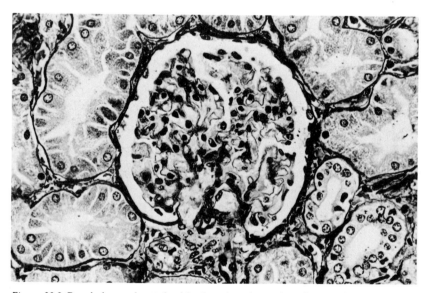

Figure 22.2 Renal glomerulus stained by Jones' methenamine–silver method demonstrating basement membrane. $2\,\mu m$ paraffin section. Original magnification $\times 100$

Method

(1) Bring sections to water.
(2) Immerse in 0.5% periodic acid for 15 minutes.
(3) Rinse well in distilled water.
(4) Place in hexamine–silver solution, preheated to 56 °C for 20–30 minutes.
(5) Rinse well in distilled water.
(6) If desired, the sections may be toned in 0.2% gold chloride for 2 minutes.
(7) Wash in water, treat with 5% sodium thiosulphate (hypo) for 2 minutes.
(8) Wash in running tap-water.

(9) Counterstain, if desired. Either haematoxylin and eosin, or 0.2% light green in 0.2% acetic acid are suitable.
(10) Dehydrate, clear and mount in synthetic resin.

Results

Basement membranes (if toned)   Black

Other tissue according to counterstain and toning.

Notes

Impregnation with the hexamine–silver solution is progressive and should be checked microscopically. It is important that this solution is preheated to the required temperature, preferably in a water-bath.

We prefer not to tone the silver impregnation. This results in a dark-brown/black deposition on the basement membranes, with other tissues staining in shades of yellow and brown. If toning is omitted, counterstaining is unnecessary.

Skin

The correct orientation of skin for microtomy is the single most important factor in producing acceptable sections. This tissue may also prove difficult to cut in the presence of hair or heavy keratinization.

Specimen

Skin specimens may be either incisional or excisional. In the former it is important that the biopsy contains a margin of normal skin adjacent to the lesion for comparative purposes (*Figure 22.3a*). The specimen must be orientated so that this is included in the

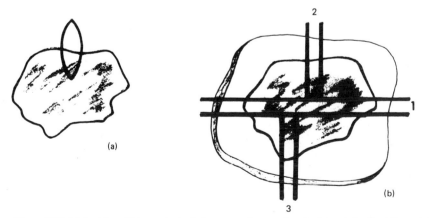

Figure 22.3 (a) Incisional biopsy to include areas of suspect pathology and adjacent normal epithelium. (b) Compromise method to show narrowest margins of clearance of an excisional biopsy

section. Excisional biopsies must answer two questions: what is the nature of the lesion and has it been completely removed? It is essential that the plane of section passes through the narrowest margin separating the lesion from the edge of the biopsy. Ideally, tissue blocks showing all margins should be processed. Where this is impractical, a compromise solution is illustrated in *Figure 22.3b*. Punch biopsies may also be received. Although small, these should not present difficulty in orientation. They may either be bisected, and the flat surfaces produced embedded face down, or the entire 'cylinder' embedded and sectioned along its longest axis.

Because of the difficulty sometimes encountered in recognizing the surface to be sectioned at the embedding stage, it is advantageous to mark the opposite side by some indelible method. A *small* amount of silver nitrate or Indian ink applied to a dried surface is suitable.

Where an ellipse has been removed to show general skin pathology, it is advisable to bisect the specimen along its length, saving one-half in fixative. The flat, cut surface should then be embedded face down. Alternatively, the whole specimen may be embedded on the curved edge and trimmed down until a nearly complete section is obtained.

It may be helpful if the biopsy, immediately on removal from the patient, is placed on a small piece of thin card. The specimen will adhere to the card when placed in fixative, producing a flat surface. A careful regimen should be established so that the laboratory is aware that the same surface is always placed in contact with the card.

If it is possible to remove excess hair present on the skin surface this should be carefully done with a sharp razor. It will be much easier to cut good sections.

Fixation and processing

Formal–saline fixation is generally suitable. If a lot of subcutaneous fat is present, secondary fixation in Carnoy's fixative makes processing and sectioning easier. Sebaceous material that may be present in many cysts hinders successful processing. Much of it should be removed. Wedge-shaped biopsies, where the epithelial surface is wider than the deepest margin, should be embedded carefully to avoid cutting obliquely through the epithelium (*see Figure 4.2*).

Microtomy

It is good practice to cut skin biopsies with the epithelial surface meeting the knife last, that is, when the underlying dermis has already passed the knife edge. If the tissue is particularly tough, it may be softened by treatment with phenol or Mollifex (BDH Ltd, Poole, Dorset, England) (Chapter 5). With a sharp knife this should only rarely be necessary. Thin sections (2–3 μm) should be cut when there is a heavy cellular infiltrate, as in lymphoma deposits.

Sections should be cut at various levels, with spare sections kept unstained from each (Chapter 5). Skin biopsies removed to assess the Kveim test should be sectioned right through to ensure that a negative result is not false. Chrome gelatin treated slides (Chapter 5) will help prevent the tendency of epithelium to lift from the slide and fold over.

Staining

Apart from the indispensable morphological features demonstrated by haematoxylin and eosin staining, the following structures may be selectively identified.

Keratin
Lendrum's phloxine–tartrazine is the method of choice. Trichromes stain keratin red/orange, and it is weakly Gram-positive. Keratin may also be demonstrated by virtue of the high concentration of disulphide (—SS—) and sulph-hydryl (—SH—) groups present. Schmorl's (page 286) is the simplest and most reliable method.

Immunoperoxidase methods using antisera to keratin and prekeratin represent the most selective means of demonstration.

Elastin
Age changes in skin and diagnosing the various dermal elastoses calls for elastic stains as described in Chapter 9. Elastotic degeneration of collagen, seen in solar keratosis, is particularly well demonstrated by synthetic orcein.

Mast cells, plasma cells and *eosinophils* may be demonstrated by appropriate methods (Chapter 24).
Pigments, especially *melanin*, are often recognized in skin sections, and it may be necessary to demonstrate the *basement membrane*.
Peripheral nerves may be demonstrated by the methods given in Chapter 20.

Immunofluorescence

Immunofluorescence is invaluable in the differential diagnosis of pemphigus, pemphigoid, dermatitis herpetiformis and lupus erythematosis. Either the direct methods, whereby frozen sections from the patient are treated with fluorescein conjugated antisera to human γ-globulin, or the indirect method, whereby normal tissue containing the desired antigen (e.g. guinea pig oesophagus) is treated with patient's serum believed to contain antibody and reactivity visualized by fluorescein conjugated antiserum to human γ-globulin, may be used (Chapter 18).

In pemphigus, patients usually have a circulating antibody that binds to the intercellular bridges of epithelial cells (*Figure 22.4a*). In pemphigoid, a circulating antibody to basement membrane is often, but not invariably, present. When pemphigoid is present in the absence of circulating antibody, immunoglobulin that has become bound to the basement membrane may be demonstrated by the direct method using conjugated antisera to IgG, IgM and IgA respectively (*Figure 22.4b*). Complement may also be present.

Dermatitis herpetiformis appears to have a high correlation with coeliac disease. The important diagnostic feature is that deposits of IgA may be demonstrated along the connective tissue papillae of clinically normal skin using direct immunofluorescence.

The immunofluorescent findings in lupus erythematosus (LE) is more complicated. The method is most useful in differentiating systemic LE (SLE) when both involved and non-involved skin may give positive results and discoid LE (DLE) in which non-involved, light protected skin is always negative. The predominant immunoglobulin is usually IgM or IgG, in contrast to dermatitis herpetiformis, when IgA is the usual finding. Patients with LE almost invariably have antinuclear antibodies circulating also.

Eye

Composed as it is of very tough and very soft tissues, sections of the eye, showing good morphological relationships between the tissues, are difficult to prepare unless great care and suitable technique is used.

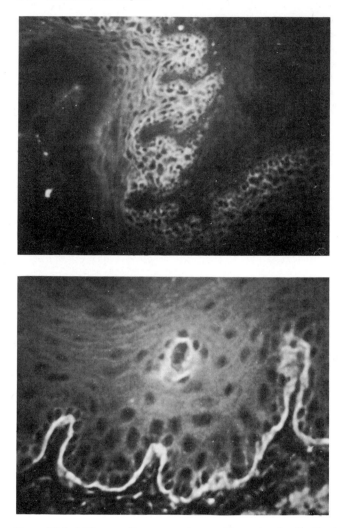

Figure 22.4 (a) Immunofluorescence in pemphigus, showing localization of circulating antibody to intercellular epithelial cell bridges. (b) Immunofluorescent localization of circulating antibody on basement membrane in pemphigoid

Fixation

Immediately on removal, the eye should be fixed by immersion in 10% neutral formal–saline. The cornea should not be allowed to dry, microtomy will be difficult enough without this artefact. After 48 hours, the eye may be very carefully sectioned using a sharp blade. It may be helpful to rapidly freeze the eye, in isopentane cooled with liquid nitrogen, before cutting, but there is a danger of artefactual separation of the various layers. The direction of the cut will normally be from the lens to the optic nerve, but occasionally a cross-section may be required. An alternative method, which we prefer, is to take off the top and bottom of the eye. This leaves the whole of the cornea, lens and optic nerve in one flat circular block. Care must be taken not to detach the retina during any stage of the technique. The eye should be returned to formal–saline for 24 hours after cutting.

Embedding

For the very best results, LVN is the embedding process of choice but double embedding will also produce acceptable results. If paraffin wax is used, a very gentle processing cycle should be carefully constructed.

Staining

Standard methods may be used to demonstrate connective tissue, myelin, neuroglia and so on.

Various components of the rods and cones of the retina may be demonstrated by iron harmatoxylin (page 162), fat-soluble stains (page 262) and PAS (page 220). The last method will also demonstrate glycogen in the retina and a web-work in the vitreous humour.

Pancreas

Biopsies or small lesions removed from the pancreas are relatively uncommon, although the advent of the needle biopsy could conceivably change this. If surgical specimens are received, they usually result from Whipple's operation and comprise a portion of stomach and duodenum with the head of the pancreas attached.

Fixation

Most routine fixatives are suitable, except that acetic acid should be avoided since it dissolves the characteristic exocrine oxyphil granules. Formal–saline and Zenker's fixative give good results with most staining methods. Since autolysis of the pancreas is rapid, tissue should be fixed as soon as possible.

Staining

For routine staining haematoxylin and eosin is adequate, but special methods are required to demonstrate specifically the A (α_2) cells, B (β) cells and the D (α_1) cells of the islets of Langerhans and the zymogen granules which are found in cells lining the alveoli. These latter are rich in tryptophan and share common staining reactions with Paneth cell granules (Chapter 24). B cells produce insulin, A cells glucagon and D cells stomatostatin, the presence of which may be confirmed by immunoperoxidase methods.

Connective tissue stains (Chapter 9) are useful differentiators, A cells staining red and B cells pale orange brown. B cells are stained positively with Gomori's aldchyde fuchsin (page 177) whilst the cytoplasm of D cells has an affinity for aniline blue and light green. Zymogen granules are acidophilic and PAS-positive.

A cells and D cells may be selectively demonstrated using silver impregnation methods (Grimelius, 1968; Hellerström and Hellman, 1960) (*see* pages 476 and 477).

Alimentary canal

The ease with which small biopsies may be obtained via the endoscope has led to an expansion in histopathological diagnosis of intestinal malignancies, Crohn's disease, ulcerative colitis, amyloidosis and other diseases. Correct orientation, so that the full depth of the epithelium and underlying connective tissue may be seen, is the major difficulty with these specimens. As it is easier to orientate fresh unfixed tissue, surgeons should be encouraged to place the specimen on a piece of card prior to fixation as described for skin, above.

Several biopsies of colon may be taken to determine the limits of the aganglionic zone in Hirschsprung's disease. In this zone there is an absence of ganglion cells and an increase in acetylcholinesterase-containing nerve fibres in the lamina propria and in the muscularis mucosae. Demonstration techniques for acetylcholinesterase allow easy recognition of ganglion cells and nerve bundles in frozen sections. The following method is recommended.

■ **Acetylthiocholine esterase method (modified from Lake *et al.*, 1978)**

Use cryostat sections of snap frozen biopsies, orientated on edge.

Reagents

Stock solutions	Strength (%)	For storing (ml)
Sodium acetate (3 H_2O)	0.82	25.2
Acetic acid	0.6	0.8
Trisodium citrate	2.94	2.0
Copper sulphate (5 H_2O)	0.75	4.0
Distilled water		4.0
	Total	36

Deep freeze four aliquots of 9 ml.

Working solution

Stock	9 ml
Acetylthiocholine iodide	5 mg
Potassium ferricyanide (0.165%)	1 ml

Filter for use. For negative control prepare as above without the acetylthiocholine iodide.

Di-aminobenzidine (DAB) in tris buffer pH 7.4

0.2 M Tris	6.25 ml
0.1 N Hydrochloric acid	10.5 ml
Water	to 25 ml
Di-aminobenzidine	12.25 mg

Method

(1) Air-dry cryostat sections.
(2) Fix in formal–calcium for 1 minute.

(3) Rinse in distilled water.
(4) Incubate in substrate (preheated at 37 °C) for 1 hour.
(5) Wash briefly in distilled water.
(6) Treat with DAB in tris buffer pH 7.4 for 30 minutes.
(7) Wash in tap-water for 15 minutes.
(8) Dehydrate, clear and mount in resinous mountant.

Results

Brown precipitate at enzyme sites.

Note

Stain may be intensified by treatment with 1% osmium tetroxide for 10 minutes at room temperature after step (7) above.

Lymph nodes

Occasionally lymph nodes may be biopsied, but more usually they are excised intact. The thorough investigation of lymphoid tissue demands special preparatory methods.

Specimen

Ideally, fresh tissue should be received by the laboratory. Imprint smears should be obtained by pressing a freshly cut surface against a clean glass slide and allowing to air-dry. These may be used for Romanowsky-type staining and spare smears stored, unfixed at -20 to -70 °C for subsequent enzyme demonstration.

A portion of tissue should be snap frozen and kept for cryostat sections and immunofluorescence.

Tissue homogenates, with viable lymphocytes present, are required for many of the cell surface marker techniques used to differentiate T and B lymphocytes.

The remainder of the tissue is fixed, including a small portion reserved for electron microscopy. The preferred fixative is 10% neutral formal–saline (Reynolds, 1982), although B-5, formalin–zinc chloride mixture has also been recommended (Elias, 1982). Lymph nodes should be cut into 3 mm thick slices prior to fixation.

Processing and cutting

This highly cellular tissue, with little supporting matrix, requires a particularly gentle and thorough processing schedule. It is important to ensure that dehydration is complete. The specimen should be embedded in a wax, without exceeding 58 °C, that permits thin (2–3 μm) sectioning. Disposable microtome blades greatly facilitate the production of thin, high quality sections. It is important that the floating out bath is maintained at 10 °C below the melting point of the wax, and that the drying oven is maintained at a similar temperature. Heat may easily cause the tissue to 'float apart'.

Resin sections are often recommended to provide the highest quality morphological detail, but with careful attention to detail, 2 μm paraffin wax sections yield equal information.

Staining

Haematoxylin and eosin stained sections remain the cornerstone of diagnostic lymph node pathology, even though the precise diagnosis may depend upon the identification of particular lymphoid cells.

Methyl green–pyronin (Chapter 24) identifies plasma cells by virtue of the intense pyroninophilia of the RNA, although in neoplastic lymphoid tissue, there are many other cell types rich in RNA.

Reticulin forms the supporting network for the cells of the lymph node. In lymphoreticular disease, this may be completely lost. Metastatic deposits, on the other hand, modify the normal pattern.

Romanowsky stains—Giemsa on sections, Leishman's stain on imprint smears—are helpful in relating the cell types present to those identified in peripheral blood or marrow aspirates, by the haematologist.

■ Giemsa method

(1) Bring sections to water.
(2) Treat with Sörensen's buffer, pH 6.8, for 15 minutes.
(3) Place in Giemsa stain diluted 1:10 with buffer for 1 hour.
(4) Differentiate, until pink, in buffer.
(5) Dehydrate rapidly, clear and mount in neutral synthetic resin.

Results

Nuclei	Blue
Neutrophil granules	Pink
Eosinophil granules	Bright red
Basophil granules	Blue
Red blood cells	Pink

■ Leishman's stain

(1) Filter undiluted Leishman stain directly onto imprint smear for 2 minutes.
(2) Dilute stain, on slide, with an equal quantity of pH 6.8 buffer for 8 minutes.
(3) Wash in buffer.
(4) Differentiate in buffer until smear appears pink.
(5) Blot and air-dry.

Results

As above (Giemsa).

Enzyme histochemistry

Chloroacetate esterase is a marker for granulocytes; promyelocytes and leukaemic cells are particularly reactive. Lymphoid cells are negative, although monocytes and histiocytes may give weakly positive results. The enzyme withstands paraffin processing.

■ **Naphthol AS–D chloroacetate esterase method (from Yam, Li and Crosby, 1971; Li, Lam and Yam, 1973)**

Reagents

Solution A

4% Pararosaniline in 2 N hydrochloric acid	0.1 ml⎱ Mix
4% Sodium nitrite	0.1 ml⎰
Sörensen's phosphate buffer, pH 6.3	35 ml

Solution B

Dissolve 20 mg Naphthol AS–D chloroacetate in 1 ml *N,N*-dimethylformamide.

Mix solutions A and B, shake and filter directly into a Coplin jar.

Method

(1) Bring sections to water.
(2) Incubate in substrate solution at room temperature for 2 hours.
(3) Rinse in water.
(4) Stain in Mayer's haemalum for 2 minutes.
(5) Blue in Scot's tap-water substitute for 2 minutes.
(6) Wash, dehydrate, clear and mount in synthetic resin.

Results

Nuclei	Blue
Chloroacetate esterase activity (neutrophils and mast cells)	Red

Non-specific esterase is a useful marker of monocytes (histiocytes or macrophages). According to Reynolds (1982), if the technique is performed at pH 6.3, monocytes become negative, but T lymphocytes show punctate positivity. The method is given in Chapter 16.

Alpha-naphthol acid esterase demonstration can be used as a T-lymphocyte marker using imprint smears or cryostat sections.

■ **Alpha-naphthol acid esterase**

Reagent

4% Pararosanaline in 2 N hydrochloric acid	1.5 ml⎱ Mix
4% Sodium nitrite	1.5 ml⎰
Sörensen's phosphate buffer (0.7 M) pH 5.0	37 ml

Adjust to pH 5.8 with 2 N sodium hydroxide (20–30 drops).

Dissolve 10 mg alpha-naphthyl acetate in 0.5 ml acetone and add to above solution and filter.

Method

(1) Fix smears or sections in 2.5% glutaraldehyde in 0.9% saline at 4 °C for 10 minutes.
(2) Wash in buffer.
(3) Incubate in substrate at 37 °C for 3 hours.

(4) Wash well in water.
(5) Counterstain lightly in 2% methyl green for $1-1\frac{1}{2}$ minutes.
(6) Dehydrate, clear and mount in synthetic resin.

Results

T lymphocytes show distinct red punctate positivity around the nucleus. There may be diffuse staining in the cytoplasm of monocytes or histiocytes and platelets are positive.

Alpha-naphthyl butyrate has some advantages as a substrate for esterases. At pH 6.3 specificity for monocytes is claimed to be made complete, whilst at pH 8.0, monocytes, T lymphocytes and null-cells are reported to display distinctive staining patterns.

Immunocytochemistry

The precise classification of lymphoid neoplasias helps indicate the prognosis of the disease and determines treatment. Immunocytochemical methods of cell identification form a major tool in achieving this objective. A detailed description of the types and functions of various leucocytes is beyond the scope of this book; the following list is but a brief account of some of the more common cells that may be identified.

Neutrophils and other cells of the *myeloid* series are characterized by their typical reaction in Romanowsky-type stains and enzyme reactions (e.g. chloroacetate esterase).

Lymphocytes may be subdivided according to derivation and function. T lymphocytes are derived from the thymus. Sixty-five per cent of these are termed *helper* cells (T_h) because of their role in helping other cells (B lymphocytes) produce antibody. The remaining 35% of T lymphocytes are either *cytotoxic* (T_c) or *suppressor* (T_s) cells. *Effector* T lymphocytes produce *lymphokine*—a macrophage activating factor.

B lymphocytes are derived from the bone marrow or Bursa equivalent. They carry surface immunoglobulins, *Fc receptors* and C_3b *receptors*. Their role is in the production of antibody, differentiating into *plasma cells*. Lymphocytes which carry neither T nor B cell markers are termed *null cells* and include the *natural killer* (NK) cells which are activated by *interferon*.

Monocytes include not only those blood-carried cells, but the wandering tissue macrophages or histiocytes and fixed macrophage type cells such as the *dendritic* cells of the spleen, *Kupffer* cells of the liver and *Langerhans* cells of the skin. Activated macrophages (*see above*) increase the T and B cell population and enhance T cell differentiation.

In the identification of selected antigens, monoclonal antibodies may be applied, where available, to cryostat sections or immunoperoxidase methods applied to paraffin processed sections. For the demonstration of cell surface immunoglobulins—to identify B lymphocytes, for example—immunofluorescence on cryostat sections is the method of choice (*see Table 22.2*).

Other methods of identification

Viable cells obtained by tissue homogenation can be used to assess the relative proportions of cell types. For example, T lymphocytes cause the red blood cells of various animals (sheep cells are commonly employed) to adhere to their surface, forming rosettes. Appropriate treatment of the red blood cells permits the detection of Fc receptors and C_3 receptors on human leucocytes.

Table 22.2 Useful monoclonal antibodies for mononuclear leucocytes

Cell type	Ortho[1]	Becton-Dickinson[2]
T cells	OKT11; OKT3	Anti-Leu 1
T_c/T_s	OKT8	Anti-Leu 2 (a and b)
T_h	OKT4	Anti-Leu 3 (a and b)
NK		Anti-Leu 11
B cells	OKIa 1	Anti-HLA-DR
Monocyte/macrophage	OKM1; OKIa 1	Anti-HLA-DR
Large granular lymphocyte		Anti-Leu 7

[1] Ortho Diagnostic Systems Inc., Route 202, Raritan, New Jersey, USA.
[2] Becton-Dickinson Monoclonal Center Inc., 2375 Garcia Ave, Mountain View, California, USA.

Bone marrow

In some laboratories, it is routine procedure to process bone marrow aspirates. As a generalization, haematologists are more adept at identifying haemopoietic cells in Romanowsky stained smears than are histologists using paraffin-wax sections. However, there are occasions, such as in the identification of tumour cells, when this method is valuable.

The marrow aspirate should be placed in Zenker's fixative in a small glass tube. Ideally, the marrow fragments should be processed in this tube so it helps if the inside is lightly smeared with glycerol. Each processing fluid is replaced using a Pasteur pipette and great care taken to ensure that no fragments are lost. Fifteen minutes is sufficient in each fluid, the tube being rapidly centrifuged in the final wax, so that on solidification, the marrow forms a small pellet at the base of the tube. The tube should be carefully broken to expose the wax block. Serial sections should be cut from the marrow.

May–Grünwald–Giemsa staining is most suitable. Other methods that may be employed include methyl green–pyronin (page 189) and Perls's method for haemosiderin (page 279).

As an alternative to the above procedure, fixed fragments of marrow may be carefully folded in tissue paper and processed in a cassette. The drawback is that tissue may be lost, particularly at the embedding stage, and it is difficult to arrange the fragments at the same level within the wax block.

Marrow trephines are sometimes performed, especially in cases where there is little marrow cellularity (as in myelofibrosis) or when a solid tumour is present—as may happen with some leukaemias. The trephine will contain bone and therefore require decalcification (Chapter 21) before processing as a routine tissue block. Methyl green–pyronin staining is rarely satisfactory on sections of decalcified tissue.

■ May–Grünwald–Giemsa method

Method

(1) Bring slides to water.
(2) Treat with pH 6.8 buffer, 30 min, at 37 °C.
(3) Stain in May–Grünwald stain diluted 1:5 with pH 6.8 buffer, 10–15 min.
(4) Rinse in buffer.
(5) Stain in Giemsa's stain diluted 1:10 with pH 6.8 buffer, 1–12 hours.

(6) Wash in buffer.
(7) Differentiate in glycerin-ether (commercial), controlling microscopically.
(8) Wash in buffer, dehydrate, clear and mount in synthetic resin.

Results

Similar to Giemsa.

References

COLODNY, A. H. and RECKLER, J. M. (1975). A safe simple and reliable method for percutaneous (closed) renal biopsies in children: results in 100 consecutive patients. *J. Urol.*, **113**, 222–224

ELIAS, J. M. (1982). *Principles and Techniques in Diagnostic Histopathology*. Noyes Publications, Park Ridge, New Jersey

GRIMELIUS, L. (1968). A silver nitrate stain for α_2 cells in human pancreatic islets. *Acta Soc. Med. Uppsala*, **73**, 243–270

HELLERSTRÖM, C. and HELLMAN, B. (1960). Some aspects of silver impregnation of the Islets of Langerhans in the rat. *Acta Endocrinol.*, **35**, 518–532

JOHNSON, C. I. and HAM, K. N. (1980). Immunoperoxidase technique for electron microscopy of renal biopsies. *Micron*, **11**, 413

JONES, D. B. (1957). Nephrotic glomerulonephritis. *Am. J. Pathol.*, **33**, 313–330

LAKE, B. D., PURI, P., NIXON, H. H. and CLAIREAUX, A. E. (1978). Hirschsprung's disease. An appraisal of histochemically demonstrated acetylcholinesterase activity in suction rectal biopsy specimens as an aid to diagnosis. *Acta Path. Lab. Med.*, **102**, 244–247

LEDER, L. D. (1964). The selective enzyme cytochemical demonstration of neutrophil myeloid cells and tissue mast cells in paraffin sections. *Klin. Wchnschr.*, **42**, 553

LI, C. Y., LAM, K. W. and YAM, L. T. (1973). Esterases in human leucocytes. *J. Histochem. Cytochem.*, **21**, 1–12

REYNOLDS, G. J. (1982). *Lymphoid Tissue*. Wright PSG, Bistol

YAM, L. T., LI, C. Y. and CROSBY, W. H. (1971). Cytochemical identification of monocytes and granulocytes. *Am. J. Clin. Pathol.*, **55**, 283–290

23

Muscle

Muscle consists of specialized groups of cells forming contractile tissue which controls movements of many kinds. There are three kinds of muscle: skeletal, cardiac and visceral. Both skeleton and cardiac muscle are striated but only skeletal is voluntary, cardiac and visceral being involuntary.

The striations seen in longitudinal views of muscle fibres are due to the orderly arrangement of the constituent actin and myosin filaments. Actin and myosin are also present in non-striated visceral muscle but the orderly arrangement is lacking, so striations are not present.

Skeletal muscle

The muscle cell is very large, 1–40 mm in length and up to 40 µm in diameter. Within the cytoplasm are found the myofibrils which consist of actin and myosin filaments. The unit of structure within the myofibril is the sarcomere extending between two Z-lines (*Figure 23.1*). The most obvious striations are the A bands (anisotropic) and the I bands (isotropic), so-called because of their optical characteristics. The Z-line traverses the I band. On closer examination it will be found that there is a lighter central zone in the A band, the H zone, which is itself bisected by the thin M line.

The contraction is accomplished by thick myosin filaments sliding between thin actin filaments which in turn are fixed to the Z-lines, thus shortening the sarcomere.

It is therefore essential to ensure that the muscle fibre is relaxed before subsequent fixation or freezing in order to observe the striations.

The myofibrils lie in the cytoplasm (sarcoplasm) along with nuclei, glycogen, mitochondria and smooth endoplasmic reticulum (sarcoplasmic reticulum).

The muscle is formed of bundles of cells with different appearances, activities and histochemical reactions and can be classified into two main groups, the slow-twitch (Type 1) and the fast-twitch (Type 2) fibres. The Type 2 fibres can be subdivided into 2A, 2B and 2C types using ATPase preincubation at pH 10.4, 4.6 and 4.3 (Brooke and Kaiser, 1970), and further divided into Types 2AB and 2AC (Ingjer, 1979).

Cardiac muscle

The ultrastructure of cardiac muscle is similar to that of skeletal muscle but differs in that mitochondria are more numerous, the nuclei are central, the sarcoplasm branches and individual cells are separated terminally by intercalated discs. The endocardium forms the internal lining of the heart.

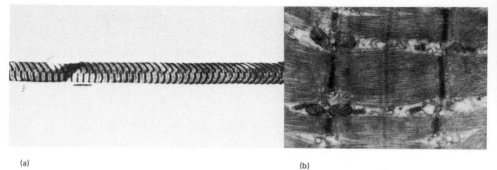

(a)   (b)

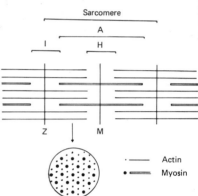

Figure 23.1 (a) Striated muscle fibre. Heidenhain's
iron haematoxylin. Light microscopy. Original
magnification × 40. (b) Striated muscle fibre. Electron
microscopy. Original magnification × 20 000. (c)
Diagrammatic representation of skeletal muscle
showing the formation of the striations in
longitudinal section (*above*) and the relationship of
actin and myosin filaments in cross-section   (c)

Visceral muscle

Smooth muscle cells are much smaller than the striated muscle cells. The sarcoplasm
contains myofibrils, an eccentric elongated nucleus and mitochondria dispersed
between the sarcomeres. The functions of smooth muscle are intermittent and
sustained contraction.

Demonstration

Histological stains

The morphology of muscle fibres is demonstrated using haematoxylin and eosin,
Verhoeff–Van Gieson and Engel and Cunningham's modification of the Gomori
trichrome method. The Verhoeff–Van Gieson, demonstrating yellow muscle and red
collagen, will also stain mitochondria, elastic and myelin black. Heidenhain's iron
haematoxylin and phosphotungstic acid haematoxylin will both demonstrate muscle
striations, the latter, requiring no differentiation, is often preferred and may be used to
demonstrate the rods in nemaline myopathy. Nerve endings are demonstrated by vital
staining with methylene blue, and cholinesterase techniques are used to demonstrate
muscle endplates.

Histochemical techniques

These are used to identify different fibre types and so demonstrate their involvement in

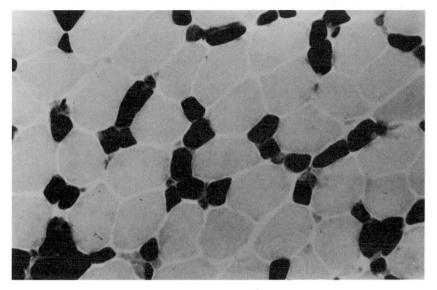

Figure 23.2 Myosin ATPase with pre-incubation at pH 4.3 identifying atrophy of type I fibres. Original magnification × 40

certain diseases (*Figure 23.2*). They will show structural changes not apparent with histological stains, for example, enzyme deficiency in central core disease, and will demonstrate deficiencies of enzymes, or deficiencies or excesses of storage products in the glycogenoses.

The techniques for lactate dehydrogenase, succinate dehydrogenase (*Figure 23.3*), NADH- and NADPH-diaphorases, phosphorylase and adenosine triphosphatase are of diagnostic value. Methods for nucleic acids and lipids, and the PAS technique are also used.

The skeletal muscle biopsy

The selection and operation procedures for muscle biopsy are well described by Dubowitz and Brooke (1973). It is essential that the specimen should be relaxed and to ensure this several techniques have been advocated. The specimen may be placed on moist gauze, on a wooden spatula, or preferably held in a relaxed state by means of a muscle clamp. Dissection of the specimen should be carried out under a stereo-microscope so that both longitudinal and transverse sections are obtained but since it is recognized that most information is derived from the transverse section, this block should take priority. The priority for processing is firstly the frozen block, secondly the block for electron microscopy and lastly material for paraffin processing.

Whilst it is desirable that the biopsy should be delivered to the laboratory as soon as possible after excision, in practice a time lag of up to 30 minutes is acceptable.

The tissue should be orientated in either 10% tragacanth gum or OCT compound (Miles Laboratories) on a cork disc. The disc is then immersed in isopentane cooled to a syrupy consistency with liquid nitrogen. It is essential that the tissue is frozen as quickly as possible in order to avoid the formation of ice-crystal artefact. The specimen should remain in the isopentane only long enough to ensure thorough freezing. Long

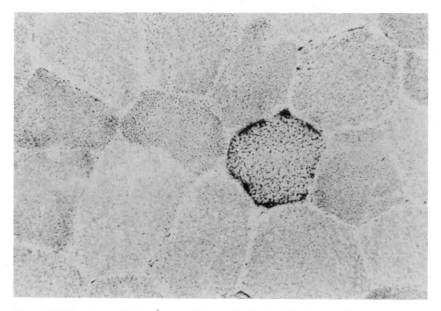

Figure 23.3 Succinate dehydrogenase. Abnormal mitochondria in so-called ragged red fibre (from modified Gomori trichrome appearance). Original magnification ×100

immersion should be avoided since cracking of the block may occur. The cork disc may then be attached to the microtome chuck with a drop of water, then frozen. The blocks attached to the cork disc may be removed from the chuck for storage in an air-tight container with ice in the deep-freeze cabinet at −70 °C.

The block for electron microscope studies should be fixed in 2.5% glutaraldehyde in 0.1 M phosphate buffer at pH 7.2 for 3 hours. Where delay is encountered Elias (1982) prefers to fix the whole specimen in 3% cacodylate buffered paraformaldehyde, then select blocks for EM and post-fix in 3% glutaraldehyde.

A suggested routine scheme for frozen sections is as follows:

Serial sections are cut at both 8 and 12 μm and mounted on slides.

8 μm sections

(1) Haematoxylin and eosin after air-drying and formal–saline fixation for 1 minute.
(2) Diastase–PAS after fixation in ethanol for up to 30 minutes.

■ (3) Modified Gomori trichrome (Engel and Cunningham, 1963)

Gomori's trichrome stain

Chromotrope 2R	0.6 g
Fast green FCF	0.3 g
Phosphotungstic acid	0.6 g
Glacial acetic acid	1 ml
Distilled water	100 ml

Raise the pH to 3.4 with 1 N NaOH.

Method

(1) Air-dry sections.
(2) Stain in Harris haematoxylin for 5 minutes.
(3) Rinse briefly in three changes of distilled water.
(4) Stain in Gomori's trichrome stain for 10 minutes.
(5) Differentiate in 0.2% acetic acid (seconds only).
(6) Rinse, dehydrate, clear and mount in synthetic resin.

Results

Myofibrils	Green (A bands darker than I bands)
Sarcoplasmic reticulum	Red
Sarcolemma	Red
Nuclei	Red/purple
Nemaline rods	Red

Note

Engel and Cunningham state that Type 1 fibres are distinguished from Type 2 fibres by their greater content of red intermyofibrillary material.

12 μm sections

■ **(1) ATPase with pre-incubation**

Reagents

Pre-incubation medium pH 4.6

Distilled water	11 ml
0.32 M CaCl$_2$	15 ml
0.1 M Acetate buffer pH 4.6	4 ml

Adjusted to pH 4.6 with NaOH or acetic acid.

Pre-incubation medium pH 4.3

For use adjust pre-incubation pH 4.6 medium to pH 4.3 using 0.1 N NaOH and 0.1 N acetic acid.

Pre-incubation medium pH 9.4

0.1 M Sodium barbiturate (2.062 g/100 ml)	20 ml
0.18 M CaCl$_2$ (1.998 g/100 ml)	10 ml
Distilled water	30 ml

Adjust to pH 9.4 with NaOH or acetic acid and make up to 100 ml with distilled water.

Substrate

0.1 M Sodium barbiturate (2.062 g/100 ml)	20 ml
0.18 M CaCl$_2$ (1.998 g/100 ml)	10 ml
Distilled water	30 ml

Add 152 mg of adenosine triphosphate disodium salt and as soon as ATP is dissolved adjust to pH 9.4 with 0.1 M NaOH. Then make up to 100 ml with distilled water. Filter if turbid.

Calcium chloride

0.32 M $CaCl_2 = 3.47$ g/100 ml distilled water

Sodium acetate buffer (pH 4.6)

0.1 M Sodium acetate (sodium acetate trihydrate—13.6 g/litre)	96 ml
0.1 M Acetic acid (0.6 ml glacial acetic acid/100 ml distilled water)	100 ml

Method

(1) Air-dry sections for 30 minutes (may be used after 5 hours air-drying). All incubations are carried out at 37 °C.

(2) Pre-incubate one slide at pH 9.4 for *25 minutes* and then incubate in substrate for *15 minutes*.

Pre-incubate one slide at pH 4.6 for *5 minutes* and then incubate in substrate for *30 minutes*.

Pre-incubate one slide at pH 4.3 for *3 minutes* and then incubate in substrate for *30 minutes*.

Note: The pre-incubation times should be staggered so that all slides will finish their incubation at the same time.

(3) Wash in three changes of 1% calcium chloride for *3 minutes*.

(4) Wash in distilled water.

(5) Wash in 2% cobaltous chloride for *3 minutes*.

(6) Wash in distilled water.

(7) Develop in 1% yellow ammonium sulphide for *2 minutes*.

(8) Wash well in distilled water.

(9) Dehydrate, clear and mount in synthetic resin.

Results

Black deposits indicate ATPase activity.

(2) Oil red O

After fixing in formal–calcium for up to 30 minutes.

(3) Phosphorylase

Air-dry sections (*see* page 322).

(4) NADH diaphorase

Air-dry sections (*see* Pearse's method, page 327).

Additionally, succinate dehydrogenase may be of value in the study of mitochondrial myopathies.

Table 23.1 Histochemical reactions of human muscle fibre types (after Dubowitz and Brooke, 1973)

Fibre type	1	2A	2B	2C
ATPase pH 9.4 pre-incubation	+	+ + + +	+ + + +	+ + + +
ATPase pH 4.6 pre-incubation	+ + + +	−	+ + + +	+ + + +
ATPase pH 4.3 pre-incubation	+ + + +	−	−	+ +
NADH-diaphorase	+ + + +	+ +	+	+ +
Succinate dehydrogenase (SDH)	+ + + +	+ +	+	+ +
PAS	+ + to + + +	+ + + +	+ +	+ +
Phosphorylase	− to +	+ + + +	+ + + +	+ + + +

Muscle biopsy for study of innervation

The chances of finding nerve endings in a random muscle biopsy are very slight. The probability of obtaining suitable material is increased when the biopsy is taken at the motor point which is localized with threshold electrical stimuli (Coërs, 1952).

The method of Ehrlich (1886), who perfused animals with methylene blue before removing organs of interest, has been modified for human application. The methylene blue is absorbed and converted to its colourless leuco dye. This is re-oxidized by oxygenation.

Although the effects of neuromuscular diseases may be adequately studied in most cases using the modern histochemical approach described in the previous section, the demonstration of nerve fibres and endings may still be of value.

■ Methods

Methylene blue technique for nerve fibres and endings (Coërs and Woolf, 1959)

(1) When the most excitable area has been located 0.03–0.05% methylene blue in physiological saline is injected, using a very fine needle until the muscle cannot be made bluer (10–30 ml).
   After 2 or 3 minutes a strip of the stained fasciculus is removed.
(2) Immediately after removal the strip is split longitudinally and placed on gauze moistened with isotonic saline in a Petri dish.
(3) Oxygen is passed through a filter funnel inverted over the specimens at 1 litre/minute for at least 1 hour. During this time the strips of muscle should be turned over occasionally.
   The oxygen should be bubbled through water to ensure the specimens do not dry, otherwise the specimens must be moistened at regular intervals with saline.
(4) When oxygenation is complete, the muscle is placed in filtered saturated aqueous ammonium molybdate at 4 °C for 24 hours.
(5) Wash thoroughly in three changes of distilled water to prevent subsequent crystallization of ammonium molybdate.
(6) Place in 10% formal–saline for 24 hours.
(7) Freeze and cut cryostat sections at 50 and 100 μm.

Results

Nerve fibres and endings   Blue

Notes

After step (5) squash preparations may be made.

■ **Cholinesterase method**

Strips of muscle, located as above, are removed before methylene blue injection.

Method

(1) Place a strip of muscle in physiological saline for 1 hour.
(2) Place in 10% formal–saline for 6 hours.
(3) Cut frozen sections at 50 µm and place in distilled water overnight.
(4) Perform a cholinesterase technique using acetyl thiocholine as substrate (page 319).

Other strips of muscle may be treated as follows:

(a) Fixed in buffered osmium tetroxide, and paraffin sections prepared for direct demonstration of myelin.
(b) Fixed in 10% formal–saline, after 1 hour in physiological saline, for routine paraffin processing and orthodox histological methods including Luxol fast blue for myelin.
(c) Bielschowsky techniques may be performed on frozen sections.

Cardiac biopsies

Non-surgical cardiac biopsies may be obtained by a needle biopsy technique but this has been largely replaced by right or left ventricular endomyocardial biopsy techniques during cardiac catheterization.

Indications for cardiac biopsy include monitoring of cardiac transplants and drug toxicity effects, and differentiation of cardiomyopathies from myocarditis.

The biopsy is taken by closing the jaws of the bioptome when in contact with the ventricular endomyocardium.

The techniques are described by Olsen (1978) and Fenoglio (1982). The handling of the biopsies is of crucial importance, they should not be grasped by forceps or cut. Fortunately the biopsies are usually small (2–3 mm) and at least three in number. It is best to freeze or fix each sample in its entirety. The order of precedence is: fix, for paraffin section, fix for electron microscopy and finally freeze for histochemistry or immunofluorescence, unless tissue for bacteriological or viral culture is indicated.

The samples should be fixed as soon as possible. If this is not possible in the cardiac catheter room, they should be placed on fine filter paper, moistened with isotonic saline at 4 °C in a Petri dish, for immediate delivery to the laboratory.

Ten per cent formal–saline or the 4CF-1G fixative of McDowell and Trump (1976) may be used to fix the sample for light microscopy.

4CF-1G fixative

Anhydrous sodium dihydrogen phosphate	1.16 g
Sodium hydroxide	0.27 g
Water	88 ml

40% Formaldehyde   10 ml
50% Glutaraldehyde   2 ml

This can be stored at − 20 °C in aliquots and brought to room temperature for use.

Fenoglio (1982) uses 2.5% phosphate buffered glutaraldehyde at pH 7.35 for both light and electron microscopy.

When there is sufficient material a third sample should be snap frozen as described under skeletal muscle biopsy.

The sample fixed for light microscopy is processed as appropriate and embedded in paraffin wax. The whole block should be sectioned serially and all the sections mounted on slides in groups of three or four. Groups of slides from at least three depths of the block are stained, the rest being retained for further techniques which may be indicated.

The routine stains employed are haematoxylin and eosin, elastic Van Gieson, diastase PAS and Masson trichrome. Congo-red stains for amyloid may be of value.

It is important to take serial sections, since orientation is often impossible and levels may contain only endocardium or only myocardium. The entire biopsy should be sectioned because many disease processes are focal.

The frozen sections are used for oil red O and PAS techniques, and many enzyme methods include SDH as a marker for mitochondrial activity (*Figure 23.4*) and acid phosphatase to assess lysosomal activity (Olsen, 1978).

Immunofluorescence studies may also be carried out on the frozen sections (Bolte, 1977). Techniques using FITC conjugated antisera to several viruses, on cold acetone-fixed (in ethanol/CO_2 bath) sections, may be of diagnostic value in myocarditis (Fenoglio, 1982).

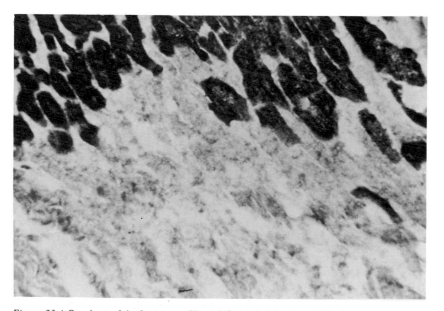

Figure 23.4 Succinate dehydrogenase. Heart infarct. Original magnification × 40

References

BOLTE, H. D. (1977). Immunologic investigation in patients with cardiomyopathies. In *Cardiomyopathy and Myocardial Biopsy*. Eds Kaltenbach, M., Loogen, F. and Olsen, E. G. J. Springer-Verlag, Heidelberg

BROOKE, M. H. and KAISER, K. K. (1970). Three 'myosin ATPase' systems: the nature of their pH lability and sulphydryl dependence. *J. Histochem. Cytochem.*, **18**, 670–672

COËRS, C. (1952). The vital staining of muscle biopsies with methylene blue. *J. Neurol. Neurosurg. Psychiat.*, **15**, 211–215

COËRS, C. and WOOLF, A. L. (1959). *The Innervation of Muscle*. Blackwell, Oxford

DUBOWITZ, V. and BROOKE, M. H. (1973). *Muscle Biopsy: A Modern Approach*. Ed. Walton, J. N. Vol. 2. Major problems in neurology. Saunders, London, Philadelphia and Toronto

EHRLICH, P. (1886). Über die Metheleneblau-reaktion der lebenden Nervensubstance. *Dtsch. Med. Wchnschr.*, **12**, 49

ELIAS, J. M. (1982). *Principles and Techniques in Diagnostic Histopathology: Developments in Immunohistochemistry and Enzyme Histochemistry*. Noyes, New Jersey

ENGEL, W. K. and CUNNINGHAM, G. C. (1963). Rapid examination of muscle tissue. An improved trichrome method for fresh-frozen biopsy specimens. *Neurology*, **13**, 919–923

FENOGLIO, J. J. (1982). *Endomyocardial Biopsy: Techniques and Applications*. CRC Press, Boca Raton, Florida

INGJER, F. (1979). Effects of endurance training on muscle fibre ATPase activity, capillary supply and mitochondrial content in man. *J. Physiol.*, **294**, 419–432

McDOWELL, E. M. and TRUMP, B. F. (1976). Histologic fixatives suitable for diagnostic light and electron microscopy. *Arch. Pathol. Lab. Med.*, **100**, 405–414

OLSEN, E. G. J. (1978). Endomyocardial biopsy. *Invest. Cell. Pathol.*, **1**, 139–157

Part VII

Cells and cell products of special interest

24

Miscellaneous cells

Paneth cells

These cells are found at the base of the glands in the small intestines—the crypts of Lieberkühn. They may also be demonstrated in the appendix and parts of the proximal colon. There is no certainty about their pathological significance, although they are known to be increased in ulcerative colitis and decreased in coeliac disease. They are involved in the metabolism of zinc and cadmium.

Fixation

Acetic acid is contraindicated, but the granules are preserved by most other fixatives including formal–saline.

Staining

The characteristic granules by which Paneth cells are demonstrated are positively stained by the p-dimethylaminobenzaldehyde-nitrate technique for tryptophan, stain blue with PTAH and are usually PAS-positive. The techniques of choice are Giemsa (page 442) by which they are stained red and the phloxine–tartrazine method.

■ Phloxine–tartrazine method (Lendrum, 1947)

Reagents

Dissolve 0.5 g phloxine in 0.5% aqueous calcium chloride.

Tartrazine-saturated solution in Cellosolve (2-ethoxyethanol).

Method

(1) Bring sections to water.
(2) Stain with Mayer's haemalum for 3 minutes.
(3) Wash in running tap-water (blue) for 10 minutes.
(4) Stain in phloxine for 15 minutes.
(5) Wash in tap-water, followed by Cellosolve.
(6) Place in tartrazine solution. This differentiates and counterstains. Examine microscopically until only red blood cells and Paneth cells are stained red.

(7) Rinse in 95% alcohol.
(8) Dehydrate, clear and mount in synthetic resin.

Results

Paneth cell granules, RBCs	Red
Nuclei	Blue
Background	Yellow

Eosinophils

In man, these cells have a bilobed nucleus and the cytoplasm contains many acidophilic granules. It is the property of these granules to stain with eosin that gives them their name. They are blood derived and migrate to the tissues via capillaries. Eosinophils are plentiful in the small intestine lamina propria, so that this forms a good control tissue for their selective demonstration. Ultrastructurally, the granules appear membrane bound, each containing at least one crystal in a granular matrix. Eosinophils are rich in the enzymes peroxidase, aryl–sulphatase, ribonuclease and cathepsin. The granules also contain the hydrolytic enzymes normally associated with lysosomes.

Eosinophils are now thought to be derived from a distinct parent cell to the neutrophil and are concerned with the immune response of allergic hypersensitivity. They are plentiful in hay fever and large numbers are also present in protozoan infections. Several mechanisms of immunological reactivity have been proposed for eosinophils, including the phagocytosis of immune complexes. They are thought to become active following the action of mast cells bearing IgE. It has recently been suggested that eosinophils act by secretion of the contents of their granules which may have a role in neutralizing mast cell products, or a direct action on protozoans.

Staining

Romanowsky-type stains are useful for differentiating eosinophils, but the method of choice for demonstration is carbol–chromotrope. Nasal polyps make good control sections.

■ **Carbol–chromotrope method for eosinophils (Lendrum, 1944)**

Reagent

Phenol crystals (melt by gentle heat, e.g. hot water)	1 g	⎫ Mix
Chromotrope 2R	0.5 g	⎬
Distilled water	100 ml	

This stain keeps for about 3 months.

Method

(1) Bring sections to water.
(2) Stain with Mayer's haemalum for 3 minutes.
(3) Wash well in tap-water (blue) for 10 minutes.
(4) Place in carbol–chromotrope solution for 30 minutes.

(5) Rinse in water.
(6) Dehydrate, clear and mount in synthetic resin.

Results

Eosinophil granules	Red
Nuclei	Blue

Prolonged staining in dilute (0.05%) aqueous eosin will also demonstrate eosinophils selectively. If overstained, the sections may be differentiated in running tap-water.

Mast cells

There is a tremendous species variation in the morphology and, especially, the staining reactivity of mast cells. Thus techniques for demonstrating mast cells in one species may give negative or even opposite results in another. Mast cells are distributed throughout the connective tissue and are similar in appearance and function to blood basophils. They are believed to be a separate cell, however.

The most striking morphological feature of mast cells is the large number of strongly metachromatic granules present in the cytoplasm. High concentrations of the sulphated mucopolysaccharide heparin are responsible for this metachromasia. Mast cells also contain the bulk of the histamine in the body, a substance which increases the permeability of blood vessels. Histamine is released in immediate type hypersensitivity, the cell degranulating when antigen and IgE antibodies become bound to the cell surface. 5-Hydroxytryptamine present in mast cells, gives a positive argentaffin reaction (Chapter 26).

Ultrastructurally, mast cells are seen to have numerous large, electron dense granules throughout the cytoplasm. The granules have a homogeneous ground substance in which whorled lamellae are seen. Although there is a well-developed Golgi complex, there is little endoplasmic reticulum and few mitochondria. The cell membrane has numerous fine projections or microvilli.

Staining

Mast cells are most commonly demonstrated by exploiting their metachromatic properties using thionin, or by using Alcian blue at low pH (Chapter 12). Depending upon their metabolic state, mast cells are often recognized in other staining procedures. For example, in the methyl green–pyronin procedure mast cells may exhibit pyroninophilia. They are readily differentiated from plasma cells on morphological features.

Plasma cells

Normal plasma cells are easily recognized in haematoxylin and eosin-stained sections. They are ovoid cells with an eccentric nucleus in a basophilic cytoplasm. The nuclear chromatin has a distinctive pattern, clumps present around the periphery giving a characteristic 'cart wheel' appearance. The cytoplasm is filled with rough endoplasmic reticulum and free ribosomes. There is a prominent Golgi present, but it is unclear what role this complex plays in plasma cell secretion. The cytoplasmic basophilia is due to the presence of large quantities of nucleoprotein, shown, by specific ribonuclease digestion, to be ribonucleic acid.

Plasma cells do not normally divide. They are derived from lymphocytes by differentiation in the connective tissue. Lymph nodes, in particular, and the lamina propria are well populated by plasma cells, the prime functions of which are to produce antibodies. At any time, a single plasma cell is concerned with the production of a single immunoglobulin only. Light and heavy chains, plus the J chain, are synthesized.

Occasionally, amorphous inclusions staining positively for glycoproteins are seen in plasma cells. These are termed Russell bodies, the inclusion presumably being composed of accumulated immunoglobulin.

Staining

Plasma cells may be demonstrated positively using the methyl green–pyronin technique, specificity being established by ribonuclease digestion. They also stain brilliantly with the fluorescent acridine orange technique. These methods are given in Chapter 10.

Specific immunoglobulins, or their component parts, may be demonstrated using immunofluorescent or immunoenzyme techniques.

In certain tumours, notably myeloma, vast amounts of immunoglobulin may be synthesized by plasma cells and this property, together with the immortality of malignant cells, has led to the development of methods for producing monoclonal antibodies. Simply, this method involves fusing malignant myeloma cells with mouse spleen derived plasma cells producing the specific antibody, culturing these hybrid cells and harvesting the immunoglobulin produced.

Corpora amylacea

This is a plural term for collections of bodies having the characteristic property of starch that they stain with iodine. They are circular or oval bodies, often with a laminar structure. Sometimes they feature calcification. Corpora amylacea is a type of hyaline degeneration, most commonly found in the central nervous system, but may also be present in prostate and lung. They are of such variable size and reactivity that they cannot be regarded as the same structures in all sites (*Table 24.1*).

Table 24.1

	Site		
	CNS	*Prostate*	*Lung*
Haematoxylin and eosin	Blue	Red	Red
PAS	Positive	Positive	Negative
Congo red	Negative	Positive	Variable
Birefringence	—	Variable dichroism	Variable dichroism

After Cook, 1974

Alcoholic hyaline (Mallory bodies)

In alcoholic hepatitis, amorphous eosinophilic aggregates may be seen within the cytoplasm of some hepatocytes. These proteinaceous bodies have a fibrillar structure when viewed by electron microscopy and may contain lysosomes and enlarged mitochondria. They stain blue with PTAH, are weakly positive with Congo red and stain with Luxol fast blue.

Juxtaglomerular cells

These cells are present in the walls of the terminal regions of the glomerular arterioles. They contain cytoplasmic granules which have a high concentration of renin. This forms part of the renin–angiotensin–aldosterone system which is of importance in the regulation of hypertension, in Addison's disease and in acute renal failure. This system is also responsible for the central stimulation of thirst.

There appears to be little significance in the demonstration of juxtaglomerular cells despite their important pathological role. The granules are not normally visible in haematoxylin and eosin-stained preparations, but they may be selectively demonstrated using Bowie's stain—a Biebrich scarlet, ethyl violet mixture.

■ **Bowie method for juxtaglomerular cell granules (1936)**

Fixation

Helly's is the fixative of choice. There is a considerable species difference in the number of granules present.

Solution

A	Biebrich scarlet	1 g
	Distilled water	250 ml
	Filter	
B	Ethyl violet	2 g
	Distilled water	500 ml
	Filter	

Add solution B to solution A slowly and with constant stirring. From time to time during the addition, place a drop of the mixture onto coarse filter paper. When no separation of colours occurs, cease adding ethyl violet. Filter and dry on filter paper. Redissolve 0.2 g of dry precipitate in 20 ml of 95% alcohol.

Method

(1) Bring sections to water.
(2) Mordant in 2.5% potassium dichromate at 40 °C overnight.
(3) Wash in tap-water then distilled water.
(4) Dilute staining solution by adding 10 to 15 drops to 100 ml of 95% alcohol. Stain at room temperature overnight.
(5) Drain and blot carefully.
(6) Dip in two changes of acetone.
(7) Differentiate in equal parts xylene/clove oil.
(8) Clear and mount in synthetic resin.

Results

Juxtaglomerular cell granules	Purple-blue
Elastin	Purple-blue
Background tissue	Red

Juxtaglomerular cell granules also fluoresce brilliantly when stained with thioflavine T (Chapter 25).

References

BOWIE, D. J. (1936). Method for staining pepsinogen granules in gastric glands. *Anat. Rec.*, **64**, 357–367

COOK, H. C. (1974). *Manual of Histological Demonstration Techniques*. Butterworths, London

LENDRUM, A. C. (1944). The staining of eosinophil polymorphs and enterochromaffin cells in histological sections. *J. Pathol. Bacteriol.*, **56**, 441

LENDRUM, A. C. (1947). The phloxine–tartrazine method as a general histological stain and for the demonstration of inclusion bodies. *J. Pathol. Bacteriol.*, **59**, 399–404

25

Amyloid and fibrin

Amyloid

Amyloid is an extracellular, amorphous, eosinophilic material most commonly arising as a consequence of chronic inflammatory disease of long standing. Spleen, liver, kidneys, adrenals, lymph nodes and pancreas are the organs usually affected. Traditionally, amyloid of this type was referred to as secondary or typical. Primary, or atypical amyloid is usually found in muscle and the cardiovascular system, but may be more conveniently diagnosed in rectal, skin or gingival biopsies. It arises in the absence of any obvious predisposing inflammatory disease.

Experimental amyloidosis has been successfully induced in animals using techniques which abnormally stimulate the protein synthesizing mechanism and reticulo-endothelial system. Recent work, reviewed by Glenner (1980a and b) and by Cohen *et al.* (1983) confirms amyloid to be composed of β-pleated sheet fibrils derived from protein, including immunoglobulin, together with a carbohydrate component. The protein content, together with the site of deposition, forms the basis of the modern classification of amyloid, a simplified version of which is shown in *Table 25.1*.

The variable protein and carbohydrate content of amyloid most probably accounts for the variable staining properties and the difficulties of making a positive identification. Whilst the demonstration of the typical fibrillar ultrastructure of amyloid by electron microscopy (*Figure 25.1*) or X-ray diffraction of the cross β-pleat structure are undoubtedly the most reliable means of identification, positive staining with Congo red together with a resultant green polarization colour is generally considered the most specific method available to the light microscopist.

Demonstration

Amyloid stains a homogeneous pale pink colour with haematoxylin and eosin and yellow to yellow/brown with Van Gieson. In fresh tissue treated with iodine (Gram's or Lugol's), amyloid stains mahogany brown, turning to blue on treatment with 10% sulphuric acid. Gottschalk (1960) has shown that the carbohydrate component contains sialic acid, which presumably accounts for the positive staining, though weak, with both Alcian blue and PAS. The DMAB–nitrite method stains most amyloid because of its tryptophan content. However, it is unreliable for diagnostic purposes as it is non-specific and unreactive with non-tryptophan containing amyloid such as endocrine type (AE) (Pearse, Ewen and Polak, 1972). It should be noted also that amyloid may be demonstrated by silver impregnation.

Table 25.1 Classification of amyloidosis

Process	Type	Designation
Acquired systemic	Primary	AL
	Secondary	AA
	Familial	AF
Organ limited	Senile	AS
Localized	Endocrine	AE

The designation AL is derived from amyloid-light chain, AA from amyloid A-protein, the others
from the type.

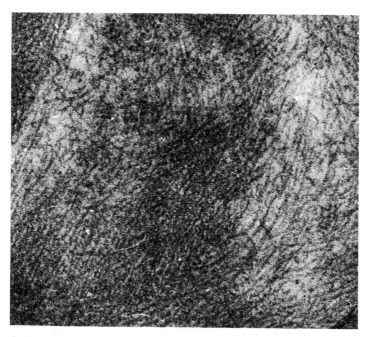

Figure 25.1 The fibrillar ultrastructure of amyloid deposits in kidney as seen by electron microscopy.
Note the discrete interlacing fibrils which are characteristic ($\times$ 120 000) (reproduced by courtesy of
Dr W. H. Chase)

Metachromatic methods

Staining with 1% aqueous methyl violet for 5 minutes, followed by differentiation with
1% acetic acid gives quite good results. Sections should be mounted in aqueous media
of high sugar or salt content to prevent diffusion of the stain. The following method
gives preparations which are stable for a number of years.

■ Lendrum's technique

Method

(1) Bring sections to water.
(2) Stain in 1% aqueous methyl violet (or 1% aqueous dahlia) for 3 minutes.

(3) Differentiate in 70% formalin (controlling microscopically).
(4) Wash in running water for 1 minute.
(5) Flood with saturated aqueous sodium chloride for 5 minutes.
(6) Rinse in water and mount in corn syrup.

Results

Amyloid   Pink to red
Other elements   Violet

Congo red methods

The specificity of methods of this type are dependent on the β-pleated sheet configuration of amyloid and the linearity of the dye molecules.

Amyloid stained with Congo red is dichroic and shows a green polarization colour. One of the rays transmitted has its green component absorbed. On recombination in the analyser, interference takes place between the two rays. Wolman and Bubis (1965) showed that the characteristic green polarization colour was not present in very thin or very thick sections and that a thickness of 5–10 μm was optimal. This thickness is necessary to produce a phase difference of half a wavelength of red light, allowing destructive interference of the red component of the white ray; resulting in the characteristic green colour.

Sirius red, with properties similar to Congo red, has proved a popular alternative dye. Toluidine blue methods are thought to depend on the same principle and not on the carbohydrate component (Cooper, 1974).

In tissue sections containing amyloid AA protein, affinity for Congo red is lost after pretreatment with potassium permanganate (Wright, Calkins and Humphrey, 1977).

■ **Bennhold's technique (1922)**

Method

(1) Bring sections to water.
(2) Stain with Ehrlich's haematoxylin for 20 minutes.
(3) Differentiate with 1% acid alcohol.
(4) Wash in running water for 1 minute to remove the acid (sections will blue in the lithium carbonate used in stage (6)).
(5) Stain with 1% aqueous Congo red for 20–30 minutes.
(6) Pour off stain and flood slide with a saturated aqueous solution of lithium carbonate; leave for 15 seconds.
(7) Differentiate in 80% alcohol until excess Congo red is removed.
(8) Wash in running water for 10 minutes.
(9) Dehydrate, clear and mount in Canada balsam or synthetic resin.

Results

Amyloid   Pink to red
Nuclei   Blue

■ **Alkaline Congo red technique (Puchtler, Sweat and Levine, 1962)**

This method has the advantage of not requiring differentiation. This is probably because the Congo red is in alkaline solution; since aqueous alkaline solutions causes sections to become detached from slides it is employed in an alcoholic solution. The addition of sodium chloride gives more intense staining.

Fixation

The best results are obtained after alcohol or Carnoy fixed tissues; however, formalin or Zenker-fixed tissues were found to stain better than with other techniques.

Reagents

(1) Alkaline salt solution. To 50 ml of 80% alcohol saturated with sodium chloride add 0.5 ml of 1% aqueous sodium hydroxide. Filter and use within 15 minutes.
(2) Stock stain solution. Use 80% alcohol saturated with Congo red and sodium chloride.
(3) Staining solution. Add 0.5 ml of 1% aqueous sodium hydroxide to 50 ml of stock stain, filter and use within 15 minutes.

Method

(1) Bring sections to water.
(2) Stain in haematoxylin for 5 minutes.
(3) Rinse well in distilled water.
(4) Pretreat in alkaline alcohol–salt solution for 20 minutes.
(5) Stain in alkaline Congo red solution for 20 minutes.
(6) Dehydrate rapidly in three changes of absolute alcohol.
(7) Clear and mount in synthetic resin.

Results

Amyloid   Deep pink to red
Nuclei   Blue
Elastic tissue Pale pink

Toluidine blue method

■ **Standard toluidine blue (Wolman, 1971)**

Method

(1) Bring sections to water.
(2) Stain in 1% toluidine blue in 50% isopropanol for 30 minutes at 37 °C.
(3) Blot and place in absolute isopropanol for 1 minute.
(4) Clear in xylene and mount.

Results

Amyloid is distinguished by its dark red polarization colour.

Fluorescence techniques

The thioflavine T technique was developed following research on a range of fluorescent dyes under varying conditions (Vassar and Culling, 1959). It is an extremely sensitive technique although not specific. Attempts have been made to increase the specificity of the method by using acid solutions (Burns, Pennock and Stoward, 1967) and by including magnesium chloride (Mowry and Scott, 1967). Thioflavine S may be substituted for thioflavine T (Schwartz, 1970).

■ Thioflavine T method (Vassar and Culling, 1959)

Method

(1) Bring sections to water.
(2) Stain in alum–haematoxylin for 2 minutes to quench nuclear fluorescence. The haematoxylin does not need to be differentiated, or blued.
(3) Wash in water for a few minutes.
(4) Stain in 1% aqueous thioflavine T for 3 minutes.
(5) Rinse in water.
(6) Differentiate in 1% acetic acid for 20 minutes.
(7) Wash in water.
(8) Mount in Apathy's medium.

Results

Amyloid and mast cells fluoresce bright yellow when examined using a BG12 exciter filter and an OG4 or OG5 barrier filter. The finest deposits can be seen using a UG1 or UG2 exciter filter with a colourless ultraviolet barrier filter.

Alcian blue method

The technique introduced by Lendrum, Slidders and Fraser (1972) was derived from the critical electrolyte concept of Scott and his co-workers (*see* page 239) and is compatible with a range of counterstains.

Fixation in formal–saline is usually adequate.

■ The sodium sulphate–Alcian blue (SAB) method

Reagents

Acetic alcohol

95% Ethanol	45 ml
Distilled water	45 ml
Glacial acetic acid	10 ml

Prepare fresh for use.

SAB solution

1% Alcian blue in 95% ethanol	45 ml
1% Aqueous sodium sulphate decahydrate	45 ml
Glacial acetic acid	10 ml

Prepare from stock solutions and stand for 30 minutes before use.

Method

(1) Bring sections to water.
(2) Immerse in acetic alcohol for 1–2 minutes.
(3) Stain in SAB working solution for 2 hours.
(4) Transfer to acetic alcohol for 1–2 minutes.
(5) Wash in water.
(6) Alkalinize in 80% ethanol saturated with borax for 30 minutes.
(7) Wash in water.
(8) Stain nuclei with Celestine blue–haemalum sequence and counterstain with Van Gieson.
(9) Dehydrate, clear and mount.

Results

Amyloid, mast cells and some colloids   Green

Fibrin

Fibrin is derived from the fibrinogen of blood plasma, being precipitated initially as fine fibres in an irregular network. It is found in acute inflammatory processes where there is a transudation of plasma from vessels.

The term fibrinoid has been used to describe various hyalin materials giving similar staining reactions to fibrin. Lendrum, Slidders and Fraser (1972) believe that much of such hyalin material is fibrin which has undergone an ageing process and will eventually end with staining properties similar to collagen (pseudocollagen). Hyalin material which has similar staining characteristics to fibrin but which can be proved immunologically not to be derived from fibrin might be described as fibrinoid.

Fibrin is eosinophilic, weakly PAS-positive, yellow with Van Gieson and red with phloxine–tartrazine.

Fibrin may be demonstrated in sections by Mallory's phosphotungstic acid haematoxylin, Weigert's modification of Gram's stain or by one of the trichrome methods. The most specific method of demonstration is by immunofluorescence using an FITC conjugated anti-human fibrinogen serum.

■ Weigert's stain for fibrin

Method

(1) Bring sections to water.
(2) Stain with 2.5% aqueous eosin at 56 °C for 10 minutes.
(3) Wash in water.
(4) Stain in 1% aqueous methyl violet for 3 minutes.
(5) Rinse in water, and treat with Lugol's iodine for 3 minutes.
(6) Blot dry with fine, fluffless filter paper.
(7) Differentiate with aniline oil and xylene (equal parts) until only the fibrin network is stained violet.
(8) Rinse well with xylene to remove aniline oil.
(9) Rinse in fresh xylene and mount in resinous medium.

Results

Fibrin, Gram-positive bacteria, hyalin degeneration   Blue-black
Other tissue constituents   Red

For routine use the most reliable methods are those developed by Lendrum *et al.* (1962). Best results are obtained after mercuric chloride fixation. Sections of tissue fixed in formal–saline should be de-waxed and rinsed with trichlorethylene for 48 hours (degreasing). After rinsing in alcohol sections are placed overnight in 3% mercuric chloride in saturated alcoholic picric acid. The MSB method stains fibrin red in material that is blue with picro–Mallory V. Older fibrin stained blue with MSB may still give a positive result for fibrin with the Masson 44/41 method. For general use the MSB method is recommended.

■ MSB method

(1) Bring sections to water.
(2) Stain nuclei with Celestine blue–haemalum sequence.
(3) Wash in running water.
(4) Rinse in 95% alcohol.
(5) Stain in 0.5% Martius yellow in 95% alcohol containing 2% phosphotungstic acid for 2 minutes.
(6) Rinse in distilled water.
(7) Stain in 1% brilliant crystal scarlet 6R (Ponceau 6R) in 2.5% acetic acid for 10 minutes.
(8) Rinse in distilled water.
(9) Treat with 1% aqueous phosphotungstic acid for up to 5 minutes. This fixes and differentiates the crystal scarlet staining.
(10) Rinse in distilled water.
(11) Stain in 0.5% soluble blue in 1% acetic acid for up to 10 minutes.
(12) Rinse in 1% acetic acid, blot, dehydrate in absolute alcohol, clear in xylene and mount in synthetic resin.

Results

Nuclei   Blue-black
Fibrin   Red
Erythrocytes   Yellow
Connective tissue   Blue

■ Picro–Mallory V method

Reagents

Yellow mordant

Orange G   0.4 g
Lissamine fast yellow 2G   0.4 g
80% Ethanol saturated with picric acid   200 ml

Differentiator

Yellow mordant   30 ml
80% Alcohol   70 ml

Method

(1) Bring sections to water and stain nuclei with Celestine blue–haemalum sequence.
(2) Stain in yellow mordant for 3–5 minutes.
(3) Wash in water for 1 minute.
(4) Stain in 1% acid fuchsin in 1% acetic acid for 5 minutes.
(5) Rinse in tap-water.
(6) Differentiate for 10–15 seconds.
(7) Rinse in tap-water.
(8) Treat with 1% aqueous phosphotungstic acid for 5 minutes.
(9) Rinse in tap-water.
(10) Stain with 1% soluble blue for 2 minutes.
(11) Rinse, dehydrate rapidly, clear and mount.

Results

Nuclei	Blue-black
Fibrin	Red
Erythrocytes	Yellow
Connective tissue	Blue

■ **Masson 44/41 method**

Method

As MSB except omit steps (4)–(6) and substitute, at step (11), 1% naphthalene blue black CS in 1% aqueous acetic acid for 30 minutes.

Results

Older fibrin is stained black, fresh fibrin red with intermediate stages.

■ **The fuchsin–Miller method (Slidders, 1961)**

This popular method is based on a combination of the principles of the Masson, and the phloxine–tartrazine method (Lendrum, 1939). Best results are obtained after mercuric chloride fixation and degreasing.

Method

(1) Bring sections to water and stain nuclei with Celestine blue–haemalum sequence.
(2) Differentiate in 0.25% hydrochloric acid in 70% alcohol. Wash.
(3) Stain with 1% acid fuchsin in 2.5% acetic acid for 10 minutes.
(4) Rinse.
(5) Treat with 1% aqueous phosphotungstic acid for 5 minutes.
(6) Rinse with distilled water, blot and rinse thoroughly with Cellosolve.
(7) Differentiate in a closed jar of 2.5% milling yellow 3G in Cellosolve. This reagent must be free from contaminants. Differentiation takes from ½–4 hours.
(8) Rinse in Cellosolve, clear in xylene and mount.

Results

Fibrin	Red
Nuclei	Black
Other tissues	Yellow

References

BENNHOLD, H. (1922). Einer spezifische Amyloid-Färbung met Kongorot. *Munch. Med. Wchnschr.*, **69**, 1537

BURNS, J., PENNOCK, C. A. and STOWARD, P. J. (1967). The specificity of staining amyloid deposits with thioflavine T. *J. Pathol. Bacteriol.*, **94**, 337–344

COHEN, A. S., SHIRAHAMA, T., SIPE, J. D. and SKINNER, M. (1983). Amyloid proteins, precursors, mediator and enhancer. *Lab. Invest.*, **48** (1), 1–4

COOPER, J. H. (1974). Selective amyloid staining as a function of amyloid composition and structure. *Lab. Invest.*, **31**, 232–238

GLENNER, G. G. (1980a). Amyloid deposits and amyloidosis. The β-fibrilloses (first of two parts). *New Engl. J. Med.*, June 5th, 1283–1292

GLENNER, G. G. (1980b). Amyloid deposits and amyloidosis. The β-fibrilloses (second of two parts). *New Engl. J. Med.*, June 12th, 1333–1343

GOTTSHALK, A. (1960). *Chemistry and Biology of Sialic Acids*, Cambridge University Press, Cambridge

LENDRUM, A. C. (1939). A new trichromic staining method. *J. Pathol. Bacteriol.*, **49**, 590–592

LENDRUM, A. C., FRASER, D. S., SLIDDERS, W. and HENDERSON, R. (1962). Studies on the character and staining of fibrin. *J. Clin. Pathol.*, **15**, 401–413

LENDRUM, A. C., SLIDDERS, W. and FRASER, D. S. (1972). Renal hyalin: a study of amyloidosis and diabetic fibrinous vasculosis with new staining methods. *J. Clin. Pathol.*, **25**, 373–396

MOWRY, R. W. and SCOTT, J. E. (1967). Observations on the basophilia of amyloids. *Histochemie*, **10**, 8–32

PEARSE, A. G. E., EWEN, S. W. B. and POLAK, J. M. (1972). The genesis of apudamyloid in endocrine polypeptide tumours: histochemical distinction from immunoamyloid. *Virchows Archiv B Zellpathologie*, **10**, 93–107

PUCHTLER, H., SWEAT, F. and LEVINE, M. (1962). On the binding of Congo red by amyloid. *J. Histochem. Cytochem.*, **10**, 355–364

SCHWARTZ, P. (1970). *Amyloidosis*. C. C. Thomas, Illinois

SLIDDERS, W. (1961), The fuchsin–Miller method. *J. Med. Lab. Technol.*, **18** (1), 36–37

VASSAR, P. S. and CULLING, C. F. A. (1959). Fluorescent stains with special reference to amyloid and connective tissues. *Arch. Pathol.*, **68**, 487–498

WOLMAN, M. (1971). Amyloid: its nature and molecular structure: comparison of a new toluidine blue polarised light method with traditional procedures. *Lab. Invest.*, **25**, 104–110

WOLMAN, M. and BUBIS, J. J. (1965). The cause of the green polarisation colour of amyloid stained with Congo red. *Histochemie*, **4**, 351–356

WRIGHT, J. R., CALKINS, E. and HUMPHREY, R. L. (1977). Potassium permanganate reaction in amyloidosis. *Lab. Invest.*, **36**, 274–281

26

Endocrine cells

Introduction

The classical endocrine system consists of several ductless glands, composed of compact masses of cells secreting hormones directly into the blood stream to act at a distant site. Included in this group of glands were pituitary, pineal, thyroid, parathyroid, pancreatic islets, adrenal, ovary and testis, secreting mainly peptide and steroid hormones.

Feyrter's discovery of 'clear cells' in several organs led to the concept of a diffuse endocrine system (1938) in which the secretions performed a local function. Pearse (1969) introduced the concept of the APUD system (amine and amine precursor uptake and decarboxylation) consisting of polypeptide secreting endocrine cells. Active peptides have been identified in the central and peripheral nervous systems and along with the diffuse endocrine system have now been unified into a single system—the diffuse neuroendocrine system (DNES) (Polak and Bloom, 1979). The enzyme, neuron-specific enolase, has been found in all components of the DNES lending support to the unified system and providing an immunocytochemical marker for the demonstration of component cells. The products of the cells of the DNES include short-chain polypeptides or amines or, predominantly, both. They are either released directly into the blood stream (endocrine) or released locally to act on neighbouring cells (paracrine). When released from nerve terminals they may act as neurotransmitters or neuromodulators.

Peptides are stored in neurosecretory granules which are usually concentrated in the basal part of the cell cytoplasm, being released from the basal areas of the cell membrane. The granules have characteristic ultrastructural appearances which have been used in the classification of the gastroenteropancreatic neuroendocrine cells by Solcia and others (1973).

Pearse (1972) divides the DNES into two divisions, the central and the peripheral. The central division includes cells found in the pineal, hypothalamus and pituitary. A much simplified list of the commoner cells of the DNES peripheral division along with their products is given in *Table 26.1*. A comprehensive list is given by Pearse and Takor (1979).

Table 26.1 Cells of the peripheral diffuse neuroendocrine system

Tissue	Cell type	Peptide	Amine
Pancreatic islets	A (α_2)	Glucagon	5-HT
	B (β)	Insulin	5-HT
	D (α_1)	Somatostatin	Dopamine
Stomach	G	Gastrin	—
	EC$_1$	Substance P	5-HT
Intestine	EC$_1$	Substance P	5-HT
	EC$_2$	Motilin	—
	H	VIP	—
	I	Cholecystokinin	—
Lung	K	Bombesin	—
Parathyroid	Chief	Parathryn	—
Thyroid	C	Calcitonin	—
Adrenal medulla	E	—	Adrenaline
	NE	—	Noradrenaline
Sympathetic	Ganglion	VIP	Noradrenaline
Skin	Melanoblast/melanocyte	—	Promelanin

VIP = Vasoactive intestinal polypeptide.
5-HT = 5-Hydroxytryptamine.

Demonstration

Methods for cells of the DNES (diffuse neuroendocrine system)

The cells of the diffuse neuroendocrine system can be demonstrated by the following:

(1) silver techniques;
(2) dye staining and histochemical reactions;
(3) fluorescent techniques;
(4) immunocytochemistry.

Silver techniques

Formaldehyde or Bouin's fluid should be used as fixatives. Alcohol should be avoided and frozen sections are not applicable since aldehyde condensation is necessary for the reaction.

Argentaffin reactions take place when the silver attaches to tissue components and is reduced to metallic silver.

Argyrophil reactions occur when the silver is attached to the tissue component but requires an external reducer for subsequent reduction.

The reactions for argentaffin cells are mainly modifications of the Masson method whilst those for argyrophil cells are derived from the Davenport, Bielschowsky and Bodian techniques.

■ Singh's modification of the Masson–Hamperl argentaffin reaction (1964)

Fixation

Formalin, Bouin or glutaraldehyde may be used but 10% formalin for at least 24 hours is recommended.

Silver solution

To 10% aqueous silver nitrate add strong ammonia drop by drop until the precipitate first-formed redissolves. Add 10% silver nitrate drop by drop until a slight opalescence persists. Dilute with nine volumes of distilled water.

Method

(1) Bring sections to water and wash in several changes of distilled water.
(2) Immerse for 15–30 minutes (until light brown) in the silver solution (preheated) at 60 °C in the dark.
(3) Wash in distilled water.
(4) Treat with 1% sodium thiosulphate for 30 seconds.
(5) If desired, counterstain with neutral red.
(6) Wash, dehydrate, clear and mount in resinous mountant.

Results

Argentaffin cells   Black

Note

Normally EC_1 and EC_2 cells are impregnated along with melanin and some lipofuscin. If glutaraldehyde is used as the fixative dopamine and noradrenaline granules are also impregnated.

■ Grimelius argyrophil reaction (1968)

Fixation

Formalin, formaldehyde–glutaraldehyde or Bouin's fluid. Grimelius recommended Bouin with reduced acetic acid.

Silver solution

1% Silver nitrate in distilled water	4 ml
0.2 M Acetate buffer at pH 5.6	10 ml
Distilled water	86 ml

Reducer

Hydroquinone	1 g
Sodium sulphate	5 g
Distilled water	100 ml

Method

(1) Bring paraffin sections to water and wash in distilled water.
(2) Immerse in preheated freshly prepared silver solution at 58–60 °C for 3 hours.
(3) Remove slides and drain.
(4) Without washing, place in preheated reducer at 40–45 °C for 1 minute.
(5) Wash, dehydrate, clear and mount in resinous mountant.

Results

Most DNES cells are positive *except* B and D cells of pancreatic islets and I cells of upper small intestine.

Notes

Counterstaining is not recommended. A weak reaction can be improved by re-impregnation in fresh silver solution for 15 minutes at room temperature followed by fresh reducing solution for 1 minute at 55 °C. Clean glassware rather than plastic should be used.

■ Hellerström and Hellman's argyrophil reaction (1960)

Fixation

Formalin or Bouin's fluid.

Silver solution

Silver nitrate   10 g
Distilled water   10 ml
95% Ethanol   90 ml

Adjust to pH 5–5.2 with dilute ammonia.

Reducing solution

Pyrogallic acid   5 g
95% Ethanol   95 ml
40% Formaldehyde   5 ml

Method

(1) Bring paraffin sections to water and wash for 1 hour.
(2) Treat with 95% ethanol.
(3) Place in silver solution at 37 °C in the dark overnight.
(4) Rinse rapidly in 95% ethanol (less than 10 seconds).
(5) Reduce for 1 minute.
(6) Rinse in three changes of 95% ethanol for 1 minute each.
(7) Rinse in absolute ethanol.
(8) Mount in resinous mountant.

Results

Granules of D (α_1) cell of pancreatic islets   Brown-black
A and B cells are negative

Notes

Counterstaining is not recommended. Use 100 ml of silver solution for no more than five or six slides.

■ **Sevier–Munger argyrophil reaction (1965)**

Fixation

Formalin or Bouin's fluid.

Silver solution

To 50 ml of 10% silver nitrate add strong ammonia drop by drop until the dark brown precipitate which forms has almost disappeared. Complete clearing should be avoided. Add 0.5 ml of sodium carbonate (8 g of $Na_2CO_3 . 10 H_2O$ dissolved in 30 ml of distilled water). Shake well. Add 25 drops of strong ammonia. Shake well and filter. (The solution should be crystal clear.)

Method

(1) Bring paraffin sections to water and wash in distilled water.
(2) Place in prewarmed 20% silver nitrate at 60 °C for 15 minutes.
(3) Wash slides through two Coplin jars of distilled water.
(4) Drain off excess water and place in a dry Coplin jar.
(5) To the ammoniacal silver solution add 10 drops of 2% formalin (2 ml 40% formaldehyde/98 ml water), shaking gently. Pour quickly over the slides in the Coplin jar. Develop for up to 30 minutes (3–10 minutes are usually sufficient).
(6) Wash well in three jars of fresh tap-water.
(7) Treat with 5% sodium thiosulphate for 2 minutes.
(8) Wash in water.
(9) Dehydrate, clear and mount in resinous mountant.

Results

Most DNES cells are positive, results are almost the same as with the Grimelius method (Grimelius and Wilander, 1980).

Notes

Counterstaining is not necessary. Celloidin treatment of sections may be necessary to avoid precipitation of silver on the section.

Dye staining and histochemical reactions

■ **Aldehyde–fuchsin (Halmi, 1952)**

Fixation

Ten per cent formal–saline or Bouin's fluid.

Stains

Aldehyde–fuchsin

Basic fuchsin	0.5 g
70% Ethanol	100 ml
Concentrated hydrochloric acid	1 ml
Paraldehyde	1 ml

Dissolve the dye in the alcohol, then add the acid and the paraldehyde. Leave at room temperature for 2–3 days. Store at 4 °C.

Counterstain

Light green	0.2 g
Orange G	1 g
Phosphotungstic acid	0.5 g
Glacial acetic acid	1 ml
Distilled water	100 ml

Method

(1) Bring paraffin sections to water.
(2) Oxidize with Lugol's iodine for 10 minutes.
(3) Rinse in tap-water.
(4) Bleach with 2.5% sodium thiosulphate.
(5) Wash in tap-water and 70% ethanol.
(6) Stain in aldehyde–fuchsin for 15–30 minutes.
(7) Wash in 95% ethanol.
(8) Wash in water.
(9) Stain nuclei with Celestine blue and haemalum.
(10) Wash in water.
(11) Differentiate briefly in acid alcohol.
(12) Wash in water and rinse in distilled water.
(13) Counterstain in light green–orange G solution for 45 seconds.
(14) Rinse briefly with 0.2% acetic acid.
(15) Rinse in 95% ethanol.
(16) Dehydrate, clear and mount in synthetic resin.

Results

Pancreatic islet cells	A	Yellow
	B	Purple-violet
	D	Green

■ Lead haematoxylin (Solcia, Capella and Vassallo, 1969)

Lead haematoxylin probably acts as a basic dye, combining with side chain carboxyl and carboxyamide groups of polypeptides.

Fixation

Formaldehyde or glutaraldehyde.

Reagent

Stabilized lead solution

5% Lead nitrate (aqueous)	100 ml
Saturated aqueous ammonium acetate	100 ml

Mix and filter then add 4 ml of 40% formaldehyde.

Lead haematoxylin solution

Mix 0.2 g haematoxylin dissolved in 1.5 ml 95% ethanol with 10 ml of stabilized lead solution. Add, with stirring, 10 ml of distilled water. Stand for 30 minutes, filter and make up to 75 ml.

Method

(1) Bring paraffin sections to water.
(2) Stain in freshly prepared lead haematoxylin for 2–3 hours at 37 °C or for 1–2 hours at 45 °C.
(3) Wash in distilled water.
(4) Dehydrate, clear and mount in synthetic resin.

Results

Endocrine cells   Blue-black

Notes

Glutaraldehyde or Helly fixed tissue require longer staining times. Acid hydrolysis may increase the depth of staining.

■ Masked basophilia (Solcia, Vassallo and Capella, 1968)

Basic dyes react with anionic carboxyl groups of polypeptides. The reaction is intensified with prior acid hydrolysis by unmasking further carboxyl groups and removing nucleotide phosphate groups which would also react. Metachromatic basic dyes may be used, the reaction being described as masked metachromasia.

Fixation

Formalin or Bouin's fluid are preferred.

Reagent

0.01% Toluidine blue in distilled water
    Buffer to pH 5 with 0.02 M McIlvaine's buffer.

Method

(1) Bring paraffin sections to water.
(2) Hydrolyse in 0.2 M HCl for 3–4 hours at 60 °C.
(3) Wash in water.

(4) Stain for 6 hours.
(5) Wash in water and blot dry.
(6) Treat with absolute isopropanol for 1 minute.
(7) Clear and mount in synthetic resin.

Results

Reacting neurosecretory granules   Blue-red

Notes

Azure A or Alcian blue may be substituted for toluidine blue.

■ Diazo method for 5-hydroxytryptamine (Gomori, 1952)

When aldehyde condenses with 5-HT a β-carboline is formed. This can couple with a diazonium salt to produce a coloured product.

Fixation

Formalin.

Reagent

1% Aqueous fast red salt B	5 ml
Saturated aqueous lithium carbonate	2 ml

Cool the stock solutions to 4 °C and use immediately after mixing.

Method

(1) Bring paraffin sections to water.
(2) Treat with fast red salt B for 1 minute.
(3) Wash in water.
(4) Counterstain lightly with haemalum.
(5) Wash, dehydrate, clear and mount in synthetic resin.

Results

Enterochromaffin granules   Orange-red

■ Schmorl's ferric ferricyanide reaction

This demonstrates enterochromaffin cells and the chromaffin reaction, in addition, demonstrates adrenaline and noradrenaline. These techniques are detailed in Chapter 14.

Fluorescent techniques

Primary and secondary catecholamines condense with formaldehyde to form dihydroisoquinolines. Indoleamines similarly condense with formaldehyde to form β-

carbolines. The reaction products are fluorescent having excitation maxima of 380–410 nm and emission maxima of 470–540 nm. The excitation and emission maxima for a range of amines is given by Pearse (1972).

The formaldehyde induced fluorescence (FIF) technique of Eranko (1955) using water phase reactions was largely replaced by gas phase reactions introduced by Falck *et al.* (1962). It is essential to ensure that the correct degree of humidity is present, too much water vapour causing diffusion of the amine, too little producing poor condensation. In the method of Falck and Owman (1965), for freeze-dried material, the block is exposed in a 1 litre container to 5 g of paraformaldehyde (equilibrated over sulphuric acid at a relative humidity of 50–70%, 500 g/litre H_2SO_4, for 10 days) at 60–80 °C for 1–3 hours. The blocks are vacuum embedded in paraffin wax (Pearse, 1972).

There have been many developments to simplify the procedure by using cryostat sections (Watson and Ellison, 1976), and vibrotome sections (Hokfelt and Ljungdahl, 1972). Water phase reactions have been developed which prevent diffusion of the amine and give more sensitive visualization, using formaldehyde/glutaraldehyde (Faglu) mixtures (Furness, Costa and Wilson, 1977; Furness, Heath and Costa, 1978), glyoxylic acid (GA) (Lindvall and Björklund, 1974) and sucrose–potassium phosphate–glyoxylic acid (SPG) mixture (de la Torre and Surgeon, 1976). Incorporation of high concentrations of magnesium ions is claimed to give enhanced fluorescence (Lorén, Björklund and Lindvall, 1977). Exposure of tissue to aluminium ions prior to or concomitant with formaldehyde treatment has also been reported to give enhanced fluorescence (ALFA) (Lorén *et al.*, 1980).

Immunocytochemistry

The immunocytochemical identification of the cells of the DNES has been approached in three ways using antibodies to:

(1) peptides,
(2) amines,
(3) enzymes.

Peptides

A wide variety of antibodies have been prepared to peptide hormones, many of which are available commercially.

Many peptide hormones are stable to formalin fixation allowing retrospective studies to be performed. Variants of Bouin's fluid are also much used. Since many peptides are water-soluble, cross-linking agents have been introduced as fixing agents, for example, *p*-benzoquinone or diethylpyrocarbonate (Pearse, 1980). Great care should be taken with glutaraldehyde since anything other than short exposure will render the peptide antigenically inactive. Chromate fixatives should be avoided.

Amines

Antibodies to noradrenaline, adrenaline and 5-HT have been prepared by Steinbusch, Verhofstad and Joosten (1978) using hapten techniques. A review of this approach by Verhofstad *et al.* (1983) is recommended to the reader.

Enzymes

Antibodies to synthesizing enzymes have been used in the study of the DNES. The enzymes may be widespread, as in the case of neuron-specific enolase, when antibodies can be used for general identification. The enzymes may be specific to the synthesis of particular amines, for example, antibodies to dopamine β-hydroxylase may be used to identify cells capable of synthesizing noradrenaline or adrenaline (Fuxe *et al.*, 1970).

The methods used are standard immunocytochemical methods using antibodies, labelled with fluorochromes or enzymes (*see* Chapters 26 and 27). Great attention must be paid to preparation of tissues and adequate controls must be used. Technical details of antibody purification and conjugation are given by Pearse (1980) and Sternberger (1979).

Methods for cells of the anterior pituitary

Although cells of the anterior pituitary are strictly part of the DNES, they have traditionally been classified separately. For convenience, they are treated separately here.

Three types of cells can be recognized in a haematoxylin and eosin-stained section, acidophils, basophils and chromophobes. The PAS–orange G and OFG methods make a more definite differentiation. Using the performic acid–Alcian blue–PAS–orange G technique the basophils can be further divided into R and S types.

The hormones associated with pituitary cells are:

Acidophils   Prolactin (LTH), Growth Hormone (STH)
Basophil-R   TSH, LH, FSH
Basophil-S   ACTH, MSH
Chromophobe None

■ PAS–orange G (Pearse, 1953)

Fixation is not critical and all types of sections may be used.

Method

(1) Bring sections to water.
(2) Perform the standard PAS haematoxylin sequence.
(3) Stain in 2% orange G in 5% phosphotungstic acid for 20 seconds.
(4) Differentiate in tap-water until only acidophils and RBCs are yellow.
(5) Dehydrate, clear and mount in synthetic resin.

Results

Basophils   Magenta
Acidophils   Orange
Chromophobes   Pale blue-grey

■ Orange–fuchsin–green (OFG) (Slidders, 1961)

Fixation is not critical but the author preferred mercuric chloride fixation.

Method

(1) Bring paraffin sections to water.
(2) Stain nuclei with Celestine blue–haemalum.
(3) Differentiate in acid alcohol.
(4) Wash in running water.
(5) Rinse in 95% ethanol.
(6) Stain in saturated orange G in 95% ethanol containing 2% phosphotungstic acid.
(7) Rinse in distilled water.
(8) Stain in 0.5% acid fuchsin in 0.5% aqueous acetic acid until the basophils are prominent.
(9) Rinse in distilled water.
(10) Treat with 1% aqueous phosphotungstic acid for 5 minutes.
(11) Rinse in distilled water.
(12) Stain in 1.5% light green in 1.5% aqueous acetic acid for 1 minute.
(13) Rinse in distilled water.
(14) Dehydrate, clear and mount in synthetic resin.

Results

Acidophils	Orange-yellow
Basophils	Magenta
Chromophobes	Greyish
RBCs	Yellow
Connective tissue	Green

▪ PFAAB–PAS–orange G (Adams and Swettenham, 1958)

Fixation

Formalin or formal–mercuric chloride.

Method

Perform PFAAB (page 274).
Perform PAS–orange G (*see above*).

Results

Acidophils	Orange
Basophil-R	Magenta
Basophil-S	Blue
Chromophobes	Grey
RBCs	Yellow

References

ADAMS, C. W. M. and SWETTENHAM, K. V. (1958). The histochemical identification of two types of basophil cell in the normal human adenohypophysis. *J. Pathol. Bacteriol.*, **75**, 95–103

DE LA TORRE, J. C. and SURGEON, J. W. (1976). A methodological approach to rapid and sensitive monoamine histofluorescence using a modified glyoxylic acid technique: the SPG method. *Histochemistry*, **49**, 81–93

ERANKO, O. (1955). Distribution of adrenaline and nor-adrenaline in the adrenal medulla. *Nature*, **175**, 88–89

FALCK, B., HILLARP, N. Å., THIEME, G. and TORP, A. (1962). Fluorescence of catechol amines and related compounds condensed with formaldehyde. *J. Histochem. Cytochem.*, **10**, 348–354

FALCK, B. and OWMAN, C. (1965). A detailed methodological description of the fluorescence method for the cellular demonstration of biogenic monoamines. *Acta Univ. Lund*, **2**, No. 7 Lund

FEYRTER, F. (1938). *Über Diffuse Endokrine Epitheliole Organe*. J. A. Barth, Leipzig, pp. 6–17

FURNESS, J. B., COSTA, M. and WILSON, A. J. (1977). Water-stable fluorophores, produced by reaction with aldehyde solutions, for the histochemical localization of catechol and indolethylamines. *Histochemistry*, **52**, 159–170

FURNESS, J. B., HEATH, J. W. and COSTA, M. (1978). Aqueous aldehyde (Faglu) methods for the fluorescence histochemical localization of catecholamines and for ultrastructural studies of central nervous system. *Histochemistry*, **57**, 285–295

FUXE, K., GOLDSTEIN, M., HOKFELT, T. and JOB, T. H. (1970). Immunohistochemical localization of dopamine β-hydroxylase in the peripheral and central nervous system. *Res. Commun. Chem. Pathol. Pharmacol.*, **1**, 627–636

GOMORI, G. (1952). *Microscopic Histochemistry*. Chicago University Press, Chicago

GRIMELIUS, L. (1968). A silver nitrate stain for α_2 cells in human pancreatic islets. *Acta Soc. Med. Uppsala*, **73**, 243–270

GRIMELIUS, L. and WILANDER, E. (1980). Silver stains in the study of endocrine cells of the gut and pancreas. *Invest. Cell. Pathol.*, **3**, 3–12

HALMI, N. S. (1952). Differentiation of the two types of basophils in the adenohypophysis of the rat and mouse. *Stain Technol.*, **27**, 61–64

HELLERSTRÖM, C. and HELLMAN, B. (1960). Some aspects of silver impregnation of the Islets of Langerhans in the rat. *Acta Endocrinol.*, **35**, 518–532

HOKFELT, T. and LJUNGDAHL, A. (1972). Modification of the Falck–Hillarp formaldehyde fluorescence method using the vibratome: simple, rapid and sensitive localization of catecholamines in sections of unfixed or formalin-fixed brain tissue. *Histochemie*, **29**, 325–339

LINDVALL, O. and BJÖRKLUND, A. (1974). The glyoxylic acid fluorescence histochemical method: a detailed account of the methodology for the visualization of central catecholamine neurons. *Histochemistry*, **39**, 97–127

LORÉN, I., BJÖRKLUND, A., FALCK, B. and LINDVALL, O. (1980). The aluminium–formaldehyde (ALFA) histofluorescence method for improved visualisation of catecholamines and indolamines. I. A detailed account of the methodology for central nervous tissue using paraffin, cryostat or vibratome sections. *J. Neurosci. Methods*, **2**, 277–300

LORÉN, I., BJÖRKLUND, A. and LINDVALL, O. (1977). Magnesium ions in catecholamine fluorescence techniques: application to the cryostat and vibratome techniques. *Histochemistry*, **52**, 223–239

PEARSE, A. G. E. (1953). *Histochemistry, Theoretical and Applied*. 1st Ed. Churchill, London

PEARSE, A. G. E. (1969). The cytochemistry and ultrastructure of polypeptide hormone-producing cells of the APUD series and the embryonic, physiologic and pathologic implications of the concept. *J. Histochem. Cytochem.*, **17**, 303–313

PEARSE, A. G. E. (1972). *Histochemistry, Theoretical and Applied*. 3rd Ed. Vol. 2. Churchill-Livingstone, Edinburgh and London

PEARSE, A. G. E. (1980). *Histochemistry, Theoretical and Applied*. 4th Ed. Vol. 1. Churchill-Livingstone, Edinburgh and London, pp. 108–112

PEARSE, A. G. E. and TAKOR, T. T. (1979). Embryology of the diffuse neuroendocrine system and its relationship to the common peptides. *Fed. Proc.*, **38**, 2288–2293

POLAK, J. M. and BLOOM, S. R. (1979). The diffuse neuroendocrine system. *J. Histochem. Cytochem.*, **27**, 1398–1400

SEVIER, A. C. and MUNGER, B. I. (1965). A silver method for paraffin sections of neural tissue. *J. Neuropathol. Exp. Neurol.*, **24**, 130–135

SINGH, I. (1964). A modification of the Masson–Hamperl method for staining argentaffin cells. *Anat. Anz.*, **115**, 81–82

SLIDDERS, W. (1961). The OFG and Br AB–OFG methods for staining the adenohypophysis. *J. Pathol. Bacteriol.*, **82**, 532–534

SOLCIA, E., CAPELLA, C. and VASSALLO, G. (1969). Lead haematoxylin as a stain for endocrine cells. Significance of staining and comparison with other selective methods. *Histochemie*, **20**, 116–126

SOLCIA, E., PEARSE, A. G. E., GRUBE, D., KOBAYASHI, S., BUSSOLATI, G., CREUTZFELDT, W. and GEPTS, W. (1973). Revised Wiesbaden classification of gut endocrine cells. *Rendiconti di Gastroenterologia*, **5**, 13–16

SOLCIA, E., VASSALLO, G. and CAPELLA, C. (1968). Selective staining of endocrine cells by basic dyes after acid hydrolysis. *Stain Technol.*, **43**, 257–263

STEINBUSCH, H. W. M., VERHOFSTAD, A. A. J. and JOOSTEN, H. W. J. (1978). Localisation of serotonin in the central nervous system by immunohistochemistry: description of a specific and sensitive technique and some applications. *Neuroscience*, **3**, 811–819

STERNBERGER, L. A. (1979). *Immunocytochemistry*. 2nd Ed. Wiley, New York

VERHOFSTAD, A. A. J., STEINBUSCH, H. W. M., JOOSTEN, H. W. J., PENKE, B., VARGA, J. and GOLDSTEIN, M. (1983). Immunocytochemical localisation of nor-adrenaline, adrenaline and serotonin. In *Immunocytochemistry*. Eds Polak, J. M. and van Noorden, S. Wright PSG, Bristol, London and Boston, pp. 143–168

WATSON, S. J. and ELLISON, J. P. (1976). Cryostat technique for central nervous system histofluorescence. *Histochemistry*, **50**, 119–127

27

Cytology technique

Exfoliative cytology is the study of superficial cells which have been exfoliated or shed from mucus membranes, renal tubules, serous membranes, etc. Cells may also be obtained by scraping or washing mucosal surfaces, for example, cervix or endometrium. Most of these techniques are employed for the rapid diagnosis of malignancy but may be used to obtain information regarding the hormonal state of the tissue or for the diagnosis of bacterial, fungal, viral or parasitic infections.

Diagnostic cytological techniques are being increasingly applied to material obtained from solid tissues by fine needle aspiration. The aspiration of superficial tissues, for example, thyroid, lymph node, etc. is carried out by direct observation while aspiration of deeper organs is usually performed under X-ray or ultrasound control, for example, lung, liver, etc. Cytology may also be successfully applied to touch preparations or smears from surgical specimens, for example, brain.

Technique

Accurate and reliable cytology depends on the quality of the cytological preparation. Material obtained by scraping or aspiration should be smeared on slides immediately and either placed at once in fixative for delivery to the laboratory or quickly air-dried, depending on the staining procedures to be used.

The clinical and nursing staff should be advised of the exact procedure to be followed to ensure that the highest quality preparations are submitted for examination. Slides with frosted ends should be used to allow reliable identification using a soft lead pencil. Smears should include all the material obtained, several slides being prepared as necessary, and the smears should be thin enough to allow reliable microscopical examination. It is often an advantage to have laboratory staff present during fine needle aspirations to prepare the smears for cytological examination.

Female genital tract

Specimens for the diagnosis of cancer and precancerous conditions of the cervix, or fungal, viral and parasitic infections, may be obtained by scraping the cervical squamocolumnar junction or by vaginal aspiration. Scraping is the recommended method for the diagnosis of malignant changes. For malignant changes in the endometrium the vaginal pool aspirate is preferred to cervical scraping but several methods of direct sampling of the endometrium have been used. Techniques using bushes, plastic samplers, direct aspiration, saline lavage, etc., are reviewed by Morse (1981).

Specimens for the assessment of the hormonal state of the patient, using karyopyknotic indices, are obtained by scraping the lateral vaginal wall.

The method of choice is to make smears and wet-fix immediately. This is done using 95% alcohol, one of the commercial spray fixatives or by dropping carbowax fixative* onto the slides.

When 95% alcohol is used for fixation a container of fixative should be used for each case. It is convenient to use plastic containers which hold two slides and which can be sealed by a hinged lid.

When a commercial spray fixative is used the spray container should not be held close to the slide but at a distance of 9–12 inches. Slides fixed by the spray and coating methods must be washed well in 80% alcohol to remove the coating. Some coating fixatives require ether–alcohol treatment for their removal, the manufacturer's instructions should be followed.

When the volume of fluid obtained from lavage is too great for direct smearing it may be centrifuged and smears made from the deposit or examined after membrane filtration.

The universally used staining technique is that of Papanicolaou.

Serous fluids

Serous fluids are obtained from pleural and peritoneal cavities or less commonly from the pericardial sac, and are usually sent to the laboratory for the identification of malignant cells.

Clots often form in these fluids and it is a matter of personal preference whether or not an anticoagulant is used. If no anticoagulant is used it is imperative that the fluid is centrifuged and any clot is fixed, processed and paraffin sections examined, as well as smears being made from the residual deposit. In our experience malignant cells have often been found in the clot while the smears from the residual deposit were negative.

If preferred, universal bottles containing anticoagulant (38 mg sodium citrate, 2 mg heparin or 20 mg EDTA) should be supplied to the ward. It is no use adding anticoagulant to the specimen after delivery to the laboratory since by that time the clot is usually present. If cell counts are to be performed anticoagulant bottles must be provided.

The normal procedure is to centrifuge the universal container and remove the supernatant fluid completely leaving the deposit with no fluid remaining, and retaining the supernatant.

Smears are made from the deposit and air-dried *instantly* for May–Grünwald–Giemsa staining. After adding a drop of supernatant to the deposit smears are made and wet-fixed in 95% alcohol for haematoxylin and eosin, and/or Papanicolaou staining.

* Carbowax fixative (carbofix)

Concentrate
Carbowax 1500	60 g
Distilled water	100 ml
Glacial acetic acid	4 ml

The carbowax is dissolved in warm distilled water, after cooling the acetic acid is added and the solution mixed. For use, dilute 6 ml of the concentrated stock with 94 ml of 95% ethanol.

If large volumes of aspirate are obtained they may be allowed to sediment in separating funnels. When the sediment is removed it can be treated as above. An alternative procedure for serous fluids is to use membrane filtration techniques (*see* page 490).

If fluids contain a large amount of blood it is often advantageous to remove the RBCs before making the smear. Haemolysing agents such as 2.5% acetic acid in 95% ethanol, saponin, etc., have been used and are assessed by Sharpe (1963). The results obtained depend on the number of RBCs present and may result in an excess of cell debris on the slide.

Sputum

Sputum specimens are usually submitted for the identification of malignant cells, but may require examination for asthmatic stigmata (Charcot Leyden crystals, Curschmann spirals and eosinophils) or organisms such as *Pneumocystis carinii*.

Early morning specimens should be obtained before teeth are brushed or food is taken. The specimen may be sampled directly or concentrated.

Direct sampling is made by selecting floccular or blood-stained particles if present. The specimen should be poured into a Petri dish if the specimen container does not allow adequate visual examination. Salivary specimens are usually not suitable but should nevertheless be examined. The smears are wet-fixed in 95% alcohol and stained by haematoxylin and eosin or Papanicolaou.

Concentration of sputum is accomplished by liquefying the whole specimen; after centrifuging, smears are made from the deposit. Two per cent Cytoclair (Sinclair Medicine, Borough Road, Godalming, Surrey, UK) (methyl cysteine), or Mucolex (Lerner Laboratories, 17 James St, Newhaven, Connecticut, USA), mucolytic agents may be used to liquefy the specimens. An equal volume is added to the specimen and incubated at 37 °C until the specimen has liquefied. This is usually accomplished in 2 hours but a longer time may be required. Various enzymes have also been used to liquefy sputum for cytological examination (Koss, 1968).

Saccomanno *et al.* (1963) described an homogenization technique in which the specimen is collected into 50% alcohol containing 2% carbowax (1540) and then blended in a high speed food blender for 6–25 seconds. After centrifugation the supernatant fluid is removed and the deposit dispersed using a vibrator. Smears are made and allowed to dry completely. The carbowax is removed by alcohol before staining by haematoxylin and eosin or Papanicolaou.

Sputum specimens should always be handled in a protective cabinet since they must be regarded as potentially tuberculous.

Pulmonary cytology may also be carried out on aerosol-induced sputum, bronchial secretions, bronchial brushings or bronchial washings.

Urine

Cytological examination of urine is usually performed to detect malignant cells arising from the urothelium or from the kidney. Occasionally it may be required to examine specimens for evidence of viral infections (polyomavirus, cytomegalovirus).

The specimen, which may be an early morning sample or a catheter specimen, should be examined as quickly as possible. If any delay is likely an equal volume of 95% ethanol (or 95% ethanol, three parts/25% acetic acid, one part) may be added to the fresh specimen. Drury and Wallington (1980) recommend the following fixative for specimens which have to travel by post:

Monoethylene glycol	350 ml
Diethylene glycol	18 ml
Borax pentahydrate	3.5 g
Glacial acetic acid	50 ml
Distilled water	570 ml

Two and a half ml of this solution is sufficient for 30 ml of urine. Specimens may be centrifuged or filtered.

Centrifuging

If the specimen is large several tubes may be centrifuged, the deposits combined, then again centrifuged.

Smears made from urine deposits are difficult to retain on the slide during fixing and staining. This lack of adherence may be overcome by placing a drop of glycerin–albumen on the slide and mixing the loop of deposit with it before making the smear. Alternatively an equal volume of carbofix may be added to the centrifuged deposit, left for 10 minutes, and, after centrifuging, smears made from the carbofix deposit.

Smears made from carbofixed material should be allowed to air-dry. When dry, the carbowax is removed by alcohol before commencing the staining procedure.

Membrane filtration

The urine specimen is filtered through a 5 μm pore cellulose acetate filter using a negative pressure of 25 mm of mercury. The temptation to use a higher negative pressure should be avoided. The vacuum pressure should be stopped before all the fluid is drawn through the filter so that the filter remains wet. The filter is fixed in 95% alcohol, stained by the Papanicolaou technique and mounted on a glass slide and coverslipped.

Cerebrospinal fluid

Cytological preparations may be made from cerebrospinal fluid in three ways; sedimentation, membrane filtration or centrifugation.

The sedimentation method developed by Sayk (1974) uses a small glass cylinder resting on a saline-moistened filter paper with a round opening the same size as the cylinder, below which is a microscope slide. The assembly is clamped together by a system of weights and CSF is placed in the cylinder (up to 1 ml). The CSF is gradually absorbed by the paper taking 20–30 minutes. During this time cells are deposited directly onto the glass slide. The disadvantage of this method is the great loss of cells.

Tutuarima, Hische and Van Der Helm (1979) developed a modification of the Sayk method. A polished Perspex cylinder is clamped directly onto a glass slide and CSF added. The CSF is absorbed from above by Sephadex G10 held in a disposable pipette tip whose orifice is covered by a Nucleopore filter. den Hartog Jager (1980) claims a 90% cell recovery using this technique.

Centrifugation techniques must be used with great care since the number of cells present is usually small and often no visible deposit can be seen. After centrifugation as much supernatant as possible is removed leaving no more than two small drops of fluid (fine bore Pasteur pipette). One smear is made from one drop of fluid and air-dried for May–Grünwald–Giemsa staining. A second drop is mixed with a small drop of glycerin–egg albumen on a microscope slide, smeared and wet-fixed immediately. This prevents loss of cells which might occur when placing the slide into the fixative.

Membrane filtration may be carried out using a modified Hemmings filter. This is a metal collar threaded at both ends to correspond with the threads of $\frac{1}{4}$ ounce Bijou bottles. The central perforated diaphragm supports a 1.7 cm membrane filter which is screwed onto the bottle containing the fluid. An empty bottle is attached to the other thread. Centrifuging at 2000 rev/min for 10 minutes causes the fluid to pass through the filter to the empty bottle leaving the cells deposited on the membrane.

Cytocentrifuges have been developed which combined the Sayk and centrifugation technique. Perspex blocks, with sample wells and either basal or lateral conical openings, are placed against microscope slides. Filter card or decanting principles are employed. Centrifugation deposits the cells directly onto the microscope slides. The fluid is either absorbed by a filter card or simply decanted depending on the method used.

Eye specimens

Conjunctival or corneal scrapes are smeared onto alcohol-moistened slides in a horizontal position. The alcohol is allowed to evaporate then the slides are placed in a container of alcohol (Naib, 1981).

Ocular chamber aspirates yield one or two drops of fluid which is smeared directly onto slides and wet-fixed, or diluted with a small amount of saline and filtered through a membrane (Wolter and Naylor, 1968).

Haematoxylin and eosin or Papanicolaou methods are used routinely. Carbol chromotrope may be preferred to demonstrate eosinophils in allergic conjunctivitis. Giemsa is recommended for the demonstration of chlamydial inclusions when the use of a green filter helps in their differentiation from melanin deposits (Naib, 1981).

Miscellaneous

Joint fluids should always be examined for crystals in addition to normal examination for assessment of the cell population (*see* Chapter 15, page 298). Wet preparations from 'hydrocele' fluids may reveal the presence of spermatozoa and so prove a diagnosis of spermatocele. Sperms will also be identified in haematoxylin and eosin or Giemsa preparations.

Cyst fluids (e.g. breast) should be centrifuged and treated with carbofix as detailed above.

When examining 'cyst fluids' from the abdomen one should be aware of the possibility of hydatid disease. Scolices and hooklets of *Taenia echinococcus* can be identified in haematoxylin and eosin preparations but the use of polarization microscopy can be used with advantage in the study of wet preparations from the centrifuge deposit since the hooklets are birefringent.

Staining methods

Smears are often stained by May–Grünwald–Giemsa or by haematoxylin and eosin. The choice of method will depend on the site involved or on personal preference, though the Papanicolaou method is universally used for routine cervical smears.

■ Papanicolaou method (1942, 1957)

The staining solutions employed in this technique may be purchased commercially (Ortho Pharmaceutical Corp., Raritan, New Jersey, USA), or prepared as follows.

Reagents

(1) Harris's haematoxylin (without acetic acid).

(2) Orange G (OG 6)

0.5% Orange G 6 in 95% alcohol	100 ml
Phosphotungstic acid	0.015 g

(3) Eosin–azure (EA 36 or EA 50)

0.5% Light green SF yellowish in 95% alcohol	45 ml
0.5% Bismarck brown in 95% alcohol	10 ml
0.5% Eosin Y in 95% alcohol	45 ml
Phosphotungstic acid	0.2 g
Sat. aq. lithium carbonate	1 drop

EA 65 uses 0.25% light green which is preferable if an excess of mucus is present in the smear.

Technique

(1) Fix smears (while still moist) in 95% alcohol for 15–30 minutes, although they may be left in the fixative for longer periods without damage.
(2) Rinse smears in distilled water.
(3) Stain in Harris's haematoxylin for 4 minutes.
(4) Wash in tap-water for 1–2 minutes.
(5) Differentiate in acid alcohol.
(6) Blue in tap-water or 1.5% sodium bicarbonate.
(7) Rinse in distilled water.
(8) Transfer to 70% then 95% alcohol for a few seconds.
(9) Stain in OG 6 for 1–2 minutes.
(10) Rinse in three changes of 95% alcohol for a few seconds in each.
(11) Stain in EA 36 for 1–2 minutes*.
(12) Rinse in three changes of 95% alcohol for a few seconds in each.
(13) Dehydrate in absolute alcohol, clear in xylene and mount in synthetic resin.

Results

Nuclei	Blue
Acidophilic cells and keratin	Red to orange
Basophilic cells	Green to blue-green
Cells or fragments of tissue penetrated by blood	Orange to orange-green

* This time will vary with different batches.

■ Fluorescent acridine orange technique (von Bertalanffy, Masin and Masin, 1956)

This method gives good differentiation of RNA and DNA, although there is doubt as to its absolute specificity. It gives a brilliant orange staining of RNA and is excellent for plasma cells and those cells actively synthesizing protein.

Reagents

(1) M/15 Phosphate buffer pH 6.0.
(2) Acridine orange 0.1% in phosphate buffer, pH 6.
(3) M/10 Calcium chloride differentiator (1.109 g in 100 ml distilled water).

Method

Smears are fixed in ether/alcohol for at least 30 minutes. Tissue sections fixed in an alcoholic fixative (formalin-fixed tissue cannot be used) are brought to water.

(1) Hydrate by passing them through 80, 70 and 50% alcohol for 10 seconds each, and rinse in distilled water.
(2) Treat with 1% acetic acid for 6 seconds, followed by rinsing in two changes of distilled water.
(3) Stain in 0.1% acridine orange for 3 minutes.
(4) Wash in M/15 phosphate buffer, pH 6.0 for 1 minute.
(5) Differentiate in M/10 calcium chloride for 30 seconds.
(6) Mount in a drop of pH 6.0 phosphate buffer, and examine under a fluorescence microscope.

Results

DNA fluoresces   Green
RNA fluoresces   Orange

■ Rapid acridine orange fluorescent method

This method has been described by Riva and Turner (1962) as a 10-second staining method for unfixed cervical smears, which can be used in offices and clinics. This method gives results comparable with the longer von Bertalanffy method, but it has not been controlled histochemically. It provides an excellent rapid method for checking preparations or smears for the presence of plasma cells, or cells with an RNA-rich cytoplasm.

Method (Riva and Turner, 1962 modified)

Staining solution 0.025% acridine orange in 2% acetic acid, to which 0.01% merthiolate has been added to prevent the growth of moulds and bacteria.

Technique

(1) Agitate unfixed or fixed smears for 5 seconds in acridine orange solution.
(2) Differentiate in 2% ethanol in physiological saline for 2 seconds.
(3) Rinse, then mount in physiological saline.

Results

As for von Bertalanffy's method.

Chromosome techniques

The culture of leucocytes from peripheral blood has become the routine method of obtaining preparations for the study of chromosomes.

■ Lymphocyte culture (modified from Moorhead *et al.*, 1960)

Culture medium

McCoy or TC199 medium	8 ml
Fetal bovine serum	2 ml
Reconstituted phytohaemagglutinin	0.2 ml

This medium should be prepared immediately before use.

Method

(1) Add 0.5 ml of patient's heparinized whole blood to freshly prepared culture medium.
(2) Incubate for 70 hours at 37 °C.
(3) Add 0.1 ml of 0.04% colcemid to the culture and continue incubation for a further 2 hours at 37 °C.
(4) Transfer the culture to a centrifuge tube.
(5) Centrifuge for 5 minutes at 1500 rev/min.
(6) Remove supernatant fluid.
(7) Resuspend the cells in 10 ml hypotonic potassium chloride (0.075 M).
(8) Centrifuge for 5 minutes at 1500 rev/min.
(9) Resuspend in 1.5 ml of 0.075 M potassium chloride.
(10) Add 10 ml of freshly made fixative (methanol three parts/acetic acid one part) whilst agitating the tube.
(11) Centrifuge for 5 minutes at 1500 rev/min.
(12) Decant supernatant fluid.
(13) Repeat steps (11) and (12) twice.
(14) Add 10 ml of fixative and store overnight at 4 °C.
(15) Centrifuge and make slide preparation from the deposit.

Skin biopsies and amniotic fluids are also used in special circumstances. The techniques of tissue culture and slide preparation are well described by Priest (1977).

Standardization in human cytogenetics was agreed at the Paris Conference in 1971. This was brought up to date as the International System for Human Cytogenetic Nomenclature (ISCN, 1978) and was followed by a supplement incorporating fine banding techniques (ISCN, 1981).

■ Aceto-orcein method

This was the original staining technique used for the examination of metaphase spreads.

Reagent

Aceto-orcein stain. Add 1–2 g orcein to 45 ml of hot acetic acid. When cool, add 55 ml of distilled water. Filter before use.

Technique

Add a few drops of stain to prepared slide, lower coverslip and apply gentle firm pressure with filter paper or glass rod. Remove excess stain by applying filter paper to the edge of the coverslip. Seal the edges of the preparation.

Results

Chromosomes   Deep purple

This method was largely replaced by the Giemsa method which in turn has been replaced by banding methods. These methods produce banding patterns along the metaphase chromosomes. A band is part of a chromosome which is clearly distinguishable from its adjacent segments appearing darker or lighter with the following methods.

Q-staining

After exposure to quinacrine derivatives human chromosomes fluoresce to different degrees ranging from faint to bright with patterns characteristic for many of the individual chromosomes, (Casperson et al., 1969). This is known as Q-banding.

■ Technique modified from Casperson

(1) Slides are stained in 0.5% quinacrine mustard for 10 minutes at room temperature.
(2) Wash in water.
(3) Mount in water, remove any air bubbles by using pressure and seal the coverglass.

C-staining

This method demonstrates centric or constitutive heterochromatin. This technique employs denaturation of DNA by alkali, renaturation and Giemsa staining (Arrighi and Hsu, 1971).

G-staining

Treatment of chromosome spreads by a variety of techniques prior to Giemsa staining has been used to produce banding patterns (G-bands) which help in the identification of individual chromosomes. Schnedl (1971) used sodium hydroxide. Sumner, Evans and Buckland (1971) compared the action of hydrochloric acid, formamide, barium hydroxide and boiling but preferred pretreatment with 0.3 M sodium chloride/0.03 M trisodium citrate. Seabright (1971) introduced a rapid method using trypsin digestion. This method is described below.

■ Rapid Giemsa banding technique

(1) Conventional air-dried preparations are flooded with 0.25% trypsin in isotonic sodium chloride for 10–15 seconds.

(2) Rinse twice in isotonic sodium chloride.
(3) Stain in Leishman stain diluted 1 in 4 with pH 6.8 buffer.
(4) Differentiate, if necessary, in pH 6.8 buffer.
(5) Blot dry.
(6) Rinse in xylene and mount in neutral mounting medium.

R-staining

The reverse Giemsa method of Dutrillaux and Lejeune (1971) demonstrates the reciprocal pattern of the G methods producing R-bands.

Fine-banding

High resolution banding involves prophase–synchronization using an amethopterin (methotrexate, Lederle) block during culture and Wright stained preparations (Yunis, 1976).

Sex chromatin

Barr body

The first demonstration of the sex chromatin body was by Barr and Bertram (1949). Moore, Graham and Barr (1953) described a simple method of chromatin testing in human skin biopsies and demonstrated the practical value of the test as a guide to chromosomal sex in ambisexual patients. Sex chromatin is seen as an intensely staining body lying against the nuclear membrane (*Figure 27.1*).

Preparations are commonly made from the buccal mucosa by scraping the inside of the cheek with a spatula, smearing on glass slides and fixing immediately in equal parts ether and ethanol for 15 minutes (Moore and Barr, 1955).

Sex chromatin is visible in haematoxylin and eosin, Papanicolaou or Feulgen preparations but is strikingly demonstrated by the cresyl echt violet method of Moore (1962) or by Guard's method (1959).

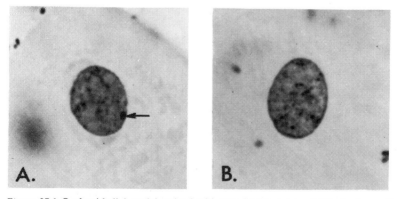

Figure 27.1 Oral epithelial nuclei stained with cresyl echt violet ×2000. A, chromatin-positive nucleus from a normal female; the arrow indicates a typical mass of sex chromatin. B, chromatin-negative nucleus from a normal male; no sex chromatin is visible. (Reproduced from Moore, K. L., and Barr, M. L. (1955), by courtesy of the Editor of *The Lancet* **2**, 57)

■ Cresyl echt violet method (Moore, 1962)

(1) Remove the slides from the fixative and pass through 70% alcohol, 50% alcohol and distilled water, 5 minutes in each, with two changes of distilled water.
(2) Immerse the slides in a 1% solution of cresyl echt violet for 5–8 minutes.
(3) Differentiate in 95% ethanol, five to eight quick dips.
(4) Continue differentiation in absolute ethanol, checking with the microscope at intervals until the details of cell structure are defined clearly. Usually this takes about 1 minute.
(5) Clear in two changes of xylene, 3 minutes in each and mount in synthetic resin.

Results

Sex chromatin is seen as a deeply stained dot in the nucleus, usually lying against the nuclear membrane.

■ Guard's method for sex chromatin (1959)

Reagents

Biebrich scarlet stain

Biebrich scarlet	1 g
Phosphotungstic acid	0.3 g
Glacial acetic acid	5.0 ml
50% Alcohol	to 100 ml

Fast Green FCF

Fast green FCF	0.5 g
Phosphomolybdic acid	0.3 g
Phosphotungstic acid	0.3 g
Glacial acetic acid	5.0 ml
50% Alcohol	to 100 ml

Method

(1) Fixation (as above).
(2) 70% Alcohol for 2 minutes.
(3) Biebrich scarlet for 2 minutes.
(4) Rinse in 50% alcohol.
(5) Differentiate in fast green FCF for 1–4 hours (usually 3 hours) until cytoplasm and nuclei are green. Pyknotic nuclei and sex chromatin are red.
(6) Rinse in 50% alcohol, leave for 5 minutes.
(7) Dehydrate, clear and mount.

Results

Sex chromatin	Bright red
Pyknotic nuclei	Bright red
Cytoplasm, nuclei and so on	Green

Y chromosome

Casperson *et al.* (1969), using fluorescent dyes to give banding of chromosomes noticed particularly bright fluorescence of the long arm of the Y chromosome. Zech (1969) described a simple technique to demonstrate the Y chromosome using quinacrine mustard. Pearson, Bobrow and Vosa (1970) used quinacrine dihydrochloride (Atebrin) to demonstrate the Y chromosome in both metaphase spreads and interphase nuclei. In the latter a characteristic fluorescent body is seen in buccal smear preparations thus providing the ideal counterpart of the Barr body or X chromosome. The recommended method is that modified from Casperson (*see above*).

References

ARRIGHI, F. E. and HSU, T. C. (1971). Localization of heterochromatin in human chromosomes. *Cytogenetics,* 10, 81–86

BARR, M. L. and BERTRAM, E. G. (1949). A morphological distinction between neurons of the male and female, and the behaviour of the nucleolar satellite during accelerated nucleoprotein synthesis. *Nature (Lond.),* 163, 676–677

CASPERSON, T., ZECH, L., MODEST, E. J., FOLEY, G. E., WAGH, U. and SIMONSSON, E. (1969). Chemical differentiation with fluorescent alkylating agents in *Vicia faba* metaphase chromosomes. *Exp. Cell Res.,* 58, 128–140

DEN HARTOG JAGER, W. A. (1980). *Colour Atlas of CSF Cytopathology.* Elsevier/North-Holland, Amsterdam, New York, Oxford

DRURY, R. A. B. and WALLINGTON, E. A. (1980). *Carleton's Histological Technique.* 5th Ed. Oxford University Press, Oxford, New York, Toronto

DUTRILLAUX, B. and LEJEUNE, J. (1971). Sur une nouvelle technique d'analyse de caryotype humain. *C. R. Acad. Sci. Paris,* 272, 2638–2640

GUARD, H. R. (1959). A new technique for differential staining of the sex chromatin and the determination of its incidence in exfoliated vaginal epithelial cells. *Am. J. Clin. Pathol.,* 32, 145–151

ISCN (1978). *An International System for Human Cytogenetic Nomenclature. Birth Defects: Original Article Series.* Vol. 14. No. 8. National Foundation, New York

ISCN (1981). *An International System for Human Cytogenetic Nomenclature. High Resolution Banding. Birth Defects: Original Article Series.* Vol. 17. No. 5. National Foundation, New York

KOSS, L. G. (1968). *Diagnostic Cytology and its Histopathologic Bases.* 2nd Ed. J. B. Lippincott Co., Philadelphia, Toronto

MOORE, K. L. (1962). The sex chromatin: its discovery and variations in the animal kingdom. *Acta Cytol. (Phil.),* 6, 1–12

MOORE, K. L. and BARR, M. L. (1955). Smears from oral mucosa in detection of chromosomal sex. *Lancet,* 2, 57–58

MOORE, K. L., GRAHAM, M. A. and BARR, M. L. (1953). Detection of chromosomal sex in hermaphrodites from skin biopsy. *Surg. Gynecol. Obstet.,* 96, 641–646

MOORHEAD, P. S., NOWELL, P. C., MELLMAN, W. J., BATTIPS, D. M. and HUNGERFORD, D. A. (1960). Chromosome preparations of leucocytes obtained from human peripheral blood. *Exp. Cell Res.,* 20, 613–616

MORSE, A. R. (1981). The value of endometrial aspiration in gynaecological practice. In *Advances in Clinical Cytology.* Eds Koss, L. G. and Coleman, D. V. Butterworths, London, pp. 44–63

NAIB, Z. M. (1981). Cytology of ophthalmological disease. In *Advances in Clinical Cytology.* Eds Koss, L. G. and Coleman, D. V. Butterworths, London, pp. 232–253

PAPANICOLAOU, G. N. (1942). New procedure for staining vaginal smears. *Science,* 95, 438–439

PAPANICOLAOU, G. N. (1957). The cancer-diagnostic potential of uterine exfoliative cytology. *CA,* 7, 124–135

PARIS CONFERENCE (1971). *Standardisation in Human Cytogenetics. Birth Defects: Original Article Series.* Vol. 8. No. 7. National Foundation, New York

PEARSON, P. L., BOBROW, M. and VOSA, C. G. (1970). Technique for identifying Y chromosomes in human interphase nuclei. *Nature (Lond.),* 226, 78–80

PRIEST, J. H. (1977). *Medical Cytogenetics and Cell Culture.* 2nd Ed. Henry Kimpton, London

RIVA, H. L. and TURNER, T. R. (1962). Further experience with fluorescence microscopy in exfoliative cytology. A ten-second acridine orange staining technique for cytologic cancer screening by fluorescence microscopy. *Am. J. Obstet. Gynecol.,* 85, 713–723

SACCOMANNO, G., SAUNDERS, R. P., ELLIS, H., ARCHER, V. E., WOOD, B. G. and BECKLER, P. A. (1963). Concentration of carcinoma or atypical cells in sputum. *Acta Cytol.,* 7, 305–310

SAYK, J. (1974). The cerebrospinal fluid in brain tumours. *Handbook of Clinical Neurology*. Eds Vinken, P. J. and Bruyn, G. W. Vol. 16. *Tumours of the Brain and Skull*. Pt 1. North-Holland, Amsterdam

SCHNEDL, W. (1971). Banding pattern of human chromosomes. *Nature, New Biol.*, **233**, 93–94

SEABRIGHT, M. (1971). A rapid banding technique for human chromosomes. *Lancet*, **2**, 971–972

SHARPE, S. H. (1963). The preparation of slides of the exfoliated cellular material in body fluids. *J. Med. Lab. Technol.*, **20**, 245–260

SUMNER, A. T., EVANS, H. J. and BUCKLAND, R. A. (1971). New technique for distinguishing between human chromosomes. *Nature, New Biol.*, **232**, 31–32

TUTUARIMA, J. A., HISCHE, E. A. H. and VAN DER HELM, H. J. (1979). An improved method for the concentration of cerebrospinal fluid cells by suction tip and sedimentation chamber. *J. Neurol. Sci.*, **44**, 61–67

VON BERTALANFFY, L., MASIN, F. and MASIN, M. (1956). The use of acridine orange fluorescence technique in exfoliative cytology. *Science*, **124**, 1024–1025

WOLTER, R. and NAYLOR, B. (1968). A membrane filter method: used to diagnose intraocular tumour. *J. Pediat. Ophthalmol.*, **5**, 36–38

YUNIS, J. J. (1976). High resolution of human chromosomes. *Science*, **191**, 1268–1270

ZECH, L. (1969). Investigation of metaphase chromosomes with DNA-binding fluorochromes. *Exp. Cell Res.*, **58**, 463

Part VIII

Special techniques

28

Quantitative methods

Quantitative assessment of tissues has long been expressed in subjective terms such as mild, moderate, severe, scanty, numerous, while histochemical reactions have been (similarly) expressed as $\pm$, $+$, $++$, etc. Methods of quantifying these assessments are now available allowing a more accurate comparison of structure and function. A mathematical approach to histopathology and histochemistry can lead to a more reliable assessment of disease processes and of the effects of treatment.

These techniques have been applied to diseases involving lung, bone, muscle, gastrointestinal tract, placenta, kidney, etc. The purpose of this chapter is to introduce the reader to the possibilities of applying these techniques to the study of tissues. Quantitative assessment may be considered according to the classification suggested in *Table 28.1*. The determination of weight is included under Morphology for convenience, while the inclusion of biochemical analysis is for completeness and will not be discussed.

Table 28.1

	Morphology	*Reaction*
Macro	Dimension Volume Weight	Biochemical analysis
Micro	Number Measurement (length, area, volume) Weight (mass, concentration)	Section analysis (histochemistry, cytochemistry)

Preparation of tissues

In order to ensure that the organ retains its shape and that changes in structural relationships are avoided special fixation may be necessary, for example, for lung. Installation of liquid into the airways tends to cause distortion of the architecture of the lung. To try to overcome this Weibel and Vidone (1961) used a formaldehyde–steam technique but Wright *et al.* (1974) preferred a closed ventilation system in order to avoid the accumulation of fluid in the air spaces which caused distortion. For other organs fixation by perfusion and immersion is the method of choice.

Morphology

Introduction

Using a statistical approach, which is dependent on probability, a number of terms require explanation.

Accuracy

This describes how closely a given measurement lies to the true value. The opposite of accuracy is error, the greater the accuracy the less the error. To determine the accuracy of a given method a more accurate method of measurement is needed to make comparisons. Consideration of the distortion and resolution of optical imaging systems and of shrinkage during fixation and processing shows that the accuracy of grid techniques, for example, is between 5 and 10% and this is considered adequate. To obtain an accuracy of better than $\pm 5\%$ would require a tremendous effort.

Precision

This describes the reproducibility of a measurement. Errors usually exceed precision by a factor of 2 to 3.

Dispersion

This is the variation of individual measurements round the mean and is measured as Standard Deviation. Random errors tend to cancel out leaving the result very near to the true value while systematic errors make the observed value differ from the true value.

The internal structure of an organ can only be investigated after destruction of the tissues. The most orderly method of destruction is sectioning. The tissue to be sampled should be uniform and selection of blocks should be random. The sample size and number of measurements made is important. Generally 50 observations will give reliable results. Smaller numbers show a higher standard deviation, whilst larger numbers will give no greater accuracy.

Macro

It is normal procedure to measure and weigh organs prior to dissection, but it is less common to obtain their volume. All these measurements must be taken accurately if the organ is to be quantified in any way. Organs must be removed intact and their volumes measured both before and after fixation in order to detect any changes and allow the incorporation of correction factors to subsequent calculations.

A convenient method of determination of volume of an organ is by simple water displacement. Where this method is not applicable volume may be estimated by using Simpson's rule for calculating the volume of an irregular solid. The organ is cut into slices of equal thickness (h). The area (A) of the cut surface on each slice is measured, by planimetry, or by a point counting, or linear intercept method (*see below*).

The number of slices (n) should be even.

Simpson's formula is

$$V = \frac{h}{3}[(A_0 + A_n) + 4(A_1 + A_3 + \ldots A_{n-1}) + 2(A_2 + A_4 + \ldots A_{n-2})]$$

This technique is usually adopted for lung or for irregularly shaped organs with attached tissues where water displacement is not practicable.

Micro

Number

Quantitative methods have been used for some time in cytology to assess hormonal status, for example, karyopyknotic index. This involves a simple differential counting method, where the whole objects are present on the slide. When counting objects in sections the following conditions must be satisfied:

(1) Objects must be randomly distributed.
(2) The structures must be well defined and must yield only one transection.
(3) The size of the structures must be small compared with the total containing volume.
(4) The section must be thin and randomly orientated.

Accurate counting is made difficult by the fact that the components are represented by random segments. A simplified correction formula derived from Abercrombie (1946) and DeHoff and Rhines (1961) can be applied to counts in unit area of tissue sections.

$$N = n\left(\frac{t}{D+t}\right)$$

N = true count
n = observed count
D = mean diameter of transections
t = section thickness

When a count of objects in unit volume is required the method of Weibel and Gomez (1962) is recommended. This is used when the dimensions of the objects are large compared with the thickness of the section, for example, alveoli. They devised a coefficient which depended on the shape of the objects being counted. This is introduced into the relationship between N and n.

$$N = \frac{n^{3/2}}{\beta\sqrt{V}}$$

N = the count per unit volume
n = number of alveolar transections per unit area
β = shape coefficient (e.g. normal alveoli 1.55)
V = proportion by volume which the objects occupy (determined by point counting, see page 507)

Measurement

Length

Many objects can be measured using an eyepiece micrometer, for example, diameter of vessels. When measuring the diameter of spheres in tissue sections the true diameter will be greater than the observed diameter. It can be shown (Aherne and Dunnill, 1982) that the expected radius of a set of transection discs $= (\pi/4)R$, where R is the true radius it follows that

$$D = \frac{4}{\pi} d$$

D = true diameter
d = observed diameter

The length of an irregular outline or perimeter can be measured by an intercept technique employing parallel lines of known distance apart superimposed on the section.

$$L = \frac{id\pi}{2}$$

L = length of perimeter
d = distance between projected lines
i = mean number of intercepts

When a number of objects are present the mean periphery can be obtained by dividing by the number of objects under the grid.

Area

Cross-sectional area   Many methods have been employed for the measurement of areas in tissue sections, much work being directed to estimating the cross-sectional area of muscle fibres. Of the methods assessed by Clancy and Herlihy (1978) one which gave accurate results was calculated by using the formula:

$$A = \frac{\pi}{4} Dd$$

A = the cross-sectional area
D = largest diameter
d = 'smallest' diameter (the greatest distance across the object at right angles to D)

Surface area   The internal surface area of a structure in an organ can be estimated by using a linear intercept technique on sections of the organ.
    The method depends on the fact that if a line of known length is superimposed on a section it will be intersected a number of times by the component whose surface area is required. The mean linear intercept (L_m) is calculated by dividing the total length of line superimposed on the structure by the number of intercepts observed. This is incorporated into the formula:

$$S = \frac{2V}{L_m}$$

S = total surface area
V = total volume of tissue enclosing the structures
L_m = mean linear intercept

This formula is applicable where a single surface is to be measured, for example, placental villus. However, in the case of lung the line crosses two alveolar surfaces and a factor of 4 has to be substituted giving:

$$S = \frac{4V}{L_m}$$

A Zeiss II graticule consisting of six parallel lines or a graticule with two lines at right angles can be used. It is convenient to use a projection microscope, the lines being drawn on an acetate sheet placed on the ground glass projection surface. Normally correction factors for changes due to fixation and processing are incorporated. In the case of lung a correction for the fraction of lung containing parenchyma is also incorporated. The lines should be cast a number of times, at random, on the object.

Volume

The Delesse (1847) principle states 'In a rock composed of a number of minerals the area occupied by any given mineral on a surface of a section of the rock is proportional to the volume of the mineral in the rock'.

In other words, by measuring area fractions on sections, volume fractions may be estimated.

The two methods most commonly used are point counting and linear analysis, the former being the most popular.

Point counting grids or graticules are geometrical arrays of points arranged at the angles of equilateral triangles, squares or hexagons. The total number of points falling within the object of interest are recorded (n) and the total number of points superimposed on the sections (both on and off the object) are noted (N).

The area function $= n/N$ and from the Delesse principle the volume fraction also $= n/N$.

In linear analysis a grid of parallel lines is superimposed on the section. The sum of the lengths of the segments of line traversing the object is calculated $(\sum 1)$. The total length of the grid line is also found (L).

The area fraction $= \sum 1/L$ and again from the Delesse principle the volume fraction $= \sum 1/L$.

Weight (mass and concentration)

The interference microscope (*see* Chapter 34) can be used to measure the dry mass of living cells (Davies, Chayen and La Cour, 1954; Barer and Joseph, 1954, 1955a and 1955b). When dealing with tissue sections the choice of the type of interference microscope will be determined by the topography within the section, since the small separation between the object beam and reference beam in polarizing interference systems might be a limiting factor (Galjaard, 1967).

If the refractive index of the object differs from that of the immersion medium then the rays passing through the object and the immersion medium respectively will have a phase difference. This difference or retardation can be measured in an interference microscope when the rays interfere on recombination.

If the area of the object and its thickness are measured then dry mass and concentration of dissolved substances can be calculated. The specific refraction increment of dissolved proteins must also be known. This is a constant which is equal to the change in refractive index with a concentration change of 1%. For dissolved protein this is taken to be 0.0018.

Dry mass

This can be calculated if the optical path difference of the object immersed in water in cm (Δ), the are in cm^2 (A) and the specific refraction increment (α) are known.

$$M = \frac{\Delta A}{100\alpha}\ \text{g}$$

Concentration

The dry mass concentration of dissolved substances in g/100 ml can be calculated if the optical retardation in cm (Δ), the thickness in cm (t) (*see below*) and the specific refraction increment (α) are known (Galjaard, 1967).

$$C = \frac{\Delta}{100\alpha \cdot t}\ \text{g/100 ml}$$

The concentration of total solids in a cell in g/100 ml can be obtained by subtracting the refractive index of water from the refractive index of the protein solution in which the cytoplasm becomes invisible and dividing the result by the specific refraction increment (Barer and Joseph, 1955b).

$$C = \frac{n_0 - n_w}{\alpha}$$

Measurement of section thickness

Measurement of thickness, necessary for the estimation of concentration (*above*), is also of great importance in quantitative histochemistry (*see below*). This apparently simple measurement is in fact one of the most difficult to make. Consequently a great variety of approaches to the problem have been used. It is simple to estimate the approximate average thickness of sections but since microtome settings cannot be relied upon and sections cut in the normal way vary in thickness some method must be used to measure the true thickness of individual sections when quantitative techniques are being used.

   Lange and Engstrom (1954) list four types of methods for measuring section thickness:

(1) focusing,
(2) stereoradiography,
(3) mechanical,
(4) interferometry.

Focusing

The fine adjustment of the microscope is used, along with a high NA objective, to focus on the bottom and top surfaces of the section. The calibration scale on the fine adjustment control being noted at each point. The accuracy of this method is not great.

Stereoradiography

This method is not recommended for thin sections.

Mechanical

Commercial devices have been used which employ a probe which traverses the section surface (Mikrokator—Glimstedt and Hakansson, 1951; Surfometer—Pearse and Marks, 1976). It is probable that the pressure of the probe, no matter how light, will cause distortion of the section giving unreliable results (Rost, 1980). Hallén (1956) used a profile microscope as a substitute for the probe and achieved great accuracy.

Interferometry

Using an interference microscope the optical retardations produced by the object when mounted in two media of known but differing refractive index can be measured. The thickness can be calculated using the following formula (Hale, 1958):

$$t = \frac{\Delta_1 - \Delta_2}{n_2 - n_1}$$

t = thickness
n_1 = lower refractive index
n_2 = higher refractive index
Δ_1 = path difference mounted in medium of lower refractive index
Δ_2 = path difference mounted in medium of higher refractive index

Butcher (1971) found that cutting at a regular normal speed produced sections of a thickness close to the setting of the microtome. Fast cutting produced thinner sections whilst slow cutting produced thicker sections. He found that the use of a motorized drive, set to a suitable speed produced sections with a very regular thickness.

Galjaard (1967) recommends cutting a material of known refractive index simultaneously with the tissue allowing calculations of thickness from the formula.

Optical path difference $= (n_0 - n_m) \cdot t$

n_0 = refractive index of material
n_m = refractive index of immersion medium
t = thickness

Reaction

Section analysis

Measurement of reaction products from either reactive groups in tissues or from the results of enzyme action on a substrate can be accomplished by optical means. The final reaction product (FRP) has been measured photometrically using electromagnetic radiation varying in wavelength from electron to infrared beams.

The essential requirements are that fixatives should not interfere with the reactivity of the substance, that there should be no diffusion of the substance or of the FRP into the fixative, the substrate or other areas of the tissue and that the FRP should be linearly proportional to the amount of the substrate present and obey the Beer–Lambert law if absorptiometry is to be used.

The criteria proposed by Stoward (1980) concerning quantitative enzyme histochemistry can be extended to other histochemical reactions, namely that the technique should give precise localization, should be reproducible, specific and valid (FRP is related to the concentration or activity of the substance being measured).

Meijer (1972) used semipermeable membranes to improve localization in enzyme histochemistry. A semipermeable membrane interposed between the incubating medium and the tissue section prevents diffusion of the large molecule enzyme whilst allowing access of the smaller substrate molecules.

Reactive groups in tissue (or isolated cells) are reacted with a reagent which binds to the reactive group to form a coloured compound which is held in place by its chemical linkage to the structural component. Such chromogenic reactions are used for nuclear studies (Feulgen) and for the quantitative analysis of reactive groups of proteins.

Enzymes convert colourless substrates into highly coloured FRPs which are related to the amount of enzyme activity.

The FRP is measured in one of a variety of ways depending on its characteristics.

Absorptiometry

The groups accepting energy from light may be present in the tissue (endogenous) or may be the results of staining or of chemical reactions.

The intensity of a light beam before and after passage through the region of interest is measured. The proportion of light absorbed depends on the amount of chromophore present.

Fluorimetry

The intensity of fluorescence can be very accurately measured because of the precise selection of excitation and emission wavelengths.

Interferometry

This method is used to measure the dry mass of a transparent reaction product.

Reflectometry

This technique is used for particulate deposits, for example, silver grains, formazan, etc.

Microdensitometry

The most widely used technique is that of microdensitometry which is, in its simplest terms, spectrophotometry carried out through a microscope. It is beyond the scope of this book to describe these techniques in detail, only a brief description of microdensitometry is given below. The reader is referred to Weid (1966), Weid and Bahr (1970), Holborow (1970), Rost (1980) and the Ciba Foundation Symposium No. 73 for more detailed descriptions.

In microdensitometry it is not the concentration of the coloured product that is measured but its mass per cell or unit area. In sections meaningful results will only be obtained if the thickness of the section can be determined accurately since mass is equal to the concentration multiplied by the volume (area × thickness) (see above).

The basis of spectrophotometry is the Beer–Lambert law relating concentration to absorbance (extinction).

$$A = \log_{10} \frac{I_0}{I} = Kcl$$

I = intensity of transmitted light
I_0 = intensity of incident light
c = concentration of chromophore
l = path length of specimen (thickness)
K = constant for the chromophore at the particular wavelength

This equation is true for dilute homogeneous solutions but in histochemistry and cytochemistry the absorbance is not uniformly distributed over the area to be measured. This is overcome by using scanning and integrating systems (Barr and Stroud, G. N.: Vickers, M85). In these systems the area to be measured is broken up by optical means into a large number of regions, each region being measured separately. The results from these regions are summed giving the integrated absorption of the specimen.

The size of the region to be measured can be varied by using masks, the diameter of the spot being chosen to ensure that each region is always optically homogeneous.

Microdensitometry of heterogeneously distributed chromophores can be precise, the potential errors becoming small or negligible if the correct conditions for the cytochemical reactions and the correct operating procedures for the micro-densitometer are observed (Bitensky, 1980).

References

ABERCROMBIE, M. (1946). Estimation of nuclear population from microtome sections. *Anat. Rec.*, **94**, 239–247

AHERNE, W. A. and DUNNILL, M. S. (1982). In *Morphometry*. Edward Arnold, London

BARER, R. and JOSEPH, S. (1954). Refractometry of living cells. Part I. Basic principles. *Quart. J. Micr. Sci.*, **95**, 399–423

BARER, R. and JOSEPH, S. (1955a). Refractometry of living cells. Part II. The immersion medium. *Quart. J. Micr. Sci.*, **96**, 1–26

BARER, R. and JOSEPH, S. (1955b). Refractometry of living cells. Part III. Technical and optical methods. *Quart. J. Micr. Sci.*, **96**, 423–447

BITENSKY, L. (1980). Microdensitometry. In *Trends in Enzyme Histochemistry and Cytochemistry*. Ciba Foundation Symposium 73 (New Series). Excerpta Medica, Amsterdam, Oxford and New York, pp. 181–202

BUTCHER, R. G. (1971). The chemical determination of section thickness. *Histochemie*, **28**, 131–136

CLANCY, M. J. and HERLIHY, P. D. (1978). Assessment of changes in myofibre size in muscle. In *CEC Seminar on Patterns of Growth and Development in Cattle*. Eds de Boer, H. and Martin, J. Nyhoff, The Hague

DAVIES, M. H. F., CHAYEN, J. and LA COUR, L. F. (1954). The use of the interference microscope to determine dry mass in living cells and as a quantitative cytochemical method. *Quart. J. Micr. Sci.*, **95**, 271–304

DeHOFF, R. T. and RHINES, F. N. (1961). Determination of the number of particles per unit volume from measurements made on random plane sections: the general cylinder and ellipsoid. *Trans. Am. Inst. Min. Met. Eng.*, **221**, 975

DELESSE, A. (1847). Procédé mécanique pour déterminer la composition des roches (Extrait). *C. R. Acad. Sci. Paris*, **25**, 544

GALJAARD, H. (1967). Sources of error in the dry-mass concentration in tissue sections. *J. R. Micr. Soc.*, **87**, 157–164

GLIMSTEDT, G. and HAKANSSON, R. (1951). Measurement of thickness in various parts of histological sections. *Nature (Lond.)*, **167**, 397–398

HALE, A. J. (1958). *The Interference Microscope in Biological Research*. Livingstone, Edinburgh

HALLÉN, O. (1956). On the cutting and thickness determination of microscope sections. *Acta Anat.*, **16**, Suppl. 25

HOLBOROW, E. J. (Ed.) (1970). *Standardisation in Immunofluorescence*. Blackwell, Oxford

LANGE, P. W. and ENGSTROM, A. (1954). Determination of thickness of microscopic objects. *Lab. Invest.*, **3**, 116–131

MEIJER, A. E. F. H. (1972). Semipermeable membranes for improving the histochemical demonstration of enzyme activities in tissue sections. I: acid phosphatase. *Histochemie*, **30**, 31–39

PEARSE, A. D. and MARKS, R. (1976). Further studies on section thickness measurement. *Histochem. J.*, **8**, 383–386

ROST, F. W. D. (1980). Quantitative histochemistry. In *Histochemistry, Theoretical and Applied*. Ed. Pearse, A. G. E. 4th Ed. Vol. 1. Churchill-Livingstone, Edinburgh, London and New York

STOWARD, P. J. (1980). Criteria for the validation of quantitative histochemical enzyme techniques. In *Trends in Enzyme Histochemistry and Cytochemistry*. Ciba Foundation Symposium 73 (New Series). Excerpta Medica, Amsterdam, Oxford and New York, pp. 11–31

WEIBEL, E. R. and GOMEZ, D. M. (1962). A principle for counting tissue structures on random sections. *J. Appl. Physiol.*, **17**, 343–348

WEIBEL, E. R. and VIDONE, R. A. (1961). Fixation of the lung by formalin steam in a controlled state of air inflation. *Am. Rev. Resp. Dis.*, **84**, 856–861

WEID, G. L. (1966). *Introduction to Quantitative Cytochemistry*. Academic Press, New York and London

WEID, G. L. and BAHR, G. F. (1970). *Introduction to Quantitative Cytochemistry II*. Academic Press, New York and London

WRIGHT, B. M., SLAVIN, G., KREEL, L., CALLAN, K. and SANDIN, B. (1974). Post-mortem inflation and fixation of human lungs. *Thorax*, **29**, 189–194

29

Autoradiography

Autoradiography is a technique used to determine the presence, and to study the distribution, of radioactive isotopes in tissue. There are three principal areas in which the technique is useful.

(1) In studying the distribution of naturally occurring, or accidentally absorbed radioisotopes in plants and animals.
(2) In studying cells and organs known to have a specific affinity for substances which are deliberately labelled with particular isotopes, for example, tritiated thymidine in mitosing cells.
(3) In studying the fate and distribution of labelled organic substances such as hormones to give information on specific metabolic pathways.

The basis of these methods is to expose photographic emulsion to tissue containing the radioisotope for a sufficient period to allow the radioactivity to reduce the silver in the emulsion. Sites of activity are visualized through the photographic emulsion overlying the tissue. For good localization, section and emulsion must be in close contact. Although methods exist to preserve soluble substances by performing the entire process, from quenching tissue to exposure of the emulsion, at temperatures below 0 °C, autoradiography is usually performed on paraffin-wax sections.

The photographic process

Photographic emulsions are presented as a suspension of silver bromide crystals in gelatin. The silver bromide is sensitive to light, exposure causing a change in the crystal which, upon treatment with a suitable developer, results in the formation of grains of metallic silver. Emulsion, or film, which has been exposed, but not developed, is said to possess a 'latent image'.

It is a feature of photographic emulsions that the silver bromide crystals are not perfect, but contain defects which give the essential property of photosensitivity. The controlled production of these defects is an essential part of the manufacturing process. They are called 'sensitivity specks' and it is at these sites that a nucleus of metallic silver forms to catalyse the conversion of the entire crystal.

Silver bromide crystals which have not been activated during exposure are removed from the emulsion by fixative during the developing process, leaving a real image, formed in metallic silver, against a clear background.

It has for long been recognized that radioisotopes are able to activate silver bromide crystals in a similar manner to light. However, the specialized needs of this technique has led to the development of emulsions dedicated to this purpose. It is easy to imagine, for example, that the grain size of film used in popular photography would be too large to be of use in high resolution microscopy. The major photographic suppliers recognized the needs of autoradiography and developed special emulsions of uniform crystal size and sensitivity for this purpose termed nuclear emulsions.

Radioisotopes in autoradiography

Radioisotopes emit either α, β or γ radiation. β-Emitters are the most important tools in autoradiography. Three properties are important.

(1) The lifespan of the radioisotope

This may be measured in fractions of a second up to thousands of years; it is a process known as decay. The decay is uniform, following an exponential time scale and constant for any given isotope. The decay of an isotope is usually measured by its *half-life*, that is, the time taken for half of its radioactivity to disappear. Examples are given in *Table 29.1*.

Table 29.1

Isotope	Half-life	Maximum energy E_{max} (keV)	Range in emulsion (μm)
H^3 (tritium)	12.3 years	18	6
C^{14}	5568 years	155	120
P^{32}	14.5 days	1701	4000
S^{35}	87.1 days	167	140
Ca^{45}	164 days	255	220
I^{131}	8.05 days	608	1000

(Taken from Ruthmann, 1970.)

(2) The activity of the radioisotope

This is measured in Curies (abbreviated to Ci), 1 Curie being equivalent to 3.7×10^{10} disintegrations/second. In biological work, isotopes are used in a much smaller range of activities, either microcuries (1 μCi $= 3.7 \times 10^4$) or millicuries (1 mCi $= 3.7 \times 10^7$). The activity obviously varies according to the concentration of the radioisotope. In 1983, the EEC adopted the Becquerel (Bq) as the standard unit of radioactivity in Europe. One Becquerel is equal to one disintegration/second. Thus 1 mCi equals 37 MBq.

(3) The energy of the radioisotope

This factor is constant irrespective of concentration and will reflect, for example, the distance over which radiations from a radioisotope will travel. This is measured as the maximum energy (E_{max}) of the isotope.

Factors affecting the resolution of autoradiographs

Radioisotopes that emit high energy β particles produce silver grains further away from the source than do low energy emitters. The result is that the 'background' count of reduced silver is greater and the separation between sites of activity will become blurred (*Figure 29.1*). It is therefore desirable to select a radioisotope of lower energy when possible. It is fortunate that tritium, one of the most useful radioisotopes in biology, is very low in maximum energy (*Table 29.1*).

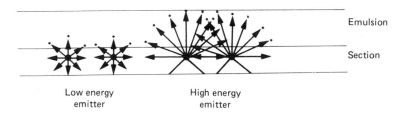

Low energy emitter   High energy emitter   Emulsion   Section

Figure 29.1 Diagram to show the absence of overlap between low energy emitters and the lack of discrimination between adjacent sources of high energy

The distance between the source and the emulsion must be kept to an absolute minimum. The slide dipping technique is superior to the film stripping technique (*see below*) in this respect. A gap between the source and the emulsion will not only reduce the chances of silver halide crystals being hit, but make the difference in distance of adjacent crystals from the source less significant, increasing the chances of their being hit. This factor is particularly important on those occasions when it is necessary to interpose a celloidin or polyvinylchloride layer between source and emulsion to prevent a direct chemical reaction between the two.

A thick section has the possibility of having several sources lying immediately below one another, or at least in close proximity when viewed from above. This will have the same disadvantage as trying to study the individual cell detail in a thick section of highly cellular tissue such as lymph node.

A similar effect can be produced by having too thick an emulsion. Grain density remains greatest immediately above the source, but the fall off in activated grains will not be as sharp as with a thinner emulsion. It should be possible to detect this artefact as the reduced silver grains will appear at deeper optical levels in the emulsion the further they are from the source (*Figure 29.2*).

As may be expected, large silver halide crystals in the emulsion will not give resolution as good as that obtained with smaller crystals. Not only may large crystals overlap, but the sensitivity speck discussed earlier in this chapter may be to one side of the crystal and its activation result in a metallic silver deposit out of line with the path of the emitted β radiation. The advent of autoradiographs for electron microscopy has led to the development of extremely small silver halide crystal emulsions. Conventional emulsions for autoradiography contain crystals of around 0.2 μm diameter, whilst those for electron microscopic autoradiography may be as small as 0.05 μm. As may also be expected, these smaller crystal sizes are achieved at the expense of some sensitivity.

Exposure times in autoradiography are usually measured in days or even weeks rather than seconds or minutes. Unfortunately, long exposure times lead to a decrease

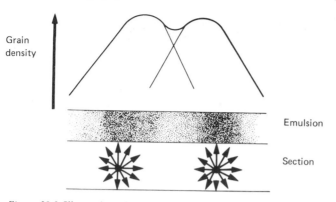

Grain
density

Emulsion

Section

Figure 29.2 Illustration of the difficulties of discriminating between sources as the emulsion thickness increases. (From Ruthman, 1970)

in resolution. Crystals lying immediately over the source may be hit more than once, but can only produce one silver grain. Therefore, with time, the density over the source cannot increase, but the density away from the source can as the chance of remote crystals being hit increases. Loss of resolution results.

Sensitivity of autoradiographs

This describes the efficiency of the system and may be summarized as the response of the emulsion relative to the number of radioactive disintegrations occurring in the source during exposure. It is easy to see that increasing sensitivity can sometimes impede resolution. Consider, for example, the following.

(1) Close proximity between section and emulsion gives good sensitivity and resolution.
(2) A thin source (section) gives good sensitivity and resolution.
(3) Few double hits give good sensitivity and resolution.

However, increasing the thickness of the emulsion will improve the sensitivity but reduce resolution.

Background contamination

The most obvious source of true contamination is the presence of light or an extraneous radioactive substance. Other causes may be rather more subtle. For example, silver halide grains may be activated by stress. Clumsy handling of unexposed film can result in fingerprints that are true images in metallic silver. More insidious is background resulting from the stress induced by drying the gelatin too quickly, usually because the emulsion is applied as too thin a coat or is too dilute when used in the dipping technique (*see below*). The inherently variable thickness of tissue sections may also give rise to spurious background during drying of the emulsion. For example, the thickness of a dewaxed section will fall to zero in the lumen of a blood vessel leading to stress in the overlying emulsion. Any line of developed silver grains which follows the natural contour of morphological structures should be interpreted with caution. The method by which emulsion is dried should be carefully chosen to avoid stress artefact. Liquid emulsion should be cooled to a temperature close to its setting point prior to application.

A background artefact peculiar to the stripping film technique (*see below*) results from the activation of silver bromide crystals by static electricity arising from the physical act of stripping the emulsion layer from its backing. This is reduced in a humid atmosphere, and if the film is very slowly 'stripped'.

Latent image fading

It has already been suggested that ionized particles hitting a silver halide crystal results in the deposition of minute particles of un-ionized silver which act as a catalyst and convert the entire crystal to metallic silver during development. High temperature, and the presence of water in the emulsion, encourage the sensitized specks of un-ionized silver to become ionized to silver bromide once more, destroying the latent image formed during exposure.

Chemography

Two opposite effects resulting from direct chemical reaction between tissue and emulsion are recognized. In positive chemography, reactive tissue groups (those with a reducing capability are obviously implicated) can produce a latent image in the silver halide. This is an unpredictable event, although more likely to occur in unfixed cryostat sections than in fixed and paraffin-wax processed tissue.

Negative chemography is the opposite effect, causing fading of the latent image. The regular, or anatomical, distribution of reactive groups can make this unpredictable artefact very difficult to interpret.

Macroautoradiographs

The whole body distribution of radioisotopes has achieved popularity in recent years, especially in toxicology. Usually, information is required on the relative distribution between organs of radioactively labelled compounds, with animals such as mice, rats and even rabbits being sectioned on special microtomes. As resolution is less critical in these procedures, β-emitters are required to activate larger grains of silver halide. X-ray film is employed because of the larger crystal diameter in the emulsion. However, X-ray film incorporates an additional layer of an anti-abrasive coating over the emulsion necessitating the use of high energy β-emitters to overcome the greater distances involved.

Techniques

General precautions

The interpretation of autoradiographs depends upon visualizing black 'specks' overlying tissue sections. It therefore follows that meticulous attention must be paid to cleanliness at all stages of the technique. Black specks of dust, perhaps easily recognizable as such in the haematoxylin and eosin sections, may be much more confusing in autoradiographs.

The usual precautions must be followed in the 'photographic' stages of the technique, that is, chemically clean glassware and distilled water should be used and metallic containers and instruments, such as forceps, should be avoided.

If quantification is to be attempted, the difficulties of producing sections of reproducible thickness should be borne in mind. Rogers (1979) suggests that paraffin sections may vary by up to 30% of stated thickness, and resin sections (1–2 μm) by up to 70% (*see* discussion on section thickness in Chapter 28). Standardized technique, a hard paraffin wax and, preferably, a motorized microtome help to produce uniformity.

Sections should be mounted on slides 'subbed' in gelatin according to the method described in Chapter 5.

Staining methods

A choice has to be made upon whether sections submitted to autoradiography are stained before or after this process. The advantages of prestaining are that in theory any staining procedure may be carried out without concern over the difficulties of penetrating an overlayer of emulsion. The disadvantages are that soluble substances may be lost in the staining process, it may interfere with the subsequent 'photographic' process (i.e. induce chemography—Celestine blue produces positive chemography) or the photographic process may affect the stain. Prestaining is not recommended unless controlled experiments have shown there is no loss of activity compared with post-staining.

Three problems arise with post-staining. The staining procedure may remove developed silver grains (unlikely), the photographic process may have altered reactive groups it is wished to demonstrate and the stain has to penetrate the emulsion layer to reach the tissue. There is the additional hazard that post-staining may detach the emulsion from the section. For most general morphological staining procedures, these disadvantages are more theoretical than real. However, care should be taken with the acid hydrolysis stage of the Feulgen reaction (Chapter 10), for example, and it is hazardous to risk heating resin sections to 60 °C when staining with toluidine blue.

For most purposes, it is sufficient to post-stain developed sections by haematoxylin alone, remembering that times need to be prolonged to take account of penetrating the emulsion layer. Methods which are contraindicated include the Feulgen reaction, PTAH, Alcian blue and resorcin–fuchsin. Flitney (1982) recommends soaking autoradiographs for 30 minutes in distilled water to soften the gelatin before staining. There is some controversy over whether autoradiographs should be dried before mounting in synthetic resin rather than dehydrating and clearing. We prefer the latter procedure.

■ Liquid emulsion 'dipping' technique (from Joftes and Warren, 1955)

This is the easier technique to perform and allows larger numbers of slides to be processed. It has the advantages of producing the closest contact between section and emulsion and thin emulsions of small crystal size can, if required, be prepared. The major drawback of this method is that emulsions cannot be guaranteed to be of uniform thickness. We have used Ilford K5 emulsion with consistent success but there are a range of emulsions available from both Ilford and Kodak and users are recommended to study the manufacturers' literature and make an appropriate choice.

If using high energy isotopes it is beneficial to coat the dewaxed section in celloidin, but with lower energy isotopes such as tritium or iodine[125] it is not recommended.

It is advisable to process several control sections which can be removed at intervals to test for adequate exposure. When a section shows optimum results, the remainder of the batch should have their exposure terminated.

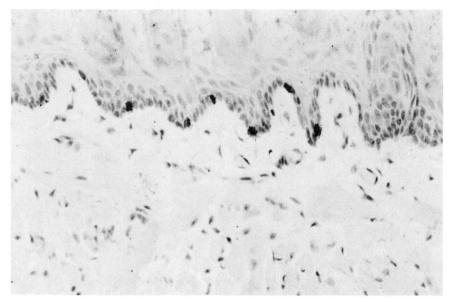

Figure 29.3 Autoradiograph showing tritiated thymidine reactivity confined to basal layer. Original magnification × 100

■ *Method*

(1) Thoroughly dewax sections and bring to water.

(2) If it is desired to prestain section (e.g. with haematoxylin), perform at this stage, wash well in distilled water and allow to dry.

(3) The following five stages should be performed in a darkroom: (a) With most emulsions, a safe-light may be used. Consult the manufacturers' literature to find a suitable filter. With K5, the Ilford 902 (light-brown) safe-light filter over a 15 watt bulb is appropriate. (b) Remove sufficient emulsion from the container for immediate use. (c) Do not remove the external wrapping from the manufacturers' container. (d) Melt the emulsion in a glass vessel in a water bath at 50 °C. (e) Stir *gently*, too much agitation will give rise to froth and air bubbles. The emulsion should not be kept at its melting point longer than a few minutes, and any unused solution must be discarded.

(4) For comparative work, a regimen must be carefully established and the details meticulously followed on each occasion. Dip the slide with section attached into the emulsion, leave for 2 seconds, remove, let drain for 2–3 seconds and stand vertically to dry (approximately 30 minutes). If thinner layers are required, the emulsion may be diluted with distilled water, glycerol or gelatin. Glycerol will reduce any stress induced background and gelatin is useful for isotopes of high activity when greater sensitivity can be achieved.

(5) Place the dry, coated slides in black plastic slide boxes and seal with black tape. If very high energy isotopes are used, the space between slides should be increased. Note the time and date and store in a refrigerator at 4 °C.

(6) Remove control slides at intervals and process. As a rough guide, 1 μCi/g of tissue requires about 20 days' exposure. Any high energy developer may be used. Ilford recommend Phenisol diluted 1 plus 4 with distilled water, Kodak recommend D72

or D19. Development time should be the shortest time necessary to achieve complete development. As a guide, the Ilford developer will take 5–15 minutes, and Kodak recommend 2–5 minutes with theirs.

(7) Treat with an acid stop bath. One per cent aqueous acetic acid for 1 minute is suitable.

(8) Fix in 30% aqueous sodium thiosulphate or a commercial fixative, for twice the time it takes the emulsion to clear. Rapid or hardening fixatives are not recommended as they are difficult to wash out.

(9) Wash in running tap-water for 15 minutes.

(10) Post-stain (assuming prestaining has not been carried out).

(11) Dehydrate, clear and mount in synthetic resin.

Results

Sites of radioactivity are shown by discrete black granules superimposed on the stained section.

■ Stripping film technique (after Pelc, 1947)

Special film bearing emulsion of predetermined thickness is supplied by the major manufacturers for this purpose. Kodak AR10 stripping film is suitable.

(1) In the darkroom, using the appropriate safe-light, score the special stripping film into oblongs with a scalpel. Remembering that the emulsion will spread on water, ensure the strips will be large enough to overlap at least two and preferably three sides of a microscope slide. Detach one corner of the strip and slowly peel from the backing plate. Hold vertically and allow the stripped film to fall face downwards onto the surface of a water-bath maintained at room temperature. Discard any cut strips that curl or crease.

(2) Immerse the slide in the water and pick up strip of emulsion so that it covers the section and overlaps at least two edges of the slide. A technique similar to that described in Chapter 5 for picking up sections is used.

(3) Stand the slide vertically to dry.

(4) Expose in a light-proof box as described for the dipping technique.

(5) Develop and stain as for the dipping technique.

The excellent textbook by Rogers (1979) is recommended further reading for those with an interest in this subject.

References

FLITNEY, F. W. (1982). In *Theory and Practice of Histological Techniques*. Eds Bancroft, J. D. and Stevens, A. Churchill-Livingstone, London

JOFTES, D. L. and WARREN, S. (1955). Simplified liquid emulsion radioautography. *J. Biol. Phot. Assoc.*, **23**, 145–150

PELC, S. R. (1947). Autoradiography technique. *Nature (Lond.)*, **160**, 749–750

ROGERS, A. W. (1979). *Techniques of Autoradiography*. 3rd Ed. Elsevier, Amsterdam

RUTHMANN, A. (1970). *Methods in Cell Research*. G. Bell & Sons, London

30

Micro-incineration

Micro-incineration, first described in 1833, is not likely ever to become a routine procedure because of the difficulty of interpreting results.

The technique is based on the preparation of parallel sections, one being incinerated, and the other stained by a routine method as a control. By this means mineral elements demonstrated in the incinerated section can be localized in the control section.

Micro-incineration has proved useful as a means of demonstrating silica in cases of silicosis of the lung. Examination of sections with the polarizing microscope before and after micro-incineration has, on occasions, resulted in a greater amount being revealed in the treated section.

Primary fixation and processing of the sections may present great difficulty since the methods employed should not detract from, or add to, the mineral content of the tissue. Aqueous fixatives are likely to dissolve certain minerals, and the use of fixing agents, such as mercuric chloride or chromic salts, may add to the mineral content: freeze-dried sections are ideal for this purpose. If the apparatus required for freeze-drying is not available, tissues should be fixed in 10% formalin in absolute alcohol, and transferred directly to fresh absolute alcohol before clearing and embedding in paraffin wax.

Technique

(1) Fix and process tissues as described above, and cut sections 3–5 μm in thickness.
(2) Float two adjacent sections on warm absolute alcohol to remove creases and transfer to clean slides. Dry in a 37 °C oven. Stain one section (the control) by the routine haematoxylin and eosin technique and treat the other section as follows.
(3) Flood with xylene for 1–2 minutes to remove wax.
(4) Transfer to absolute alcohol for 30–60 seconds.
(5) Drain off alcohol and allow the section to dry.
(6) Place the glass slide carrying the test section on to a quartz slide of equal size and inset it into a special muffle furnace (if a slide touches the sides of the oven it will crack).
(7) Raise the temperature of the oven slowly, reaching 100 °C during the first 10 minutes. During the next 25 minutes, slowly raise the temperature to 650 °C (the oven should be red-hot during the last few minutes). Switch off oven.
(8) When the slides have cooled, but before they are cold, remove them from the oven with previously heated forceps (to avoid cracking) and transfer them to a sheet of asbestos.
(9) Cover the incinerated section with a No. 1 coverslip using great care not to disturb

the tissue ash. The coverslip, which is to protect the section and prevent moisture being absorbed from the air, is then ringed with paraffin wax or cement. For most purposes, no mounting medium is used. However, glycerin may be applied if not contraindicated by subsequent examination.

(10) The section is examined by the methods described below, in parallel with the control stained by haematoxylin and eosin.

Fenton, Johnson and Zimmerman (1964) have described a method of micro-incineration that does not call for a muffle furnace and is quite satisfactory for most purposes.

(1) Mount sections on glass slides that will not break on heating.
(2) Place slide on asbestos, or similar heat resisting board. Heat directly with blue Bunsen burner flame. Direct the flame downwards onto the section. It will turn brown, then white before almost disappearing.
(3) Cover slide with metal utensil that will rest on the asbestos board around the section. This will help ensure slow cooling of the slide.

Methods of examination of section ash

The recognition and identification of minerals in these sections require a great deal of experience, and even then positive identification is not always possible. The following techniques may be employed:

(1) The use of low-power objectives with *oblique light* to determine the disposition and colour of deposits may be helpful.
(2) Birefringent (anisotropic) minerals rotate the plane of polarized light (e.g. silica) under polarizing microscopy.

Some minerals have a characteristic colour and appearance under dark ground illumination; for example, calcium and magnesium form a dense white ash.

Various chemical tests can be applied; for example, the formation of gypsum crystals by calcium as a result of treatment with 3% sulphuric acid.

Sections may be pretreated chemically to assist in the identification of specific elements; for example, treatment with hydrogen sulphide will convert lead to lead sulphide, which has a characteristic colour and appearance.

Some minerals are fluorescent and these show characteristic colours when examined by fluorescent microscopy.

Reference

FENTON, R. H., JOHNSON, F. B. and ZIMMERMAN, E. (1964). The combined use of microincineration and the Prussian blue reaction for a more sensitive histochemical demonstration of iron. *J. Histochem. Cytochem.*, **12**, 153–155

31

Museum technique

Preparation, colour maintenance, fixation and storage of specimens

The mounting of pathological specimens in Perspex containers, for long regarded as the prerogative of the larger teaching hospitals, is now becoming commonplace in many of the smaller hospitals.

Even small museums, in addition to their teaching value, play a part in recording the history of medicine, since the common diseases of today may well be the rarities of tomorrow. To fulfil such a purpose it is essential that the original shape and colour of such specimens is retained and that accurate records of the patient's medical history and, if possible, relevant photographs and radiographs, are readily available. The presentation, labelling and cataloguing are of equal importance. Lack of interest in a museum can almost always be traced to poor presentation and documentation of specimens: nothing is more uninteresting than a large number of dirty, badly labelled specimens crowded into a series of cupboards.

Preparation of the specimen

Good museum specimens are generally only obtained and preserved by care and planning at the time of autopsy, and careful treatment after removal. Indiscriminate examination of organs in the post-mortem room, and the careless removal of sections for histological examination can easily ruin a potentially valuable specimen.

Cut surfaces should be smooth and even and this is achieved by using a continuous stroke with a long-bladed, sharp knife. The usual type of brain knife may be used, but a butcher's knife with a 14-inch blade is preferred because even large organs may be cut with one long stroke; also, such knives are usually much cheaper than brain knives.

Tissue for histological examination should either be taken from the back of specimens intended for preservation, or neatly removed from the front with a scalpel so that when stained slides accompany the specimen their position in relation to the rest of the specimen can easily be seen.

Specimens should be put into a fixative almost immediately. If the specimen is allowed to dry, a permanent darkening will result.

Specimens from the operating theatre will, if properly treated, provide the best museum specimens, and containers with formal–saline should always be readily available to theatre staff.

Methods of colour maintenance

The fixing fluid to be used will depend on the technique employed, but 10% formal–saline can always be used for primary fixation and the specimen transferred to a special fixative afterwards.

The technique most widely used, and still by far the best available, is a modification of the method described by Kaiserling (1900).

The original technique employed three solutions: the first for fixing, the second for restoring colour and the third a mounting fluid in which the colour should be maintained. Pulvertaft (1936) described a method of restoring colour to tissues by the addition of a reducing agent (sodium hydrosulphite) to the mounting medium. The original specimens mounted by Pulvertaft's technique show remarkably little fading even after 35 years.

■ Pulvertaft–Kaiserling method

Solutions

(1) Kaiserling's fluid I—fixing fluid

Formalin	400 ml
Potassium nitrate	30 g
Potassium acetate	60 g
Tap-water	to 2000 ml

Specimens may be transferred to this fluid after fixation in formal–saline, or they may be directly fixed in it.

(2) Kaiserling's fluid II

80% Ethyl alcohol

This fluid may be used to restore colour in an emergency (e.g. for colour photography) but it is not necessary when using a sodium hydrosulphite mounting fluid. If colour is restored with 80% alcohol the time should be carefully controlled, since once the full colour has been restored (30 minutes–4 hours, depending on the size of the specimen), continued immersion in alcohol has a permanent bleaching effect and the colour so lost is not afterwards restored by the mounting fluid.

(3) Pulvertaft–Kaiserling mounting fluid III

Glycerin	300 ml
Sodium acetate	100 g
Formalin	5 ml
Tap-water	to 1000 ml

Sodium hydrosulphite, 0.4%, is added immediately before sealing the jar.

Dissolve the sodium acetate in warm tap-water, add the glycerin and formalin, and make up the volume with cold tap-water. If the reaction is more acid than pH 8, a few drops of N/1 sodium hydroxide should be added.

If the solution is not crystal clear it should be filtered through a paper pulp filter. Cloudiness of the solution is usually due to impurities in the sodium acetate. On rare occasions, simple filtration will fail to produce the desired clarity, in which case 30 ml of a saturated solution of camphor in alcohol should be added to 1 litre of the solution; refilter as before.

The use of camphor will always produce a fluid of sparkling clarity, but the overwhelming smell of camphor in the curator's room is a decided disadvantage.

Israel and Young (1978) used pure liquid paraffin as the final mountant after colour restoration with alcohol. This procedure reduces discoloration of the mounting fluid by pigments in the specimen (*see* Iodine technique *below*).

■ Wentworth methods (1938, 1939, 1942, 1957)

In a series of papers Wentworth described modifications of the Pulvertaft method which dispensed with the alcohol step for colour restoration, using only sodium hydrosulphite, and omitted glycerol from the final mountant (because of wartime scarcity).

■ The 1957 method

Solutions

(1) Liq. formaldehyde (40%)   100 ml
    Sodium acetate   40 g
    Water   1000 ml

(2) Liq. formaldehyde (40%)   10 ml
    Sodium acetate   40 g
    Sodium phosphate tribasic $Na_3PO_4 . 12 H_2O$ 1 g
    Water   1000 ml
    This fluid will have a pH of about 9.5

(3) Liq. formaldehyde (40%)   10 ml
    Sodium acetate   100 g
    Sodium phosphate Na_2HPO_4 1 g
    Glycerin   200 ml
    Water   1000 ml
    This will have a pH of about 7.5

Method

Thorough fixation is required for at least 1 month in solution (1).

When ready to mount, the pH of the fluid is determined. If the pH is greater than 6.5 or the specimen contains fat, the specimen is placed directly into solution (3). If the pH is less than 6.5 the specimen is placed in solution (2), which has a pH of 9.5, and should remain there, changing the fluid regularly, until the pH remains constant, at least 8.5.

The specimen is placed in solution (3) and the pH checked after a few days. If it is at least pH 7.5 the specimen is mounted in fresh solution (3) to which is added sodium hydrosulphite in the proportion of 3 g/1000 g of specimen immediately before sealing.

■ Schultz's carbon monoxide technique (1931)

The Schultz method employs carbon monoxide to convert haemoglobin into the more stable compound carboxyhaemoglobin. It has two main disadvantages:

(1) the colours are unrealistic; and
(2) there is a danger of explosion during processing. There is no place for this technique in modern museum practice. The method is given for historical interest.

The technique, based on Kaiserling's method, is as follows.

(1) Bubble carbon monoxide (or coal gas) through Kaiserling's fixing fluid I containing the fixed specimen. This stage must be carried out in a fume cupboard with a good draught.
(2) When the specimen shows the characteristic colour change it is mounted in Pulvertaft–Kaiserling fluid (without the addition of sodium hydrosulphite) which has been saturated with carbon monoxide.

Fixation of specimens

Certain additional rules should be observed in the fixing of museum specimens:

(1) To ensure adequate fixation, specimens should always be injected with fixative if this is possible. Whole brains *must* be fixed in this manner by injection into the basilar artery, after first washing through with saline solution to remove the blood. After injection of the fixative, the basilar artery is tied off with a long length of linen thread; the brain is then transferred to a bucket containing fixative and suspended by the thread from a glass or wooden rod laid over the top of the bucket so that the brain (which almost floats) remains suspended in the centre of the fixing fluid. Lungs, whole limbs and kidneys are more easily and speedily fixed by injection.
(2) Specimens containing much blood must not be washed in water at any time, either before or after fixation. If excess blood or mucus is to be removed, the specimen should be washed in saline solution or formal–saline. *Figure 31.1* shows two halves of a fixed kidney, one washed in saline solution and the other in running tap-water. The half washed in water is gelatinous and in ordinary light is almost completely obscured by haemolysis.
(3) Fresh specimens should lie on a thick layer of cotton wool covered by lint since contact with the container may alter their contours.
(4) The specimen, together with its attached structures, must be fixed so that it is in the position in which it is to be finally displayed. Membranes, skin, intestine and so on may be pinned to cork boards which are then floated (specimen downwards) on the fixing fluid; the pins used must be rustless (glass or stainless steel) to avoid marking the specimen.
(5) Cystic cavities, if unopened, are inflated with fixative; or if opened are packed with cotton wool soaked in fixative so as to maintain their natural shape.
(6) Bile-stained or bile-containing specimens must be fixed and stored separately or they will stain other specimens.

Storage of specimens

The storage of potential display specimens forms an important part of museum technique since the supply of these specimens usually exceeds the number actually mounted, the latter being governed by the type of specimens currently required, the space available for display and the technical assistance to mount them.

The method of storage must permit easy and certain identification of each specimen. A reference book should be kept to record necessary details of the specimens. The specimens should be stored in separate containers to avoid damage which may be

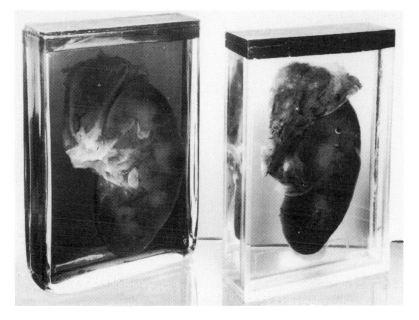

Figure 31.1 Two halves of the same kidney. The half shown on the left was washed overnight in running water after fixation, following which both specimens were mounted in routine mounting fluid. Note the haemolysis in the specimen shown on the left (by courtesy of the Editor of the *Journal of clinical Pathology*)

caused by contact with other specimens. The containers should be adequately labelled on the outside and a label should be tied to the specimen with linen thread.

Mounting of museum specimens

When specimens are brought from storage they will usually require some final attention before being actually mounted.

Slight irregularities may have developed in the surface of the specimen during fixation and it may need to be recut. In such cases, only a minimum amount of tissue should be removed since, owing to the uneven penetration of the fixative, the removal of a thick slice will reveal a surface which recolours in a concentric pattern of differing shades.

If specimens of membranes, skin or intestine have been pinned out on cork boards, the outer edges will require trimming.

If, after the removal of cotton-wool packing from cavities, the specimen will not remain in a natural position by normal mounting methods, such cavities should be filled with arsenious acid–gelatin*. Unopened cysts and cavities may, if thin-walled,

---

* *Arsenious acid–gelatin*—Boil 20 g of arsenious acid in 1 litre of water, using a reflux condenser, for at least 2 hours. Cool the solution, make up the volume to 1 litre and add 120 g of gelatin. Dissolve the gelatin by steaming for 1–2 hours, and filter while hot through chardin filter paper, or sand and paper pulp. Add 100 ml of glycerin.

To render the gelatin almost colourless, add 0.5% Victoria blue (or 1% methylene blue) drop by drop until the bulk is faintly blue, but appears colourless in a $6 \times \frac{5}{8}$ inch test tube. Bottle and store in the dark.

Add 0.5% formalin before use: this converts the gelatin to an irreversible gel.

need to be supported by the injection of gelatin, after removal of injected fixative.

Coloured Perspex arrows or rods may be used to identify anatomical details. A loop of black horse hair may be used in the same way for delicate structures.

Specimens which are particularly friable may be covered with a thin layer of arsenious acid–gelatin, and it may also be used locally to hold fragments such as blood clot in position.

Bile-stained specimens will colour the mounting fluid for some time after mounting. It has been suggested that the soaking of specimens in a saturated solution of calcium chloride for 24 hours will obviate discoloration. Although this reduces the degree of colouring, it will not prevent it and frequent changes of fluid are necessary to keep the discoloration of fluid at a minimum.

Museum jars or boxes

Perspex boxes are used almost universally today, and the technique described will be that which applies to their use. Methods of mounting in other containers are described at the end of the chapter.

Perspex boxes are available commercially, or may be made in the laboratory. The prices of commercially-made boxes may appear to be high, but it will generally be found that if the cost of Perspex sheeting and labour is estimated, laboratory-made boxes are quite often more expensive. The method employed commercially to join the sides is far superior to the cementing process described below, and gives the boxes a much longer life. Early boxes now show a whitening of the joints which eventually give way, and this has been shown to be due to a breakdown of the cement used.

For the benefit of those who prefer to make their own boxes, however, the technique described below has the advantage that such boxes may be designed to fit each specimen exactly.

Perspex boxes may be made quite simply by cutting four sides, a top and a bottom from Perspex sheeting and cementing them together with Perspex cement. An alternative and better method is to bend a strip of Perspex to form the top and sides of the box. This is done as follows.

There are several methods of heating a Perspex strip for bending. A simple one is to use a finely drawn Pasteur pipette as a gas jet and draw it across the Perspex strip on both sides at the desired place. An alternative is to use two copper rod heating elements connected with a transformer so as to pass a high current of 700 amp at $\frac{1}{2}$ V. This heats the Perspex to a state of flexibility in about 5 minutes, when it may be bent to any angle. A framework is used to ensure that the angle is square, and the Perspex is then held or clamped in this position until cold.

Bend a rectangular strip of 3 mm Perspex at right-angles at two points to form the top and sides of the box, and trim the edges accurately with a circular saw. Soak one edge in ethylene dichloride or chloroform for 10 minutes by propping the strip on three pieces of fine wire or nylon thread laid on a glass slab and run chloroform or ethylene dichloride around the lower edge to form a pool of the fluid. When the edge is softened it is applied to a roughly cut sheet of 3 mm Perspex to form one face of the box, gentle pressure being applied by weights. In 10–15 minutes the joint is firm enough to permit manipulation; the other face is cemented by the same process. Weights up to 6 kg should then be applied and left overnight. On the following day the face edges are cut off, flush with the sides of the box, sandpapered and polished on the buffing machine. The bottom of the box is sawn, squared and sandpapered, leaving an even rim to which the base is fixed. A rectangular slab of 6 mm Perspex is cut and polished to form a base, and a 3 mm hole is bored in it through which the box can finally be filled with mounting fluid.

Mounting of specimens

The specimens should be laid on a flat, waterproof (preferably formica covered) bench. The position in which they are to be mounted is decided upon, and this should, as far as possible, be anatomically correct to enable students to recognize the various structures. The specimen is then measured, allowing a 1 cm clearance at the top and sides and 2 cm at the bottom. The extra clearance at the bottom is to enable a label to be fitted without obscuring part of the specimen. The depth of the specimen is measured, and approximately 5 mm added for the centre plate. A suitable box is then taken from stock, ordered or made.

Centre plates

One of the great advantages of mounting in Perspex is its flexibility when heated, since it can be moulded or bent to satisfy the requirements of individual specimens. In spite of this fact, however, it has been found that the great majority of specimens may be simply stitched to a flat sheet of Perspex which just fits into the box with about 5 mm clearance at the top (the centre plate). Commercial boxes may be obtained already fitted with centre plates.

Coloured opaque Perspex centre plates may be used to enhance the colour of the specimen or to enable specimens to be attached to both sides.

Special methods of mounting are dealt with later in the chapter.

Attaching specimens to centre plate

The specimen is arranged in the desired position, and crosses are made on the centre plate with a scribe where stitches are to be placed. With solid specimens the number of stitches will depend on the weight and consistency of the tissue: for example, half a kidney is adequately supported with a stitch at each pole. Hollow or cystic organs, or organs with attached structures, may require stitches to hold the specimen in the correct position in addition to providing support: for example, the oesophagus and stomach may require up to 12 stitches. Attached structures may need to be stitched to the main organ or to each other to hold them in position. Stitches must not be placed through pathological lesions if this is avoidable.

When the centre plate has been marked, holes, 1–2 mm in diameter, are drilled at those points. If linen thread with a glass bead is to be used, one hole is drilled at each point; if nylon thread, two holes, 1 mm in diameter, are necessary. Nylon thread has the advantage of being almost unbreakable, but is so hard it tends, in time, to cut through specimens and for this reason linen thread may be preferred. Lengths of linen thread are cut and a small clear glass bead is threaded on and tied in the centre; the bead should be slightly larger than the hole in the centre plate since it acts as a retainer for the tie.

The centre plate is thoroughly washed in a detergent, and dried on a fluffless cloth. The specimen is stitched on by passing first one end of a tie and then the other through the centre plate and the specimen, pulling on both ends until the glass bead is tight against the centre plate. The threads should emerge from the specimen about 1 cm apart, so as to form a V of tissue on which to tie. A reef knot is tied with sufficient tension to cut slightly into the tissue, so that with the ends cut the knot is hardly discernible.

With soft tissue, such as brain, 1 cm squares of celluloid, in which two holes have been made, are threaded on to the ties on top of the tissue; the knot is then made on the celluloid to avoid cutting the tissue, and it should be made as a simple reef knot, except that instead of passing the left thread over the right once, it is passed over twice, then pulled tight and finished by passing the right thread over the left. Such a knot gives a tight tie which will not slip, and must always be used with nylon thread which will otherwise become loose.

An alternative method of attaching soft tissue to the centre plate is to cement spikes of Perspex, made from Perspex rod, to the centre plate in suitable positions, then press the specimen on to the spikes. On slipping the centre plate into the box the specimen will be retained in position.

Fixing the centre plate

The centre plate, with specimen attached, is put into the box, and marks are made with a grease pencil if 'stops' are required to hold the centre plate in position. If the box is of the correct depth there will be no movement of the specimen, but if a deeper box has been used (as for a thin membrane) two rectangles of 3 mm Perspex measuring 5 mm square, with polished edges, are cemented to the wall of the box to keep the centre plate in position. These 'stops' may be used to hold centre plates that have been bent in any desired position.

Filling and sealing

When the specimen is in position, museum fluid, to which 0.4% sodium hydrosulphite has been added, is run in to within 1 cm of the top. Air bubbles trapped between the specimen and centre plate are released with a broad-bladed spatula.

A hole, 3 mm in diameter, is drilled in one corner of the lid, though which is introduced the remaining mounting fluid.

The top of the box is wiped dry and Perspex cement applied with a Pasteur pipette; ethylene dichloride may be used in place of Perspex cement. After 30 seconds the lid is laid lightly in position, surplus Perspex cement being carefully removed. After a further 30 seconds, a lead weight is applied and left for at least 1 hour, preferably 2–3 hours. A short length of Perspex rod, 3 mm in diameter, is tapped lightly into the hole in the lid and the specimen left for 24–48 hours to remove residual air bubbles. The Perspex plug is removed, and the box filled with museum fluid by means of a Pasteur pipette. When the last bubble is removed, the Perspex plug is replaced and tapped firmly into position and, when dried, a small amount of Perspex cement is applied.

It will be found that large specimens develop air bubbles over a period of 2–3 weeks after mounting; these may be removed by drilling a fresh hole, filling up and replugging, but it is advisable to wait 2–3 months before removing this residual air.

An alternative method is to tap the hole and plug it with a nylon screw. This allows the fluid to be easily changed avoiding the necessity of drilling further holes.

The screw may be on either the top or the bottom of the box. If on the bottom, Perspex feet should be cemented in place in order to give clearance for the head of the screw.

Mounting in glass jars

Specimens may be mounted in glass jars on Perspex centre plates, as described above, or on glass centre plates if the mounting medium dissolves Perspex (e.g. Spalteholz fluid). The specimens are mounted as described above except that holes are drilled with an engraver's tool (a metal rod with a diamond-shaped end) in a hand drill, using camphor dissolved in turpentine as a lubricant. When drilling such holes the glass sheet must be on an absolutely flat surface. An alternative but inferior method of holding the specimen is to bend glass rod to form a frame which just fits into the jar, the specimen then being stitched to the frame.

Glass jars are sealed with an asphaltum–rubber compound (Picein) which must be applied to a perfectly dry ground-glass surface. It is best to wash the empty jar, dry it thoroughly with a cloth and then gently apply a Bunsen burner flame to the ground-glass edges until they turn white. One edge of the Picein should then be warmed in the flame and scraped along the edge of the jar until there is an even amount all round. Flame with a Bunsen burner until the Picein runs and completely covers the ground edge, but does not run over the edge. Place the specimen in the jar and fill with mounting fluid to within 1 cm of the top; if glass jars are completely filled they will crack with atmospheric changes. Hold the lid in a pair of forceps, heat it and the Picein on the jar gently with a Bunsen burner, then press the lid firmly into position on top of the jar with a cloth. When set remove the excess Picein with a hot knife. These jars look neater if, after sealing, the edges are painted with black enamel or asphaltum varnish.

Gelatin embedding

Delicate or intricate structures (e.g. the circle of Willis) which are difficult if not impossible to stitch, may be embedded in a thin layer of arsenious acid–gelatin on a centre plate, and then mounted by the routine method. A trough is formed by applying Sellotape around the edge of the centre plate to a depth of 0.1–1 cm and filled with gelatin. The Sellotape is removed after the gelatin has set. Although after 4–5 years this layer tends to become detached from the centre plate, it is so easily replaced that the method is worthwhile.

Specimens may be mounted in a solid block of gelatin by fixing the specimen in position with a thin layer on one surface of the jar. When this layer is set, the jar is filled to within 1 cm of the top with gelatin, which is allowed to set before the top is affixed. This method was popular with glass containers since they were easily broken and the gelatin protected the specimen and avoided the sudden release of a glycerin solution. It has the disadvantage that the gelatin tends to become yellow with age, and also to undergo liquefaction with the resultant formation of air bubbles. The durability of Perspex boxes offers most of the advantages of the old method of gelatin embedding without its disadvantages.

Embedding in solid plastic blocks

Embedding in a solid block of plastic would appear to offer the ideal method of presenting museum specimens, but unfortunately there is as yet no method available which preserves the colour of soft tissues. Such methods while adequate for hard tissues (certain insects, plants and so on) are useless for the normal pathological museum specimen.

Special methods

Macerated specimens of bones

Cutting the surface

Macerated specimens of bones, like all others, should have a clean-cut even surface. This is best achieved by cutting the specimen on a circular saw or a band-saw, by which method slices as thin as 3 mm may be cut. The specimens are easiest to cut if they have been frozen hard in a deep-freeze cabinet before cutting, since the soft tissue then has a similar consistency to the bone. Specimens of soft tissue may also be cut into thin even slices by the freezing technique.

Maceration

Maceration is used to demonstrate bony lesions, such as are produced by osteogenic sarcomas, osteomas and the effects of chronic osteomyelitis and tuberculosis.

The technique employed will depend, to a degree, on the type of lesion present. The finer spicules of bone in an osteogenic sarcoma are easily damaged or dissolved, whereas an osteoma will withstand comparatively harsh treatment.

The method which will preserve even the finest spicules of bone is that of putrefaction, where the bone and soft tissue is put into a tank of water and left for several months, but this method is almost completely impracticable owing to the nauseating smell.

As a routine method, the specimen, after trimming off the excess soft tissues, may be boiled in tap-water or very dilute (N/100) sodium hydroxide. At intervals during the boiling, the bone is removed from the fluid and the softened tissue removed with forceps, care being taken not to damage the specimen.

A gross method for hard compact bone is autoclaving in N/10 sodium hydroxide for 5 minutes. This will effectively remove all the soft tissue, but will also remove the fine spicules of bone.

Degreasing and bleaching

Following removal of the soft tissue by one of the methods described above, any fat is removed by immersion of the bone in chloroform for 3–4 hours. Specimens are then dried in an incubator and bleached in hydrogen peroxide.

Mounting

Macerated bones are mounted dry, either on a centre plate as described for routine mounting, or with Perspex supports designed for individual specimens (*Figure 31.2*). When tied to a centre plate, nylon thread should be used, employing a double knot; a drop of Perspex cement should be applied to the knot and to places where the specimen touches the centre plate to give added support to the specimen.

Calculi

Calculi are often presented by either (a) dry mounting in boxes with removable glass lids or (b) mounting in gelatin to which formalin has been added. The disadvantages of these older methods are that in the former the specimens became very dirty and in the

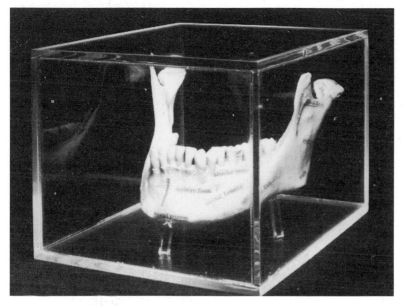

Figure 31.2 Method of mounting dry specimens (by courtesy of the Editor of the *Journal of clinical Pathology*)

latter the gelatin slowly dissolved. Several methods were tried in an endeavour to meet the following requirements.

(1) Laminations must show clearly.
(2) It should be possible to see both surfaces of the calculus.
(3) Variants of one particular type should be mounted together to allow of easy comparison, and the method of labelling should be such that the observer's knowledge can be tested.
(4) Containers should be dust-proof.
(5) Students should be able to handle the specimens.

It was obvious that the last two conditions would be the most difficult to satisfy with any one method; it was decided, therefore, to utilize both halves of calculi by polishing and mounting one half and labelling the other half with Indian ink, the latter being kept for students to handle and study more closely at lectures.

The polished specimens are cemented halfway through a sheet of Perspex which, in turn, is cemented into the box, thus ensuring a minimum of disturbance. The stencilling is done on a sandpapered rectangle (*Figure 31.3*).

Technique

(1) Stones are cut in halves with a fine fretsaw, or coping saw, and the cut surfaces polished with sandpaper, using grade 1 at first and then grade 0. The polishing may be completed on a fine oil stone, but this is not usually necessary.
(2) The calculi are assembled in their appropriate groups, and the size of the museum jar decided upon, allowance being made for a label under each specimen.

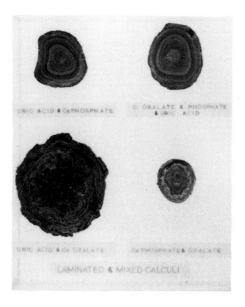

URIC ACID & CaPHOSPHATE

C OXALATE & PHOSPHATE & URIC ACID

URIC ACID & Cc OXALATE

CaPHOSPHATE & OXALATE

LAMINATED & MIXED CALCULI

Figure 31.3 Method of mounting cut and polished calculi. Although the wording can be seen it is sufficiently obscured to test the observer's knowledge

(3) A centre plate of 3 mm clear Perspex sheeting is cut to fit exactly the inside of the museum jar, and the edges are polished.

(4) The stones are arranged on the centre plate and the outlines of the stones, and rectangles for the labels, drawn with a metal scribe.

(5) The outline of each stone is cut round with an 'Amprofile' in a hacksaw frame, and filed until the stones fit tightly when pressed halfway through.

(6) The label rectangles are sandpapered to give a ground glass appearance on both sides of the Perspex the scribed line giving a clean edge, a metal shield being used to protect the remainder of the Perspex. The object of preparing both sides of the Perspex is merely to prevent the stencilled label from being seen too easily from the front. The metal shield is easily made from a piece of tin cut to an appropriate shape.

(7) The museum number or details of the composition of the calculi are stencilled on to the rectangle (*Figure 31.3*).

(8) The stones are pressed gently into position and cement applied to the edge of the centre plate touching the calculi.

(9) The cement is allowed to harden overnight, having been covered to keep the specimen free from dust.

(10) On the following day the centre plate is placed in a museum jar with the cut surface of the stones tight to the face of the jar. Being a close fit, one drop of cement halfway down each side of the centre plate is sufficient to hold it firmly in place.

(11) The lid of the museum jar is cemented on in the usual manner and allowed to stand with a light weight on it for 1–2 hours.

An alternative method is to mount calculi in a Perspex box, the back and sides of which should be black. The cut surface of one half, and the outer surface of the other are secured to the bottom with Perspex cement so as to show both surfaces from above.

Transparent specimens

The techniques used in the preparation of transparent specimens are dependent on the replacement of the tissue fluids by fluids of a higher refractive index.

Such techniques are usually employed to demonstrate either the bones of embryos or circulatory systems (*Figures 31.4* and *31.5*).

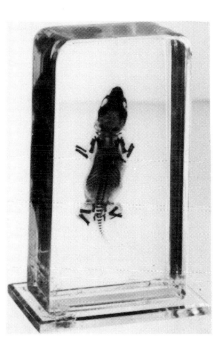

Figure 31.4 Mouse embryo treated by Dawson's alizarin technique (by courtesy of the Editor of the *Journal of clinical Pathology*)

■ Dawson's technique (1926)

Dawson's technique is excellent for the demonstration of bone in embryos or small animals, and depends on clearing the soft tissues in potassium hydroxide, the staining of bone with alizarin and the replacement of body fluids with glycerin.

Method

(1) Fix embryos, or small animals, in 95% alcohol for 48–72 hours. Prolonged fixation in alcohol renders the tissues less liable to maceration in the caustic potash solutions.

(2) In specimens prepared by this method, any fat present is partially saponified and appears in the cleared material as opaque white masses. Therefore extract fat immediately after fixation by treatment in acetone for 2–4 days. Return the specimen to 95% alcohol for 12–24 hours.

(3) Place the tissue in 1% potassium hydroxide until the bones are clearly visible through the muscle. Transfer to a solution of 0.1% alizarin red S in 1% potassium hydroxide.

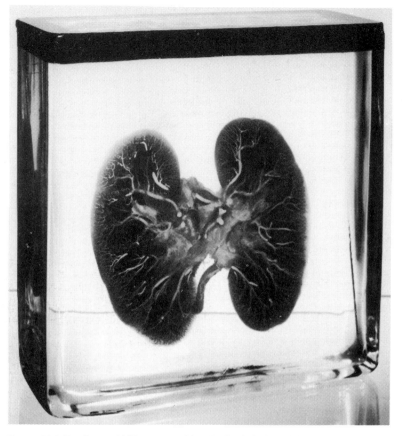

Figure 31.5 Specimen of kidney treated by the Spalteholz technique after injection of chrome yellow in gelatin (by courtesy of the Editor of the *Journal of clinical Pathology*)

(4) Leave the specimens in the alizarin red S solution until the bones are stained the desired colour. If the dye is absorbed from the solution before the maximum intensity is obtained the specimen can be transferred to a fresh solution of stain. If clearing in the initial caustic potash solution has progressed to the proper stage, nothing but the bone will take up the stain. If the clearing was not complete the muscles and other tissues take up the stain almost as readily as the bone itself.

(5) Following the staining, place the tissues in the following fluid:

Potassium hydroxide	1 g
Distilled water	79 ml
Glycerin	20 ml

(6) When properly cleared the tissues are passed through increasing concentrations of glycerin and finally stored and mounted in pure glycerin (*Figure 31.4*).

■ Spalteholz technique (1911)

This technique, which completely clears the soft tissues, is excellent for the demonstration of the circulatory system after injection with coloured pigments. Its success depends on the complete dehydration of the specimen with graded alcohols, and replacement of the tissue fluids with benzyl benzoate and oil of wintergreen.

Method

(1) Fix specimens in 10% formal–saline.
(2) Bleach in 10 vol. hydrogen peroxide for 1–2 days.
(3) Transfer to 50% alcohol for 14 days, followed by immersion in 60, 70, 80 and 90% alcohol, each for 14 days.
(4) Transfer to absolute alcohol for 14 days.
(5) Transfer to fresh absolute alcohol with a layer of anhydrous copper sulphate at the bottom of the container covered with five layers of filter paper, for a further 14 days.
(6) Transfer to benzene for 14 days.
(7) Transfer to fresh xylene for a further 14 days.
(8) Transfer to benzyl benzoate for 14 days.
(9) Transfer to fresh benzyl benzoate for a further 14 days.
(10) Mount in a mixture of equal parts of benzyl benzoate and oil of wintergreen. If the specimen is not completely clear at this stage it should be left in this fluid until clearing is completed.

Since the mounting fluid is a Perspex solvent, the specimens must be mounted in glass museum jars, and Spalteholz cement used to seal the lid.

Spalteholz cement

Powdered gum arabic	50 g
Sugar	50 g
Sodium silicate (waterglass)	2 g
Formalin	1 ml

All the ingredients are mixed into a paste with as little water as possible.

The specimen, fixed on a glass centre plate or frame, is placed in the jar which is filled with mounting fluid to within $\frac{1}{2}$ inch of the top. Dry the top of the jar and apply the cement evenly to the ground-glass edge. Place the lid in position and apply pressure with a lead weight. Leave undisturbed for 24–48 hours. (The specimen shown in *Figure 31.5* was injected with 5% gelatin containing finely ground chrome yellow.)

Amyloid

Amyloid degeneration may be stained deep brown with iodine, or bright red with Congo red.

■ Iodine technique

Method

(1) Place slices of formal-fixed tissue in Lugol's iodine to which 1% sulphuric acid has been added; leave for 1–2 hours.
(2) Wash in running water overnight.
(3) Mount in liquid paraffin. The colour will fade in ordinary mounting fluid.

■ Congo red technique

Method

(1) Place slices of formal-fixed tissue in 1% Congo red for 1 hour.
(2) Transfer to a saturated aqueous solution of lithium carbonate for 2 minutes.
(3) Differentiate in 80% alcohol until only the amyloid (and arteries and veins) are coloured red.
(4) Mount in normal mounting fluid.

Haemosiderin (iron)

Haemosiderin in gross specimens may be demonstrated by the Prussian blue reaction.

Method

(1) Specimens are fixed in formal-saline, taking care to avoid contamination with rust.
(2) Place in a solution of equal parts of 10% hydrochloric acid and 5% potassium ferrocyanide until, after a few minutes, the specimen develops a blue colour.
(3) Wash overnight in running water.
(4) Mount in 5% formal-saline. The colour diffuses out of the specimen in normal mounting fluid.

Notes

(1) Specimens fade after several months, but the colour is completely restored by treatment with hydrogen peroxide.
(2) The fluid of haemochromatosis specimens becomes milky and the colour diffuses after a few months; this seems to be unavoidable.

Staining of specimens

Fat in gross specimens may be demonstrated by staining with Sudan III, followed by differentiation in 70% alcohol. The specimen may be counterstained with Ehrlich's haematoxylin to show infiltration with malignant tissue.

Gough and Wentworth paper mounted sections

By the Gough and Wentworth (1949) technique thin sections of entire organs are mounted on paper. Such a method lends itself to the storage of a large number of such sections in the form of a book, with a great saving in space; they may be examined as transparencies and compared and demonstrated side by side with the corresponding radiographs. The organ most commonly treated is the lung, but the liver, the kidney and the heart may also be used.

The most convenient machine for cutting the large sections is the MSE 'Large Section' Microtome.

Technique

(1) Remove the lungs from the body whole and without rupturing the pleura. If there are dense adhesions remove the parietal pleura with the lung (a few small tears do

not matter except where there are large emphysematous bullae). One or both lungs may be used; one may be reserved for bacteriological and chemical investigation.

(2) Cut off at the hilum and fully distend by running the following solution in to the major bronchi, by means of a tube and cannula from a reservoir about 4 feet above the lung.

Liq. formaldehyde (40%)	500 ml
Sodium acetate	200 g
Tap-water	to 5000 ml

There is no need to tie the bronchi after expansion. The amount necessary to distend the lung varies up to about 2 litres and the containers used by Gough and Wentworth contained a further 3 litres.

(3) Place the lung in a container of fixative large enough for it to float freely with no distortion from pressure. Cover with a cloth wetted with the fixative.

(4) Fix for 2 days or longer and then cut a slice about $\frac{3}{4}$ inch in thickness; this may be in any direction but a sagittal one is most convenient. Good results are usually obtained after a few days' fixation, but in the absence of any urgency the slice is allowed to continue to fix for some weeks to reduce proteolytic enzyme activity.

(5) Wash the slice in running water for at least 72 hours to remove the formalin. Use a syphon system and have a drip of copper sulphate solution or nitric acid running into the washing water to give a dilution of 1:500 000 to 1:1 000 000. The copper or acid reduces enzyme action which—especially in summer—may digest the gelatin in the next stage of the technique.

(6) Place the slice in the following solution.

Gelatin	250 g
Cellosolve (ethylene glycol monoethyl ether)	40 ml
Capryl alcohol	5 ml
Tap-water	850 ml

Note: In the USA gelatin of the specification 80–100 bloom should be used.

Remove the air from the slice to assist penetration by the gelatin. To do this, place the slice in a jar containing the gelatin solution heated to about 60 °C, and put under a bell jar connected to a vacuum pump. A solution of agar is useful as a seal around the jar. With an efficient glass pump sufficient air can be removed within an hour, during which time the gelatin remains fluid at ordinary room temperature.

(7) Place the specimen, still in the gelatin solution, in an incubator at 35 °C for 48 hours, in a container in which it can lie flat and be completely immersed.

(8) Cast the gelatin and specimen into a block by allowing the gelatin to set in a container with a loose bottom.

(9) Remove the block by pushing out the loose bottom of the container.

(10) Fix the block to the microtome holder by warming the latter and then put weights on top of the block. The undersurface of the gelatin melts and as it resets the block sticks to the holder. Put in an icebox at −15 °C for several hours, preferably overnight.

(11) Cut as thawing takes place; a warm cloth rubbed on the surface hastens thawing. Do not try to cut sections until the block is thawed sufficiently to cut easily. For lungs the optimum thickness is 400 μm. For solid organs like liver somewhat thinner sections of 300 μm are usually preferable.

(12) Put the sections into 10% formalin–sodium acetate solution for 24–48 hours to harden the gelatin.
(13) Wash in cold water for 1–2 hours to remove the formalin.
(14) Pour some fresh solution of the following over a sheet of Perspex.

Gelatin   75 g
Glycerin   70 ml
Cellosolve   40 ml
Water   805 ml

Note: Perspex is an acrylic resin. Other plastics would probably work as well. Glass cannot be used for this purpose as the sections would then adhere to the glass and not to the paper.

(15) Trim the surplus gelatin from the edges of a section, place it flat on the Perspex and cover with a sheet of Whatman's No. 1 filter paper.
(16) Run a rubber roller squeegee lightly over the paper to remove surplus solution and air bubbles.
(17) Stand the Perspex sheet on end for 15–30 seconds and then lay flat until the gelatin sets.
(18) While still wet, place in a radiograph drying cabinet, and when thoroughly dry strip the paper with the section attached from the Perspex. If no 'dryer' is available, dry as thoroughly as possible at room temperature, and when there are no wet patches left, complete the drying at 37 °C.

Note: Sections can be stiffened by applying water permeable cellophane to the surface using the final gelatin solution (Gough, 1967).

References

DAWSON, A. B. (1926). A note on the staining of the skeleton of cleared specimens with alizarin red S. *Stain Technol.*, **1**, 123–124

GOUGH, J. (1967). *Twenty Years' Experience of the Technic of Paper Mounted Sections: The Lung.* International Academy Monograph No. 8, pp. 311–316

GOUGH, J. and WENTWORTH, J. E. (1949). The use of thin sections of entire organs in morbid anatomical studies. *J. R. Micr. Soc.*, **69**, 231–235

ISRAEL, M. S. and YOUNG, L. F. (1978). Use of liquid paraffin in the preservation of pathological specimens. *J. Clin. Pathol.*, **31**, 499–500

KAISERLING, C. (1900). Über Konservierung und Aufstellung pathologischanatomischer Präparate für Schau und Lehrsammlungen. *Verh. Dtsch. Pathol. Ges.*, **2**, 203–217

PULVERTAFT, R. J. V. (1936). Colour fading in chloroma and other museum specimens. *J. Tech. Methods*, **16**, 27

SCHULTZ, I. H. (1931). Eine Spechstundenprüfung des Zeitsinnes. *Klin. Wchnschr.*, **10**, 1864

SPALTEHOLZ, W. (1911). *Über das Durchsichtigmachen von Menschlichen und Tierischen Präparaten.* Leipzig

WENTWORTH, J. E. (1938). A new method of preserving museum specimens in their natural colours. *J. Tech. Methods*, **18**, 53–56

WENTWORTH, J. E. (1939). The hydrosulphite method of preserving museum specimens. *J. Tech. Methods*, **19**, 79–82

WENTWORTH, J. E. (1942). The preservation of museum specimens in war time. *J. Pathol. Bacteriol.*, **54**, 137–138

WENTWORTH, J. E. (1957). The hydrosulphite method of museum mounting. *J. Med. Lab. Technol.*, **14**, 194–195

32

Photomicrography

Introduction

There is an increasing need for the photography of microscopical preparations. These are used for recording, teaching and for publications. In teaching, colour transparencies are invariably used. The high cost of colour reproduction, however, ensures that black and white photomicrographs are still widely used.

The traditional equipment was the optical bench. The camera, microscope and illuminator were mounted on a rigidly mounted and accurately aligned heavy steel bed. Other components, such as filters, could be inserted or removed as the need arose. The image was accurately focused on a ground-glass screen which was removed, then replaced by the photographic plate or flat film holder. The apparatus was usually installed in a darkroom to facilitate focusing on the screen and mounted on a heavy bench to reduce vibration. The procedure took a considerable time.

The introduction of 35 mm camera equipment speeded up the process. There are many versions of photomicrographic apparatus on the market usually allowing routine microscopy to be undertaken with the camera in position. Beam splitters allow light to enter both camera and ocular simultaneously but have the disadvantage of reducing the light reaching the camera. The disadvantages of the fixed prism system were overcome by the introduction of movable reflectors or prisms so that all available light could be deflected from one path to another.

Modern photomicrographic apparatus contains a fixed photoelectric cell so that the light intensity can be measured and the exposure set automatically.

Preparation of sections

Sections which may be adequate for teaching or diagnosis will often be unsuitable for photomicrography. Sections must be free of all fixation, cutting and staining artefacts. Fixation deposits, if present, must be removed. There should be no chatters, scores or folds and dust and squames must be avoided. Thick sections are often preferred for low power photomicrography but for high power work the sections should be thin in order to ensure that the section is in perfect focus. The eye makes allowances for slight imperfections but the camera does not. Staining should be of good contrast for colour work whilst contrast may be improved in black and white photomicrography by the use of filters. Perfectly flat section mounting must be obtained otherwise variations will produce areas which are not in focus.

Optics

Flat field apochromatic objectives should be used and aplanatic condensers will give superior results. If high power dry apochromatic objectives are used best results will be obtained if a correction collar is incorporated to allow compensation for coverglass thickness.

The field should be evenly illuminated and the microscope should be accurately adjusted for Kohler illumination (*see* Chapter 33). The focusing eyepiece will have the ability to focus double lines or circles (reticles) which are seen in the field of view. These must be in sharp focus along with the object and will allow for variations between observers.

Illumination

Light sources emit either a continuous spectrum or a line spectrum.

A continuous spectrum emission consists of energy of all wavelengths in the visible range. Examples of such sources are daylight, and tungsten filament or tungsten–halogen lamps.

A line spectrum, or discontinuous spectrum, emission consists of peaks of energy and corresponding gaps denoting that at certain wavelengths no light (or much less light) is emitted. A line spectrum light source is unsuitable for general colour photomicrography but is used in fluorescence photomicrography.

Tungsten light sources are preferred for colour work and have a colour temperature of either 3200 or 3400 K. It is essential that lamps are run at the correct voltage. As voltage increases, current increases and the colour temperature of the lamp rises, the colour of the light moves from yellowish to bluish. Lamp manufacturers indicate the colour temperature of their lamps when operated at a specific voltage and current (Vetter, 1974a).

Black and white photomicrography

The visual contrasts visible to the observer will not be obvious in the photograph. Orthochromatic film is not sensitive to red light, so panchromatic film should be used. Contrast may be emphasized by using filters so that certain colours appear as light tones on the finished print whilst others appear in dark tones. Contrast filters are always used in black and white photomicrography. The general rule is to select a filter of the complementary colour to the structure which is to appear dark in the print. In

Table 32.1 Complementary filters

Subject	Filter
Red	Green
Orange	Blue
Yellow	Violet
Green	Red
Blue	Orange
Violet	Yellow

practice when dealing with haematoxylin and eosin-stained preparations both the blue and the pink are intensified by using an orange/yellow and a green filter. The preparation should show as much contrast as possible between stained and unstained elements or between elements stained in different colours.

Colour photomicrography

The exact proportion of each spectral colour varies with different light sources. Daylight contains more blue light than artificial light which itself is reddish. This spectral composition can be measured. The light source can be compared with the light emitted from an incandescent 'black body'. When both are emitting light of the same colour, the temperature of the 'black body' in degrees Kelvin (K) is said to be the colour temperature of the illumination. The 'black body' is essentially a theoretical concept in physics, although an apparatus with such properties can be set up in the laboratory. For tungsten filament lamps the colour temperature is approximately 50 K above the actual temperature of the filament.

Every colour temperature has an associated Mired value (microreciprocal degree).

$$\text{The Mired value} = \frac{10^6}{T}$$

T = colour temperature in K

Mired values simplify the calculation of the colour correction required, and therefore the selection of the correct colour correction filters.

Table 32.2 Mired values

(K)	0	100	200	300	400	500	600	700	800	900
2000	500	476	455	435	417	400	385	370	357	345
3000	333	323	312	303	294	286	278	270	263	256
4000	250	244	238	233	227	222	217	213	208	204
5000	200	196	192	189	185	182	179	175	172	169
6000	167	164	161	159	156	154	152	149	147	145

Certain filters have the property of converting the radiation of a light source from one colour temperature to that of another. Colour correction filters possess a specific Mired-shift value.

$$\text{Mired-shift value} = \left(\frac{1}{T_2} - \frac{1}{T_1} \right) \times 10^6$$

T_1 = colour temperature of the original light source
T_2 = colour temperature required for the film emulsion

The Mired-shift value will be either positive or negative.

Brownish filters lower the colour temperature and raise the Mired-shift value and are therefore positive.

Bluish filters raise the colour temperature and lower the Mired-shift value and are therefore negative.

For example:

(a) Type B film is balanced for a colour temperature of 3200 K. To expose this to tungsten light of 3400 K:

$$\text{Mired-shift value} = \left(\frac{1}{3200} - \frac{1}{3400}\right) \times 10^6$$

or from *Table 32.2* $= 312 - 294$

$$= +18$$

From *Table 32.3*, use a Wratten 81 A filter.

Table 32.3 Mired-shift value of Wratten filters

Positive (towards yellow)		Negative (towards blue)	
81	+9	82	−10
81 A	+18	82 A	−21
81 B	+27	82 B	−32
81 C	+35	82 C	−45
81 EF	+52	80 B	−112
85 C	+81	80 A	−131
85	+112		
85 B	+131		

Filters may be combined, e.g. 82 A + 82 C = −66.
Note: A filter which makes a significant change in the colour temperature is called a conversion filter, e.g. the Kodak 80 and 85 series. One which is used for only minor adjustments is called a light-balancing filter, e.g. the Kodak 81 and 82 series.

(b) To use daylight film (5500 K) with tungsten light of 3400 K:

$$\text{Mired-shift value} = \left(\frac{1}{5500} - \frac{1}{3400}\right) \times 10^6$$

or from *Table 32.2* $= 182 - 294$

$$= -112$$

From *Table 32.3*, use a Wratten 80 B filter.

Colour films

Colour reversal films are supplied by several manufacturers each having their own particular characteristics and their use is often a matter of personal preference. Daylight film (5500 K) is often used with tungsten light and the appropriate colour correction filter. Films balanced for tungsten light are available for colour temperature of 3400 K (Type A) or for 3200 K (Type B).

The ASA speed rating for reversal colour film is based on the speed of the exposures needed to give minimum and maximum useful densities appropriate to a colour transparency. In general the faster the film (higher the ASA value) the coarser will be the grain.

If the transmitted light from the stained section is between the bands of colour provided by the three colours used in colour photography, it will not be well reproduced. This obtains with eosin and may be overcome by using a neodymium filter (Koster, 1964).

Microscope lamps run at the correct voltage to produce the correct colour temperature often produce light of too high an intensity for the speed of the emulsion being used. It must not be reduced by adjusting the rheostat, otherwise the colour temperature will be altered. To reduce the intensity of light without altering the colour temperature neutral density filters must be used.

Reciprocity law failure

Reciprocity law states that the photographic effect is independent of either time or intensity of light as long as the product of the two remains the same.

Exposure = intensity × time

The concept that changes in image brightness can be compensated by exposure time no longer holds good when either intensity or time are very small or very large.

In practical photomicrography failure of this law is due to time only. Therefore when exposure times are excessive, a correction factor must be employed. Data sheets are available from manufacturers giving proper exposure indices for extended exposure times.

With black and white films when exposures of 1 minute or so are needed some extra time of exposure is given and because of the latitude of the film no problem is encountered.

With multilayer colour film, not only is additional exposure required but for exposures longer than 2 seconds a colour filter* may be needed to counteract uneven

* Colour compensating filters are used when changes in the colour balance are required. They may be used to compensate for deficiencies in the spectral characteristics of the light source or to counteract the effects of reciprocity failure, e.g. Kodak CC20Y is a yellow filter used to absorb excess blue.

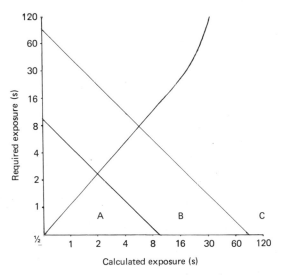

Figure 32.1 Compensation for reciprocity failure for colour reversal film. Such films are normally balanced for ½ second exposure (Langford, 1974). A, no correction required; B, colour correction filter zone; C, beyond full colour correction

reciprocity failure between the emulsions. Over 8 seconds filters will not correct adequately (*Figure 32.1*).

The two areas where difficulties may be encountered are in polarizing and fluorescence photomicrography.

If the bright material occupies at least 50% of the field exposures can be determined in the usual way (Vetter, 1974b). Some photomicroscopes are equipped with exposure meters that will measure the light over small areas of the field. In practice with polarizing microscopy it is often convenient to rotate the analyser slightly from the 90 degree position and so lighten the background sufficiently to allow a reasonable exposure time.

It is pointed out by Vetter (1974b) that increasing the intensity of the exciting light in order to decrease the exposure time may only result in increasing the rapidity with which the fluorescence is quenched, so gaining nothing photographically.

The only solution is to use high speed film and forced processing, the exposure for a certain combination of filters and fluorochromes having been assessed by trial and error.

References

KOSTER, L. W. (1964). The didymium glass filter in photomicrography. *J. Biol. Photo. Assoc.*, **32**, 59–64

LANGFORD, M. J. (1974). *Advanced Photography*. The Focal Press, London and New York

VETTER, J. P. (1974a). A systematic approach to colour photomicrography. 1. The microscope: its optics and alignment. *Med. Biol. Ill.*, **24**, 74–85

VETTER, J. P. (1974b). A systematic approach to colour photomicrography. 2. Cameras and photographic techniques. *Med. Biol. Ill.*, **24**, 140–152

Part IX

Microscopy

33

Microscopy

General microscopy

The microscope is the most commonly used piece of apparatus in the laboratory, and yet it is probably the instrument about which least is known by its users. It is generally thought that the microscope can be used effectively without any knowledge of its limitations or construction, but this is, of course, a complete misconception. An ill-adjusted, badly illuminated microscope can, when one is using high-power objectives, give completely misleading information as to the structure of an object. For this reason it is advisable to gain a knowledge of how the magnified images are produced by the microscope before attempting to assess the information obtained by its use.

The first part of this chapter is devoted to the lens and its faults, after which the component parts of the microscope, its use and maintenance are discussed.

Lens

A lens is the name given to a piece of glass or other transparent material, usually circular, having the two surfaces ground and polished in a specific form in order that rays of light passing through it shall either converge (collect together) or diverge (separate).

A lens is called positive when it causes light rays to concentrate or converge to form a real image (*Figure 33.1a–d*); or it is negative, in which case light rays passing through will diverge or scatter and positive or real images will not be seen (*Figure 33.1e–g*). These two types are easily differentiated since positive lenses are thicker at the centre than at the periphery, whereas negative lenses are thinner at the centre and although the shapes may vary considerably, these characteristics remain (*Figure 33.1a–g*).

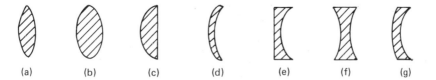

(a)	(b)	(c)	(d)	(e)	(f)	(g)

Figure 33.1 Types of lenses: (a–d) positive lenses; (e–g) negative lenses

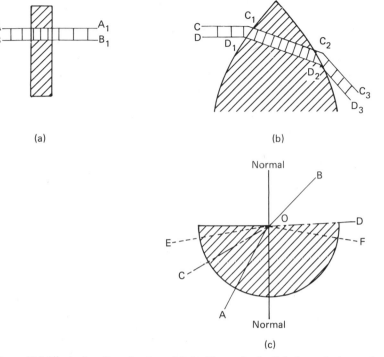

Figure 33.2 Illustrating the refraction of light. The path of a light beam is shown through (a) plane glass; and (b) the periphery of a positive lens; (c) shows the conditions of total internal reflection (EF)

Refraction of light rays

The effect of a lens on a ray of light is due primarily to the density of the glass (or other material) which reduces the speed at which light travels through it. (Light is usually considered as a vibration in the ether—a hypothetical substance which fills the whole of space). In a dense medium (e.g. glass) the light rays are retarded, or slowed down. If a beam of light containing two parallel rays (AB, A_1B_1 Figure 33.2a) strikes a sheet of plane glass at right-angles, its speed of travel through the glass will be reduced, but its direction unchanged. If it strikes the plane glass or the curved surface of a lens at an angle (CD, C_3D_3 Figure 33.2b) its speed will be reduced and its direction changed. The bending of light rays, known as refraction, is due to the fact that one part (D) strikes the surface of the glass first (D_1) and is retarded while the other part (C) is still travelling at normal speed, thus causing the ray to be bent and its direction altered. From C_1 the two portions travel in the same direction at a common reduced speed until C emerges from the dense medium (C_2) and travels at its original speed while D is still retarded in the dense medium, causing a further bending of the light ray. After D emerges from the dense medium (D_2), the two portions travel in the new direction at their original speed.

It will be obvious that the degree of refraction will be dependent not only on the angle of the surface of the lens to the light ray, but also on the optical density of the material from which the lens is made. The optical density of a substance is indicated by its refractive index (RI), which is the ratio of the velocity of light in air to the velocity of light in that substance.

The behaviour of a beam of light passing from one medium to another can be estimated from the rule that light entering a more dense medium bends towards the 'normal' (AO in *Figure 33.2c*), and when entering a less dense medium it bends away from the normal (OB in *Figure 33.2c*).

Light can always enter a lens, no matter what the angle at which it strikes, but it is not always possible for it to leave. As the angle between the beam of light leaving and the 'normal' (the angle of incidence) increases the emerging beam is bent closer and closer to the surface of the glass, until it is parallel with the surface (COD in *Figure 33.2c*). Any further increase in the angle of incidence will result in the beam being reflected from the surface instead of emerging—a condition known as total internal reflection (EOF in *Figure 33.2c*).

Focus

If, through the centre of one side of a box, a pinhole is made, so small that only one ray of light can pass through it in each direction, then the image of an object outside the box will be formed on the back of the box (*Figure 33.3a*). The ray of light from each point of the object entering the box is very narrow and it can only travel in a straight line. Therefore, each point of the object will have a corresponding point in the image (*Figure 33.3a*), and since the light rays from the bottom of the object form the top of the image, and vice versa, the image will be inverted. Similarly, variations of brightness and colour will be reproduced. Such a box may be used as a camera, though not a very efficient one; a long exposure would be needed owing to the small amount of light allowed to enter. To enlarge the hole and fit a lens would result in the production of a much brighter image, owing to the fact that instead of only one light ray entering from each point of the object, a large number will enter through the fitted lens (*Figure 33.3b*).

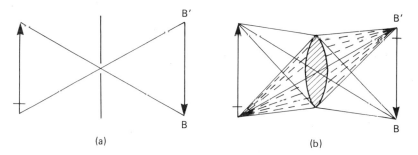

(a)   (b)

Figure 33.3 Production of (a) image through pinhole aperture, and (b) brighter image by using a lens instead of a pinhole

A notable difference in the production of images by a pinhole and a lens is that a pinhole will produce an image, regardless of the depth of the box or the nearness of the object, whereas in the case of a lens the screen and the object must be in exactly the correct positions, or the image will be indistinct and hazy. The lens will cause the light rays to converge to a single point at only one position (BB', *Figure 33.4*), and at either side of that position each point of the object will be represented by a solid circle of light; each circle being overlapped by the adjoining ones (CC', *Figure 33.4*).

When a lens concentrates the light rays to form a clear sharp image of an object, the

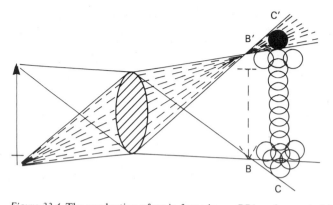

Figure 33.4 The production of an in-focus image BB′, and an out-of-focus image CC′

object is said to be in focus. The terms 'focus' or 'principal focus' are used to indicate the position in which a lens will form a sharp, clear picture of a distant object, such as the sun. (The word focus originally meant burning place, and was used to indicate the point at which a lens concentrated the sun's rays to form a sharp image having the power to burn.)

In addition to the principal focus, a lens also has conjugate foci; these are two points, one on each side of the lens, in one of which a clear image will be formed on a screen of an object placed in the other. The positions of the conjugate foci vary: as an object is moved away from the lens, so the image will be formed closer to it and vice versa (*Figure 33.5a* and *b*); and any pair of such positions are called conjugate focal planes. The magnification of the lens is affected by this movement of the lens or object since the farther away from the lens the image is formed, the larger it appears (*Figure 33.5a* and *b*) and, consequently, the greater the magnification.

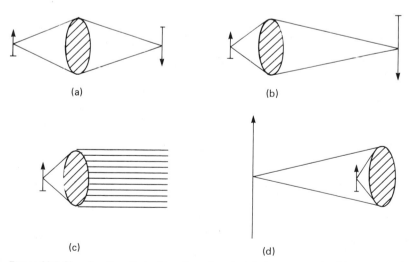

(a)

(b)

(c)

(d)

Figure 33.5 Showing the effect of moving a lens in relation to a static object (reproduced from *The Microscope* by courtesy of R. and J. Beck Ltd)

Images, as those described, which can be seen on a screen, are known as real images. As the object is brought closer to the lens, the image will move further away until it reaches infinity and cannot be seen (*Figure 33.5c*). If the object is brought still closer, the image will reappear on the opposite side of the lens—that is, the same side as the object—but it will be a ghost image which can be seen only by looking through the lens, and which cannot be focused on a screen. The image has undergone a further change in that the image will appear the right way up (*Figure 33.5d*). This is known as a virtual image.

Defects of a lens

For a microscope to be efficient, it must not only produce a magnified image, but one which will be clear and well defined. To use a simple lens of the type described will not give such good results because: (a) white light is not a single vibration but is composed of a series of vibrations of differing wavelengths; and (b) faults are inherent in its shape.

Chromatic aberration

When white light is split into its component parts, each part vibrates to a different degree, producing to the eye a different colour. These colours (red, orange, yellow, green, blue, indigo and violet) are known as the primary spectrum, and are seen in the rainbow, or through a spectroscope. Red has the longest wavelength, with a vibration of 700 nm, blue 450 nm and violet 350 nm.

It will be seen that the vibrations of red light are twice the length of those of violet light.

Since light rays cannot vibrate as easily in a dense medium as in a rare medium, it follows that the various colours will be affected by a lens to differing degrees, the colours with shorter wavelengths, such as blue violet, being affected to a greater degree than those having a longer wavelength, such as red and orange. It is for this reason that rays of white light, having passed through a prism, emerge as a spectrum, each ray having been refracted to a different degree, and each emerging at a different point. Violet and blue are refracted to a greater degree than red and orange.

In *Figure 33.6*, W represents a point source of white light entering a lens which, on emerging, forms a different point of focus for each of the component colours, blue (B) being focused at a point nearer the lens than red (R).

A screen placed at R will show a red point surrounded by the colours of the spectrum, having a blue edge; at B a blue point with a red periphery will appear. This colour defect is called chromatic aberration, and its correction is known as achromatism.

Since different types of glass have different optical properties, chromatic aberration can be corrected to within useful limits by using a two-component lens. A positive lens

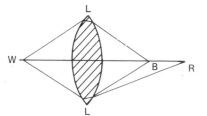

Figure 33.6 Chromatic aberration

(of greater magnifying power than is finally required) is combined with a negative lens made of glass producing a greater chromatic aberration, but with the same refractive index. The negative lens corrects the chromatic aberration in the positive lens, and only partially neutralizes its magnifying power. This method will correct a thin positive lens for any two colours, leaving a small error in the intermediate colours (secondary spectrum). This type of lens is known as an achromatic lens.

If fluorspar is incorporated in the glass of the achromatic lens, three colours can be brought to the one focal point, and the amount of chromatic aberration visible in the image will be negligible. Such lenses are known as apochromatic lenses.

Since the correction of an apochromatic lens involves the use of a larger number of lenses, its other defects are corrected at the same time so that the final lens, provided that it is correctly used, will show hardly any defects.

Spherical aberration

Spherical aberration is a further defect of a single lens, due to the fact that it has a curved surface.

Since the angle at which light rays enter (and leave) the surface of a lens varies with each part of the lens, those rays passing through the periphery (AA) will be refracted to a greater degree than those travelling through the central area (CC, *Figure 33.7*). There is

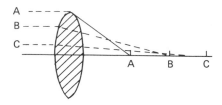

Figure 33.7 Spherical aberration

no position, therefore, where the light from a point source will be in sharp focus, and since each point is hazy the composite image is bound to be indistinct. This fault could be minimized by using only the central area of a lens, but since a microscope objective must have a short working distance and a high magnification, a large angle of light is required from each point of the object, and the correction of this aberration is most important.

The degree of spherical aberration will depend on the actual shape of the lens, and by varying the shape, although the focus may be the same, the spherical aberration will vary. The method of correction follows the same pattern used in correcting achromatism, namely, that of using a powerful positive lens and partially neutralizing its magnifying power with a negative lens made of glass having a greater relative aberration. Complete correction is extremely difficult and the above account presents the problem and its solution only in a very simple form.

Chromatic and spherical aberration are the two principal faults to be found in lenses; there are others, but since correction is achieved by similar means—variation in shape and composition, and the distance apart of component lenses—they will not be discussed in detail. Some idea of the complexity of various lens systems may be gathered from *Figure 33.8*.

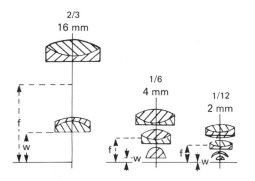

Figure 33.8 Lens arrangement of the common objectives showing the relative focal lengths and working distances: f=focal length, w=working distances (by courtesy of R. and J. Beck Ltd)

Component parts of a compound microscope

A simple microscope is composed of one or several lenses mounted closely together, as in the case of a hand lens, whereas a compound microscope is composed of two widely separated lenses, or sets of lenses, capable of producing greatly enlarged images.

The standard microscope (*Figure 33.9*) is composed of two main parts:

(1) the microscope proper, incorporating the body tube with the objective at one end and the eyepieces at the other; and
(2) the stand, which includes the supporting, adjusting and illuminating apparatus.

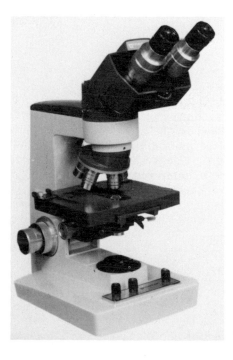

Figure 33.9 Modern light microscope with inclined binocular head, rotatory objective holder, mechanical stage and integral light source. (Courtesy of Reichert–Jung (UK) Ltd)

Optical components

The eyepieces (or oculars)

These are designed to further magnify the primary image from the objective, they also limit the field of view as seen by the eye. They may be used to correct residual errors in the objective lenses and may then be either: *undercorrected*, when a blue ray of light will be refracted to a greater degree than the red, this can be identified by the blue fringe that is seen around the edge of the field diaphragm; or *overcorrected*, when the reverse is the case and an orange fringe may be seen at the edge of the field diaphragm. Compensated eyepieces are usually overcorrected.

There are two basic types of eyepieces, as follows.

(1) With the *negative* eyepiece the focus is within (between) the lenses of the eyepiece. It is composed of two lenses; the lower or field lens collects the image that would have been formed by the objective (virtual image plane) and cones it down to a slightly smaller image at the level of the field stop (or field diaphragm) within the eyepiece (*Figures 33.10a and 33.16*); the upper lens then produces an enlarged virtual image which is seen by the microscopist. An engraved scale placed in the field stop will be superimposed (in focus) on the image (*see* the section on Micrometry on page 570).

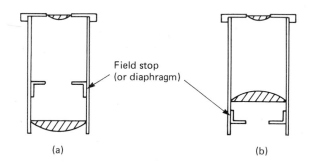

Field stop
(or diaphragm)

(a)   (b)

Figure 33.10 Basic types of eyepieces (or oculars): (a) negative type (Huygenian); (b) positive type (Ramsden)

(2) With the *positive* eyepiece the focus is outside the eyepiece lens system; for this reason it may be used as a simple microscope. The field stop (or diaphragm) is outside the eyepiece, from which the virtual image (from the objective) is focused and magnified by the entire eyepiece (*Figure 33.10b*). As with the negative type of eyepiece, a scale placed on the field stop will be superimposed (in focus) on the image formed by the objective.

Huygenian eyepieces

These eyepieces (*Figure 33.10a*), originally designed by Huygens for the telescope, are the type most commonly used in microscopy. They are negative, undercorrected (*see above*), and are best suited for use with achromatic objectives.

Ramsden eyepieces

As will be seen in *Figure 33.10b*, these are positive oculars. It will be noted that the lower lens has its plane side towards the object. Most of the compensated eyepieces are of the

Ramsden type, having doublet or triplet lenses instead of the single lenses shown in *Figure 33.10b*. Ramsden oculars are preferred for micrometer eyepieces as they impart less distortion to scales.

Wide field eyepieces

Improvements in ocular design have enabled manufacturers to produce lenses which give a large flat field of view which are particularly valuable in the biological laboratory.

High-eyepoint oculars

These have been introduced primarily for microscopists who wear spectacles, and are sometimes engraved with a diagram of a pair of spectacles. With normal eyepieces, the distance between the top of the eyepiece and the exit pupil (eyepoint) is so small as to prevent the wearing of glasses, but the high eyepoint of these special oculars make this possible. It is advised that the rubber guards supplied with such eyepieces be used to prevent the scratching of the spectacle lenses. Such eyepieces may be used by all microscopists, but some practice is needed before their use (with the head being held slightly higher than usual) becomes familiar and comfortable.

Compensating eyepieces

These eyepieces were originally intended for use with apochromatic objectives only, and were not recommended for use with achromats. They are *now recommended for use with all modern objectives*. English-speaking countries mark them 'Comp', while German lenses are designated by the letter 'K'.

Field of view

Some eyepieces are marked with their field of view number from which can be calculated the actual diameter of the specimen being viewed (the field of view number, divided by the magnification of the objective, equals the field of view in millimetres).

Magnification

Eyepieces always receive the 'virtual image' from the objective in the same plane and therefore magnify it to a constant degree, independent of other factors such as body tube length, and so on. They are consequently marked with their magnifying power and may vary from ×4 to ×50. As will be seen in the following pages it is generally inadvisable to employ powers in excess of ×12.5.

The objective

The objective screws into the lower end of the body tube by means of a standard thread, thus all objectives are interchangeable. They are usually designated, not by their magnifying power but by their focal length (from 2–50 mm); this is because their actual magnifying power will depend on the tube length at which they are used. Some confusion has arisen in the past by the terms 'focal length' and 'working distance' in relation to objectives. Whereas with a simple lens these are identical, with compound lenses such as those in an objective they are different.

The 'working distance' is simply the distance from the object to the outer surface of the front lens, whereas the 'focal distance' is that from the object to a point roughly midway between the component lenses (*Figure 33.8*). The latter is correct only when the objective is used at the standard tube length of 160 mm. If the tube length is altered the focal distance will also be altered and the object will need to be refocused.

Most instrument manufacturers mark objectives with the appropriate magnifying power, usually because they produce a microscope which has no draw tube, the tube length being a standard 160 mm.

The aperture

The first objective consisted of a single lens, and its defects were overcome by the use of a pinhole aperture, but since only a small cone of light could enter from each point of the object, the image, although greatly magnified, showed very little detail. It is apparent, therefore, that the amount of detail seen is dependent not, as commonly believed, on the magnification but on the size of the cone of light that can be collected from the object.

The ability of a lens to define detail is known as its resolving power, and this is measured by the distance apart of two lines or dots, or the number of lines to the inch, that can be visually separated from each other; for example, a lens that has a resolution of 30 000 lines to the inch has a greater resolving power than one separating only 20 000 lines to the inch. This will be appreciated by viewing *Figure 33.11a* from a distance of 10 feet, when only a single line will be seen. On closer examination it will be found that there are, in fact, five lines. Even when the image is magnified (*Figure 33.11b*) and viewed from 10 feet it still has the appearance of being a single line.

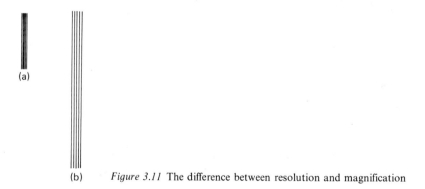

(a)

(b)   *Figure 3.11* The difference between resolution and magnification

Resolution is restricted by two factors:

(1) the numerical aperture of the lens; and
(2) the wavelength of light employed.

The relationship is as follows.

$$R = \frac{1.2\,\lambda}{2\,\mathrm{NA}}$$

where R is the resolution (the smallest distance between the closest two lines or dots that can be defined separately) and λ is the wavelength of the light employed. NA is the numerical aperture.

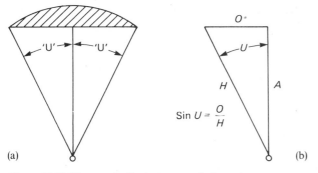

Figure 33.12 Diagram to illustrate numerical aperture

The numerical aperture

The apertures of the early microscope lenses were at first measured by the actual angle of aperture; that is, the angle formed by the outer edges of the lens, and a point on the object (*Figure 33.12a*). The aperture of oil-immersion lenses, however, depends on the refractive index of the medium between the object and the lens and for this reason may vary. This is because the cone of light, emerging from a glass coverslip into air, is refracted away from the lens face and a much smaller cone of light enters than if there was glass, or a medium having the same refractive index as glass, between the lens and the object. In *Figure 33.13a* it will be seen that the angle of the cone of light, from a point source of the object, actually entering the lens when used dry, is only 78 degrees, compared with an angle of 120 degrees when immersion oil is between them (*Figure 33.13b*). To take account of this factor, and to be able to express a lens aperture as a

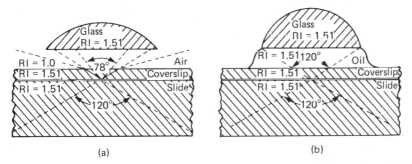

Figure 33.13 Diagram illustrating the effect of the interposing medium on the angle of light entering the objective

simple figure, the term numerical aperture (NA) is used, which may be expressed as follows.

$$NA = n \sin u$$

where n is the refractive index of the medium between the lens and object, and sin u is the sine of half the angle of aperture (*Figure 33.12a*). Since the sine of an angle is opposite over hypotenuse (O/H) (*Figure 33.12b*), it may also be roughly expressed as half the diameter of the lens over the distance from the periphery of the lens to the object. Since the highest NA theoretically possible when a lens is used dry (air RI = 1.0) must be 1.0, and with immersion oil (RI = 1.51) 1.51, it will be appreciated that modern high-power objectives (dry NA = 0.95; oil immersion NA = 1.32) approach very closely to the theoretical maxima.

The effects of a high numerical aperture

Whilst a high numerical aperture increases the resolution of an objective, it has the following disadvantages: (a) it reduces the depth of focus, that is, the ability to focus on more than one layer of an object at the same time; and (b) it reduces the flatness of the field, so that the edges are out of focus.

It will be seen, therefore, that if depth of focus and flatness of field are important, then increased magnification should be obtained with high-power eyepieces, although as a general rule a change to a higher power objective, giving increased magnification and resolution, is preferred.

Types of objective

All objectives are engraved with the information needed to obtain their maximum performance as well as any possible limitations. Such an engraving might read:

Plan   40/0.65
        160/0.17

which indicates that it is a planachromat; $\times 40$ magnification at a tube length of 160 mm (for its best performance), has a numerical aperture of 0.65 and should be used with a coverglass of 0.17 ± 0.01 mm in thickness (this /0.17 may instead be / = insensitive to coverglass thickness or /0 = for use with unmounted specimens).

Achromatic objectives

These objectives are the type most commonly used and the modern well-corrected lenses are more than adequate for routine microscopy in pathology and biology laboratories.

Apochromatic objectives

When apochromatic objectives are employed, their high degree of correction is wasted unless they are used in conjunction with a highly corrected aplanatic or achromatic condenser, and compensating eyepieces. The latter compensates for peripheral chromatic aberration due to the differing magnifications of the various coloured images. These eyepieces together with the objectives form a recombined single image free from coloured fringes even at the periphery.

Apochromatic objectives should always be used for photomicrography. To get the maximum light with high-power objectives having numerical apertures above 1.0, oil-immersion condensers should be used with an NA at least equal to that of the objective, and immersion oil between the condenser and the slide as well as between the objective and the slide.

These objectives are also highly corrected for the other lens aberrations (spherical, coma and so on).

Fluorite objectives (neofluor)

Fluorite or semi-apochromatic objectives have fluorite incorporated into the lens system to give better colour correction. They are corrected for three wavelengths of light in the yellow-green of the spectrum, and are free of colour fringes. They are generally more highly corrected in all other respects than the achromats and represent a quality of image midway between that of the achromat and apochromat.

Planachromat objectives

Planachromats are principally designed to give a perfectly flat field, with the whole field in focus at the same time. They are used mainly for photomicrography.

Polarizing objectives

Designated POL, these are strain-free objectives for use on the polarizing microscope.

Phase objectives

These objectives contain a phase-plate for use in phase-contrast microscopy (*see* page 592). They are designated Ph with a number which refers to the matching annulus.

Coverglass thickness

It will follow that oil-immersion objectives do not have coverglass restrictions since they will have the same refractive index as the immersion oil. The coverglass thickness is only important if high-power 'dry' objectives are being used, when No. 1 coverglasses should be used, or an objective with a correction collar may be employed which allows a range of thickness of coverslip from 0.12 0.22 mm to be used. To check the setting for a particular specimen (where the coverslip thickness is unknown) first focus upon a high contrast area, then determine whether changing the collar setting increases or decreases the contrast. If the coverglass thickness is known it can be set directly upon the engraved scale above the collar.

Mechanical components

The body tube

The body tube is attached to the limb of the microscope which, in turn, is attached to the base either directly or by a hinged joint. Since the aberrations, or faults, of a lens can only be corrected for one tube length, for critical microscopy it should always be set to the standard 160 mm if a draw tube is fitted; if there is no draw tube, the body tube will, of course, be correct.

The body tube may rarely contain a draw tube, being a telescopic tube by means of which the distance between the eyepiece and objective may be varied. The draw tube usually contains a fixed diaphragm at its lower end to cut off reflections from the inside of the body tube. Such a draw tube is useful in micrometry (page 570).

A carrier or nosepiece for a number of objectives is usually fitted at the lower end of the body tube; it rotates on a central pillar, and is designated by the number of objectives it carries; for example, double, triple or quadruple nosepiece. The nosepiece should bring each objective into its correct position; that is to say, centred on the optical axis, and at the correct tube length. An increase in magnification is simply a matter of rotating the nosepiece, which is optically better than changing the eyepiece since a large aperture is being used; the oil-immersion lenses are, of course, an exception since the body tube needs to be raised to place oil on the slide.

The depth of the nosepiece will affect the tube length and this is generally 18 mm in depth, the actual length of the body tube being only 142 mm. If, for any reason, the nosepiece is removed, it must be replaced by a compensating ring of the same depth.

For accurate centring of objectives another type of objective changer may be used, a female slide being fitted to the bottom of the body tube, and each objective screwed into a male slide which has three centring screws. Owing to the improved design of modern nosepieces such attachments are now rarely seen.

Adjustment

On old models the body tube was attached to the supporting structure by two slides which were the site of the adjustment controls. This was followed by placing the slides (and controls) on the base, which entailed the controls moving the whole superstructure (body tube and limb) which caused increased wear and shorter life, but it was felt that the convenience of having the controls at almost bench level outweighed this disadvantage. Modern microscopes, however, have a fixed body tube, limb and base, the adjustment slide or slides being connected to raise and lower the stage and substage; this has the dual advantage, the controls being conveniently placed with little weight bearing on them, which gives longer life and lessens the likelihood of their 'slipping' (*Figure 33.9*).

The mechanism of the slides is such that one of them, working by rack and pinion, enables the stage and substage to be moved rapidly up and down, and is called the coarse adjustment; the other, working by micrometer screws, and levers or cams, enables the stage and substage to be moved slowly and accurately and is called the fine adjustment. Although the designs of the latter may vary, they are based on the same general principle: the movement by a lever or cam to a steel plate fixed on the back of the coarse adjustment slide (*Figure 33.14*). The coarse adjustment therefore moves the

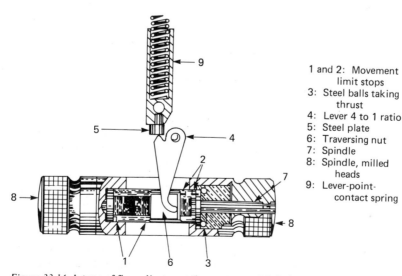

1 and 2: Movement limit stops
3: Steel balls taking thrust
4: Lever 4 to 1 ratio
5: Steel plate
6: Traversing nut
7: Spindle
8: Spindle, milled heads
9: Lever-point-contact spring

Figure 33.14 A type of fine adjustment (by courtesy of C. Baker of Holborn Ltd)

stage and substage, but the fine adjustment moves both the stage and substage and the coarse adjustment slide. As these slides wear, a degree of play will develop and cause slackness in focusing; most manufacturers, therefore, fit screws which may be adjusted to compensate for this slackness, but they should be adjusted with care as over-tightening will cause excessive wear.

The binocular microscope

The light rays emerging from the objective in the binocular microscope are equally divided between the two eyepieces. It is not sufficient simply to insert a single prism and divert one half of the rays, since this would cause eye-strain due to both the observer's eyes being focused on a single point a short distance away, and the advantage of a binocular microscope is that long periods may be spent viewing through it with the minimum amount of eye fatigue. The modern binocular microscope achieves this by the use of four prisms. It will be seen from *Figure 33.15* that the eyes are receiving two parallel beams of light. The lower central prism consists of two prisms cemented

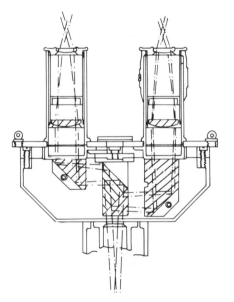

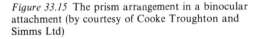

Figure 33.15 The prism arrangement in a binocular attachment (by courtesy of Cooke Troughton and Simms Ltd)

together, at the interface of which there is a semi-silvered surface: this silvering is a very special process, fine grains of silver being deposited so that alternate light rays are differentially treated, one being reflected to the right (*Figure 33.15*) and the other passing into the upper prism.

The light rays passing through the semi-silvered surface to the upper prism travel through a greater thickness of glass than those that are reflected—having the effect of retarding them—and this is compensated for by making the right-hand prism with an extra thickness of glass as will be seen by comparing the two outside prisms in *Figure 33.15*.

An additional advantage of this system is that the eyepieces, with the prisms attached, can be easily moved together or apart, and the interocular distance adjusted to suit individual requirements.

One of the eyepieces (the one on the right in *Figure 33.15*) is fitted with an adjustment to compensate for the slight variation of focus occasionally required.

With a binocular body on a microscope, the optical tube length may be increased from 160 to 240 mm, and since the objectives are corrected for the shorter tube length, a compensating lens is incorporated to overcome this factor; the lens is also necessary to re-focus the virtual image for the new tube length. The increase of tube length also has the effect of increasing the magnification, and binocular attachments may have their magnifying factor engraved on them which, since the tube is usually increased by one half, is × 1.5.

Magnification changers may be sited in the body tube above the objective on a rotating mount. The magnification increase is engraved at each position, for example, × 1.25, × 1.5, etc.

Stage

At the lower end of the limb supporting the body tube and adjustments is a platform, or stage, on which the objects to be examined are placed. The stage may be plain or mechanical. A mechanical stage will give even steady movement of the object in two directions by means of two micrometer threads. The standard type of mechanical stage takes a 3 × 1 inch slide and moves over an area approximately $3\frac{1}{2}$ × $1\frac{1}{4}$ inches so that a whole slide may be examined, but special stages are available to take very large slides and Petri dishes. Circular rotating stages are also available if preferred (e.g. the polarizing microscope).

Most mechanical stages are fitted with a Vernier scale for recording the position of the slide in each direction, and they may be very useful if a particular field is to be found quickly at a later re-examination. By noting the reading on each scale, the slide can be replaced in much the same position almost immediately. One scale will be graduated, for example, from 0 to 80, and the other from 80 to 110 in order that the two readings will not be confused. Opposite these graduations will be the smaller Vernier scale, marked from 0 to 10. These 10 graduations, being equal to 9 in the main scale, enable each of the latter to be subdivided by 10.

Illuminating apparatus

The substage

Below the stage, and usually attached to it, is an adjustable substage which can be moved up and down by a helical screw or rack and pinion (as in the coarse adjustment).

The substage consists of: (a) the condenser to focus the light on the object when using objectives with a focal length of 16 mm or less; (b) an iris diaphragm to control the cone of light entering the condenser; (c) a filter carrier; and (d) a mirror, flat on one side and concave on the other, which is mounted in gimbals so that light may be directed into the condenser from almost any angle, or more commonly a built-in light source with a fixed mirror.

The condenser

The condenser should form a perfect image of the light source, and have the same numerical aperture as the objective with which it is being used.

The two-lens Abbé condenser is in common use but is not very efficient, forming only an imperfect image of the light source. It should not be used with apochromatic or fluorite lenses (page 560). To obtain perfect results with such objectives, a condenser with a lens system equal to that of the objective being used should be employed: a three-lens aplanatic or a more highly corrected achromatic condenser will give a crisp image with good resolution. Such condensers are usually fitted with a swing-out front lens (or the front lens may be unscrewed) to illuminate the whole field for low-power lenses. By swinging out the front lens the numerical aperture of the condenser is reduced to 0.3–0.4. For critical microscopy with objectives having an NA exceeding 1.0, immersion oil should be applied between the condenser and the slide, as well as between the objective and the slide.

The iris diaphragm

Light which passes through the object but does not enter the objective is unnecessary, and may interfere with those light rays which are intended to form the image.

The iris diaphragm is employed to limit the angle of the cone of light passing through the object so that it will just fill the front lens of the objective. Its proper name is the *aperture diaphragm*.

The intensity of illumination should always, if possible, be reduced by using light-absorbing filters, or a variable resistance, not by closing the diaphragm and never by racking down the condenser.

The filter carrier

The filter carrier is usually a recessed metal ring, pivoting on a screw to facilitate the easy removal of filters.

The mirror

The two-sided mirror is plane on one side and concave on the other, and is fitted about 4 inches below the stage. A concave mirror has a focus since it causes the light rays, which have been reflected, to converge together and form an image. The focus is approximately 4 inches (its distance from the object) and is intended to take the place of a condenser when using very low-power objectives since these require a large area of the object to be illuminated.

The plane mirror must always be used with the condenser since the latter can only be used efficiently if the whole of the back lens is filled with light.

Microscopes with built-in light sources have mirrors fixed in the base.

Illumination

Although daylight may be used to illuminate the field, it will generally be found inconvenient owing to its inconstancy. Artificial illumination supplied by an electric filament lamp is therefore most commonly employed.

The lamp may be either a simple pearl bulb, or a high intensity lamp used in conjunction with a condenser and an iris diaphragm.

The source of illumination should be:

(1) uniformly intense;
(2) should completely flood the back lens of the condenser with light when the lamp iris diaphragm is open; and
(3) make the object appear as though it were self-luminous.

(1) Uniform intensity of illumination is most difficult to obtain since the solid sources of light—a tungsten arc (where a small sphere of tungsten glows white), or a carbon arc—present great difficulties if used over long periods. The difficulty is overcome by using a closely wound filament with a diffusing screen, although for routine work with a monocular microscope a 60 watt pearl bulb will suffice. Kohler illumination may be used.

(2) The source of light should be sufficient to enable its rays when directed by the plane side of the mirror to flood the back lens of the condenser uniformly. The high intensity type of lamp has an optical axis and must be correctly aligned for use, and the distance from the microscope at which it is used adjusted so that the lens magnifies the lamp image to the correct size, a built-in light source has been so adjusted.

Where separate, the lamp and the microscope should be connected so that accidental movement of one or the other will not upset the alignment. If the manufacturers do not supply such a connexion, the lamp, the microscope and the transformer (if needed) may be mounted on a wooden base.

(3) The object will behave as if self-luminous if the opal bulb or the image of the lamp condenser is focused in the object plane with the substage condenser (*see below*).

Setting up the microscope

The bench on which the microscope is mounted should be free from vibration and be in such a position that microscopist works with his back to the window; a light screen, the back and sides of which are finished with a flat black paint to minimize back-scatter of light, is a great advantage.

Illumination by Nelson or Kohler methods

These are the two universally recognized methods for correct illumination.

Nelson method

For this method the light source should be homogeneous and no lamp condensers used. It is normally employed with a bare light source. The light source should be focused on the object plane by racking the substage condenser up or down.

Kohler method

For this method to be used the light source does not have to be homogeneous, but a lamp condenser is essential to project an image of the lamp filament on to the substage iris diaphragm. In this system the lamp condensing lens (which is evenly illuminated) functions as the light source. This method must be used with compound lamps, and should always be used for photomicrography.

■ Technique

(1) The lamp should be positioned opposite the microscope (the high intensity compound light being fixed), and a blue daylight filter inserted in the filter carrier to absorb the excess yellow given by artificial light.

(2) Position the lamp so that the light strikes the centre of the mirror, and adjust the mirror so that the light is directed upwards into the condenser. Modern microscopes have in-built lamps, condensing lenses and mirrors.

(3) With a compound lamp focus the condensing lens so that an image of the source of light is formed on the substage iris diaphragm (aperture diaphragm); if necessary hold a piece of white paper at this position so that the image is visible.

(4) Focus on an object on the stage and ensure that the field is evenly illuminated.

(5) With the object in focus, rack the substage condenser up or down until a sharp image of the lamp iris diaphragm (the field diaphragm) appears.

(6) Centre the image of the field diaphragm using the substage centring controls.

(7) Open the field diaphragm until its circle of light is just larger than the field of view. This reduces glare to the minimum.

(8) Remove an eyepiece and adjust the substage iris diaphragm until two-thirds of the back focal plane of the objective is illuminated. Replace the eyepiece. The microscope is now ready for use.

For critical microscopy and photomicrography, the field diaphragm may need to be centred each time the objective is changed.

One cardinal rule for the microscopist is always to rack the objective down near the object before looking through the eyepiece and then to focus on the object by racking the objective up and away from the object. This will avoid damaging the object or the front lens of the objective, and is particularly important when using oil-immersion objectives, which have very short working distances. This is good practice even when using objectives with safety retracting front lenses.

■ Summary

(1) In Nelson or critical illumination the light source and the object are in focus.

(2) In Kohler illumination the light source is focused on the aperture diaphragm, and the field diaphragm and object are in focus.

Cleaning and maintenance

It must be remembered that the microscope is an exceedingly complicated and delicate piece of apparatus, and a great deal of experience is required to completely service and maintain it. Component parts should be returned to the manufacturer when faulty, since amateur attempts at repair usually result in further damage: apart from cleaning the outer surface of their lenses objectives are best left alone. Prisms should never be touched, and cleaning should be confined to blowing off the dust with a rubber bulb fitted with a small-bore metal tube, since the slightest disalignment of the prisms will cause enormous eye fatigue. Lenses should be wiped only with fresh lens tissue or cotton wool, otherwise they may be scratched. Immersion oil should be removed immediately after use, although old oil can be removed with lens tissue or cotton wool damped with xylene or, preferably, ether, because of its higher volatility.

Daily cleaning routine

(1) The microscope should be dusted daily, and the outer surface of the lenses of objectives polished with lens tissue or cotton wool.

(2) The top lens of the eyepiece should be polished to remove dust or fingermarks, and the microscope set up for correct illumination.
(3) Rotation of the eyepiece will show if any dust is still present, in which case the eyepiece may need to be dismantled and both lenses cleaned.
(4) The substage condenser and the mirror are cleaned in a similar manner: dust on the condenser will be apparent when this is racked up and down, since it will come in and out of focus.

A little attention to cleaning the microscope daily will, by the removal of chemically-active and sharp pieces of grit and foreign matter, prolong the life of the instrument and make the weekly cleaning task a short and simple one.

Weekly cleaning routine

(1) The slides of the coarse adjustment, the mechanical stage and the substage condenser should be wiped with a cloth dampened with xylene to remove dust which would otherwise damage the slides. A little oil (as supplied for lubricating microscopes) is applied and the slides replaced: later models do not require this treatment.
(2) The lens system should be checked and cleaned.
(3) Clean the eyepieces as described in (2) and (3) of the daily routine, and then trace dirt in other places by a similar system.
(4) Dust is removed from the back lenses of objectives by use of the rubber bulb described above.
(5) Interocular adjustment slides will usually require cleaning only once a month, and great care should be taken not to damage or disturb the prisms during this operation.

Magnification

The magnification of a lens will depend on its conjugate foci (page 552); that is, the distance from the object to the lens and that from the lens to the image. In the microscope the objective forms a real inverted image in the upper part of the body tube, which is then further magnified by the eyepiece. Therefore, the magnification of the microscope is the product of the magnifications of the objective and the eyepiece, and is dependent on the following three factors:

(1) the focal length of the objective;
(2) the distance between the focal plane of the objective and the image it produces (since the optical tube length and the mechanical tube length are approximately the same, the latter is always used (*Figure 33.16*);
(3) the magnification of the eyepiece.

Magnification therefore equals:

$$\frac{\text{Tube length}}{\text{Focal length of objective}} \times \text{Eyepiece magnification}$$

To take an example: the magnification obtained with a 16 mm objective, used with a × 10 eyepiece at the standard tube length of 160 mm would be:

$$\frac{160}{16} \times 10 = 100$$

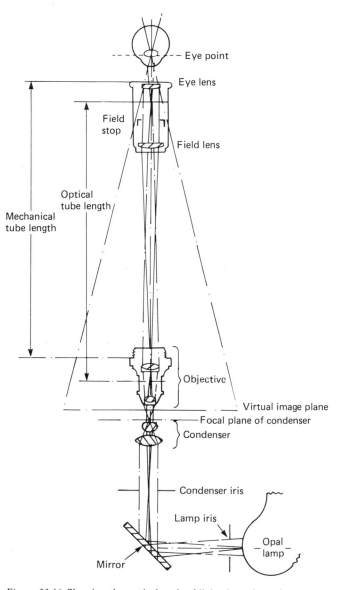

Figure 33.16 Showing the optical path of light through a microscope

Where the magnification is marked on an objective it is only correct when used at the standard tube length. Total magnification is then calculated by multiplying the magnification of the objective by the magnification of the eyepiece. It should be remembered that this magnification is a linear one, and in the example above the object will be magnified 100 times in all directions; the actual area magnification will be $100 \times 100 = 10\,000$ times.

Micrometry

The standard unit of measurement in microscopy is a micrometre (µm), which is 0.001 mm.

To measure microscopic objects an eyepiece micrometer scale is used in conjunction with a stage micrometer. The eyepiece micrometer scale is usually a disc on which is engraved an arbitrary scale. This is placed inside the Huygenian eyepiece, resting on the field stop (*Figure 33.16*). Eyepiece micrometers may be purchased with the scale permanently in position; these are usually Kellner eyepieces which have a focal plane below their bottom lens. They give a sharp image of the scale and have a greater eye clearance; they are an advantage (without a scale) for general work if spectacles are worn.

The stage micrometer consists of a 3×1 inch slide on which a millimetre scale is engraved in $\frac{1}{10}$ and $\frac{1}{100}$ graduations.

An object may be measured by the following method.

(1) Insert a micrometer eyepiece scale and place the stage micrometer on the stage.
(2) Select the objective to be used when measuring the object, and focus on the stage micrometer scale.
(3) Determine the number of divisions of the eyepiece scale equal to an exact number of divisions of the stage micrometer scale. A draw tube is useful at this stage since a slight alteration in magnification by increasing or decreasing the size of the stage micrometer scale, may greatly simplify calculations.
(4) Remove the stage micrometer, focus on the object to be measured and determine the number of eyepiece divisions exactly covered by the object.

Calculate the size of the object as follows, assuming that 100 eyepiece divisions were equal to 10 small stage divisions, and that the diameter of the object was exactly covered by 12 eyepiece divisions.

$$100 \text{ stage divisions} = 1 \text{ mm} = 1000 \text{ µm}$$

$$100 \text{ eyepiece divisions} = 10 \text{ stage divisions}$$

Therefore $100 \text{ eyepiece divisions} = 100 \text{ µm}$

Therefore $1 \text{ eyepiece division} = 1 \text{ µm}$

Therefore $12 \text{ eyepiece divisions} = 12 \text{ µm}$

The diameter of the object, therefore, was 12 µm.

Darkground microscopy

For an object to be examined microscopically, it must first be visible. Visibility is dependent on contrast, as is illustrated by the fact that a black cat is invisible in a coal cellar because there is no contrast between the object and the background. For the same reason, a spider's web is difficult to see against the sky, yet stands out clearly when viewed against a dark background with the sun shining on it; this is because the fibres reflect the rays of light from the sun and give the web the appearance of being self-luminous, the dark background increasing the contrast.

Most objects examined microscopically are naturally transparent, but in general they reflect or scatter light rays, and if, as in darkground illumination, oblique light is thrown upon them which does not enter the objective, they will appear as self-luminous objects on a dark background.

Objects examined by darkground illumination give a misleading impression of size; fine particles appear to be much larger than they are, owing to their light-scattering properties. This factor is of advantage when examining fine structures such as spirochaetes which are clearly visible by this method, yet when stained (by Giemsa's stain) are difficult to see. This will only apply if the object is alone or nearly alone in the field of view; therefore, preparations must be as thin as possible; if such objects are examined in a mass of light-reflecting material the contrast will be lost. Although it is impossible to completely isolate cells and organisms, extraneous refractile material such as air bubbles, red blood cells and oil droplets must be avoided and a thin preparation used.

Objectives and condensers

Low-power objectives work at some distance from the object and therefore darkground illumination is obtained simply by inserting a small circle of black paper (pasted on glass) in the filter carrier. The central rays which would normally pass through the object and into the objective are cut off and the peripheral rays from the condenser pass through the object, but do not enter the objective; the only light entering the objective will be that scattered by the object.

High-power objectives, having a much shorter working distance require a special condenser which will accurately focus a hollow cone of light at an acute angle. This angle is so acute that if oil is not used between the condenser and slide the light rays are reflected back into the condenser (total internal reflection, *see* page 550). Immersion oil must be used between object and objective to ensure that the maximum amount of reflected light from the object enters the objective. To get the best results the condenser must be accurately centred, otherwise peripheral light rays will enter one side of the objective; similarly, the condenser must be accurately focused to get the maximum amount of light on the object without its entering the objective.

Because of the very acute angle of light required, very few darkground condensers can be used with an objective having a numerical aperture (NA) in excess of 1.0. A 2 mm objective having a NA 1.3 can be used if a funnel stop (a small metal tube) is inserted in the back which reduces the working aperture to less than 1.0. Alternatively, a $\frac{1}{7}$-inch oil immersion lens may be used without modification. The most convenient type of 2 mm objective is one incorporating an iris diaphragm, since this can be closed just sufficiently to stop any direct light.

The fixed-focus type of darkground condenser (*Figure 33.17*) is most common, but this can only be used with extra-thin glass slides and coverslips (No. 1). Focusing darkground condensers (*Figure 33.18*) are available which will allow a variety of slides and coverslips to be used.

Since only reflected or scattered light forms an image of the object, the source of light should be an intense one, to ensure the maximum amount of light passing through the object. A Pointolite tungsten arc lamp probably gives the best results, although the modern high intensity lamp will give almost equally good results.

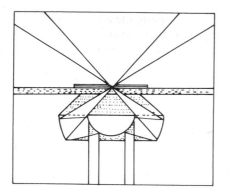

Figure 33.17 A fixed focus dark-ground condenser. (Reproduced from *The Microscope* by courtesy of R. and J. Beck Ltd)

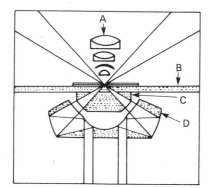

Figure 33.18 A focusing dark-ground condenser. (Reproduced from *The Microscope* by courtesy of R. and J. Beck Ltd)

Setting up the darkground microscope

■ **Method**

(1) Make a thin preparation, using a thoroughly clean thin slide and coverslip, and taking care not to have air bubbles in the preparation.
(2) Direct, or adjust, light through the condenser so that it is evenly distributed.
(3) Rack the condenser down; place a drop of immersion oil on the top lens of the condenser and on the lower side of the slide. Place the slide on the microscope stage and slowly rack up the condenser until the two surfaces of the immersion oil meet without forming air bubbles; such bubbles would reflect light in all directions.
(4) Focus on the object with a low-power objective such as the 16 mm.

Note: If the condenser is correctly focused a small point of light will illuminate the object on a dark background. If a hollow ring of light is seen the condenser is above or below its point of focus and should be adjusted.

(5) With the centring screws, adjust the condenser until the point of light is in the centre of the field.
(6) Place a drop of immersion oil on the coverslip and focus the object with the high-power oil immersion objective. Perfect darkground illumination should result if a funnel-stop objective is used; if an iris diaphragm is incorporated in the objective it

is adjusted to give the maximum performance. Occasionally the objectives are not par-central and the condenser may need a slight adjustment to get a perfect result.
(7) After use the oil should be carefully cleaned off both the condenser and objective.

The following errors are the most common causes of difficulty in setting up the microscope.

(1) The slides or coverslips are too thick.
(2) The preparation has too many air bubbles present.
(3) Condenser is not properly focused or centred.
(4) Lighting is not sufficiently intense.

Fluorescence microscopy

In 1852 Stokes first used the word 'fluorescence' to describe the reaction of fluorspar to ultraviolet light: in 1903 R. W. Wood devised a filter which would absorb visible light and transmit only ultraviolet light. These two events led to the first 'fluorescence microscope' described by Lehmann in 1911. Little use was made of this apparatus until 1935 when Max Haitinger pioneered and developed the technique of staining histological preparations and smears with fluorescent dyes. It is probably to him that most of the credit for the modern development of fluorescence techniques belongs. In 1937 Hageman applied fluorescent dyes to organisms, and probably the first routine use of fluorescent microscopy was the staining of acid fast bacilli. In 1941 Coons, Creech and Jones described a technique for labelling protein with a fluorescent dye, which led to the now almost routine technique of fluorescent antibody staining. A further advance was the introduction by Ploem (1967) of dichromatic mirrors for incident illumination (epi-illumination).

Fluorescence

When a quantum of light is absorbed by an atom or molecule, an electron is boosted to a higher energy level. When this displaced electron returns to its original ground state it may emit a quantum of light (*Figure 33.19*). If this light is emitted only during the time of exposure, or for a very short time afterwards (about 9–10 seconds) it is known as *fluorescence*; if this emission persists after the exciting light is cut off it is called *phosphorescence*. Since a certain amount of energy is lost as heat before the electron returns to its ground state the fluorescent (or phosphorescent) light is at a longer wavelength (lower energy) than the original exciting light. In fluorescence microscopy ultraviolet light (which is not visible to the human eye) may be used as the exciting light with the resulting fluorescence (of a longer wavelength) being in the visible range. Thus an object is illuminated with 'black' light and, when fluorescent, appears as a bright object on a dark background. In practice, short wavelength visible light is often used. It should be remembered that while an enormous number of compounds are fluorescent to some degree, only relatively few give sufficiently brilliant fluorescence that they may be detected in small quantities by their autofluorescence, or used as fluorescent dyes. Certain dyes, marked in catalogues as fluorescent, are virtually useless because of their poor fluorescence. Furthermore some compounds and dyes, while brilliantly fluorescent as pure compounds, may lose their power to fluoresce when bound to other

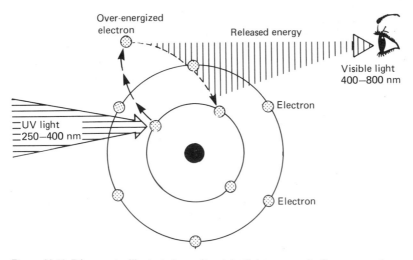

Figure 33.19 Diagram to illustrate how ultraviolet light may excite fluorescence in a molecule

structures. This is known as *quenching* of fluorescence. This latter is sometimes a useful property, since non-specific fluorescence can be quenched to give greater contrast (*see* use of haematoxylin to quench nuclear fluorescence, page 469).

Equipment

The early workers in this field used quartz condensers and slides to bring the maximum concentration of ultraviolet light on to the object. With modern optical glass (which transmits light with a wavelength of over 300 nm) it has been found that almost any condenser may be used for this purpose.

Slides should be checked for obvious fluorescence (those made of green glass being avoided); but most good brands of slides are suitable.

Illumination

The most commonly used light sources for fluorescence microscopy are tungsten–halogen, high-pressure mercury (HBO) and high-pressure xenon (XBO) lamps.

Tungsten–halogen lamps

These lamps emit a continuous spectrum in the entire visible range and have been used in immunofluorescence and for tetracycline and acridine orange fluorochromes. Although they are convenient to use, their comparative low intensity has caused them to be superseded by the HBO range (*Figure 33.20a*).

HBO high-pressure mercury lamps

These lamps emit a spectrum whose characteristics are ideal for excitation in the near ultraviolet, violet or green range. Their background emission is also sufficient for blue excitation. Several types are available principally the HBO 50, HBO 100 W/2 and HBO 200 W/4. The HBO 50 is widely used as a source for incident light fluorescence and can be used for most techniques including FITC staining. The 100 and 200 versions have similar line spectra (*Figure 33.20b*).

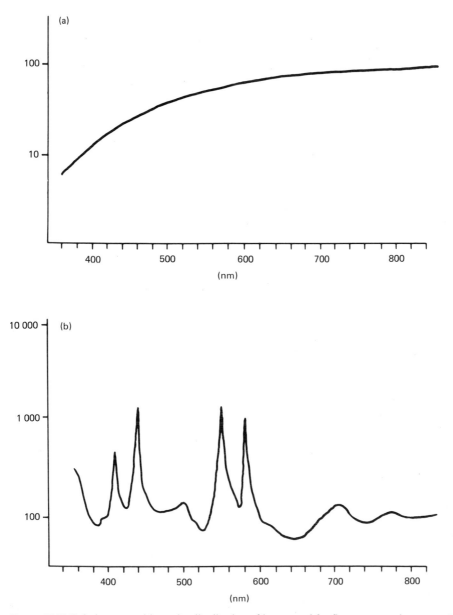

Figure 33.20 Relative spectral intensity distribution of lamps used for fluorescence microscopy. (a) Tungsten–halogen lamp; (b) HBO 50;

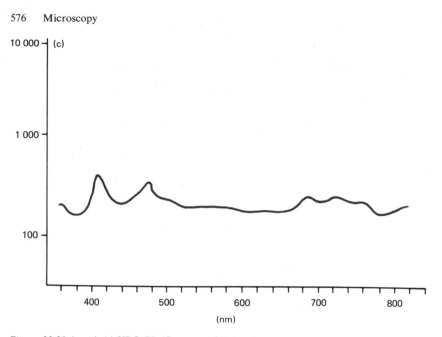

Figure 33.20 (cont.) (c) XBO 75. (Courtesy of Zeiss (Oberkochen) Ltd, West Germany)

XBO high-pressure xenon lamps

These lamps emit a spectrum similar to daylight giving an intense illumination. They are used in projection microscopes and are available as XBO 75 W/2, XBO 150 W/1 and XBO 450 W versions. The XBO 75 type is recommended for use in measurement of excitation and emission spectra (*Figure 33.20c*).

A record of the use of HBO and XBO lamps should be kept and they should not be used past the manufacturers' recommended lifetime. Nevertheless, the life of the lamp is partly determined by the number of times it is switched on and off. The lamp should certainly be replaced if it becomes dim or flickers. An adjustable reflector is usually situated behind the lamp which produces an image of the lamp. This should be focused with the original arc and centred alongside it, but should not overlap it.

Normally these lamps should not be re-ignited until they have cooled but Zeiss advise that the XBO series may be re-ignited when hot. The manufacturers' instructions for each lamp should be carefully followed.

Filter systems

A heat filter system is essential with any intense source of illumination. The heat filter is usually located in the lamp housing between the lamp and the collecting lens. The filter normally used is the KG1.

In addition, two basic filter systems are necessary for transmission fluorescence microscopy. For incident light illumination a dichromatic beam splitter is also required.

Exciter filters

The early exciter filters used in fluorescence microscopy were 'dyed-in-the-mass' glass filters and were designated UG or BG along with a number.

Schott BG 12 transmits light of 325–500 nm and a Schott UG 1 transmits light of 275–400 nm.

Modern exciter filters are designated by letter and numbers: G = dyed-in-the-glass; BP = band pass.

The number now indicates the wavelength of the transmission. They are characterized by their wavelength of maximum transmission, for example, G 405, by their centre wavelength and half the band width, for example, BP 405/6, or by the short- and long-wave half value width, for example, BP 400–440.

The transmission curves of some of the older Schott filters and of examples of the modern filters are shown in *Figures 33.21* and *33.22*, respectively.

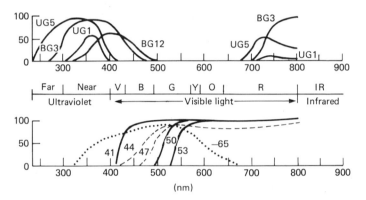

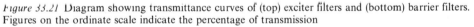

Figure 33.21 Diagram showing transmittance curves of (top) exciter filters and (bottom) barrier filters. Figures on the ordinate scale indicate the percentage of transmission

Barrier or contrast filters

These are so named because they are used primarily to protect the eyes of the observer from the damaging effects of ultraviolet light (*Figure 33.23*). By the use of different filters, with varying absorption and transmission characteristics non-specific background fluorescence may be extinguished, giving greater contrast. For example, when examining tissue stained by a yellow or orange fluorescent dye, Schott filters OG 4 and 5 (Zeiss 47 and 50) may be used to absorb the blue autofluorescence of the tissue. This will result in bright yellow staining of the tissue against a black background. The numbers of the older Zeiss filter referred to the wavelength at which they transmitted light, for example, 47 transmits light with a wavelength of 470 nm and above.

Filters are now identified with letters and numbers. LP indicates Long-pass, for example, LP 495 is a filter which transmits light above 495 nm with 50% transmission at 495 nm (*Figure 33.22*). Leitz use the prefix K for their barrier filters for transmitted light fluorescence.

The barrier filter must be chosen so that its transmission lies completely outside that of the exciter filter, but includes the fluorescence emission. Some exciter filters transmit

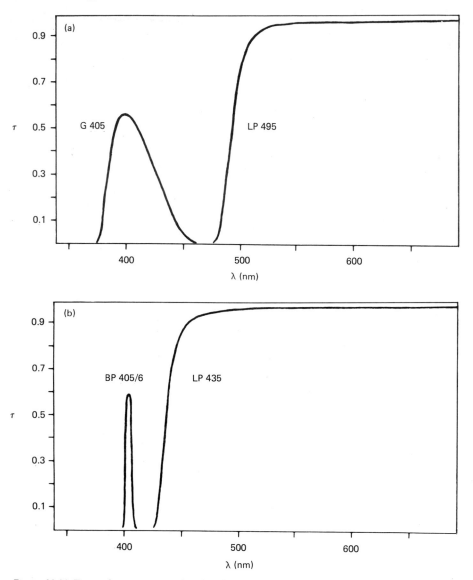

Figure 33.22 Transmittance curves of exciter filters and their appropriate LP (light passing) barrier filters for fluorescence microscopy. (a) Blue violet glass filter; (b) narrow band pass filter;

red light in addition to short wavelength light (*Figure 33.21*). Suppression filters may be used to remove this light, for example, BG 38, Zeiss – 65.

Dichromatic beam splitters

Dichromatic beam splitters reflect almost all the desired short wavelength light towards the object. The longer wavelength fluorescence radiation emitted from the specimen is almost completely transmitted to the observer (*Figure 33.24*).

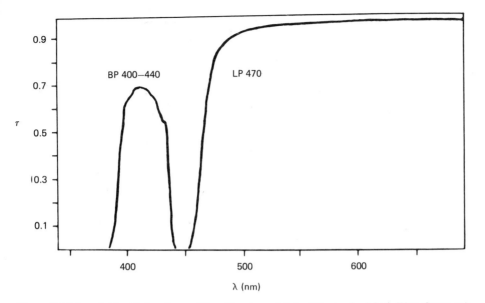

Figure 33.22 (cont.) (c) wide band pass filter. (Courtesy of Zeiss (Oberkochen) Ltd, West Germany)

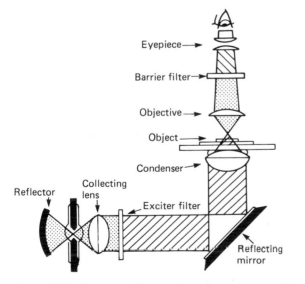

Figure 33.23 Diagram to illustrate the component parts of the fluorescent microscope. The lamp gives out mixed ultraviolet and visible light (darkened area); the visible light is filtered out by the exciter filter. The object gives rise to visible light which is mixed with ultraviolet light (darkened area); the ultraviolet light is filtered out by the barrier filter, so that only visible light reaches the observer's eye

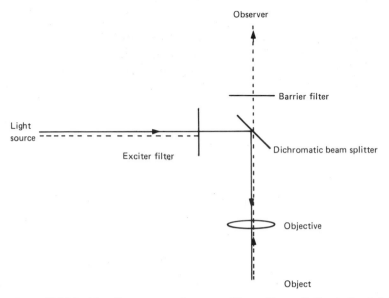

Figure 33.24 Incident fluorescence microscopy. The exciting radiation is directed downwards by the dichromatic beam splitter through the objective which acts as a condenser. The fluorescent emission passes up through the objective and on through the dichromatic beam splitter and the barrier filter to the observer. —— short wave length component; ––– longer wave length component

Filter sets are supplied by the major manufacturers, each set consisting of exciter filter, dichromatic mirror (beam splitter) and barrier filter. The dichromatic beam splitters are identified by letters and numbers. The number refers to the wavelength below which light is reflected, for example, FT 510 (Zeiss, W. Germany), RKP 510 (Leitz) and DS 510 (Reichert).

Filter combinations

A comprehensive list of excitation and emission maxima of fluorochromes is given by Rost (1980). Filter combinations for various applications are given in manufacturers' publications (Zeiss, Leitz and Reichert–Jung). A selection of filters for the most common applications is given in *Table 33.1*.

Table 33.1

		Exciter	*Barrier*
Acridine orange	Blue	BP 450–490	LP 520
Auramine	Blue	BP 450–490	LP 520
FIF catecholamines	Violet	BP 405/6	LP 435
FIF 5-HT	Ultraviolet	UG 1 + BG 38	LP 435
FIF 5-HT	Violet	BP 405/6	LP 435
FITC	Blue	BP 485/20	BP 520–560[1]
Quinacrine mustard	Blue/violet	G 434	LP 520
Lissamine rhodamine B 200	Green	BP 510–560	LP 590
Tetracycline	Blue	BP 475–495	LP 520
Thioflavine T	Blue	BP 450–490	LP 520

[1] Blue excitation with selective band transmittance of barrier filter.

Microscope

Any good microscope may be used for fluorescence microscopy. It is often convenient to purchase the lamp (HBO 200) from the manufacturer of the microscope being used since there will probably be convenient points of attachment to set the lamp in the correct position (distance).

Mirror

This should be of a front surface reflecting type (polished metal) to avoid loss of ultraviolet by double surface reflection (e.g. glass face and mirror face) and to avoid the possible absorption of ultraviolet, by the glass. However, it will be found that a large number of normal microscope mirrors will give satisfactory results.

Condenser

A *light type condenser* may be used, particularly with low-power objectives; a *darkground condenser*, however, is almost mandatory for oil immersion objectives, since it gives a darker background and allows a thinner exciter filter to be used. The disadvantage of a darkground condenser is that oil must be used between condenser and slide but this is found to be far outweighed by the advantages.

Contrast–fluorescence condenser

This is a combined fluorescence–phase condenser. The specially designed condenser annulus (the whole of which passes ultraviolet light) permits examination by phase contrast, fluorescence or a mixture of the two. It is most useful as a means of identifying the source and location of fluorescence in smears and sections.

Exciter filter attachment

Exciter filters may be as follows.

(1) Placed in a filter carrier below the condenser.
(2) Inserted in fitted slides carrying several filters, in front of the colleging lens of the illumination system and protected by the heat absorbing KG 1 filter.

Barrier filter attachment

Barrier filters may be as follows.

(1) Inserted into the eyepiece by removal of the top lens, or they may be screwed into the bottom of the eyepiece.
(2) Inserted in the body tube by means of specially fitted slides (carrying one, or a number of filters), or by placing a single filter in a convenient location.
(3) Incorporated in a rotary filter changer (such as that supplied by Zeiss) which is fitted below the binocular attachment.

If the microscope is used for a variety of purposes type (3) will be found the most convenient, since filters are easily and quickly changed. Since two rotating discs each carry three filters and one blank space, one can use a variety of filters, either alone or in combination.

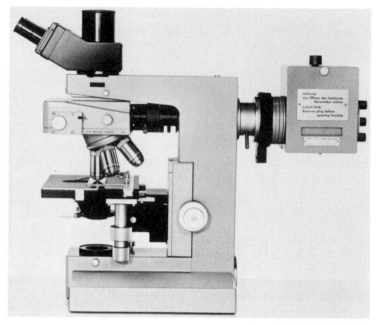

Figure 33.25 Microscope equipped for both bright field transmitted and fluorescence incident illumination. (Courtesy of E. Leitz (Instruments) Ltd)

Dichromatic filter system

The dichromatic filter sets or clusters, comprising the exciter filter, dichromatic beam splitter and barrier filter are situated in a special holder sited above the objective in line with the illuminating beam (*Figure 33.25*).

Objectives

Any non-fluorescent objective may be used. Achromats are generally preferred to apochromats as they rarely fluoresce and their colour correction is usually adequate. A high numerical aperture (NA) is preferred to ensure the maximum transmission of fluorescent light from the object. The oil immersion objective should be fitted with an iris diaphragm (or funnel stop) when using a darkground condenser.

Microscopic preparations

Microscope slides

These should be thin and of even thickness (not of green glass). Special ultraviolet transmitting slides may be purchased, but unless a quartz condenser is used it is pointless to employ them. Optical glass (as used in condensers) will only transmit light of 300 nm and over, and at this range thin glass slides have an adequate transmission.

Section adhesives

Thinly applied routine section adhesives do not interfere with preparations.

Mountants

Cleared preparations may be mounted in HSR (Harleco synthetic resin) or Depex. Fluormount will probably give the best results.

Aqueous mounts

These may be mounted in Apathy's media (*see* page 147) with the exception of acridine orange or fluorescent antibody stained preparations.

Fluorescent antibody preparations

These are mounted in glycerin to which 10% phosphate buffered saline (pH 7.1) has been added.

Acridine orange stained preparations

These are mounted in buffer only.

Autofluorescence (primary fluorescence)

The ability of some naturally occurring compounds to fluoresce is on occasion a great advantage in identification. Autofluorescent material can present a great hazard to the inexperienced microscopist, because, dependent on its structure, it may fluoresce any colour and thus appear to have been stained by the technique employed. For this reason unstained smears, identically prepared in all other respects, should always be used as controls of fluorescent stains.

Preparation of material

For the specific study of autofluorescence, unfixed smears or cryostat cut sections of unfixed tissue should be used. It may be found subsequently that fixation does not interfere with the specific fluorescence; 95% alcohol (ethyl) or ether–alcohol are usually satisfactory. Formalin should generally be avoided if possible as it tends to increase the blue autofluorescence of tissue. However, with 5HT (*see below*) it is essential

Specific autofluorescence

The number of naturally occurring autofluorescent compounds is enormous and for a more complete list of them the reader is referred to *Fluorchemistry* by De Ment (1945) (Chemical Publishing Co.), or *Fluorescent Analysis in UV Light* by Radley and Grant (1951) (Chapman and Hall). Those dealt with below are considered the most likely to be encountered.

Tissue

Generally tissue fluoresces a bright blue, although this may be absorbed by use of a yellow or orange filter.

Elastic fibres

Fluoresces an intensely brilliant blue while unstained, and may be easily seen even in a haematoxylin and eosin-stained section.

Ceroid and riboflavin

These fluoresce in shades of yellow.

Lipids and lipochromes

Many of these fluoresce in shades of yellow.

Vitamins

Many vitamins are fluorescent in shades of yellow, green and blue.

Porphyrin

This group (and chlorophyll) are among the very few compounds with an intense red fluorescence. This characteristic has been made use of by adding a drop of concentrated H_2SO_4 to blood stains (or suspected stains), the H_2SO_4 takes the iron out of the haemoglobin forming haematoporphyrin which gives a brilliant red fluorescence. There is a small accessory lachrymal gland (Harderian) in the corner of the eye of some animals which, having a high porphyrin content, gives this characteristic fluorescence.

Nissl substance

This fluoresces a bright yellow colour in formalin-fixed unstained sections.

5-Hydroxytryptamine

This gives golden yellow fluorescence (in argentaffin or enterochromaffin cells) after formalin treatment (see page 482).

Drugs

Certain drugs give a characteristic fluorescence. The ability of tetracyclines to form bright yellow fluorescent foci in malignant tumours has been investigated (Vassar, Saunders and Culling, 1960). This antibiotic (since it is bound by calcium) is used to show areas of new bone formation in tetracycline-fed animals.

Hydrocarbons

The carcinogenic compounds, in particular, have been found to be strongly fluorescent. Vassar, Culling and Saunders (1960) utilized this method to demonstrate their presence in histiocytes in sputum from heavy smokers. 3:4 Benzpyrene has been used by Berg (1951) to demonstrate even the finest lipid granules.

Fluorescence techniques

Apart from the phenomenon of autofluorescence, fluorescence microscopy is used in histopathology in the following ways.

Induced fluorescence

Pretreatment of tissue causes a reaction with the component under investigation producing a reaction product which is fluorescent. For example, formalin induced fluorescence of 5-hydroxytryptamine (*see* Chapter 26).

Secondary fluorescence

Many tissue components can be stained by fluorescence dyes in the same way non-fluorescence dyes are used. For example, amyloid stained with thioflavine T. The method using fluorescence dyes are detailed under sections dealing with individual components.

Immunofluorescence

A number of fluorescent compounds may be conjugated to antibodies so that their reaction with the appropriate antigen may be visualized, for example, fluorescein isothiocyanate. The methodology is detailed in Chapter 18.

Polarizing microscopy

Theoretical aspects

Light is assumed to be due to a wave motion, to the upward and downward vibration of ether particles. These do not move along in the direction of the light ray (*Figure 33.26*, A to B), but vibrate at right angles to it (*Figure 33.26*, C to E), and when the light ray ceases they return to their original position (*Figure 33.26*, D). Ether is supposedly a homogeneous medium and there is no reason therefore to believe that these particles will vibrate in any one direction more than another. To explain polarized light it is necessary to suppose that light normally vibrates in all planes; that is, in *Figure 33.27* from C to E, F to G, H to I and J to K. It is difficult to imagine a particle oscillating in all

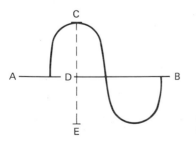

Figure 33.26 Sine curve representing a wave of light. AB = direction of travel; CDE = direction of vibration

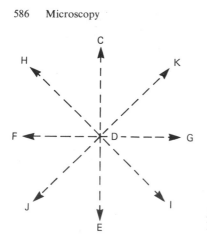

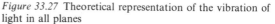

Figure 33.27 Theoretical representation of the vibration of light in all planes

planes at one time, but it is possible to imagine that it moves—at right angles to the direction of the light ray—in all planes in such rapid succession so as to act as if it were moving in all these planes at one time.

While this theory is not strictly accurate, it is sufficiently correct to explain the behaviour of polarized light.

If a dot drawn on a sheet of white card is viewed through a block of glass laid on top, only one dot will be visible from above (*Figure 33.28a*). If the block of glass is replaced by a polished block of crystal, such as Iceland spar, two dots will be visible. Such a crystal is described as being birefringent or anisotropic; it has split each light ray from the dot into two rays which emerge from the crystal at different points (*Figure 33.28b*).

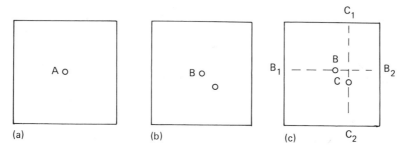

(a)   (b)   (c)

Figure 33.28 Optical effect of (a) block of glass and (b and c) birefringent material when laid on a single dot

This splitting of light rays by certain crystals is due to their uneven optical density. It is known that light rays are retarded when travelling through an optically dense medium such as glass, but since the molecules in glass are evenly spaced in all directions only a simple retardation or slowing takes place. The molecular structure of a crystal differs from glass in that although its molecules are regularly spaced they are closer together in one direction than in another; they are therefore unevenly dense. There are many types of crystalline structure, but most have the common property of being more dense in one direction than in another.

Figure 33.29 shows a downward view of a series of posts through which wind is

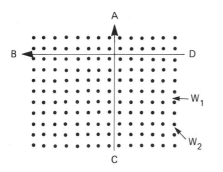

Figure 33.29 Diagram illustrating the theoretical effect of birefringent material in splitting of a beam of light (or wind) into two beams (CA, DB)

blowing from directions W_1 and W_2. It will follow that from whatever angle the wind is blowing it can only leave in the direction of A or B. The intensity of the wind emerging at points A or B will depend on the angle at which it enters. If it enters from W_1 then almost all the wind will emerge in direction B; if the wind enters from W_2, an almost equal amount will emerge in each direction. If we now substitute the words 'crystalline structure' for 'posts driven into the ground', and 'light rays' for 'wind', an understanding may be gained of what happens when a light ray passes through a crystal: the ether particles are vibrating in all directions at right-angles to the line of propagation when it enters, but two rays emerge, and each of these causes ether particles to vibrate in one plane only (A to C, or B to D in *Figure 33.29*; these two planes always being at right-angles to each other).

Light when entering a dense medium is retarded in speed. Further, being an unevenly dense medium, the crystal will retard the two rays to a differing degree, and since refraction is partly dependent on density, the two rays will be refracted or bent to differing degrees. This is known as double refraction or birefringence and explains the phenomena described above (*Figure 33.28*). A ray of light entering such a crystal will be converted into two rays (*Figure 33.28*, B and C) which will emerge at different points, and the emergent light rays will be polarized; that is, all the vibrations in one ray (B) will be in one single direction (B_1-B_2); in the other ray (C) in another single direction (C_1-C_2), and these directions will be at right-angles to each other.

The Nicol prism

Just over 100 years ago, Nicol devised a prism from which light rays, having passed through, would emerge vibrating in a single plane, that is, as polarized light. The single direction in which the light is vibrating when it emerges is known as the 'optical path' of the prism.

The prism is composed of a crystal of Iceland spar, cut to the shape shown in *Figure 33.30*, slit in half and the halves cemented together with Canada balsam along the line CB–CB. On entering the prism, a light ray (A) is divided into two rays (B and C) which are refracted differently, ray C being refracted to one side. Owing to the difference in the refractive index between Canada blasam and the calcite spar crystal, ray C on meeting the surface CB–CB at a greater angle than ray B, is totally reflected out of the prism. Ray B passes through the prism and emerges vibrating in the direction of the optical path of the prism only and is polarized light.

It will follow that if another Nicol prism is placed above the first one (*Figure 33.31*), the polarized light ray B will pass through the upper prism if their optical paths are

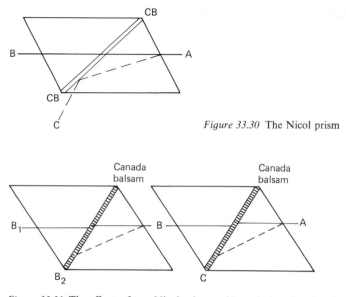

Figure 33.30 The Nicol prism

Figure 33.31 The effects of two Nicol prisms, with optical paths aligned (ABB$_1$) and optical paths crossed (ABB$_2$)

aligned (B$_1$) but if the upper prism is rotated through 90 degrees so that the optical paths of the prisms are crossed, then ray B will be totally reflected out of the upper prism (B$_2$). Such prisms are said to be crossed and it will be seen that no light will normally emerge from crossed Nicol prisms. If the upper prism is slowly rotated it will be seen that the amount of light passing through will vary with their relative positions. At a rotation of 45 degrees, from alignment of the prisms, approximately half the light will pass through the prism and so on. In practice, it will be found that with an intense light source some light will pass even through crossed Nicol prisms, but with light of moderate intensity the field will appear black.

Polaroid discs

In 1935 'polaroids'—glass or celluloid covered discs with the ability to polarize light— were first made available for use in place of Nicol prisms. They act as a single crystal of herapathite which is not only birefringent, but has the ability to absorb the ordinary ray (which would be refracted out of Nicol prism (*Figure 33.30*, C), only the extraordinary ray (*Figure 33.30*, B) being transmitted.

Polaroids are made by suspending ultramicroscopic crystals of herapathite in nitrocellulose. All the crystals in the suspension are orientated so that their optical paths are aligned. This suspension when mounted between two glass plates or celluloid sheets acts as a single crystal.

One glass plate is made to fit into the substage filter carrier, and the other has a metal mount to hold it in place on top of the eyepiece. The celluloid sheet may be cut with scissors and used in a similar manner. For all practical purposes they may be used as Nicol prisms.

Applications to microscopy

It has been shown that certain crystals have the power to convert a single ray into two
rays of light vibrating in planes at right-angles to each other. If such a crystal is placed
on the rotating stage of a microscope having a polarizer in the substage and an analyser
above the object plane the effects will be as shown in *Figure 33.32*.

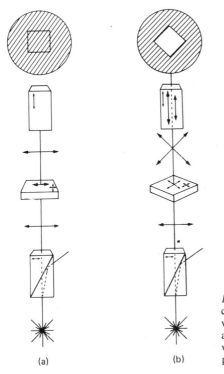

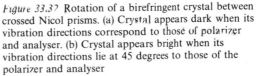

Figure 33.32 Rotation of a birefringent crystal between
crossed Nicol prisms. (a) Crystal appears dark when its
vibration directions correspond to those of polarizer
and analyser. (b) Crystal appears bright when its
vibration directions lie at 45 degrees to those of the
polarizer and analyser

(a)   (b)

With crossed polarizer and analyser, and the vibration directions of the crystal
corresponding to the vibration direction of the polarizer, the crystal will appear dark
on a dark background (a). If the vibration directions of the crystal do not correspond to
the vibration direction of the polarizer, the two rays transmitted by the crystal will be
resolved in the analyser and the crystal will appear bright on a dark background (b).

The appearance of the crystal is caused by the interference of the two rays
recombined in the analyser and will depend on the phase difference between the two
rays which in turn depends on the difference in the two refractive indices of the crystal
(its birefringence) and on its thickness.

In the case of monochromatic light, the light emerging from the analyser is plane
polarized AA' (*Figure 33.33*) and on entering the crystal is resolved into two beams, VV'
and WW' with amplitudes OC' and OC". If these waves have no phase difference they
will pass through O together and reach their crests C' and C" simultaneously. When
combined in the analyser the vertical components OX and OY are equal and opposite
and undergo destructive interference, the crystal appearing dark.

If there is a phase difference of half a wavelength, when one wave reaches its crest at

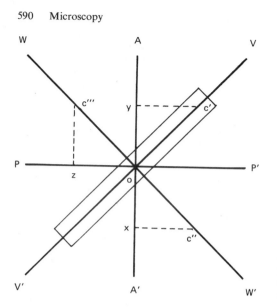

Figure 33.33 The effects of the phase difference produced by a birefringent crystal between crossed polarizer and analyser. For explanation *see* text

C' the other will be at its crest at C'''. When combined in the analyser the vertical components OY and ZC''' are equal and of the same sign and will undergo constructive interference producing a wave of increased amplitude. The crystal will therefore appear bright on a dark background.

In the case of white light, composed of light of different wavelengths, if there is a phase difference, destructive interference will occur for some wavelengths whilst other wavelengths will reinforce each other. The result with increasing phase difference will be a series of interference colours, Newton's series. This series is organized into orders each of which ends with red. The first order starts with black, proceeds to dark grey, light grey, white, yellow, orange then red. The second order proceeds from red to blues, greens, yellows, oranges and finally red again. The colours of the second order are the most brilliant, those of subsequent orders becoming progressively less brilliant.

In the case described in *Figure 33.32a* the crystal is extinguished on the axis of the polarizer and is brightest at 45 degrees. Some crystals do not extinguish on the axis and the degree to which this varies from the axis may be used to assist in the identification of a crystal. A rotating stage and graduated rotating analyser will allow the angle to be measured.

Crystals which change the plane of vibration clockwise are called 'dextrorotatory', and anticlockwise 'laevorotatory'.

Types of birefringence

As was shown above, birefringence is due to some sort of asymmetrical and orientated spatial arrangement of particles. These particles carry resonating charges capable of interacting with the oscillations of light waves. Birefringent material may show one or more than one type of such arrangement; the more common types may be characterized as follows.

Intrinsic or crystalline birefringence

This refers to a type of anisotropy due to an asymmetrical alignment of chemical bonds, ions or molecules. Many crystals display this type of birefringence, it is also common in biological objects such as collagen and muscle fibres, and chromosomes.

Intrinsic birefringence in a specimen is independent of the refractive index of the immersion medium which is probably due to the fact that the orientated elements are of close structure between which the medium does not penetrate.

Form birefringence

This is found in mixed bodies, wherein asymmetrical particles of one refractive index are dispersed in a specially orientated manner in a medium having a different refractive index. At least one dimension of the particles must be small in relation to the wavelength of light employed. These dispersed particles may be filaments, sheets and so on, and they may be dispersed in a liquid, gas or solid; they can give rise to birefringence even if separately either or both are isotropic. Tests for form birefringence depend upon causing media of varying refractive index to penetrate between the particles when, at the appropriate RI, form birefringence will disappear. (Examining objects mounted in a variety of mountants with differing RI, e.g. water, glycerol, HSR and so on.)

Strain birefringence

When a dielectric substance is subjected to mechanical stress, the bonds within the substance can be distorted and give rise to a pattern which will result in birefringence. This is most simply demonstrated by twisting clear plastic (Perspex) between crossed polaroids when a birefringent spectrum of colour is produced. Similarly, glass or elastic tissue fibres under stress show birefringence.

Positive and negative birefringence

An object that appears bright on a dark field when viewed between crossed polarizer and analyser is said to be birefringent. This does not allow the determination of direction of the fast and slow axes of the doubly refracting material. Having two different refractive indices, one light ray will be retarded (slow) in relation to the other (fast) and will correspond to some distinguishing dimension of the object.

In a collagen fibre the slow axis of transmission, corresponding to the higher refractive index, is parallel to the long axis of the fibre. The fibre is thus said to show positive birefringence with respect to its long axis. Conversely, a chromosome shows negative birefringence with respect to its long axis.

To determine the sign of birefringence in a fibre or crystal, for example, to differentiate between the sodium urate crystals of gout, and the calcium pyrophosphate crystals of so-called pseudo-gout, a retardation plate is required. A retardation plate is a crystal slice whose birefringence and sign are known. When a birefringent object is placed on the stage the phase difference of the object is combined with that of the retardation plate. There may be an increased total phase difference or a decreased total phase difference depending on the orientation of the fast and slow directions of the crystal with respect to the retardation plate. If the result is equalization of the two phase differences the retardation plate may be properly described as a compensator.

Compensation will only occur fortuitously with a quarter wave plate or with a first order red plate. Compensators have the facility of adjustment of the phase difference, for example, by tilting the plate to increase the thickness through which the light passes (Berek or Ehringhaus compensators) or by sliding a wedge laterally (quartz wedge) in the light path. Of the several compensators available the first order red plate is most convenient for histopathology use. It is located in a slot in the body tube of the microscope at 45 degrees to the vibration direction of the polarizer. Its vibration direction is marked on it and is usually length fast (Zeiss). Its birefringence imparts a reddish-mauve polarization colour to the whole field. If the birefringent object is now rotated so that its length corresponds to the slow axis of the retardation plate it will appear either blue or yellow depending on its fast and slow directions. If the fast direction of the object corresponds with the fast direction of the plate the phase difference due to the object will be added to that due to the plate and the interference due to the increased phase difference will result in the object appearing blue on a reddish background, for example, urate (length fast = lower RI = negative birefringence).

In the case of calcium pyrophosphate, when the length of the crystal corresponds to the fast direction of the plate, the crystal appears yellow. There has been a reduction in the combined phase difference because the fast and slow directions of the crystal and the plate are opposed, calcium pyrophosphate being length slow (higher RI = positive birefringence).

Dichroism is also detected by the use of a polarizing microscope (*see* page 467).

Application

Polarizing microscopy has many applications in histopathology (Wolman, 1975), some examples of which are given below:

(1) Artefacts. Formalin pigment, sutures, starch.
(2) Crystals. Talc, urate, pyrophosphate, silica, etc.
(3) Lipids. Myelin.
(4) Bone structure. Osteoid seams, woven bone.
(5) Protein. Collagen, amyloid, keratin.
(6) Miscellaneous. Muscle striations, Charcot–Leyden crystals, hydatid hooklets.

Phase-contrast microscopy

Phase-contrast microscopy is a technique which enables us to see very transparent objects, which are almost invisible by ordinary transmitted light, in clear detail and in good contrast to their surroundings, and to see very small differences in thickness and density within the object.

This is accomplished by converting these slight differences in refractive index and thickness into changes of amplitude (or brightness).

Professor Zernicke, who was awarded the Nobel prize for his work on phase contrast, first applied his original work on telescopes to the biological microscope in 1935, but it was not until 1945 that a commercial model was available in Great Britain.

These microscopes are now being widely used.

Principles

Without going too deeply into the theory of phase contrast, the first part of this chapter is intended to explain the broad principles underlying its use. To understand these principles it is necessary to recall some of the properties of light rays.

Light, arising from a point source, may be represented by straight lines or, since it is propagated in waves, by *sine* curves. These curves are a useful method of representation since they can be made to show not only amplitude and wavelength but the retardation of one ray in relation to another. *Figure 33.34* shows the method by which amplitude and wavelength may be represented using the *sine* curve. Retardation of one light ray in relation to another is shown in *Figure 33.35* where the lower ray, having passed through a block of glass, is retarded by half a wavelength. It will be appreciated that the eye is sensitive to changes in amplitude (or brightness) and to changes in wavelength (which are changes in colour) but not to changes in phase, where one wave is retarded in relation to another.

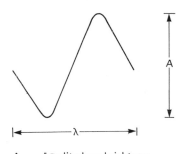

A   Amplitude or brightness
λ Wavelength or colour

Figure 33.34 Sine curve representing a ray of light

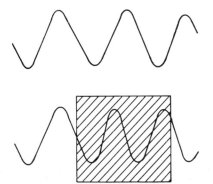

Figure 33.35 Retardation of lower light ray by a block of glass

One further property of light that must be considered is that of interference (*see Figure 33.36*). If two rays of light strike a screen at the same point, as in *Figure 33.36a*, the resultant light on the screen will be the sum of the amplitude of the two rays (b) and (c) as shown in the *sine* curve (d). If one of the two rays (arising from the same point source) had passed through a block of glass, of an exact thickness to retard that ray by half a wavelength, instead of getting an increase in light there would be no light. This is because coherent light rays have the property of interfering with each other. This interference may (as shown in *Figure 33.36c*) result in complete extinction of the light or in a reduction of it depending on the relative amplitudes of the light rays. If, for instance, in *Figure 33.36* the direct ray in (e) had the amplitude of (d) and the retarded ray the

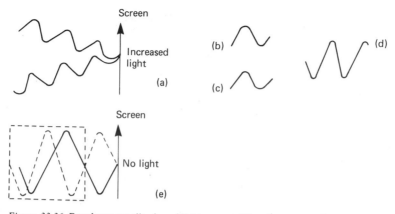

Figure 33.36 Resultant amplitudes of light rays striking the same point on a screen, in phase (a); out of phase (e)

amplitude of (b) instead of extinction of the light, there would have been light of the amplitude of (c). For practical purposes it may be said that when coherent light rays interfere the amplitude of the resultant ray can be obtained by subtracting the amplitude of one from the other. Fractional phase differences (e.g. $\frac{3}{4}$ or $\frac{1}{4}$ of a wavelength) between rays will result in partial interference and in this way an image of an unstained object may be built up.

If an annulus is placed in the substage condenser an image of that annulus will be formed in the back focal plane of the objective, and an object possessing slight non-homogeneities (such as unstained living cells) placed in the object plane will produce a halo of light both inside and outside the annular image. This halo is composed of light rays which have been diffracted by the object and are $\frac{1}{4} \lambda$ out of phase with the direct light rays.

It will follow that if the diffracted rays of light could be retarded a further $\frac{1}{4} \lambda$, then the phase difference between the direct and diffracted rays would be $\frac{1}{2} \lambda$ and interference would take place in the final image plane, building up a picture, in light and shade, of an unstained specimen. Zernicke devised the 'Z' plate, now known as the phase plate, which, placed at the back focal plane of the objective, brought this about. The phase plate consists of an optically plane glass disc out of which is cut a channel to coincide with the image of the light annulus. The depth of the channel must be the exact depth to retard the diffracted rays, which travel through the full thickness of the plate, by a $\frac{1}{4} \lambda$ in relation to the direct rays which travel through the channel (*Figure 33.37*).

Although interference will now take place, the great difference in amplitude (or brightness) between the two sets of rays will prevent the maximum contrast from being obtained. To overcome this factor light-absorbing material is deposited in the area of the channel which reduces the amplitude of the direct light without affecting the diffracted light, thus permitting the maximum contrast to be obtained.

A broad summary of these principles is illustrated in *Figure 33.38*; (a) a ray of direct light from the annulus, on passing through the object (b) gives rise to a diffracted ray (dotted line), which is retarded by $\frac{1}{4} \lambda$; (c) on passing through the phase plate the diffracted ray, retarded by a further $\frac{1}{4} \lambda$ is now in a position to interfere with the direct light ray: (a) the amplitude of the direct light ray is reduced after passing through the light-absorbing material and better contrast is obtained. Although in the illustration, for the sake of clarification, (c) and (d) take place separately, in practice they occur

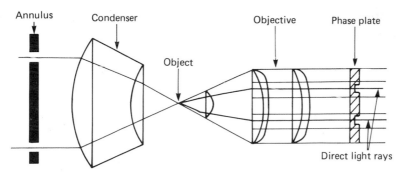

Figure 33.37 Passage of light rays through the optical components of the phase-contrast microscope

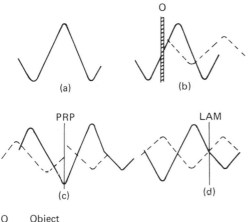

O   Object
PRP   Phase retarding plate
LAM   Light absorbing material

Figure 33.38 Diagrammatic summary of the theory of phase-contrast microscopy

almost simultaneously, and interference, of course, does not take place until the images are once again combined at the real image plane in the eyepiece.

The foregoing theory should only be true if monochromatic light is used as an illuminant, since white light would be split into its component colours when diffracted; in practice, however, white light may be used but better contrast is obtained by using a mercury green filter in conjunction with a compound high intensity lamp.

Equipment

Lamp

An intense source of illumination should be used, such as a high intensity compound lamp, with a mercury green (Wratten 62) filter.

Annulus

A different sized annulus will be required for each objective. These may be inserted separately, but a rotary changer carrying a set of annuli, one for each objective, mounted below a special condenser is more convenient; each of these annuli can be centred by means of two centring screws.

Objectives

Objectives are supplied with phase plates already fitted, and since the phase plates affect their performance only slightly when used in a normal manner, they may be used without an annulus for routine microscopy.

Auxiliary telescope

The auxiliary telescope is used in place of an eyepiece for examining the back focal plane of the objective and ensuring that the objective phase plate and the condenser annulus are properly aligned.

Setting up the microscope

(1) The microscope is set up in the usual way (page 566), ensuring that there is no annulus in the substage.
(2) Focus on the object, closing the iris diaphragm if necessary.
(3) Rotate the annulus changer until the appropriate annulus is in position. Without disturbing the focus remove the eyepiece and replace it with the auxiliary telescope.
(4) Adjust the auxiliary telescope to bring the image of the phase plate into sharp focus.
(5) If the image of the light annulus does not coincide with the grey ring of the phase plate, it is adjusted with the centring screws until its image is concentric with, and completely covered by, the grey ring of the phase plate; the condenser may need to be raised or lowered slightly to adjust the size of the image of the light annulus. If the light annulus is not evenly illuminated the light should be adjusted.
(6) The auxiliary telescope is replaced by the eyepiece and a phase contrast image will be observed.

Note

This procedure should be repeated each time the objective is changed.

Differential interference contrast microscopy

Equipment for differential interference contrast microscopy was designed by Nomarski (1952). It relies on the interference of a pair of wavefronts to generate contrast.
    The equipment comprises:

(1) a polarizer;
(2) a condenser with a modified Wollaston prism; and
(3) a beam splitting slide consisting of a modified Wollaston prism orientated at 45 degrees to an attached analyser, mounted in an adjustable carriage and accommodated in the analyser slot between the objective and the eyepiece.

Polarized light passes through the prism below the condenser. The prism below the condenser acts as a compensator. Every interference fringe of the upper prism is correlated with an interference fringe of the same order but opposite sign in this 'compensator'. The two rays pass in turn through the condenser, the object and the objective before passing through the second prism and analyser. The upper prism can be moved laterally enabling the rays to be displaced laterally, or sheared, before being recombined in the analyser when they undergo interference.

A simplified explanation is shown in *Figure 33.39*. The object is seen in relief-like contrast. High resolution is obtained and contrast can be varied to suit the object by moving the upper prism. The equipment has many applications in biology when both stained and unstained objects may be examined (*Figure 33.40*).

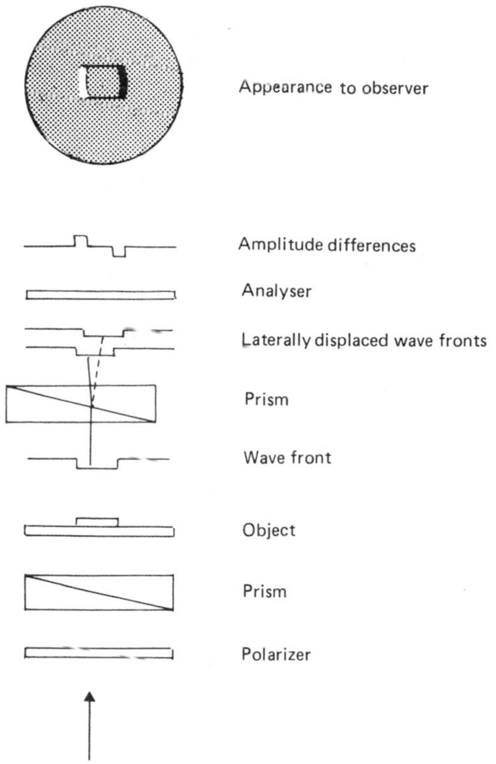

Appearance to observer

Amplitude differences

Analyser

Laterally displaced wave fronts

Prism

Wave front

Object

Prism

Polarizer

Figure 33.39 Diagrammatic representation of differential interference contrast microscopy (Nomarski)

Interference microscopy

Numerous types of interference systems have been designed for use in microscopy. Hale (1958) classifies these as (a) multiple beam systems, and (b) double beam systems, and describes the many systems proposed. Most of these have objections and few are commercially produced.

The basic difference between the interference microscope and the phase-contrast

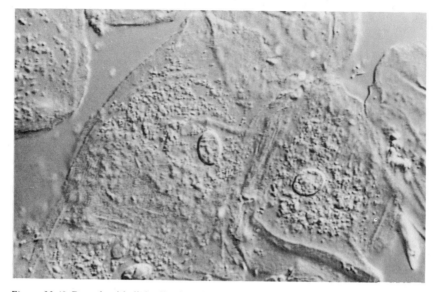

Figure 33.40 Buccal epithelial cells viewed by the Nomarski method. Original magnification × 40

microscope is that the former does not rely on diffraction by the object for interference, but generates mutually interfering beams which produce the contrast. It is this feature which enables very small phase changes to be seen and measured. The two rays, which eventually combine to produce the final image are formed by a plate of birefringent material placed immediately above the condenser. These two rays having passed through the object plane are recombined by a similar plate of birefringent material placed below the front lens of the objective (*Figure 33.41*). Both these rays will have arisen from the same point of the light source (coherent light), which is essential if interference is to take place in the final image. One ray passes through a point in the object and the other through an area adjacent to it (the reference or comparison area). Each point in the final image is a compound one made up of two mutually interfering rays. By using polarized light and an analyser the phase relationship between the two rays can be adjusted and measured.

If white light is used as an illuminant, the various phase relationships appear as different colours which change as the system is adjusted. If monochromatic light is used, an amplitude contrast image is produced allowing the phase difference between the object and the reference area to be measured.

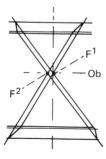

Figure 33.41 Shearing system: Ob = object plane, F′ = object beam focus; F^2 = reference beam focus

Uses

The microscope can be used for two purposes.

(1) As an infinitely variable phase-contrast microscope with which individual parts of living cells may be studied with maximum detail, in any of a wide variety of interference colours.
(2) As a highly accurate optical balance, it may be used for estimating dry mass down to 1×10^{-14} g. The discovery that an increase in refractive index of 0.0018 is due to a 1% increase in concentration of the solid substances contained in cells, and the fact that the refractive index of cell components can be estimated from the phase difference between them and the reference area (usually the fluid in which they are suspended) has made this possible.

References

BERG, N. O. (1951). Histological study of masked lipids; stainability distribution and functional variations. *Acta Pathol. Microbiol. Scand.*, Suppl. 90

BURCH, C. R. and STOCKS, J. P. P. (1942). *J. Sci. Instr.*, **19**, 71

HALE, A. J. (1958). *The Interference Microscope in Biological Research*. Livingstone, Edinburgh and London

LEITZ PUBLICATION 513-519. *The Leitz Filter System for Fluorescence Microscopy*. Ernst Leitz D-6330, Wetzlar, West Germany

NOMARSKI, G. (1952). *Brevet Français*, No. 1,059,123

PLOEM, J. S. (1967). The use of a vertical illuminator with interchangeable dichroic mirrors for fluorescence microscopy with incident light. *Z. Wiss. Mikr.*, **68**, 129–142

ROST, F. W. D. (1980). In *Histochemistry, Theoretical and Applied*. Ed. Pearse, A. G. E. 4th Ed. Vol. 1. Churchill-Livingstone, Edinburgh, London and New York

VASSAR, P. S., CULLING, C. F. A. and SAUNDERS, A. M. (1960). Fluorescent histiocytes in sputum related to smoking. *Arch. Pathol.*, **70**, 649–652

VASSAR, P. S., SAUNDERS, A. M. and CULLING, C. F. A. (1960). Tetracycline fluorescence in malignant tumours and benign ulcers. *Arch. Pathol.*, **69**, 613–616

WOLMAN, M. (1975). Polarized light microscopy as a tool of diagnostic pathology. *J. Histochem. Cytochem.*, **23**, 21–50

ZEISS PUBLICATION 41-350-e. *Fluorescence Microscopy*. Carl Zeiss D-7082, Oberkochen, West Germany

Part X

Electron microscopy

34

The electron microscope

Brian Amer, FIMLS
Department of Pathology, Southmead Hospital, Bristol, UK

Transmission electron microscopy (TEM)

The transmission electron microscope has been widely used in routine histopathology in recent years, particularly in the fields of renal disease, tumour pathology and virus infections. Scanning electron microscopy is also used in some instances and when employed in conjunction with analysis systems can identify substances by their chemical composition.

The light microscope lens systems have been perfected to such a degree that resolution is limited by the physical properties of image formation rather than the properties of the lenses themselves. From the discussion of optical theory it was seen that the resolution of any optical system is limited by the wavelength of light employed, and that an object that is smaller than this wavelength will cause so little perturbation of the light beam that it will not be resolved in the image. The best light microscopes are, therefore, limited to a resolution of about 200 nm. The ultraviolet microscope, by using wavelengths about one half that of white light, achieves a resolution of 100 nm.

By using an electron beam instead of light rays, the electron microscope gives much better resolution (*Figure 34.1*). The wavelength of moving electrons depends on their velocity. At an acceleration of 50 000 V they have a wavelength of about 0.001 nm, and one may expect to resolve images of about this order. Due to lens defects which can be corrected in the light microscope but have not so far been corrected in the electron microscope, the resolution is limited to about 0.4 nm, which is still several orders of magnitude better than the best optical microscopes.

Tissue to be examined in the transmission electron microscope must be processed so that sections of approximately 50 nm thickness can be cut. These very thin sections are necessary because of the poor penetrating properties of the electron beam: the usual sections prepared for light microscopy, having a thickness of 4–5 µm would be completely opaque. Preparative techniques have been developed which make section cutting a relatively easy procedure. These techniques are similar to those used in routine histopathology laboratories for preparation of sections from paraffin-wax embedded tissue, namely fixation, dehydration and embedding prior to sectioning. Sectioning is carried out using a specially designed microtome, an ultramicrotome. The thin sections are flattened on water prior to collection on grids, dried then stained with solutions of heavy metals such as uranium and lead before being examined in the electron microscope.

Before describing these techniques more fully, some elementary principles of electron microscopy will be reviewed.

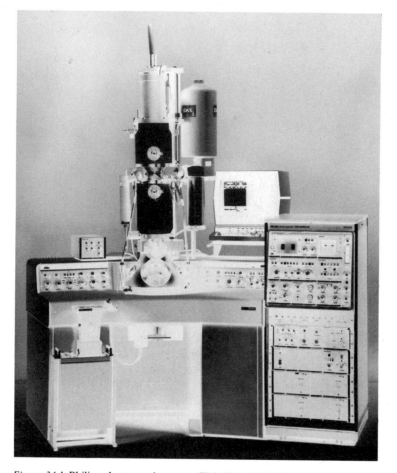

Figure 34.1 Philips electron microscope EM 420 with STEM and X-ray analysis systems. (Reproduced by kind permission of Philips)

Theory and construction of the TEM

The convergence of a light beam by a convex glass lens has its counterpart in the convergence of an electron beam as it passes through the core of a circular magnetic field. Most electron microscopes use electromagnetic lenses. The convergence of an electron beam is shown producing an image; the image and object distances are related to the focal length of the lens in exactly the same way as in light optics (*see* page 551). The electron microscope is, therefore, constructed on the same optical principles as the light microscope, and the same formulas can be used to correlate magnification and focal distances (*Figure 34.2*).

The electron beam is obtained from a heated tungsten filament which is surrounded by a metal cylinder known as the Whenalt cap. This cap serves to shape the electron beam. Just beyond the Whenalt cap is the anode which has an aperture through whieh the electron beam passes. A large voltage is passed between the cathode (the tungsten filament) and the anode, which gives the electrons their high velocity. They pass

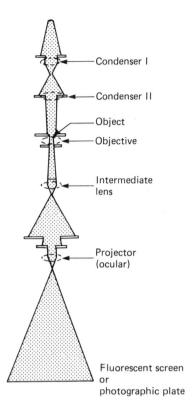

Condenser I

Condenser II

Object

Objective

Intermediate
lens

Projector
(ocular)

Fluorescent screen
or
photographic plate

Figure 34.2 Diagrammatic illustration of optical path of the
electron microscope

through the rest of the microscope without any further acceleration. The Whenalt cap is
given a voltage slightly lower than the filament, and this voltage is usually variable so
that the flow of electrons from the cathode can be controlled. This is known as the bias
voltage.

The electron beam first passes through the condenser lens. As in the light microscope
this lens serves to focus the beam on the object, and so provide 'illumination'. One must
remember that the magnetic lenses of an electron microscope can have different powers
depending on the amount of current flowing in the electrical coils. In the light
microscope the lens powers are fixed, but the lenses are made movable with respect to
the object so that the image can be focused and proper conditions of illumination
obtained. In the electron microscope all lenses are rigidly fixed, but their focal points
are variable by adjusting the lens currents. Thus the 'illumination' of the object is
achieved by varying the current to the condenser lens.

The imaging system of the electron microscope usually consists of three lenses; the
objective, the intermediate and the projector lenses. This gives three stages of
magnification and makes it possible to achieve high magnification in a reasonable
amount of space. The objective lens is placed with its focal point close to the object.
Intermediate images are formed between each lens. The projector throws its image onto
a fluorescent screen which may be substituted by a photographic plate to make a
permanent record (*Figure 34.3*). The entire illuminating and imaging system is usually
referred to as the microscope column and is constructed upside down compared with
the light microscope; that is, the electron gun and condenser lens are placed above and

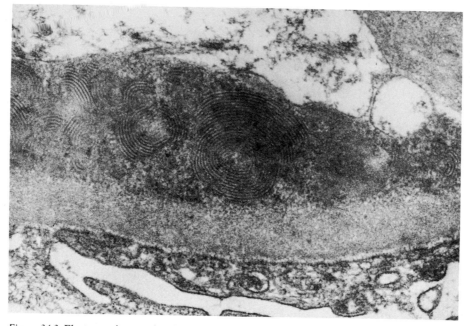

Figure 34.3 Electron micrograph ×90 000 showing 'fingerprint' whorls in electron dense deposit (immune complex), in a glomerular capillary. A characteristic feature of lupus erythematosus, lamellae are approximately 17 nm apart

the image formed below (*Figures 34.1* and *34.2*). An exception is the AEI Corinth electron microscope. The column is very rigidly constructed and is maintained at high vacuum since air molecules would deflect the electron beam. Because the specimen must be placed inside the microscope, it is not possible to examine living material in the electron microscope.

Electron optics are essentially similar to light optics. One important difference, however, is that the formation of an image is due to scattering of electrons by molecules of the specimen and this scattering depends solely on mass densities. Elements of high atomic weight such as lead and uranium cause marked electron scatter and appear very dense in the electron image, hence their use in staining. The lighter elements such as carbon, oxygen and nitrogen cause little electron scatter and have poor contrast. In the light microscope, the image is due to absorption of light which depends more on molecular structure than atomic weights. Histological stains depend on absorption of certain wavelengths of light due to their molecular structure and are composed mainly of carbon, nitrogen and hydrogen atoms. Since these are all of low atomic weight they have little electron scattering power and are not generally useful as stains for electron microscopy. Unstained tissues have very poor contrast in the electron microscope, but may be stained by a variety of heavy metal salts. Most such 'electron stains' are relatively non-specific and one does not have the battery of stains which are so useful in studying tissues in the light microscope.

Preparation of tissues for TEM

The general principles are the same as those in the routine histological laboratory, namely, fixation, dehydration, embedding, sectioning and staining.

Fixation

The fixatives most commonly used are solutions of osmium tetroxide, glutaraldehyde and paraformaldehyde.

Osmium tetroxide

Osmium tetroxide is normally used at a concentration of 1% and a pH value of 7.3. Osmium tetroxide is supplied in glass ampoules containing either 0.1, 0.5 or 1.0 g; the preparation of osmium containing fixatives should be carried out in a fume cupboard by dropping a cleaned ampoule of osmium into a bottle, shaking the bottle to break the ampoule, then adding the required volume of buffer solution or water.

Osmium tetroxide fumes are extremely toxic; avoid breathing the fumes or getting any solution on the hands.

There are many formulas for osmium tetroxide fixatives, for example, Palade (1952), Rhodin (1954).

■ Palade's fixative

Stock buffer

Sodium barbitone	14.7 g
Sodium acetate	9.7 g
Distilled water to make	500 ml

Working solution

Stock buffer	5 ml
0.1 N Hydrochloric acid	5 ml
Distilled water	2.5 ml
2% Osmium tetroxide	12.5 ml

■ Rhodin fixative

Stock solution A

Sodium acetate	1.94 g
Sodium barbitone	2.94 g
Distilled water to make	100 ml

Stock solution B

Sodium chloride	8.05 g
Potassium chloride	0.42 g
Calcium chloride	0.18 g
Distilled water to make	100 ml

Working solution

Stock solution A	10 ml
0.1 N Hydrochloric acid	11 ml
Stock solution B	3.4 ml
Distilled water to make	50 ml
Osmium tetroxide	0.5 g

Glutaraldehyde

Glutaraldehyde fixation was introduced in 1963 by Sabatini, Bensch and Barrnett as a method for electron microscopy. It is probably one of the most commonly used fixatives at present, being customarily used as a primary fixative to be followed by post-fixation with osmium tetroxide.

■ **Buffered glutaraldehyde (pH 7.3–7.4) (Karlsson and Schultz, 1965)**

Sodium dihydrogen phosphate ($NaH_2PO_4 . H_2O$)	3.31 g
Disodium hydrogen phosphate ($Na_2HPO_4 . 7H_2O$)	33.77 g
Distilled water	925 ml
25% Glutaraldehyde	100 ml

Paraformaldehyde

Paraformaldehyde based fixatives are now being used in electron immunochemistry when immunoglobulins are to be demonstrated.

■ **Buffered paraformaldehyde pH 7.4**

Solution A

Paraformaldehyde	2 g
Distilled water	25 ml

Heat to 60 °C with continuous agitation in a closed beaker. (This is best carried out in a fume cupboard.) Then add molar sodium hydroxide drop by drop until the solution clears—one to five drops are usually sufficient.

Solution B

0.2 M Sodium cacodylate	50 ml
0.1 N Hydrochloric acid	2.7 ml
0.5 M Calcium chloride	1.0 ml

Working solution

Solution A	25 ml
Solution B	25 ml

Since these fixatives penetrate very slowly into tissues, it is essential that the tissue blocks be cut into very small pieces approximately 1 mm^3. This must be done quickly, as soon as tissues are removed. Delayed or inappropriate fixation gives rise to artefactual changes in cell and organelle structure which, although invisible at the light microscope level, seriously impairs interpretation in the electron microscope. Mito-chondria are particularly susceptible to fixation artefact. Specimens are best cut on dental wax with a clean sharp razor blade so as to avoid compressing the tissue.

Fixation time is dependent on block size and type of tissue but is usually in the range of 1–4 hours at 4 °C.

Tissues fixed in osmium tetroxide are washed well with distilled water and may then be stored in 70% alcohol until processing is carried out.

Tissues fixed in aldehyde fixatives are washed in buffer solution or with buffered sucrose, in which solutions they may be stored prior to being post-fixed with osmium tetroxide.

When electron microscopy study has to be undertaken on specimens from distant sources, the choice of fixatives and the technical expertise at that source are important to the quality of the final result. In such circumstances, provided that the technical expertise is on hand, fixation can be carried out using the fixative of choice and the fixed specimen subsequently transferred to the electron microscopy laboratory in buffer or 70% alcohol. If this cannot be done, provided the specimen can reach the laboratory in 24 hours, an aldehyde fixative should be used.

Dehydration

After fixation, dehydration can be carried out using acetone or more usually ascending concentrations of alcohol, 5–15 minutes in each concentration, in glass tubes. If blocks need to be trimmed further it is best carried out at the 70% alcohol stage.

The use of 2.2 dimethyloxypropane as a rapid means of dehydration has been described by Muller and Jacks (1975), complete dehydration takes from 2–5 minutes. This may prove of value in cases where urgency is of prime importance.

Embedding

In order to cut the thin sections (50 nm) which are necessary for most electron microscopes, tissues have to be embedded in a substance which is firm enough to allow sectioning with ease. Both methacrylate and epoxy resins have been used in electron microscopy, the methacrylates infiltrate well and the blocks are easy to section, but the resin evaporates in the electron beam with the result that the section disintegrates.

Methacrylate resins have taken second place to epoxy resin in electron microscopy, but have more recently enjoyed increased popularity in the field of resin sections for light microscopy, the technique for which has been described elsewhere in this book.

Epoxy resins are usually a mixture of four components, resin, hardener, accelerator and plasticizer. Changes in the ratio of these components will alter the properties of the resin, for example, hardness increases as the volume of hardener is increased.

■ **Spurr (1969) resin**

Vinylcyclohexane dioxide (VCD)	38.8 ml
Diglycidyl ether of polypropylene glycol (DER)	8 ml
Nonanyl succinic anhydride (NSA)	104 ml
Dimethylaminoethanol	2.6 ml

Mix together thoroughly and store in glass bottles at −20 °C.

■ **Durcopan resin (Fluka)***

A	Epoxy resin	5 ml
B	Hardener 964	5 ml
C	Accelerator	0.5 ml
D	Plasticizer	0.75 ml

* Fluorochemical Ltd, Dinting Vale Trading Estate, Dinting Vale, Glossop, Derby, England.

It is usual to use a link agent, such as propylene oxide, after dehydration but before embedding in epoxy resin. Some workers take this a stage further and use a mixture of propylene oxide and resin (1:1) before finally embedding in resin.

Embedding is carried out by decanting the propylene oxide and replacing it with freshly prepared epoxy resin for 1 hour at 50 °C. (Durcopan may begin to polymerize if this time is exceeded.)

The embedded blocks are 'blocked out' by transferring the blocks from the resin using a swab stick, to a suitable capsule (gelatin or polythene) containing approximately 0.5 ml of fresh resin and a label or some other means of identification. The capsules must stand vertically in a rack which is then placed in an incubator or oven at 60 °C to polymerize for at least 24 hours. It is a wise precaution to examine the capsules after 30 minutes to make sure that the blocks have descended to the base of the capsules, if they have not then some encouragement in the form of a stiff wire is used to push the blocks gently to the base or point of the capsule.

Automatic tissue processors are widely used in routine histopathology and have advanced their design to meet the needs of the modern laboratory. Automatic processors are now available for resin embedding in electron microscopy, giving relief from the tedious task of manual processing. These processors, like the new generation of routine histology processors, can be operated by a preprogrammed computer. They are very expensive to buy and to run so that a high work load is necessary to justify their purchase.

The introduction of safety standards and codes of practice has created a greater awareness of the possible hazards to workers using resins. There is a lot of work being carried out by many workers to produce a resin which will infiltrate rapidly and evenly, polymerize well, allow easy sectioning and good staining. Many resins are now supplied in kit form, the components of which have only to be mixed together, thereby avoiding the need for weighing or measuring. When handling resins it is essential to wear protective gloves; in this laboratory volumes are measured using disposable plastic syringes.

The reagents used in processing of tissues for electron microscopy do present hazards to health and safety. The threshold limit (TLV) for osmium, glutaraldehyde, paraformaldehyde and propylene oxide are respectively 0.0002 ppm, 0.25 mg/m³, 2 ppm and 100 ppm. Such reagents are best handled in a fume cupboard.

■ **Processing schedule for 1 mm³ blocks**

Fixation

(1) Put in 2.5% glutaraldehyde at 4 °C for 1–4 hours.
(2) Wash in buffer.
(3) Store in sucrose solution.

Post-fixation

(1) 1% Osmium tetroxide at 4 °C for 1 hour.
(2) Wash in water.

Dehydration

(1) 50% Alcohol (74 °OP) for 5–15 minutes.

(2) 70% Alcohol for 5–15 minutes.
(3) 90% Alcohol for 5–15 minutes.
(4) Absolute alcohol for 5–15 minutes.
(5) Absolute alcohol for 5–15 minutes.
(6) Absolute alcohol for 5–15 minutes.

Transition solution (link agent)

(1) Propylene oxide for 15 minutes.
(2) Fresh propylene oxide for 15 minutes.

Impregnation

Epoxy resin for 45–60 minutes.

Blocking out

Epoxy resin in capsules.

Polymerization

Place capsules in oven/incubator at 60 °C for 24 hours.

This process can be speeded up in cases where urgency of report is essential. Rowden and Lewis (1974) have described a technique whereby biopsies may be processed in 3 hours; time is saved by polymerizing at 100 °C.

If polymerization at high temperature is contemplated, be certain that the capsules used for blocking out will withstand these high temperatures.

Frequently the need for electron microscopy is not realized until after paraffin-wax sections have been examined, or at least until after the specimen has been fixed in formalin. In such cases much information can be revealed by taking a piece of the formalin-fixed tissue, washing well in buffer solution to remove the formalin, post-fixing in osmium tetroxide and proceeding to embed the tissue as previously described for electron microscopy. This can be particularly useful in identifying some anaplastic tumours.

Tissue which has been embedded in paraffin wax may also be processed for electron microscopy. After removal of the wax, using a suitable solvent, the tissue is rehydrated, the blocks trimmed and then post-fixed, etc.

Stained paraffin sections can be treated in a similar manner, the results will show many artefacts, and morphology will be disrupted due to the embedding in paraffin wax, but can be rewarding particularly in cases of virus infections (*Figure 34.4*). The following technique is recommended.

■ **Technique for removing cells/sections from slides (light microscopy preparations) for EM study**

(1) Mark cell or cells on coverglass.
(2) Accurately mark reverse of slide (use diamond).
(3) Remove coverglass. (Soak in xylene or similar solvent to remove all traces of mountant.)
(4) Rehydrate section.

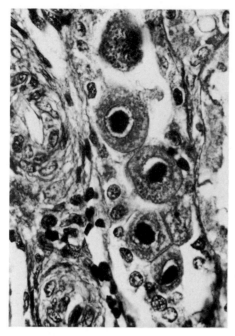 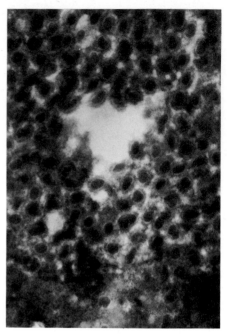

Figure 34.4 (a) Photomicrograph showing inclusion bearing cells, ×750. (b) Electron micrograph showing inclusions to be composed of viruses. ×90 000

(5) Refix with 1% osmium tetroxide for 10–15 minutes at room temperature.
(6) Wash in distilled water.
(7) Dehydrate as for sections.
(8) Soak in propylene oxide for 5–10 minutes.
(9) Put in propylene oxide/resin (1:1) for 5–10 minutes. (Take care that the section does not dry out between stages (8) and (9).)
(10) Resin 10 minutes at 60 °C.
(11) Locate capsule over the area marked, and fill with resin. (Plastic capsules have their tips removed and either end heat flattened against a hot microscope slide. This provides a good seal against the slide, preventing leakage of resin.)
(12) Polymerize at 60 °C.
(13) Remove polymerized capsule from slide by repeated short immersions in liquid nitrogen.
(14) Remove capsule from block.
(15) Examine face of block microscopically to identify cell or cells and mark accurately.
(16) Trim to form a pyramid or mesa.
(17) Prepare ultrathin sections.
(18) Stain with uranium and lead then examine.

(Not all resins are suitable for this technique, Durcopan can be recommended.)

Ultramicrotomy

There are a number of microtomes designed specifically to produce the very thin sections necessary for examination in the electron microscope, these are termed ultramicrotomes.

For the operation of the different types of ultramicrotome, the reader is recommended to refer to the appropriate manufacturers' handbook. An understanding of the basic principles of microtomy is advantageous, together with an unlimited supply of patience.

Conventional steel microtome knives will not produce a sufficiently sharp edge to cut ultrathin sections of resin embedded tissue; the fractured edge of plate glass is usually employed. Diamond knives can be used also—although their use is usually reserved for particularly hard tissue. The introduction of glass knife making machines has greatly facilitated the preparation of first class glass knives and at the same time decreased many of the frustrations of the ultramicrotomist.

Preparation of glass knives

A strip of plate glass, appropriate to the machine, is placed on the deck of the breaker, clamped in position, scored with a glass-cutter's wheel, then broken by exerting upward pressure from beneath the score, to produce a square or rhombus shaped piece of glass. (The position of the scored line should be such that it does not reach the edges of the glass strip.)

These squares or rhombi are now placed on the deck and clamped in position, scored 1–2 degrees off the diagonal and broken as before, to produce two knives. (The position of the scored line ends 1 mm from the corner of the glass, allowing a 'free break' to occur.) (*Figure 34.5*.)

Section cutting

With the knife and resin embedded block affixed to the ultramicrotome, the surface of the block is trimmed to expose the tissue. Care must be taken not to remove too much

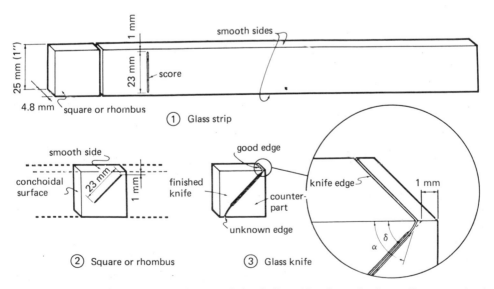

Figure 34.5 Diagram illustrating the features of glass knife making. δ=angle of score line; α=angle of break. (Reproduced by kind permission of LKB Instruments Ltd)

resin at one cut or the block may shatter. When sufficient tissue has been exposed, a section 1 μm thick is cut and the section transferred with a pair of fine toothed forceps or an eyelash fixed to an orange stick, onto a drop of water on a clean microscope slide. The slide is placed on a hot-plate and the water allowed to dry, without boiling, to flatten the section. This section is then stained with 1% toluidine blue in 1% borax on the hot-plate for 30 seconds. The stain is washed off with distilled water and the section examined with a light microscope to check for the presence of the required cells.

When a suitable area has been identified, the block is shaped into a flat topped pyramid approximately 0.2–0.3 mm² to include the cells required. Rough trimming and pyramid cutting can be carried out 'free hand' using a single edged razor blade, but this requires a great deal of skill.

A new knife, onto which a small reservoir has been fixed and sealed with dental wax, is placed in the microtome. These reservoirs can be made from insulation tape. More recently re-usable metal troughs and disposable plastic troughs have become available (*Figure 34.6*).

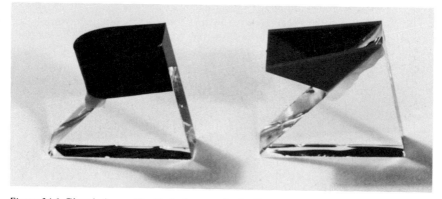

Figure 34.6 Glass knives with attached reservoirs for floating out sections

For sectioning they are filled with clean distilled water to the level at which the sections will float from the knife edge directly onto the surface of the water which must be dust free.

The thickness of the section is adjudged by its interference colour when floating on the water. Ultramicrotomes use either a mechanical or thermal advance system for advancing the block to the knife. Sections which are silver to pale gold in colour are of suitable thickness for transmission electron microscopy. The sections, when flat, are collected on suitable metal grids and allowed to dry. Grids are available in different mesh size and type (*Figure 34.7*) and must be clean and grease-free for use.

Staining

Unstained sections have little contrast and are subsequently stained with heavy metal salts such as uranium and lead, although phosphotungstic acid and silver have been used. Staining is somewhat empirical, many workers incorporate uranyl acetate in one of the alcohols used for dehydration (block staining). Others prefer double staining of the sections with uranyl acetate and lead citrate.

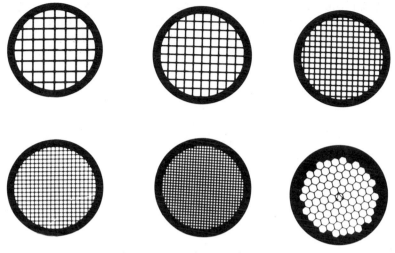

Figure 34.7 A selection of grids used in electron microscopy

■ Staining solutions

(1) Uranyl acetate   0.5–2.0 g
     Glass distilled water   100 ml

(2) Uranyl acetate   5 g
     50% Alcohol   100 ml

(3) Lead citrate (Reynolds, 1963)
     Lead nitrate   1.33 g
     Sodium citrate   1.76 g
     Distilled water   30 ml

Place the above in a 50 ml volumetric flask, shake for 1 minute, then intermittently for 30 minutes. Add 8 ml N sodium hydroxide and make up to 50 ml with distilled water, mix by inversion. Staining times vary from 2 to 60 minutes with uranyl acetate and from 2 to 30 minutes for lead citrate. The following procedure is used routinely in our laboratory.

Technique

The grids are placed section side down onto a drop of filtered, saturated uranyl acetate in 50% alcohol, on a square of dental wax in a closed Petri dish. Staining is allowed to continue for 20 minutes. The grids are picked up and held in a pair of jeweller's forceps, whilst they are washed in distilled water, then placed section side up onto a piece of filter paper to dry.

Next place the grids, section side down, onto a drop of filtered lead citrate (Reynolds, 1963) in another Petri dish and leave to stain for 15 minutes. Take the grids in forceps as before, rinse briefly in 0.01 N NaOH, wash in distilled water, dry and store in a suitable container prior to examination in the electron microscope.

Filtration is carried out using Millipore Millex or Swinnex (Millipore (UK) Ltd, 11/15 Peterborough Rd, Harrow, England) filters pore size 0.22 μm.

Lead carbonate forms quickly when lead citrate is used for staining, leaving an unacceptable precipitate on the sections. This can be minimized by placing a few drops of concentrated NaOH around the inside of the Petri dish used for staining.

Commercially prepared stains are available together with automatic staining machines.

Special techniques for TEM

Negative staining

Negative staining is used mainly in the fields of virology and microbiology where rapid identification of organisms is carried out. This method is especially useful as whole organisms are visualized in the electron microscope rather than sections through them. This obviously makes identification easier.

Small quantities of suspensions of virus or micro-organisms are mixed with an equal volume of 4% phosphotungstic acid. A drop of this mixture is placed onto a Formvar coated grid, allowed to settle and the excess stain/suspension removed with filter paper. The grid is allowed to dry and is then ready for examination in the microscope. *Because of the nature of the specimens examined by negative staining, it is imperative that strict aseptic technique is observed.*

Preparation of Formvar coated grids

Place a cleaned microscope slide into a Coplin jar containing 0.5% Formvar in ethylene dichloride, and leave for 1 minute. Remove the slide, allow to dry in a vertical position in a dust free area, cut around the slide 1 mm from its edges with a sharp razor blade or scalpel. Slowly immerse the slide, at an angle of 45 degrees, into a container of clean distilled water. The Formvar film should become detached from the slide and float onto the surface of the water. Gently drop onto this film some cleaned grids. Take another cleaned slide, place its end on the Formvar film, then quickly, completely immerse the slide trapping the grids between the slide and the Formvar film. Remove the slide and grids from the water and allow to dry. When dry, the grids are examined for complete coverage by Formvar.

Electron immunology

Immunofluorescent techniques have become commonplace in routine histopathology and are now being superseded in some instances by immunoperoxidase techniques. The latter being electron dense has opened up a much wider application in the immunological field.

The labelling of various protein substances with ferritin has been used to demonstrate surface immunoglobulins on cells, and with increased use of peroxidase labelling, exact localization of immunoglobulins in the glomeruli of patients suffering from various forms of glomerulonephritis has been described by Davies *et al.* (1977).

Cryotransfer

The examination of frozen, hydrated sections necessitates the use of a modified ultramicrotome (cryo-ultratome). This apparatus is adapted to provide a knife cooled with liquid nitrogen and a cooling system for freezing the block of tissue to the microtome.

The ultrathin sections are collected on grids and may be examined as stained or unstained preparations. These grids are placed in a cryotransfer holder for introduction into the microscope column. To maintain the sections at low temperature the cryotransfer holder is cooled by pumping dry nitrogen gas, cooled with liquid nitrogen, through the grid holder.

This technique is particularly useful for the analytical examination of specimens, when the artefacts of fixation and staining are to be avoided.

Scanning electron microscope (SEM)

This type of microscope differs from TEM in that the beam of electrons is made to scan the specimen in a raster. The secondary electrons 'reflected' from the surface of the specimen are collected by a secondary electron detector, passed through a photo-multiplier tube and onto a cathode ray tube where the image is displayed.

Back-scattered electrons are also 'reflected' from the surface of the specimen, these are electrons with less energy loss than secondary electrons. The information content of back-scattered electrons is based on the average atomic number differences in the specimen rather than the topographical information carried by secondary electrons.

Biological specimens are largely non-conductive, so it is necessary to impart conductivity. Gold, platinum and carbon are some of the substances used for this purpose.

Preparation of tissues for SEM

The preparative technique for SEM is similar to that used in other forms of microscopy (fixation, dehydration, drying and then metal coating). The fixatives recommended are those used in TEM. Dehydration can be carried out, as previously described, using ascending concentrations of alcohol before allowing the specimen to dry out in air or under vacuum. This technique causes a great deal of shrinkage which is variable throughout the specimen.

Another method, more popular, and extensively used, is critical-point drying (CPD). Using this technique the specimen is fixed, dehydrated with alcohol then transferred to acetone. The specimens are then put into suitable cassettes/baskets in a pressurized chamber of the critical-point dryer where the acetone is replaced by liquid carbon dioxide. The temperature of the carbon dioxide is slowly raised, by applying gentle heat, thereby increasing the pressure inside the chamber until the 'critical point' is reached.

The critical point of a liquid is defined as that point at which the liquid/gas interface disappears (i.e. all the liquid is instantly converted to gas and can be removed from the tissue causing minimum distortion), and is a combination of pressure and temperature (*see* Chapter 4).

The vessel is maintained at just above the critical point for 10–15 minutes to make certain that drying is complete before slowly reducing the pressure to atmospheric and subsequent coating.

Coating

The dried specimen is mounted on an aluminium stub appropriate to the microscope. A simple adhesive such as Durofix may be used, but better conductivity is achieved by using silver dag. The specimen is placed in the chamber of a sputter coating unit and the air evacuated. This is assisted by purging the chamber with argon at $2\,lb/in^2$ for 2 minutes. When a vacuum of 0.1 Torr (13.3 Pa) is attained, gold is discharged from a target situated above the specimen, and deposited on the surface of the sample. The layer of gold must be of sufficient thickness to allow examination of surface morphology without 'charging'. If the layer of gold is too thick no information will be obtained due to plating of the sample.

The thickness of the layer of gold is determined by the distance of the specimen from the target, the period of time taken to sputter and the strength of the current applied to the target.

Cryopreservation

Many artefacts occur in histological preparations and the competent histologist recognizes such artefacts. The same is true in the field of electron microscopy and ways of minimizing these artefacts is a continuous process. One such development is cryopreservation. We know from our experiences in light microscopy that cryostat frozen sections do not show the artefacts visualized in sections of dehydrated and embedded tissue. There are now cryosystems which interface directly to the SEM, which allow fresh tissue to be frozen rapidly with liquid nitrogen, sputtered with gold or carbon coated and then examined in the SEM while still frozen. This eliminates the artefacts associated with fixation, dehydration and embedding. These cryosystems comprise:

(1) a slushing chamber, usually remote from the microscope, for freezing specimens; and
(2) a low temperature preparation chamber in which specimens may be fractured, have the ice sublimed from their surface and be coated. This preparation chamber can be fitted directly to the SEM or may be a separate unit depending on the manufacturer.

When using a cryosystem the stage of the microscope has to be modified so that it can be maintained at very low temperatures. This is achieved by using a special stage cooled with liquid nitrogen, either by conduction through a braided copper rope from a Dewar of liquid nitrogen or by pumping through the stage dry nitrogen gas cooled by passing through liquid nitrogen. An anticontaminator also cooled to liquid nitrogen temperature is fitted between the stage and the final aperture.

The frozen samples are transferred to the microscope by means of specially designed transfer devices. The temperature of the preparation chamber is held at $-160\,°C$ or lower and the stage at similar temperatures, but provision is made to be able to heat the stage to sublime any surface ice and to hold the specimen at optimum viewing temperature.

Scanning transmission electron microscope (STEM)

Many of the modern high resolution TEMs have an extra optional facility in the form of a STEM unit, which enables a scanning image to be obtained from a transmission electron microscope. The column arrangement differs from conventional TEM in so far as the electrons originating from the filament are formed into a small probe which is made to scan the specimen in a rectangular raster in a similar way to SEM. The resulting transmitted signal is collected by a detector below the specimen, situated near the viewing chamber, and relayed to the cathode ray tube (viewing monitor) of the STEM unit. The contrast obtained is due entirely to the average atomic number differences of the constituent elements.

The specimen holder for STEM is similar to that used for TEM, and the sections may be examined stained or unstained.

Surface topography can also be obtained from a TEM using a STEM unit. The beam of electrons is made to scan the specimen in a rectangular raster as for pure STEM. The secondary electrons 'reflected' by the specimen are collected by a secondary electron detector situated above the sample, and are then processed in the same way as in a dedicated SEM. The scanning image is displayed on the monitor of the STEM unit.

Specimens to be examined with this form of microscope have to be treated in the same way as those for dedicated SEM. The size of the specimen that can be examined is limited by the type of holder used and is usually in the order of 10×5 mm. The maximum height permissible is 3 mm, as it becomes mechanically impossible to produce an image of a taller specimen.

Analytical systems

X-ray dispersive analysis

The analysis of certain specimens to provide identification of constituent elements such as aluminium, copper, gold and asbestos, which may be present as the result of a pathological process can be carried out using TEM, SEM or STEM in conjunction with an attached X-ray dispersive system.

When an electron beam strikes a specimen there is an electron shift in the atoms and the specimen will emit X-rays which are different for each element present.

Standard systems will detect elements ranging from sodium to uranium. When an element is to be detected the appropriate energy range (window) is selected and the emitted X-rays are analysed and displayed in graphical form. (Special detectors are necessary to detect elements lower than sodium.)

Electron energy loss spectroscopy (EELS)

This is a new concept in chemical analysis of specimens using TEM and STEM. The contrast of the image formed is due to the average atomic number of the constituent elements.

Electrons with varying degrees of energy loss, arising from the passage of the primary electron beam through the specimen, are passed through a magnetic sector and focused onto a detector. These energy loss peaks can be recorded and quantitative data on the elemental composition of the specimen can be obtained. This is calculated from the difference in energy peaks of elements that show a maximum peak (no energy loss) and heavy elements (maximum energy loss). This technique may be of use for light element analysis, for example, carbon, fluorine and lithium.

For more information on specific topics the reader is referred to more specialized textbooks.

The EM section of the Royal Microscopical Society has produced some guidelines which should be considered before choosing an electron microscope and these can be found in the *Proceedings of the Royal Microscopical Society* (1983), Vol. 18, Pt 2, pp. 98–100.

References

DAVIES, D. R., TIGHE, J. R., WING, A. J. and JONES, E. F. (1977). Immunoglobulin deposition in membranous glomerulonephritis. Immunofluorescence and immunoelectron microscopy findings. *Histopathology*, **1**, 39–52

KARLSSON, U. and SCHULTZ, R. L. (1965). Fixation of the CNS for electron microscopy by aldehyde perfusion. Preservation with aldehyde perfusates versus direct perfusion with osmium tetroxide with special reference to membrane and the extracellular space. *J. Ultrastruct. Res.*, **12**, 160–186

MULLER, L. L. and JACKS, T. J. (1975). Rapid chemical dehydration of samples for electron microscopic examinations. *J. Histochem. Cytochem.*, **23**, 107–110

PALADE, G. E. (1952). A study of fixation for electron microscopy. *J. Exp. Med.*, **95**, 285–298

REYNOLDS, E. S. (1963). The use of lead citrate at high pH as an electron opaque stain in electron microscopy. *J. Cell Biol.*, **17**, 208–212

RHODIN, G. (1954). Correlation of ultrastructural organisation and function in normal and experimentally changed proximal convoluted tubule cells of the mouse kidney. Thesis. Karolinska Institutet, University of Uppsala, Stockholm, Sweden

ROWDEN, G. and LEWIS, M. G. (1974). Experience with a three hour biopsy service. *J. Clin. Pathol.* **27**, 505–510

SABATINI, D. D., BENSCH, K. and BARRNETT, R. J. (1963). Cytochemistry and electron microscopy. The preservation of cellular structure and enzymatic activity by aldehyde fixation. *J. Cell Biol.*, **17**, 19–58

SPURR, A. R. (1969). A low viscosity epoxy resin embedding medium for electron microscopy. *J. Ultrastruct. Res.*, **26**, 31–43

Index